POSITRON EMISSION TOMOGRAPHY – CURRENT CLINICAL AND RESEARCH ASPECTS

Edited by **Chia-Hung Hsieh**

Positron Emission Tomography – Current Clinical and Research Aspects
Edited by Chia-Hung Hsieh

Published by InTech
Janeza Trdine 9, 51000 Rijeka, Croatia

Publishing Process Manager Martina Durovic

Technical Editor Teodora Smiljanic

Cover Designer InTech Design Team

Additional hard copies can be obtained from orders@intechopen.com

Positron Emission Tomography – Current Clinical and Research Aspects,
Edited by Chia-Hung Hsieh
p. cm.
ISBN 978-953-307-824-3

For EU product safety concerns:
IN TECH d.o.o., Prolaz Marije Krucifikse Kozulić 3, 51000 Rijeka, Croatia,
info@intechopen.com or visit our website at intechopen.com.

Meet the editor

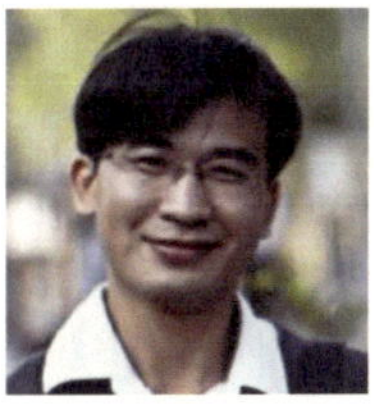

Dr Chia-Hung Hsieh is an associate professor at the Graduate Institute of Basic Medical Science, Faculty of Medicine, China Medical University in Taichung, Taiwan. He obtained both his MS and PhD degree from the National Yang Ming University, Taipei, Taiwan. Dr. Hsieh has held positions second lieutenant as Medical Officer in the Armed Forces at Taichung General Hospital and as post doctoral fellow at Academia Sinica. His research experience is focused primary on Molecular Imaging and Medicine, Molecular Cell Biology, Nuclear Medicine, Tumor and Radiation Biology, as well as on Radiation Science and Radiological Technology. His research interests include Molecular Imaging, Molecular Therapy, Molecular Mechanism of Cancer Biology, and Radiation Oncology.

Contents

Preface

Positron emission tomography (PET) is a molecular imaging technology for examining the molecular basis of normal biological functions of cells and their failure from diseases. By using radio-labelled tracers, four-dimensional (4D) images can be reconstructed by a computer. This computer shows the concentration and location of the tracer of interest, and noninvasively observes the changes of interesting molecular targets in living subjects. Therefore, PET plays a critical role in the era of molecular medicine because it allows for earlier diagnosis and better management of patients with various diseases, such as cancer, neurodegenerative diseases, mental diseases, and metabolic disorders.

This book's stated purpose is to provide a discussion of the technical basis and clinical applications of PET, as well as their recent progress in nuclear medicine. It also summarizes current literature about research and clinical science in PET. The book is intended not only for scientists, but also clinicians seeking recent information regarding PET imaging processing, kinetic modelling, free software, radiopharmaceuticals, clinical application, and diagnosis. The authors are qualified experts in the fields of physics, chemistry, technology, and medicine. They introduce each concept clearly, and they provide new research data and valuable experiences in their respective areas. We hope that both clinicians and scientists find this work useful and stimulating.

Finally, I would like to acknowledge the contributions of the authors and the team of the Publishing Process Management at InTech - Open Access Publisher. Additionally, I would like to thank Ms. Jean Hung and Dr. Chi-Wei Chang for review assistance.

Dr. Chia-Hung Hsieh, PhD
Associate Professor,
China Medical University and Hospital,
Taiwan

Part 1

Imaging Processing, Kinetic Modeling and Software

1

Virtual PET Scanner – From Simulation in GATE to a Final Multiring Albira PET/SPECT/CT Camera

M. Balcerzyk[1,5], L. Caballero[3], C. Correcher[3], A. Gonzalez[2,3], C. Vazquez[4], J.L. Rubio[4], G. Kontaxakis[4], M.A. Pozo[5] and J.M. Benlloch[2]

[1]*National Accelerators Center, University of Seville*
[2]*I3M, CSIC, Valencia*
[3]*Oncovision, Valencia*
[4]*Technical University of Madrid*
[5]*Complutense University of Madrid*
Spain

1. Introduction

Simulation of the Positron Emission Tomography (PET) camera became a useful tool at the level of scanner design. One of the most versatile methods with several packages available is Monte-Carlo method, reviewed in (Rogers 2006). It was applied in GEANT4 code (Agostinelli *et al.* 2003) used in nuclear physics applications. Other codes used in medical physics and medicine are EGS (for review see (Rogers 2006)), FLUKA (Andersen *et al.* 2005), MCNP (Forster *et al.* 2004), PENELOPE (Sempau *et al.* 2001).

The simulations of PET scanners are done in GATE software (Jan *et al.* 2004) which extensively uses GEANT4. This versatile package offers the possibility of simulation of radioactive source decays. It allows tracking of the individual γ events resulting after positron-electron annihilation. They can be absorbed by photoelectric event in the detector crystal or scattered in the phantom. It allows also simulation of detector electronics including paralyzed mode of the amplifiers. Coincidences can be monitored if they are true or random. The software is now available in version 6.1. Part of the simulations were performed in version 3.0, part in vGate 1.0 (containing version 6.0 via virtualization software for Linux).

GATE was used in simulation of SPECT and CT systems (see papers citing (Jan et al. 2004)). Among PET systems for example Siemens PET/CT Biograph 6 scanner (Gonias *et al.* 2007), GE Advance/Discovery LS (Schmidtlein *et al.* 2006), Philips Gemini/Allegro (Lamare *et al.* 2006), Philips Mosaic small animal PET (Merheb, Petegnief and Talbot 2007) or purely *in-silicon* (van der Laan *et al.* 2007) were used for simulation or design of new detectors and systems.

After the initial electronic designs of the camera, its geometry and number of detectors, one can successfully simulate the data collection process including a wide variety of radioactive sources. Data can be classified to individual interactions in the detector (photoelectrically absorbed, scattered), at the coincidence level (true coincidences, scattered coincidences or random coincidences). Singles and coincidences are processed in digitizer module which simulates event collection from initial gamma absorption, via photon generation and reflection within the crystal (not implemented in current simulation), electronic pulse formation, amplification with dead times of the amplifiers, forming of singles and coincidences and then reconstructed into an image of the measured source.

We started from simulating an existing PET scanner called Albira with one ring formed by eight detectors and compared with actual measurements of point sources, animal NEMA phantoms and source grids. As the simulations reproduced very well the actual data in terms of coincidence and single rates, and also in terms of image quality, we moved forward to two and three rings scanner composition, which were at this time only in the design phase. As the electronic modules were to be the same it was a perfect case for simulation.

In the development of new electronics, the depth of interaction was to be included and, this implementation was also simulated in GATE prior to preparation of electronics. This data allow us to observe how the image quality is influenced by the particular implementation of such correction.

On the base of PET camera design and simulation, the multiring version of a breast PET tomograph (MAMMI) was also introduced into the simulation. Again, the simulated data were the base of design modifications and allowed to prepare a reconstruction software long before first real data were taken with a prototype.

2. Methods

We thoroughly modified the simulation of 1-ring Albira scanner prepared by Aurora Gonzalez for her Master thesis on the base of the benchmark of a PET scanner simulation included in Gate release (Gonzalez 2008).

Generally, the simulation of the PET scanner contains the following modules and submodules:

1. *Main module,* containing calls to submodules.
2. *Visualization module,* which defines the way the simulation, is presented during run.
3. *Camera module,* which defines tomograph size, crystal dimensions and grouping.
4. *Phantom module,* which defines phantom inserted in the scanner. The phantom can be a geometrical structure or a pixelated phantom, based on 3D image.
5. *Physics module,* which defines the processes to be included in the simulation.
6. *Digitizer module,* which defines how the γ particle detection is processed. It can be very detailed, i.e. storing information on individual interactions in stopping process, then how photons of the scintillation process are reflected in the crystal, how they are detected by the photomultiplier. Then the amplification stage is simulated with energy windows, dead times of the amplifiers, if they are paralysable or not, etc. This

leads to detection of a single event, which can also be stored, and then processed in several coincidence processors, with individual energy (or signal height) windows, and delays.

7. *Sources module,* which defines sources in geometrical or point form. Sources may be also masked with the phantoms, which allow more complicated geometries, like Derenzo phantom, animal pixelated phantoms, etc.

The listing of the Gate macro with corresponding submodules is provided in Appendix 1 (Section 9.1) of this chapter. The macro is based on benchmarkPET.mac macro provided with Gate 3.0.0. Additional materials used in Gate (in a form readable by Gate) are provided in Appendix 2 (Section 9.2). The file used in Root program (bundled with Gate) to calculate ist mode files and statistics can be obtained from the corresponding author (MB, see Appendix 3, Section 10.3)). This program is based on benchmarkPET.C provided with Gate 3.0.0.

The Albira camera mounts one to three rings formed by eight detectors, each containing only one single crystal fit to a position sensitive photomultiplier (PSPMT). One can see the details in Fig.1, Fig.2 and Fig.7. Such large crystal coupled to the PSPMT allows one to additionally detect the depth of interaction of the annihilation gamma ray in the crystal (Lerche *et al.* 2005; Lerche 2006). The position detection resolution in this continuous crystals are 1.9±0.1 mm in plane of the PSPMT (i.e. axial and tangential directions), and about 3.9±1.5 mm in depth direction (i.e. radial). The errors of these values resulted from variation of these values in the crystal space. The largest errors appear in the edges and corners whereas and smallest errors are located in the center of the crystal, as expected.

General characteristics of the simulated Albira camera are as follows:

- 8 tapered center-pointing trapezoid crystals of 9.8 mm thickness (1-ring scanner), or 12 mm thickness (2- and 3-ring scanner).
- Albira crystals are made of LYSO $(Lu_{0.95}Y_{0.05})_2SiO_5:Ce$
- The process and stored area of each detector is 40×40 mm.
- Dead time for singles is 0.4 μs paralysable and then 2 μs in non-paralysable mode, for coincidences is 1.8 μs non-paralysable mode.
- For simulations we used a mouse phantom and a point-like source at the center of the FOV according to NEMA standard.
- The separation of multiple rings is 4.4 mm. Crystal separation (bore) along the scanner diameter is 112 mm.
- For verification of the 1 ring simulation we placed the "real" mouse phantom in the center of the FOV of the actual scanner and loaded the tube with 237 μCi of 18-FDG. For a point source measurement, an eppendorf with a droplet of a few tens of μl (18-FDG) was centered placed. The measurements were performed for about 16 hours to end up at the activities of around 1μCi, as suggested also in NEMA standards.
- Radioactivity of ^{176}Lu was not included in the simulations. In the crystals of Albira we estimate the abundance of ^{176}Lu (2.59% naturally, 3.78×10^{10} years half-life) to be 280Bq/ml (Moszynski *et al.* 2000).

The sketch of 2-ring scanner is shown in Fig.1

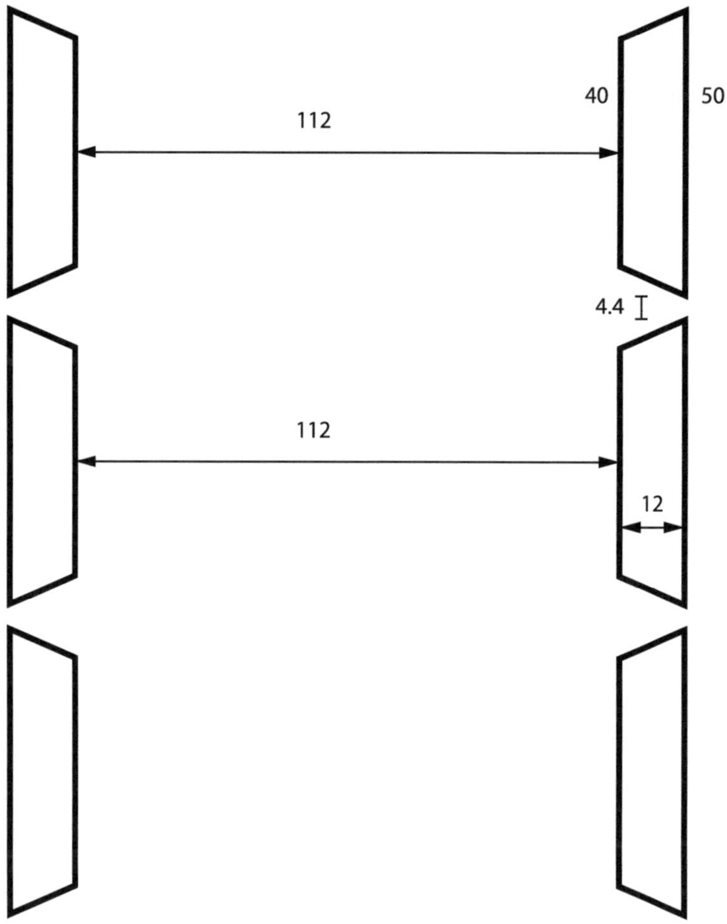

Fig. 1. Sketch of the dimensions of 2-rings camera in a horizontal plane. All dimensions are in mm. For 1-ring scanner the main difference is that the crystals are 9.8 mm thick, instead of 12 mm for 2- and 3-ring scanner. In simulations, 12 mm crystals were used, in actual production they are of 10 mm.

3. Validation of simulation for a one-ring scanner with the measurement of mouse phantom

We simulated six different activities for a mouse phantom, exactly the ones that were measured with the phantom. A view of scanner with the mouse phantom and source during the simulation is depicted in Fig.2.

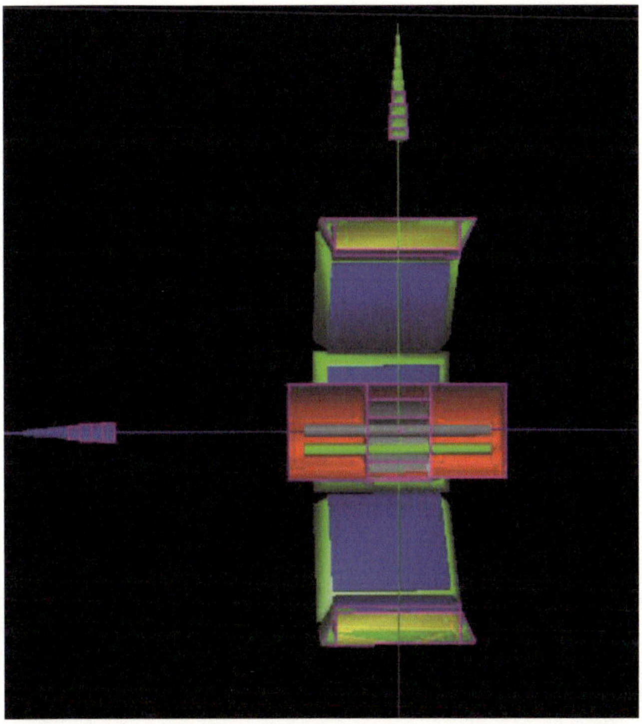

Fig. 2. Simulated 1-ring Albira scanner at a cross section at x=0 plane. XYZ axes are coded as x in red (not seen in the image), y in green and z in blue. The green cylinder in the image represents the location of the tube with radioactive material. In the camera, green structures refer to the crystals.

The simulations were initially done for 1 s acquisition, while the measurements were taken in 10 s frames, and the values of singles and coincidences were counted with a customized Albira application. The comparison between the simulated and acquired real data is shown in Fig.3 and Table 1.

One can see from Fig.3, that coincidence rate is particularly well reproduced almost in the whole activity range down to 1.5 μCi (-10% error) and reduces to about 20% below 1 μCi levels.. Single rates are well reproduced down to 100 μCi, while below this activity the correspondence is quite poor. We would not underestimate the discrepancies for low activities, as this may be the source of artifacts in the images in animals in the areas of low injected activity.

One possible explanation of the effect is the background activity of ^{176}Lu. The estimate gives the rate of ^{176}Lu decay events of about 270 cps per ccm, which translates into about 45 kcps in all detectors, and about 2700 cps in one detector at ±30% energy window (see background spectrum of LSO:Ce in Figure 1 of (Moszynski et al. 2000). 1 ring Albira scanner has 33% solid angle coverage (Balcerzyk et al. 2009). 0.92 μCi (32 kBq) source generates about 770 singles in a detector. If, as calculated, ^{176}Lu background is about 2700 cps in a single crystal, we would simulate only about 770/(770 + 2700) = 22% which corresponds well with 29% shown in Fig.3.

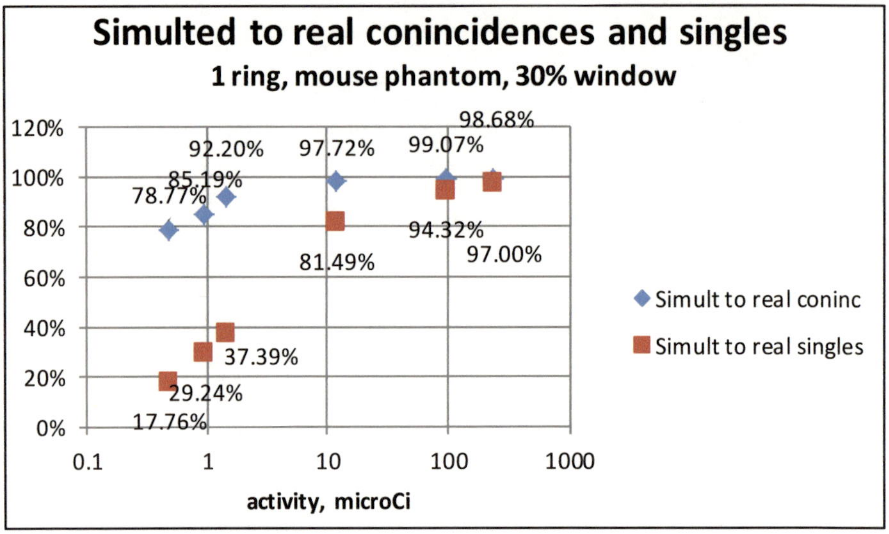

Fig. 3. Comparison between simulated and real coincidences and singles in the 1-ring Albira scanner geometry. Diamonds show the ratio of simulated to real coincidences. Squares show the analogous ratio but for singles. Coincidences are well reproduced (i.e. above 90% agreement) down to 1.5 μCi, while singles agree well for activity values higher than about 50 μCi. Data labels indicate detailed values of these ratios.

Activity, kBq	Measured coincidences rate, 1 ring	Measured singles rate, 1 ring	Simulated coincidences rate, 1 ring	Simulated singles rate, 1 ring
8769	30197	901229	26743	835574
7892	28866	845677		
7015	27969	792326		
6138	26603	728288		
5261	24924	652691		
4384	22577	575520		
3507	20024	489651	18068	441574
2630	16700	392602		
1753	12283	280864		
877	6938	156013		
438	3640	87008	3295	67749
263	2266	58374		
175	1549	43782		
88	799	29248		
53	500	23526	431	8414
35	337	19878	267	5552
17	196	16525	141	2799

Table 1. Detailed comparison between single and coincidence rates for 1-ring scanner, used to calculate the diagram in Fig.3 for a mouse phantom. Note that for activites below 1.5μCi there is a slight discrepancy between simulated and registered singles.

A 5 ns coincidence window should translate into about 1 to 2 cps in coincidences, which is the measured rate in empty scanner. We see in Table 1 that for all very low activities there is about 50 cps coincidence differences between measured and simulated ones. For the same activities, the singles difference is about 15 kcps, which increases to about 70 kcps for high activities. 15 kcps difference in singles treated as randoms yields about 2.3 cps in coincidences (from $R=2\tau S^2$ relation, R being randoms, S singles rate, τ coincidence window (Balcerzyk et al. 2009)).

With the above in mind, one can tell, that background activity of ^{176}Lu is rather not responsible for discrepancy between simulation and experiment in coincidences but only for singles. One possible reason may be the singles (and hence coincidences) discarded from the tapered region of the crystals. In simulation, the distinction for the localization is very sharp, as we do not simulate photon transport. In real measurement some of the signal from the tapered area may probably leak into the detected area.

Background activity of ^{176}Lu is now used in Albira scanner for internal tests of detectors upon initialization of the instrument.

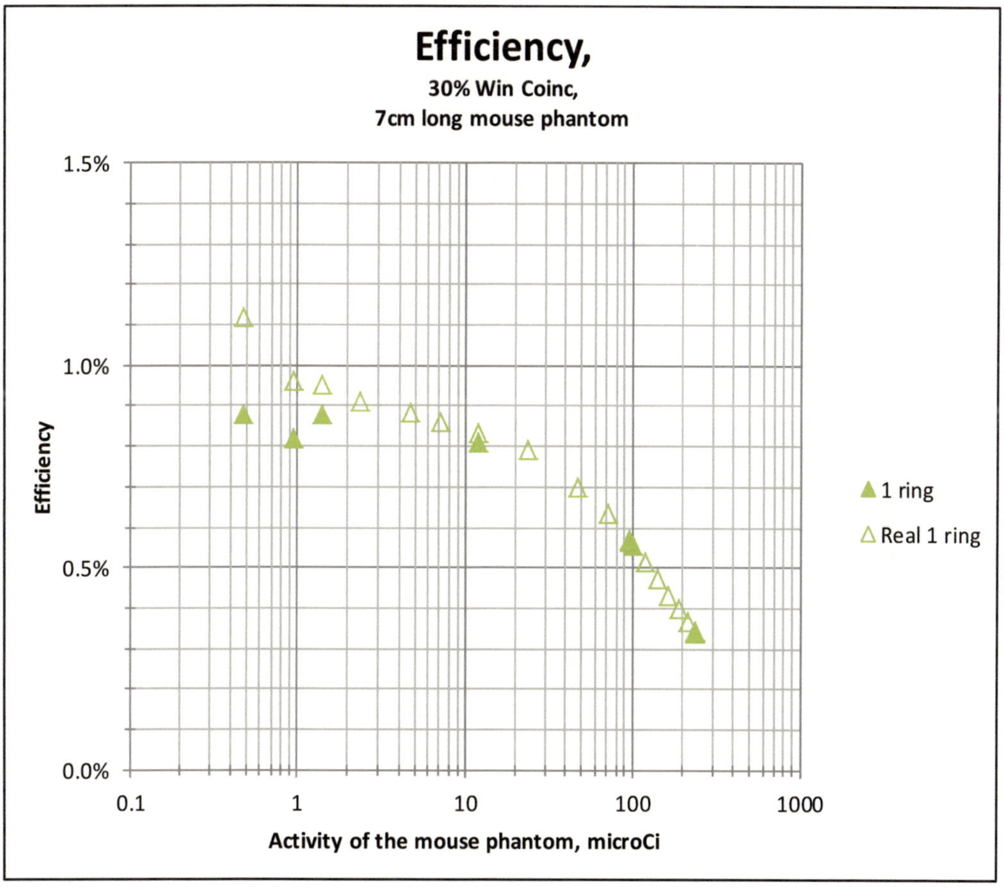

Fig. 4. Efficiency for a mouse phantom simulated (filled symbol) in 1-ring camera compared with measured data (open symbol).

The efficiency for low activities stabilizes at about 0.9% regarding measurement and simulates mouse phantom data. Those activities may serve as a reference for saturation and dead time level calculations. For mouse phantom, an activity of 1 μCi may be taken as a reference, especially for saturation estimations.

The simulation result of a cylindrical phantom for Ø10×10mm and 3.7 MBq 18F activity is shown in Fig.5 for a cross section perpendicular to 1 ring scanner axis. One can see that true scattered and random coincidences contribute little to the image quality, as their total level is about 10% at NEC maximum. In Fig.6 one can see the contribution of each coincidence type to NEC.

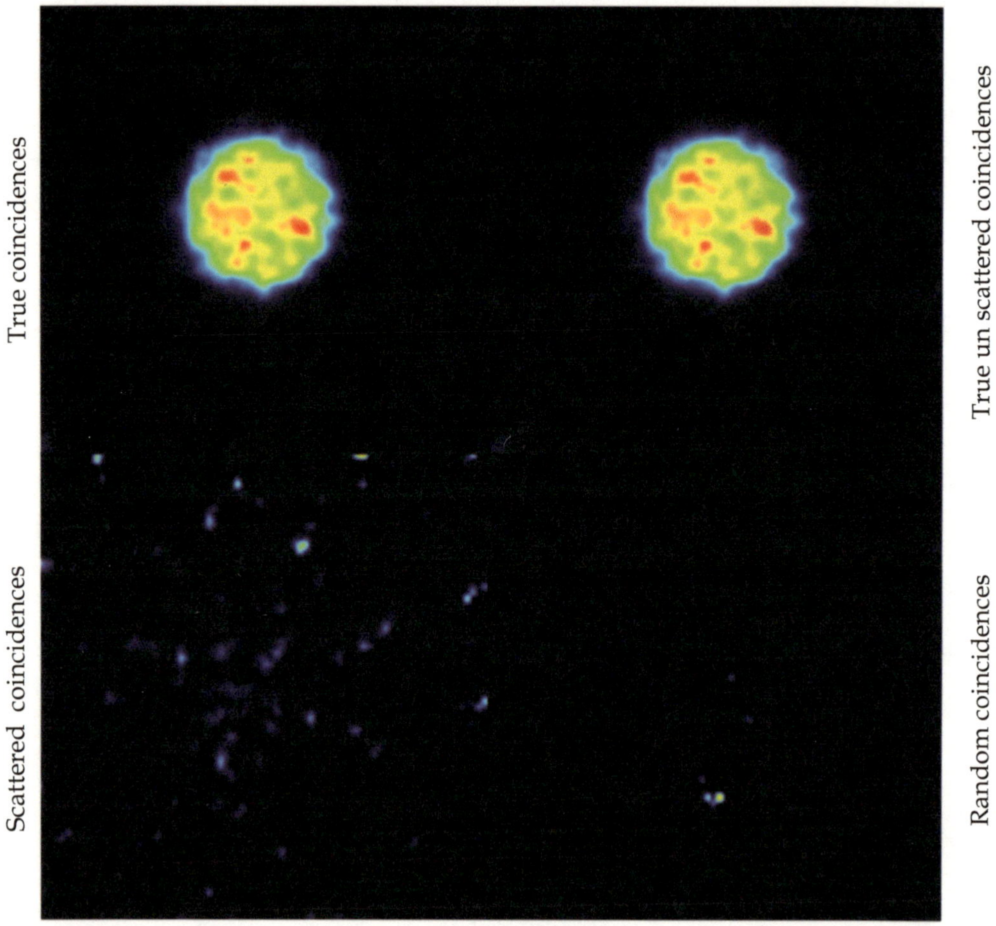

Fig. 5. Gate simulation of Ø10×10mm phantom with a solution of 3.7 MBq of ^{18}F in water obtained with the 1 ring Albira scanner. Contribution of each type of coincidences is described on the left and right margins. Gate simulated events were converted to four separate list mode files and reconstructed in Albira reconstruction program.

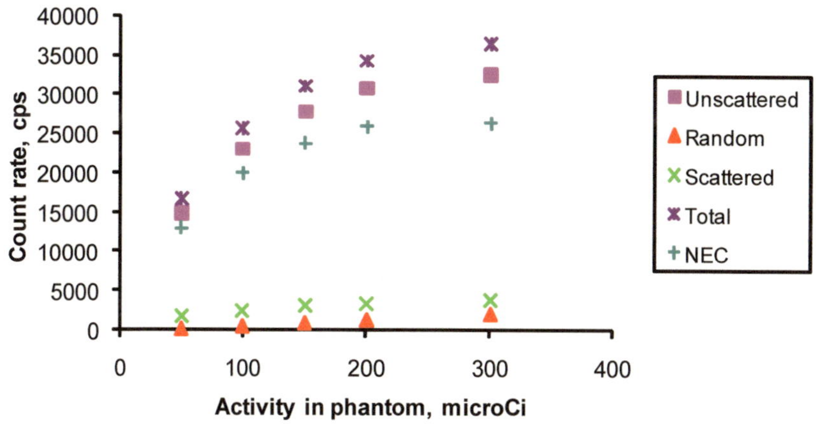

Fig. 6. Simulated NEMA mouse phantom rates for true unscattered, true scattered, random and total coincidences and noise equivalent counts (NEC) for 1 ring Albira scanner. Scatter fraction is constant and about 9% for the whole activity range. NEC has its maximum at 8.8 MBq of the described mouse phantom.

4. Three- and two-ring scanner simulation

The 3D renders of the 2- and 3-ring scanner with the mouse phantom inside the camera are shown in Fig.7.

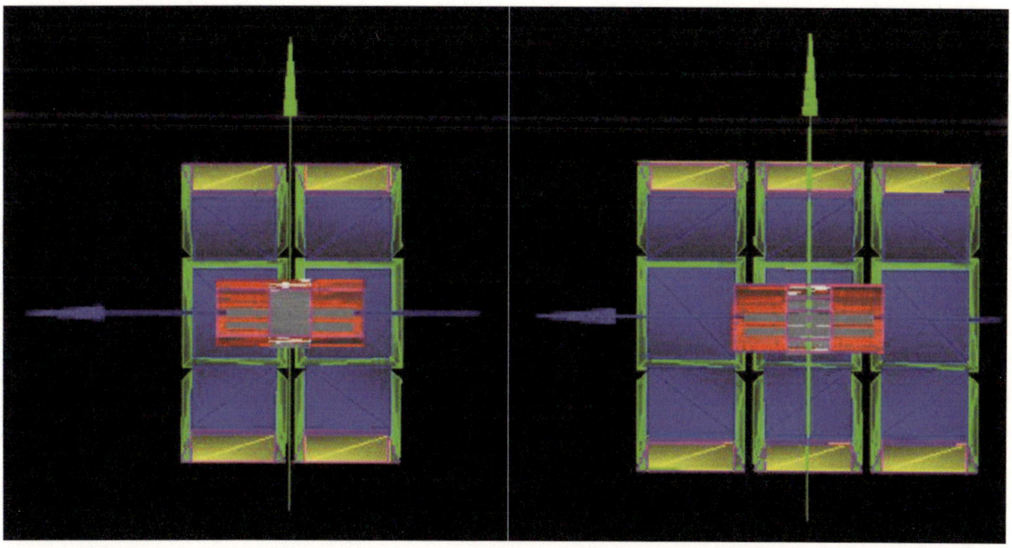

Fig. 7. The cross section view at around x=0 of the simulated 2- and 3-ring scanner with the mouse phantom inside. The coding of the colors is the same as in Fig.2, disregard extra shapes inside the red mouse phantom.

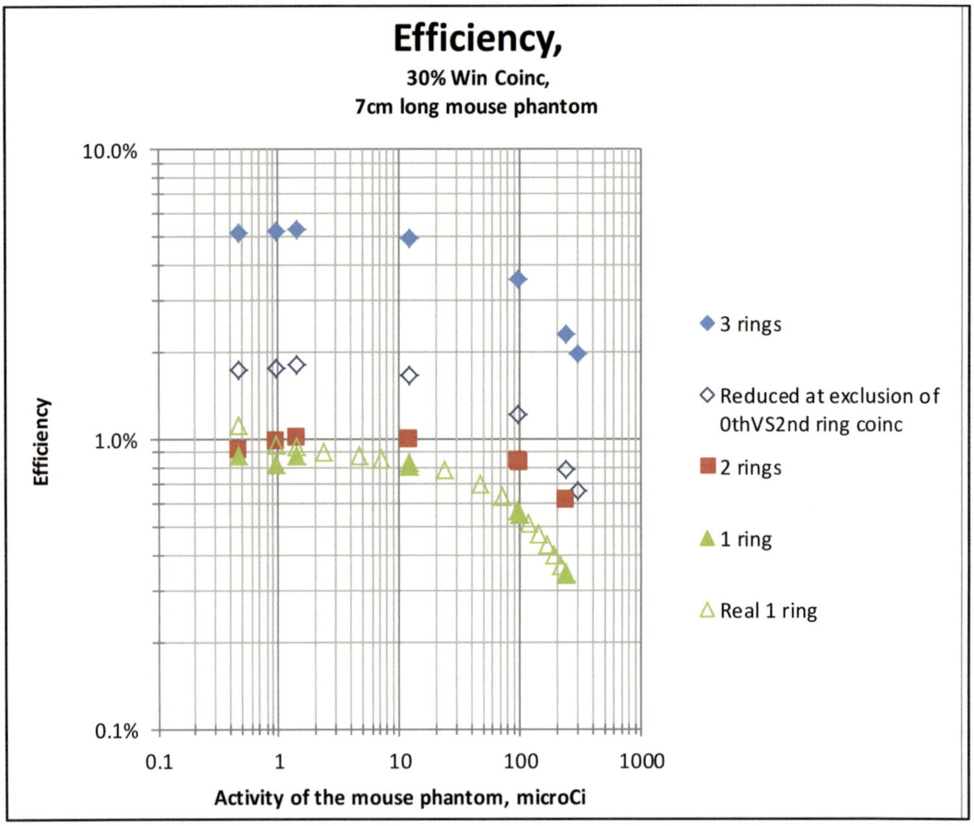

Fig. 8. Efficiency in 30% energy window of coincidences for 1-, 2- and 3-ring scanner. Blue shows 3-ring scanner, squares 2-rings and triangles 1-ring geometry. Open diamonds show the efficiency for a 3-ring scanner with removed coincidences between 0th and 2nd ring (border rings).

5. Efficiency

Fig.8 shows the efficiencies for coincidences for 30% energy window for 1-, 2- and 3-ring scanner for simulations with closed symbols. 1-ring values are the same as in Fig.4. In this picture one can see the power of a 3-ring scanner, where all coincidences are stored. With a mouse phantom the efficiency reaches 5.3% for low activities. Assuming the proper simulation of 1-ring camera, one can expect the same efficiency for a measured mouse phantom, and for real animal measurements.

With open diamonds we show the efficiency in the projected 3-ring scanner with omission of the coincidences between border rings 0th and 2nd. In one of the first projects, such design was considered. It was estimated by analysis of first 50 coincidences from that scanner for the pair of detectors which form the coincidence. Once can generate such ASCII output in a table from Gate. The coincidences between rings 0th and 2nd include about 34% of all detected coincidences. The line of response is at small angle towards z-axis of the scanner, so one can expect large parallax errors for this pair of detectors. That effect suggested to include the depth of interaction encoding, which was considered in the final version.

5.1 Saturation level

Saturation levels for multiring scanners are shown in Fig.9. They heavily relay on the choice of the two activities for which the efficiency is constant within 5%, being around 1µCi. However, some simulations there is higher efficiency at 0.5 µCi activity. The difference may be due to fluctuations of small numbers, as the coincidence count for these activities is around a few hundreds. In this only aspect 2-ring scanner is better than 1- and 3-ring scanner. The saturation of 50% for 1- and 3-ring scanner is at the level of about 120 µCi, while for 2-ring scanner it is about 320 µCi. We do not see the reason for 2-ring scanner to behave so well in terms of saturation. It is possible that it is a geometrical effect of having smaller fraction of the phantom within FOV of each ring in this geometry (see Fig.7).

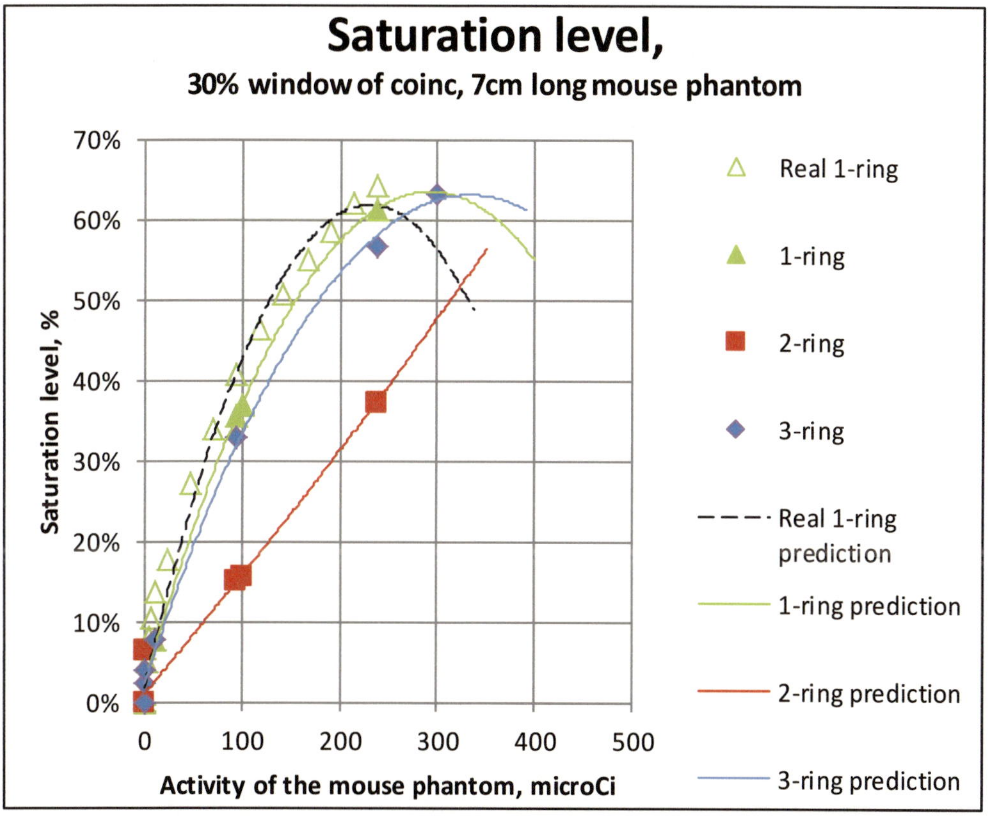

Fig. 9. Saturation levels for multiring scanners. For the 3-ring scanner with omitted 0th vs. 2nd ring coincidences, the saturation curve would be the same as for 3-ring geometry, as the efficiency is calculated as a fraction of valid coincidences for all activities. As the number of points for simulation is limited, we added the trend lines (2nd order polynomials) to look for expected evolution at higher activities.

We drew also prediction lines using simple polynomial 2 curves level. The predictive value of this curve is low, but it shows, that the expected 50% saturation level for 3-ring scanner is higher than for 1-ring scanner.

5.2 Omission of 0^{th}vs 2nd ring coincidences in 3-ring scanner

The reader may have already found that we try to encourage the designers to drop the idea of excluding 0th vs. 2nd ring coincidences. It would result in the loss of 34% of detected coincidences. In Gate, there is no straightforward way to exclude the mentioned coincidences from the simulation. The only way we perceive it, is to post-hoc exclude them from simulated 3-ring scanner during the creation of list mode files. The problem is that there will be false overestimation of saturation, dead times for coincidences and others during the simulation, so the resulting list mode file will have an artificially lower coincidence level.

6. Point source

The proper way (NEMA standard) to measure the efficiency is to place a point source of activity corresponding to saturation level of less than 5% in the center of FOV. The simulations were done for exactly 0.95 μCi source, which roughly fulfills the requirement and the results are shown in Fig.10 in comparison with the real study in 1-ring scanner. The real scanner measurement was done using a droplet of few tens of μl of about 10μCi of 18-FDG placed in the eppendorf tube and at the center of FOV. For the 1-ring scanner the measured value is 2.49%, while simulation returns 3.2% being in reasonable agreement with expected 10% saturation level at 10 μCi. Again, one can see the superiority of 3-ring scanner reaching 9.35% efficiency. This value may be further increased to about 12.9% if the tapered areas of the crystal are used for the coincidence detection. This would require most likely sophisticated point-spread function inclusion in the reconstruction besides other technical challenges regarding position calibration of such impinging events.

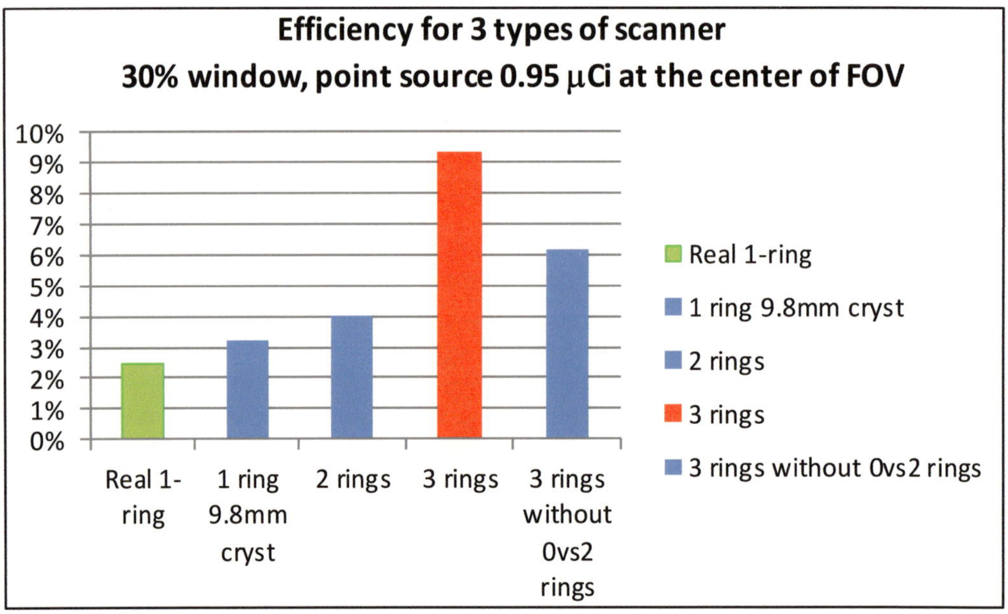

Fig. 10. Efficiency for a real 1-ring scanner and simulated multiring scanners for the low activity (0.95 μCi) point source placed in the center of FOV.

7. Depth of interaction

For the sources or phantom parts far radially from the center of the field of view, the resolution is deteriorating, mainly due to the so-called parallax error. To correct it, if possible, depth of interaction (DOI) of the detection of annihilation 511 keV γ photon needs to be recorded, and not only planar coordinates in plane of the photomultiplier. In the Albira detector, the DOI is estimated from the scintillation light spread into the position sensitive photomultiplier as shown in Fig.11.

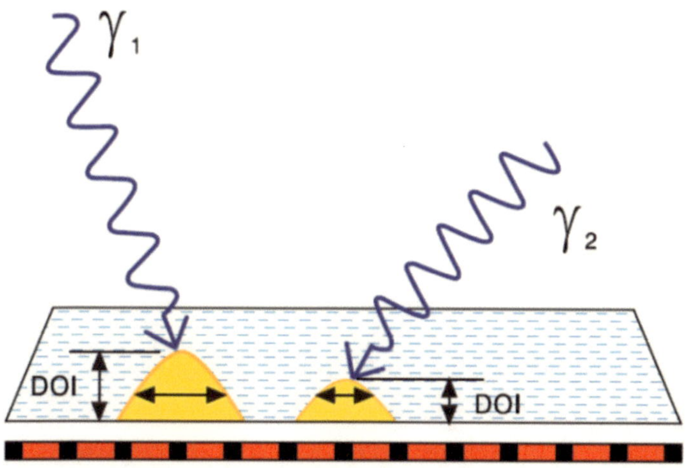

Fig. 11. Scheme of DOI detection in Albira PET detector. From (Oncovision).

In the current Albira 3 ring scanner the DOI is included, but not in the simulations. The DOI is included in the following way: the exact line of response is calculated for each detected coincidence connecting the point corresponding to detected blue arrow in Fig.11 to the interaction point in second detector. The cross section point with the surface optically coupled to the photomultiplier is then re-calculated. This corresponds to already stored LOR for planar detectors. One can see that this sort of DOI for very oblique angles of LOR may result in cross sections with neighboring detectors.

The simulation did not include DOI corrections. The interaction point on the plane of PMT corresponded to the planar simulated coordinates.

8. Conclusion

Surprisingly for a point source there is little (from 3% to 4%) increase in efficiency for 2 ring scanner compared to 1-ring (see Fig.10). The larger difference appears with the inclusion of a third ring and, moreover, if coincidences among all rings are allowed, resulting in a efficiency increase up to 9.35%. Higher values reaching 12.9% efficiency would be expected if the events impinging the tapered parts of the crystals are also used for reconstruction.

Upon the simulations results, some managerial decisions in Oncovision have been made. Namely, for 3 ring scanners, coincidences in between all three rings were included in the final product. Depth of interaction correction was introduced as well. For future versions, inclusion of all coincidences, also from the tapered region of the crystal would be available, as it considerably increases the detector total efficiency.

9. Acknowledgements

We thank Aurora Gonzalez for initial adaptation of benchmarkPET.mac macro to one ring Albira scanner.

10. Appendices

10.1 Appendix 1: Albira macro files listing for 3 ring scanner Gate simulation

Note that that all files must be in one directory. All lines in *.mac files end with Linux LF end of line character only. In the listing above, long lines are continued in the following one, with the first having hanging indent. Macro is based on benchmarkPET.mac provided with Gate 3.0.0 and Gate 6.0 (Jan et al. 2004).

10.1.1 Main macro

```
# /control/execute *.mac calls the lower level macro
#/vis/disable
/control/execute visu.mac

/gate/geometry/setMaterialDatabase ../../GateMaterials.db
# LYSOAlbira and Nylon added

#        W O R L D
/gate/world/geometry/setXLength 150. cm
/gate/world/geometry/setYLength 150. cm
/gate/world/geometry/setZLength 150. cm

/control/execute camera.mac
/control/execute phantom.mac
/control/execute physics.mac

#        INITIALIZE
/gate/run/initialize

/control/execute digitizer.mac
# digitizer.mac OK, except for deadtimes 1 and 2 for singles, LES and HES for trapezoid
crystalSD

#        SOURCE
/control/execute sources.mac
#sources.mac OK with A
```

```
#        VERBOSITY
#/gate/verbose Physic   0
#/gate/verbose Cuts     0
#/gate/verbose Actor    0
#/gate/verbose SD       0
#/gate/verbose Actions  0
#/gate/verbose Step     0
#/gate/verbose Error    0
#/gate/verbose Warning  0
#/gate/verbose Output   0
#/gate/verbose Core     0

/run/verbose 0
/event/verbose 0
/tracking/verbose 0

#        OUTPUT
#ASCII output is disabled
/gate/output/ascii/disable
/gate/output/ascii/setOutFileHitsFlag 0
/gate/output/ascii/setOutFileSinglesFlag 0
/gate/output/ascii/setOutFileCoincidencesFlag 0
#/gate/output/ascii/setOutFiledelayFlag 0

/gate/output/root/enable
/gate/output/root/setFileName AlbiraARS
/gate/output/root/setRootHitFlag 0
/gate/output/root/setRootSinglesFlag 0
/gate/output/root/setRootCoincidencesFlag 1
#/gate/output/root/setRootdelayFlag 1

#        RANDOM
#JamesRandom Ranlux64 MersenneTwister
/gate/random/setEngineName Ranlux64
#/gate/random/setEngineSeed default
#/gate/random/setEngineSeed auto
/gate/random/setEngineSeed 123456789
#/gate/random/resetEngineFrom fileName
/gate/random/verbose 1

#        START
/gate/application/setTimeSlice    1. s
/gate/application/setTimeStart    0. s
/gate/application/setTimeStop     1. s
#/gate/application/startDAQ
```

```
# the # sign may be omitted in the above line to run the macro automatically, otherwise, the above line must be introduced manually in Gate to run the simulation.
#exit
```

10.1.2 Visualize macro: Visu.mac

```
#          VISUALISATION
# requires OpenGL graphic card
/vis/open OGLSX
/vis/viewer/set/viewpointThetaPhi 25 45
/vis/viewer/zoom 7
/vis/drawVolume
#/vis/viewer/flush
#/tracking/verbose 0
/tracking/storeTrajectory 1
#/vis/scene/add/trajectories
/vis/scene/endOfEventAction accumulate
```

10.1.3 Camera description macro: Camera.mac

```
#-------------------oooooOOOOO00000OOOOOooooo---------------------#
#                                   #
#   DEFINITION AND DESCRITION       #
#     OF YOUR PET DEVICE          #
#                                   #
#-------------------oooooOOOOO00000OOOOOooooo---------------------#

#insert 3 axes this does not work in vGate 1.0
#/gate/world/daughters/insert 3axes

#
#          CYLINDRICAL : The cylindralPET system is dedicated
# for PET device !
#
/gate/world/daughters/name PETscanner
/gate/world/daughters/insert cylinder
/gate/PETscanner/setMaterial Air
/gate/PETscanner/geometry/setRmax 70 mm
/gate/PETscanner/geometry/setRmin 55.8 mm
/gate/PETscanner/geometry/setHeight 150 mm
/gate/PETscanner/vis/setVisible 0

# PETscanner1 is daughter of PETscanner to correctly place the trpd shape
/gate/PETscanner/daughters/name PETscanner1
/gate/PETscanner/daughters/insert cylinder
/gate/PETscanner1/setMaterial Air
/gate/PETscanner1/geometry/setRmax 70 mm
/gate/PETscanner1/geometry/setRmin 55.8 mm
```

```
/gate/PETscanner1/geometry/setHeight 150 mm
/gate/PETscanner1/vis/setVisible 0

/gate/PETscanner/daughters/name LYSO
/gate/PETscanner/daughters/insert box
/gate/LYSO/geometry/setXLength 12 mm
/gate/LYSO/geometry/setYLength 40 mm
/gate/LYSO/geometry/setZLength 40 mm
/gate/LYSO/setMaterial LYSOAlbira
/gate/LYSO/vis/setColor yellow
/gate/LYSO/vis/forceWireframe
# we repeat the block 3x lineary
/gate/LYSO/repeaters/insert cubicArray
/gate/LYSO/cubicArray/setRepeatNumberZ 3
/gate/LYSO/cubicArray/setRepeatVector 0.0 0.0 54.4 mm

#
#        TRPD (level1): Trapezoid LYSO (not used for the moment)
#
/gate/PETscanner1/daughters/name trapezoid
/gate/PETscanner1/daughters/insert trpd
/gate/trapezoid/geometry/setX1Length 50 mm
/gate/trapezoid/geometry/setY1Length 50 mm
/gate/trapezoid/geometry/setX2Length 40 mm
/gate/trapezoid/geometry/setY2Length 40 mm
/gate/trapezoid/geometry/setZLength 12 mm
/gate/trapezoid/setMaterial LYSOAlbira
/gate/trapezoid/vis/setColor green
/gate/trapezoid/vis/forceWireframe
/gate/trapezoid/placement/setTranslation 0. 0. 62. mm

#
#        LEVEL3 : in your crystal unit !
# (front end nylon to be a phantom)
# Nylon is missing in GateMaterial.db, add it
#
# FrontPad was a daughter of PETscanner
/gate/world/daughters/name FrontPad
/gate/world/daughters/insert box
/gate/FrontPad/geometry/setXLength 1.9 mm
/gate/FrontPad/geometry/setYLength 40. mm
/gate/FrontPad/geometry/setZLength 40 mm
/gate/FrontPad/placement/setTranslation 54.85 0. 0. mm
/gate/FrontPad/setMaterial Nylon
/gate/FrontPad/vis/setColor blue
/gate/FrontPad/vis/forceWireframe
/gate/FrontPad/repeaters/insert cubicArray
/gate/FrontPad/cubicArray/setRepeatNumberZ 3
```

```
/gate/FrontPad/cubicArray/setRepeatVector 0.0 0.0 54.4 mm
/gate/FrontPad/repeaters/insert ring
/gate/FrontPad/ring/enableAutoRotation
/gate/FrontPad/ring/setRepeatNumber 8

#       REPEAT YOUR BLOCK (TRPD)
# IN YOURSCANNERPET (8 detectores)
# LYSO box is repeated around z axis
/gate/LYSO/repeaters/insert ring
/gate/LYSO/ring/enableAutoRotation
/gate/LYSO/ring/setFirstAngle 270 deg
# the above line sets the first detector at 12 hour
/gate/LYSO/ring/setPoint1 0. 0. 0. mm
/gate/LYSO/ring/setPoint2 0. 0. -1. mm
/gate/LYSO/ring/setRepeatNumber 8

#trapezoid is repeated around x axis
/gate/trapezoid/repeaters/insert ring
/gate/trapezoid/ring/enableAutoRotation
/gate/trapezoid/ring/setFirstAngle 270 deg
# the above line sets the first detector at 12 hour
/gate/trapezoid/ring/setPoint1 0. 0. 0. mm
/gate/trapezoid/ring/setPoint2 1. 0. 0. mm
/gate/trapezoid/ring/setRepeatNumber 8
/gate/trapezoid/repeaters/insert cubicArray
/gate/trapezoid/cubicArray/setRepeatNumberX 3
/gate/trapezoid/cubicArray/setRepeatVector 54.4 0.0 0.0 mm
/gate/PETscanner1/placement/setRotationAxis 0 1 0
/gate/PETscanner1/placement/setRotationAngle 90 deg

#       ATTACH SYSTEM : definition of your global detector
/gate/systems/PETscanner/level1/attach LYSO
#/gate/systems/PETscanner1/level1/attach trapezoid

#       ATTACH LAYER SD :
# definition of your sensitive detector
# for trapezoid, below SD must be for trapezoid
/gate/LYSO/attachCrystalSD

# update the view manually
/vis/drawVolume
```

10.1.4 Mouse phantom description macro: Phantom.mac

```
#       PHANTOM 1
/gate/world/daughters/name phantom1
/gate/world/daughters/insert cylinder
```

```
/gate/phantom1/geometry/setRmax  15 mm
/gate/phantom1/geometry/setRmin  0. mm
/gate/phantom1/geometry/setHeight 70 mm
/gate/phantom1/setMaterial Polyethylene
/gate/phantom1/vis/setColor red
/gate/phantom1/vis/forceWireframe

#         PHANTOM 2
/gate/phantom1/daughters/name phantom2
/gate/phantom1/daughters/insert cylinder
/gate/phantom2/geometry/setRmax  1.75 mm
/gate/phantom2/geometry/setRmin  0. mm
/gate/phantom2/geometry/setHeight 60 mm
/gate/phantom2/placement/setTranslation 0 -5.9 0 mm
/gate/phantom2/setMaterial Plastic
/gate/phantom2/vis/setColor green
/gate/phantom2/vis/forceWireframe

#         PHANTOM 3
/gate/phantom2/daughters/name phantom3
/gate/phantom2/daughters/insert cylinder
/gate/phantom3/geometry/setRmax  1.05 mm
/gate/phantom3/geometry/setRmin  0 mm
/gate/phantom3/geometry/setHeight 60 mm
/gate/phantom3/setMaterial Water
/gate/phantom3/vis/setColor green
/gate/phantom3/vis/forceWireframe

#         ATTACH PHANTOM SD
/gate/phantom1/attachPhantomSD
/gate/phantom2/attachPhantomSD
/gate/phantom3/attachPhantomSD
/gate/FrontPad/attachPhantomSD
#FrontPad is defined in camera.mac
```

10.1.5 Physical processes description macro: Physics.mac

```
#     PHYSICS
#
/gate/physics/addProcess PhotoElectric
/gate/physics/addProcess Compton
/gate/physics/addProcess GammaConversion
/gate/physics/addProcess LowEnergyRayleighScattering

/gate/physics/addProcess ElectronIonisation
/gate/physics/addProcess Bremsstrahlung
/gate/physics/addProcess PositronAnnihilationStd
```

```
/gate/physics/addProcess MultipleScattering e+
/gate/physics/addProcess MultipleScattering e-

/gate/physics/processList Enabled
/gate/physics/processList Initialized
#     CUTS
#
#/gate/phantom1/attachPhantomSD
#/gate/phantom2/attachPhantomSD
#/gate/phantom3/attachPhantomSD
#/gate/FrontPad/attachPhantomSD
#FrontPad is defined in camera.mac, phantomN in phantom.mac

# Cuts for particle in phantoms
/gate/physics/Gamma/SetCutInRegion     phantom1 1.0 cm
/gate/physics/Electron/SetCutInRegion  phantom1 1.0 cm
/gate/physics/Positron/SetCutInRegion  phantom1 1.0 cm

/gate/physics/Gamma/SetCutInRegion     phantom2 1.0 cm
/gate/physics/Electron/SetCutInRegion  phantom2 1.0 cm
/gate/physics/Positron/SetCutInRegion  phantom2 1.0 cm

/gate/physics/Gamma/SetCutInRegion     phantom3 1.0 cm
/gate/physics/Electron/SetCutInRegion  phantom3 1.0 cm
/gate/physics/Positron/SetCutInRegion  phantom3 1.0 cm

/gate/physics/Gamma/SetCutInRegion     FrontPad 1.0 cm
/gate/physics/Electron/SetCutInRegion  FrontPad 1.0 cm
/gate/physics/Positron/SetCutInRegion  FrontPad 1.0 cm
```

10.1.6 Digitizer description macro: Digitizer.mac

```
#        ADDER
/gate/digitizer/Singles/insert adder

# ENERGYBLURRING
/gate/digitizer/Singles/insert blurring
/gate/digitizer/Singles/blurring/setResolution 0.14
/gate/digitizer/Singles/blurring/setEnergyOfReference 511. keV

# DEADTIME
/gate/digitizer/Singles/insert deadtime
/gate/digitizer/Singles/deadtime/setDeadTime 400. ns
/gate/digitizer/Singles/deadtime/setMode paralysable
/gate/digitizer/Singles/deadtime/chooseDTVolume LYSO
```

```
/gate/digitizer/Singles/name deadtime2
/gate/digitizer/Singles/insert deadtime
/gate/digitizer/Singles/deadtime2/setDeadTime 2000 ns
/gate/digitizer/Singles/deadtime2/setMode nonparalysable
/gate/digitizer/Singles/deadtime2/chooseDTVolume LYSO

# THRESHOLDER
/gate/digitizer/Singles/insert thresholder
/gate/digitizer/Singles/thresholder/setThreshold 357.7 keV
/gate/digitizer/Singles/insert upholder
/gate/digitizer/Singles/upholder/setUphold 664.3 keV


# Singles for energy spectrum:
/gate/digitizer/name LESingles
/gate/digitizer/insert singleChain
/gate/digitizer/LESingles/setInputName Hits
/gate/digitizer/LESingles/insert adder
/gate/digitizer/LESingles/insert blurring
/gate/digitizer/LESingles/blurring/setResolution 0.14
/gate/digitizer/LESingles/blurring/setEnergyOfReference 511. keV
/gate/digitizer/LESingles/insert deadtime
/gate/digitizer/LESingles/deadtime/setDeadTime 400. ns
/gate/digitizer/LESingles/deadtime/setMode paralysable
/gate/digitizer/LESingles/deadtime/chooseDTVolume LYSO
/gate/digitizer/LESingles/name deadtime2
/gate/digitizer/LESingles/insert deadtime
/gate/digitizer/LESingles/deadtime2/setDeadTime 2000. ns
/gate/digitizer/LESingles/deadtime2/setMode nonparalysable
/gate/digitizer/LESingles/deadtime2/chooseDTVolume LYSO
/gate/digitizer/LESingles/insert thresholder
/gate/digitizer/LESingles/thresholder/setThreshold 10. keV
/gate/digitizer/LESingles/insert upholder
/gate/digitizer/LESingles/upholder/setUphold 664.3 keV

# Singles for proper +/-20% coincidences to use:
/gate/digitizer/name HESingles
/gate/digitizer/insert singleChain
/gate/digitizer/HESingles/setInputName Hits
/gate/digitizer/HESingles/insert adder
/gate/digitizer/HESingles/insert blurring
/gate/digitizer/HESingles/blurring/setResolution 0.14
/gate/digitizer/HESingles/blurring/setEnergyOfReference 511. keV
/gate/digitizer/HESingles/insert deadtime
/gate/digitizer/HESingles/deadtime/setDeadTime 400. ns
/gate/digitizer/HESingles/deadtime/setMode paralysable
```

```
/gate/digitizer/HESingles/deadtime/chooseDTVolume LYSO
/gate/digitizer/HESingles/name deadtime2
/gate/digitizer/HESingles/insert deadtime
/gate/digitizer/HESingles/deadtime2/setDeadTime 2000. ns
/gate/digitizer/HESingles/deadtime2/setMode nonparalysable
/gate/digitizer/HESingles/deadtime2/chooseDTVolume LYSO
/gate/digitizer/HESingles/insert thresholder
/gate/digitizer/HESingles/thresholder/setThreshold 408.8 keV
/gate/digitizer/HESingles/insert upholder
/gate/digitizer/HESingles/upholder/setUphold 613.2 keV

# COINCI SORTER
#Check what is the default multiple coincidence sorter policy, that is:
/gate/digitizer/Coincidences/MultiplesPolicy takeAllGoods
/gate/digitizer/Coincidences/setWindow 5. ns
/gate/digitizer/Coincidences/minSectorDifference 3

/gate/digitizer/name Coincidences2
/gate/digitizer/insert coincidenceChain
/gate/digitizer/Coincidences2/addInputName Coincidences
# no or second chain for coinc
/gate/digitizer/Coincidences2/insert deadtime
/gate/digitizer/Coincidences2/deadtime/setDeadTime 1800. ns
/gate/digitizer/Coincidences2/deadtime/setMode nonparalysable
/gate/digitizer/Coincidences2/deadtime/conserveAllEvent true

# 20% window of HESingles used to create real coincidences of Albira
/gate/digitizer/name HECoincidences
/gate/digitizer/insert coincidenceSorter
/gate/digitizer/HECoincidences/MultiplesPolicy takeAllGoods
/gate/digitizer/HECoincidences/setWindow 5. ns
/gate/digitizer/HECoincidences/minSectorDifference 3
/gate/digitizer/HECoincidences/setInputName HESingles

/gate/digitizer/name HECoincidences2
/gate/digitizer/insert coincidenceChain
/gate/digitizer/HECoincidences2/addInputName HECoincidences
/gate/digitizer/HECoincidences2/insert deadtime
/gate/digitizer/HECoincidences2/deadtime/setDeadTime 1800. ns
/gate/digitizer/HECoincidences2/deadtime/setMode nonparalysable
/gate/digitizer/HECoincidences2/deadtime/conserveAllEvent true
```

10.1.7 Source file in sources.mac

```
/gate/source/addSource SourceF
/gate/source/SourceF/setActivity 0.0000009467 Ci
/gate/source/SourceF/gps/particle e+
```

```
/gate/source/SourceF/setForcedUnstableFlag true
/gate/source/SourceF/setForcedHalfLife 6586.2 s
/gate/source/SourceF/gps/energytype Fluor18
/gate/source/SourceF/gps/type Volume
/gate/source/SourceF/gps/shape Cylinder
/gate/source/SourceF/gps/radius 1.05 mm
/gate/source/SourceF/gps/halfz 30. mm
/gate/source/SourceF/gps/angtype iso
/gate/source/SourceF/gps/centre 0. -5.9 0. mm
#/gate/source/SourceF/gps/confine phantom2_P
/gate/source/list
```

10.2 Appendix 2. Gatematerials.db file additional materials

```
LYSOalbira:  d=7.2525 g/cm3; n=4 ; state=Solid
    +el: name=Lutetium ; f=0.725820
    +el: name=Yttrium ; f=0.031097
+el: name=Silicon; f=0.063166
    +el: name=Oxygen; f=0.179918
Nylon: d=1.15 g/cm3; n=4 ; state=Solid
    +el: name=Carbon ; f=0.636853
    +el: name=Hydrogen ; f=0.097980
    +el: name=Oxygen; f=0.141388
    +el: name=Nitrogen; f=0.123779
Polyethylene: d=0.96 g/cm3 ; n=2
+el: name=Hydrogen ; n=2
    +el: name=Carbon  ; n=1
```

10.3 Appendix 3: Root program for preparation of list mode files for reconstruction in Albira program

The file can be received from corresponding author (MB) by request. Its size exceeds the allowed size of this publication.

11. References

Agostinelli, S., J. Allison, K. Amako, J. Apostolakis, H. Araujo, P. Arce, et al. (2003). GEANT4 - A simulation toolkit. *Nuclear Instruments and Methods in Physics Research, Section A: Accelerators, Spectrometers, Detectors and Associated Equipment,* Vol. 506, No. 3, pp. 250-303, ISSN 0168-9002

Andersen, V., F. Ballarini, G. Battistoni, F. Cerutti, A. Empl, A. Fassò, *et al.* (2005). The application of FLUKA to dosimetry and radiation therapy. *Radiation Protection Dosimetry,* Vol. 116, No. 1-4, pp. 113-117, ISSN 0144-8420

Balcerzyk, Marcin, George Kontaxakis, Mercedes Delgado, Luis Garcia-Garcia, Carlos Correcher, Antonio J. Gonzalez, *et al.* (2009). Initial performance evaluation of a high resolution Albira small animal positron emission tomography scanner with monolithic crystals and depth-of-interaction encoding from a user's perspective.

Measurement Science and Technology, Vol. 20, No. 10, pp. 104011, ISSN 0957-0233-1361-6501.

Forster, R. Arthur, Lawrence J. Cox, Richard F. Barrett, Thomas E. Booth, Judith F. Briesmeister, Forrest B. Brown, *et al.* (2004). MCNP™ Version 5. *Nuclear Instruments and Methods in Physics Research Section B: Beam Interactions with Materials and Atoms,* Vol. 213, No. 0, pp. 82-86, ISSN 0168-583X.

Gonias, P., N. Bertsekas, N. Karakatsanis, G. Saatsakis, A. Gaitanis, D. Nikolopoulos, *et al.* (2007). Validation of a GATE model for the simulation of the Siemens biograph™ 6 PET scanner. *Nuclear Instruments and Methods in Physics Research, Section A: Accelerators, Spectrometers, Detectors and Associated Equipment,* Vol. 571, No. 1-2 SPEC. ISS., pp. 263-266, ISSN 0168-9002

Gonzalez, A. 2008. M.S. Thesis, Technical Univerisity of Madrid, Madrid.

Jan, S., G. Santin, D. Strul, S. Staelens, K. Assié, D. Autret, *et al.* (2004). GATE: a simulation toolkit for PET and SPECT. *Phys Med Biol,* Vol. 49, No. 19, pp. 4543-4561, ISSN 0031-9155-1361-6560.

Lamare, F., A. Turzo, Y. Bizais, C. C. L. Rest &D. Visvikis. (2006). Validation of a Monte Carlo simulation of the Philips Allegro/GEMINI PET systems using GATE. *Phys Med Biol,* Vol. 51, No. 4, pp. 943-962, ISSN 0031-9155

Lerche, C. 2006. Depth of Interaction Enhanced Gamma-Ray Imaging for Medical Applications, Departamento de Fisica Atomica, Molecular y Nuclear, Universidad de Valencia, Valencia.

Lerche, C., J. Benlloch, F. Sanchez, N. Pavon, N. Gimenez, M. Fernandez, *et al.* (2005). Depth of interaction detection with enhanced position-sensitive proportional resistor network. *Nucl. Instr. Meth. A,* Vol. 537, No. 1-2, pp. 326-330, ISSN 01689002.

Merheb, C., Y. Petegnief &J. N. Talbot. (2007). Full modelling of the MOSAIC animal PET system based on the GATE Monte Carlo simulation code. *Phys Med Biol,* Vol. 52, No. 3, (Feb 7) pp. 563-76, ISSN 0031-9155 (Print) 0031-9155 (Linking).

Moszynski, M., M. Balcerzyk, M. Kapusta, D. Wolski &C. L. Melcher. (2000). Large size LSO:Ce and YSO:Ce scintillators for 50 MeV range γ-ray detector. IEEE *Trans. Nucl. Sci.,* Vol. 47, No. 4, pp. 1324-1328, ISSN 0018-9499.

Oncovision. 2011. *AlbiraARS brochure* [cited 2011-8-18 2011]. Available from http://www.gem-imaging.com/descargas/productos/albira.pdf.

Rogers, D. W. O. (2006). Fifty years of Monte Carlo simulations for medical physics. *Phys Med Biol,* Vol. 51, No. 13, pp. R287-R301, ISSN 0031-9155

Schmidtlein, C. R., A. S. Kirov, S. A. Nehmen, Y. E. Erdi, J. L. Humm, H. I. Amols, et al. (2006). Validation of GATE Monte Carlo simulations of the GE Advance/Discovery LS PET scanners. *Medical Physics,* Vol. 33, No. 1, pp. 198-208, ISSN 0094-2405

Sempau, J., A. Sánchez-Reyes, F. Salvat, H. Oulad Ben Tahar, S. B. Jiang &J. M. Fernández-Varea. (2001). Monte Carlo simulation of electron beams from an accelerator head using PENELOPE. *Phys Med Biol,* Vol. 46, No. 4, pp. 1163-1186, ISSN 0031-9155

van der Laan, D. J., M. C. Maas, H. W. A. M. de Jong, D. R. Schaart, P. Bruyndonckx, C. Lemaître, *et al.* (2007). Simulated performance of a small-animal PET scanner based on monolithic scintillation detectors. *Nucl. Instr. Meth. A,* Vol. 571, No. 1-2, pp. 227-230, ISSN 0168-9002.

2

Rationale, Instrumental Accuracy, and Challenges of PET Quantification for Tumor Segmentation in Radiation Treatment Planning

Assen S. Kirov[1], C. Ross Schmidtlein[1], Hyejoo Kang[2] and Nancy Lee[1]
[1]Memorial Sloan-Kettering Cancer Center, New York,
[2]Northwestern Memorial Hospital, Chicago,
USA

1. Introduction

In the past few decades, radiation therapy of cancer has reached a high level of dosimetric and spatial accuracy due to the strong efforts of both science and industry. This has led to the emergence of today's precise radiation therapy procedures, such as stereotactic radiosurgery and stereotactic body radiation therapy, whose very names indicate a resemblance to surgical precision. This resemblance stems from the high precision with which a dose can be delivered relative to the calculated value in a treatment plan, which is typically within a few percent. However, there are still limits to this precision arising from the technical limitations of the delivery machines and due to the finite errors caused by patient motion and the positioning uncertainties during patient set-up for treatment (LoSasso, 2003; Palta & Mackie, 2011). In addition, one needs to consider the finite penumbra of a radiation therapy beam. Although the dose gradient is fairly steep (at a depth of 10 cm in water, the dose falls off by more than a factor of 10 at less than 5 mm distance from a 1-mm diameter 6 MV pencil beam), photon scatter in the patient and in the accelerator head leads to low-dose but long-range wings of the dose kernel (Kirov et al., 2006). Hence, despite radiation therapy's high dose delivery precision with respect to the planned dose, it is still a relatively blunt instrument when compared to surgery.

As an added difficulty, while the precision of matching the delivered to the planned dose in radiation therapy is well known, the boundaries of the tumor target are not. One of the reasons for this is that the high-resolution imaging modalities—computed tomography (CT) and magnetic resonance imaging (MRI)—are unable to identify the metabolically active or molecularly relevant parts of the tumor. In contrast, positron emission tomography (PET) offers an important advantage by defining the tumor based on its molecular properties (Ling et al., 2000; Schöder & Ong, 2008). In fact, PET has one of the highest sensitivities and specificities in detecting metabolically active tumor tissue (Gambhir et al., 2001). As a result, PET is now widely used for cancer staging and to supplement traditional imaging systems that are used to define the target volume for radiation therapy (i.e. CT and MRI) (Gregoire & Chiti, 2011; Gregoire et al., 2007; Nestle et al., 2009).

However, despite PET's ability to identity metabolic and molecular activity, delineating gross tumor volume (GTV) with PET is problematic due to uncertainties in the biological and physiological processes governing tracer uptake and the instrumental inaccuracy of PET images. These biological and physical uncertainties lead to significant ambiguity of the position of the tumor boundary in images generated by PET in PET/CT and PET/MRI scanners, which in turn leads to uncertainty as to where to aim the precise beam of modern radiotherapy.

In this chapter, which is aimed as an introductory review, we address in order the following questions:

i. What does radiation treatment planning (RTP) need from imaging?
ii. What can PET provide for RTP?
iii. What are the artifacts of PET images and how do they affect RTP?
iv. What are the primary challenges of PET-based tumor segmentation?

Within the context of these questions and the RTP process, we describe the effects of the factors that are mainly responsible for degradation of the PET image, including limited resolution, photon attenuation, scatter, noise, and image reconstruction. In addition, we specifically address the impact of potential inaccuracies of the current artifact correction strategies on segmenting lesions in PET images.

2. The imaging requirements of radiation treatment planning

In radiation therapy (RT), the prescribed dose can be delivered to a phantom and verified with precision better than 5% for most points within a patient, even for very large and non-uniform intensity modulated radiation therapy (IMRT) fields (Kirov et al., 2006). Furthermore, with the introduction of image guidance and respiratory gating techniques, both before and during treatment, similar precision can be achieved for dynamic treatments in which the target is moving. As a result, high treatment delivery precision is becoming standard today for more and more tumor types and disease sites ('A Practical Guide To Intensity-Modulated Radiation Therapy,' 2003; Palta & Mackie, 2011). This high RT dose delivery precision sets high accuracy and precision requirements in imaging for both tumor boundary definition (segmentation) and for activity concentration determination for dose painting (Ling et al., 2000), as described in Section 3 below.

This leads to the question: how accurately are GTV contours currently drawn? At present, tumor boundaries are drawn by radiation oncologists using CT images, in which the tumor may or may not be clearly seen, in a process resembling art. Using PET images in the treatment planning process is becoming more common since it provides additional functional information (Gregoire et al., 2007; Nestle et al., 2009). The use of PET images in treatment planning has led to better agreement among physicians on target definition (Fox et al., 2005; Steenbakkers et al., 2006) and is hypothesized to improve the outcome of therapy. However, CT and PET have vastly different resolution and noise properties. As a result, when CT images are combined with PET images, which have much poorer resolution, an additional source of uncertainty is introduced into the segmentation process. Thereby, the uncertainties in PET images are translated into uncertainty of the RTP contours. Here it is also worth mentioning that many studies that show large discrepancies between PET-derived GTV and CT-derived GTV are performed without intravenous (IV) contrast. The routine use of IV contrast during PET/CT is expected to enable the clinician in further refining the GTV (Haerle et al., 2011).

Ideally, drawing target contours with an accuracy of the order of 1 mm is desirable to match the precision of contemporary dose delivery. While this is achievable with CT and MRI, it is still a challenge for PET. Lastly, GTV is also derived based on clinical examination. Because all imaging modalities (PET, CT, or MRI) have limitations in defining mucosal involvement, the value of a physical examination by a radiation oncologist cannot be underestimated.

Currently, due to the limited resolution of PET and its poorly known quantification accuracy, defining the target for radiation therapy by segmenting PET images is problematic. For this reason, it is important to understand and try to minimize the potential image degrading factors for each patient PET scan (Kang et al., 2009).

3. What can PET provide to radiation treatment planning?

PET reveals functional information about elevated cell metabolic activity, including proliferation or molecular processes that may help localize the most active or potentially radiation-resistant parts of a tumor as well as cancerous metabolic activity not visible in CT images (Erdi et al., 2002; Zanzonico, 2006). Fig. 1 shows an example of how fluorodeoxyglucose [FDG-]PET (red contour) can lead to alteration of a CT-defined GTV and the final planning treatment volume (PTV). This illustrates the substantial difference between the use of PET for diagnostic and RTP purposes. Whereas the goal of diagnostic PET is to detect the presence of a tumor by its abnormal uptake, the goal of using PET in RTP is to delineate cancerous from normal tissue with high accuracy. This poses new challenges for PET. The physical basis for these challenges is discussed in section 5 of this chapter.

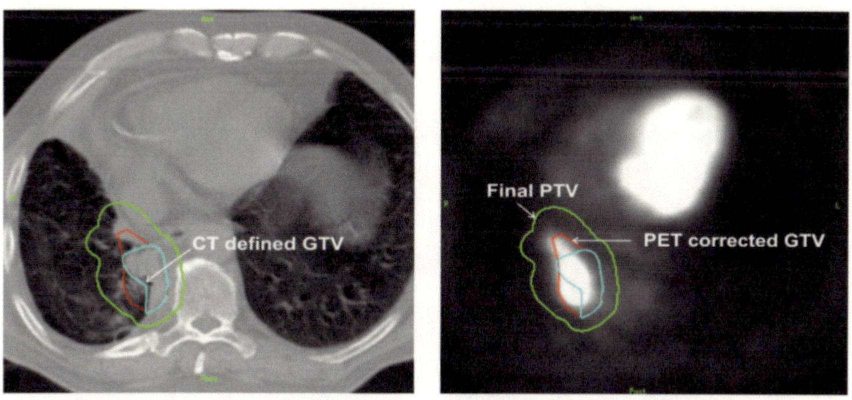

Fig. 1. CT (blue) and FDG-PET (red) gross tumor volume (GTV) and planning target volume (PTV, green) contours drawn around a lung lesion that is positioned close to the spinal cord.

This discussion cannot be considered complete without addressing the various relationships between the actual tumor volume, its estimate as outlined by the physician (GTV), the established margins for both the clinical target volume (CTV) and PTV, the physician's prescription, and the delivered dose (Mackie & Gregoire, 2010; Palta &

Mackie, 2011).Traditional imaging techniques, such as CT and x-ray, attempt to identify volume in a binary (tumor/no tumor) fashion via anatomical abnormalities because they do not supply any functional or metabolic information about the tumor cells or sub-regions. As a result, most radiation therapy planning and delivery is based on irradiating a homogenous target and avoiding the surrounding tissue. These plans are designed to maximize the likelihood of tumor control while minimizing the likelihood of normal tissue complications constrained by the properties of radiation, by the dose delivery precision and by the tumor position uncertainties. The lack of in-vivo biological information about the tumor at voxel size scale requires assuming homogeneity of the target, which implies that the dose delivery should also be homogeneous in order to maximize the probability of tumor control.

In this case, the uncertainty in subclinical disease and delivery is dealt with by extending margins from the estimated GTV to account for the subclinical disease (CTV) and delivery uncertainty (PTV). The beam penumbra leads to a gradual fall off on the edge and outside of these margins. However, the segmentation's boundary, physician's prescription, and treatment plans are based on a hard boundary. The dose is effectively delivered to a soft boundary where that dose may or may not fall off proportionally with the tumor cell density. Quantitatively accurate PET images using tracers that capture the appropriate tumor information have the potential to make the definition of these soft boundaries more explicit and thus, more conformal to the targeted tumor function.

Currently there is an increased interest in using PET to define highly aggressive or radiation-resistant parts of the tumor and selectively treat them with a higher dose in order to increase tumor control probability (TCP) without increasing normal tissue complication probability (NTCP). This treatment approach is known as "dose painting" (Ling et al., 2000; Lee et al.,2008; Aerts et al.,2010; Petit et al., 2009; Bentzen & Gregoire, 2011). Fig. 2 shows how PET has been used for dose painting by increasing the dose to physician-selected regions by using information from the fused PET/CT image as well as from other sources.

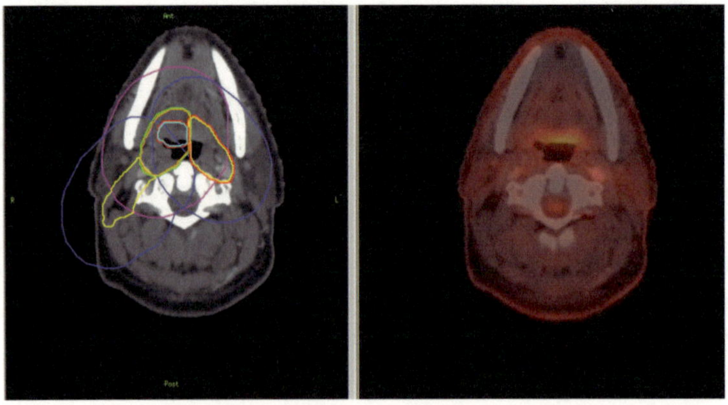

Fig. 2. Example of "dose painting by regions" using PET/CT: CT scan with dose contours (left) and fused CT and FDG-PET (right). The inner contours, some of which encompass the PET avid regions seen, are irradiated to higher doses.

Due to the recently observed highly complex spatial distribution of various tissue properties probed with different tracers on a micro-environmental scale, it was suggested that treatments can be prescribed and delivered on a voxel-by-voxel basis with a technique known as "dose painting by numbers" (Petit et al., 2009; Bentzen & Gregoire, 2011). However, although PET has the potential to provide this type of information, there are difficulties, which need to be addressed for the implementation of such treatments. Among the main challenges are: the limited spatial resolution and signal-to-noise ratio of the imaging system; the dynamic nature of the tumor microenvironment, which can shift between planning and treatment; the fact that there are few tracers that can reliably provide the needed biological information about the relevant molecular processes, and those that do exist require further validation; and the finite setup and delivery uncertainties in radiation therapy.

4. PET uncertainties

The accuracy of the PET segmentation task is limited by the uncertainties of the PET image. As described in a paper by Boelaard (Boellaard, 2009) the factors leading to uncertainty in PET can be divided into three groups: biological (e.g., glucose levels, inflammation, patient comfort, heterogeneity of tumor composition, perfusion, etc.), physical (e.g., positron annihilation physics, detector limitations, reconstruction method), and technical (e.g., activity specification and injection errors, residuals, injection time). The uncertainty contributed by each of these factors can be quite large —up to tens of percent—and these estimates are often approximate or reflect observed maximum deviations. As an example of one technical factor, Fig. 3 shows an illustration of the uncertainty in administered activity.

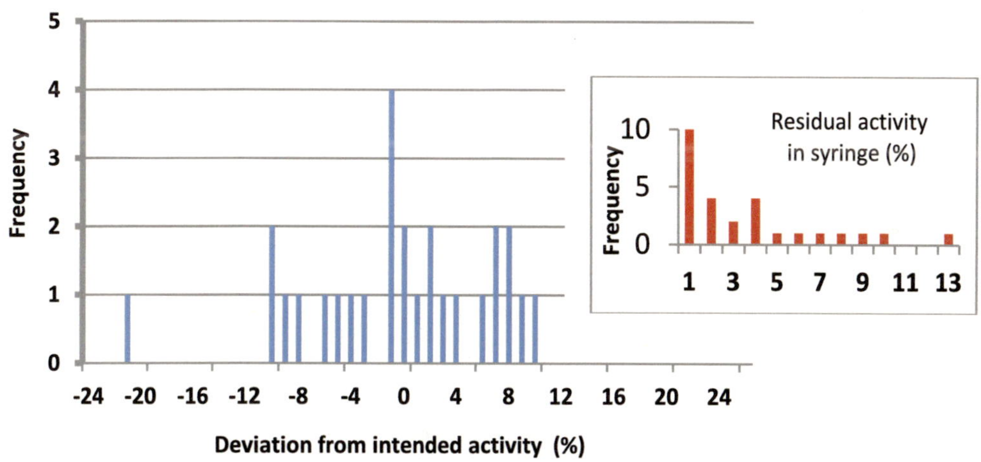

Fig. 3. Deviation of injected activity from intended in percent as observed for 23 patients who were participants in different clinical protocols.

Compared to the accuracy of dose delivery that is achievable in RT today (of the order of a few percent), further efforts are necessary to better quantify the uncertainty contributed by each PET image degrading factor. This is especially true if dose-painting by numbers is considered. In the next section, we address in more detail the physical factors.

5. Physical PET image degrading factors and their effect on segmentation

The activity distribution in a PET image differs from the actual tracer activity distribution due to physical limitations of the PET scanners (Surti et al., 2004; Cherry et al., 2003) and the physical processes summarized in Table 1. In this section we briefly describe the effects of these processes and provide some insight on how each of them may affect the accuracy of PET segmentation even after correction. An illustration of some of the physical phenomena based on a realistic Monte Carlo simulation of a PET scan is presented in Fig. 4.

No.	Factor	Brief Description
1	PET Resolution	Smearing of activity obtained with PET due to physical and detector phenomena (see Table 2)
2	Photon Attenuation	Loss of photons due to scatter or absorption in the patient
3	Photon Scatter	Deviation of photons from their original trajectory due to scatter (see Fig. 8)
4	Random Coincidences	Accidental coincidences from photons originating from the decay of different atomic nuclei
5	Arc Effects	For lines of response close to the periphery of a PET scanner, the effective detector face is smaller and the effective detector thickness is larger due to the curvature of the detector ring
6	Electronics Dead Time	Loss of counts due to overloading the electronic modules with too many events
7	Image Reconstruction	Mathematical reconstruction of the PET data from a patient scan to produce three dimensional images of the activity distribution (this image is dependent on the reconstruction method and its parameters)
8	Registration with the Attenuation Image	Alignment between the PET and CT images in a PET/CT scan
9	Motion	Movement of the tumor and of neighboring tissues due to patient or organ motion

Table 1. Summary of the main physical factors involved in the degradation of PET images

In the above table are listed only the physical phenomena and factors affecting the PET image. It does not include the technical factors, which may cause inaccurate determination of the Standard Uptake Value (SUV) related to activity measurement and injection inaccuracies, and the biological uncertainty factors as listed by Boellaard (Boellaard, 2009), since they are not subject of the present chapter.

5.1 Resolution

The factors affecting PET resolution (Cherry et al., 2003; Tomic et al., 2005) are summarized in Table 2. The finite resolution of PET scanners degrades quantification accuracy and can make small objects invisible if they are comparable or smaller than the Full Width at Half Maximum (FWHM) of the point spread function (PSF). It can also lead to loss of contrast for larger objects due to blurring. The effect is known as partial volume effect (PVE). Various PVE correction methods exist, which apply the correction either at a region or at a voxel level (Soret et al., 2007), during or post reconstruction. Most of the post-reconstruction correction methods lead to variance increase and often use anatomical images (CT or MRI) to control noise amplification. Since PET images are functional and therefore do not need to match the anatomical structures, PVE corrections which do not use anatomical images were also explored (Boussion et al., 2009; Kirov et al., 2008). Fig.5 shows PET images before and after applying one of these approaches. A straightforward and promising approach implemented by some vendors is to incorporate the point-spread function in the reconstruction process (Alessio & Kinahan, 2006). For isotopes with higher positron energy (e.g. ^{13}N and ^{82}Rb) the positron range contribution to the PET PSF is greater and its spatial variance becomes important (Alessio & MacDonald, 2008).

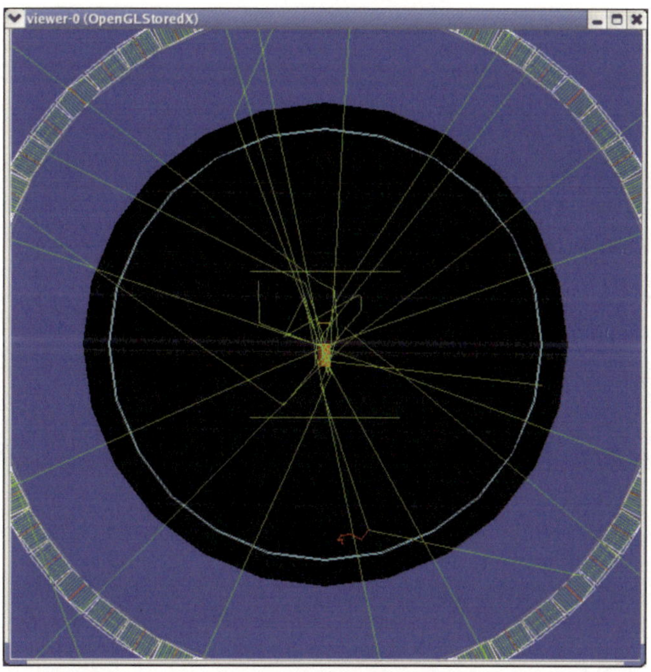

Fig. 4. Annihilation photons originating from a FDG cylinder placed next to an air cavity (short yellow lines close to center) in a water cylinder (horizontal green lines) within a model of the GE Discovery LS PET scanner (Schmidtlein et al., 2006) as simulated by the GATE Monte Carlo code (Jan et al., 2004). Many photons are seen to scatter in the phantom and one even scatters in air, producing a delta electron (red). Some photons are absorbed in the phantom or scattered outside the solid angle of the scanner. A simulation result from this arrangement is shown in Fig.12.

No.	Factor	Brief Description
1	Positron Range	Distance the positron travels prior to annihilation, typically up to about 3 mm for the most often used radioactive isotopes (Zanzonico, 2006)
2	Detector Size and Distance to Detector	PET spatial resolution usually cannot be less than half the size of the face of detector elements; increasing the diameter of the detector ring decreases its efficiency and increases the effect of photon non-colinearity
3	Photon Non-colinearity	Photons are not emitted exactly back-to-back since the positron is not fully stopped at the time of annihilation
4	Block Effect	Scattering of photons in neighboring detectors broadens resolution; also the block readout scheme or detector coding can affect resolution
5	Depth of Interaction	Photons may protrude from one detector without interaction and interact within a neighboring detector
6	Under-sampling	In addition to finite detector size, the angular sampling interval and selected voxel size also impose a limit on resolution
7	Reconstruction	Smoothing functions are applied to data during or after reconstruction to suppress noise in the data

Table 2. Summary of the main factors affecting PET resolution

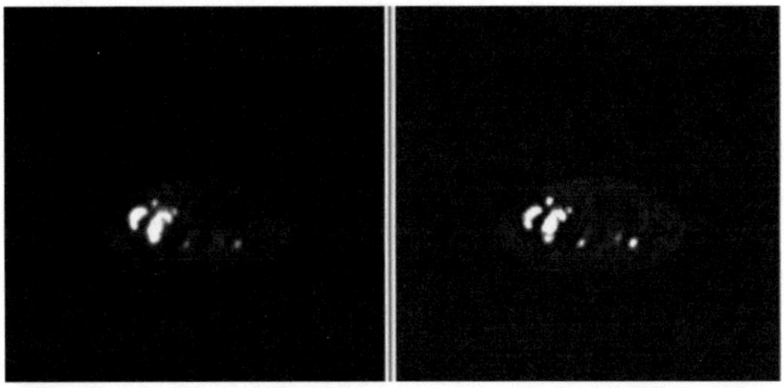

Fig. 5. Effect of a post-reconstruction resolution correction(Kirov et al., 2008) as seen on a PET image before (left) and after (right) PVE correction. Improved contrast is observed especially for the small lesions, but there are modifications of the image related to the Gibbs phenomenon that require further investigation.

The smearing of the tracer distribution due to the finite PET resolution affects segmentation. This is in addition to any biological effects, which may lead to variable gradients of the tumor cell density or metabolism on the tumor periphery and thereby also blur the tracer uptake distribution. PVE related blurring leads to a size dependent variation of the optimal segmentation threshold. This is addressed by using adaptive threshold methods where the threshold is a function of the size of the lesion, as was shown for spherical objects (Erdi et al., 1997; Lee, 2010). The reconstruction parameters (number of iterations, filter types) affect the resolution and their effect on the segmentation threshold has been demonstrated by several groups (Daisne et al., 2003; Ford et al., 2006). Some of the more advanced auto-segmentation approaches combine a resolution correction step within the segmentation process using either deconvolution (Geets et al., 2007), or convolution (De Bernardi et al., 2009) operations.

5.2 Attenuation correction

The attenuation correction (AC) (Zaidi & Hasegawa, 2003) may cause inaccuracies (Mawlawi et al., 2006) due to:

i. incorrect attenuation caused by streaking CT artifacts in proximity to metallic implants
ii. movement resulting in loss of registration between the CT and PET images
iii. use of contrast media, which may cause an overestimation of the AC especially for older bilinear AC algorithms (Nehmeh et al., 2003)
iv. truncation - for large or mis-positioned patients, part of the patient may be outside the CT Field of View (FOV). Unaccounted attenuation results in underestimation of the SUV and will produce streaking artifacts at the edge of the CT images - a rim of high activity at the edge of the CT FOV

Dual energy CT attenuation correction methods have been proposed for reducing (iii) above (Kinahan et al., 2006; Rehfeld et al., 2008)

Each of the mechanisms listed above can affect quantification within the images. As a result, they can alter the basic data that automated segmentation approaches use for determining the probability for assigning a voxel to a certain class. The effects of streaking artifacts in CT due to metallic implants are difficult to quantify due to the gross mismatch between the estimated attenuation coefficients and the actual amount of attenuation in the data. This can cause an artificial increase of uptake in the reconstructed images in some regions and reduction in others. Because of the statistical nature of iterative reconstruction and of the irregularity of the CT artifacts, it is difficult to determine where these effects will be seen. Some vendor software smoothes or redefines regions in the images to remove these CT artifacts, which allows the reconstruction of more reliable PET images. In Fig.6. is shown an artifact that was caused by inaccurate attenuation correction due to CT streaking artifact. The non-AC corrected image indicates this artifact to be clearly visible just above the prosthesis.

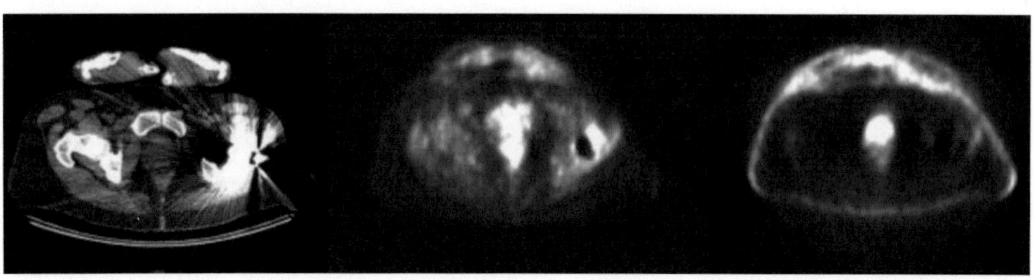

Fig. 6. PET attenuation correction (AC) artifact caused by hip prosthesis: CT streaking artifact (left), and PET with (center) and without (right) AC and scatter correction.

PET and CT misregistration causes systematic shifts in the intensity within the PET images. This may cause similar systematic shifts in the boundaries of the various segmentation schemes. These intensity shifts are especially noticeable in the lung, where small shifts in the patient's position can shift bone into lung and vice versa. In general regions in the patient that were dense during the CT and then less dense during the PET acquisition will show artificially elevated uptake. This effect is demonstrated in Fig. 7. for Monte Carlo simulated PET images of a female thorax, for which the correct position of the AC map is known (Kang et al., 2009). In practice, most vendors use heavily smoothed CT images for AC in the reconstruction process, which smooth these effects but do not eliminate them especially for larger misalignments.

In addition, scatter correction estimates rely on the attenuation map from the CT to estimate the contribution of the scatter events and can therefore be offset because of attenuation correction misalignment, as discussed in more detail in the next section.

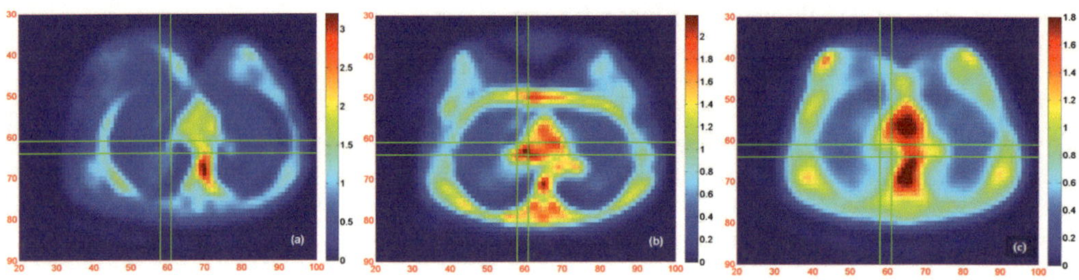

Fig. 7. Reconstructed images of true coincidences with an attenuation correction (AC) map, shifted by 15 mm in positive X (right; a) and Y (down; b) directions, show pronounced changes in activity distribution compared to correctly aligned AC (c). The activity is plotted in relative units.

5.3 Scatter corrections

Photon scatter can lead to erroneous lines of response (LOR, Fig. 8). In the top right inset one can see that photons Compton scattered up to 50 degrees will fall inside a coincident photon energy window above 375 keV. 3D PET provides much higher sensitivity, but also results in a higher fraction of scattered events compared to 2D PET. In Fig.9 is illustrated how scattered photons obtained from Monte Carlo simulation can contaminate the PET energy window. It should be noted that 2D PET systems are in the process of being phased out by the manufacturers, however, a large number of these scanners are currently in use.

Various methods for evaluation of scatter exist (Bailey, 1998; Surti et al., 2004; Zaidi & Koral, 2004) and can be performed at different levels of accuracy: uniform, in which the number of scattered photons across the sinogram is approximated by a smooth function, or more detailed and based on the attenuation correction (AC) image. Historically scatter correction strategies included uniform sinogram tail fitting methods which are outdated and may perform well for uniform phantoms. Experimental approaches using dual or multiple energy windows to separate scatter events have also been investigated (Grootoonk et al., 1996; Trebossen et al., 1993).

Vendors currently use CT based scatter correction schemes and apply the corrections so that they are invisible for the user. Calculating the scatter from the AC image was initiated by

Olinger (Ollinger, 1996) and can be performed either analytically using the Klein-Nishina formula for single scattered photons, which is becoming the industry standard, or using Monte Carlo. The latter is a more accurate method, but it is very time consuming and currently different groups are working on improving the efficiency of these calculations.

There are three main mechanisms through which scatter can affect the quantitative accuracy of the reconstructed images: i) inaccurate modeling of the scatter distribution; ii) inaccurate scatter fraction that is used for scaling the correction in some of the correction approaches; and iii) a shift of the location of the distribution.

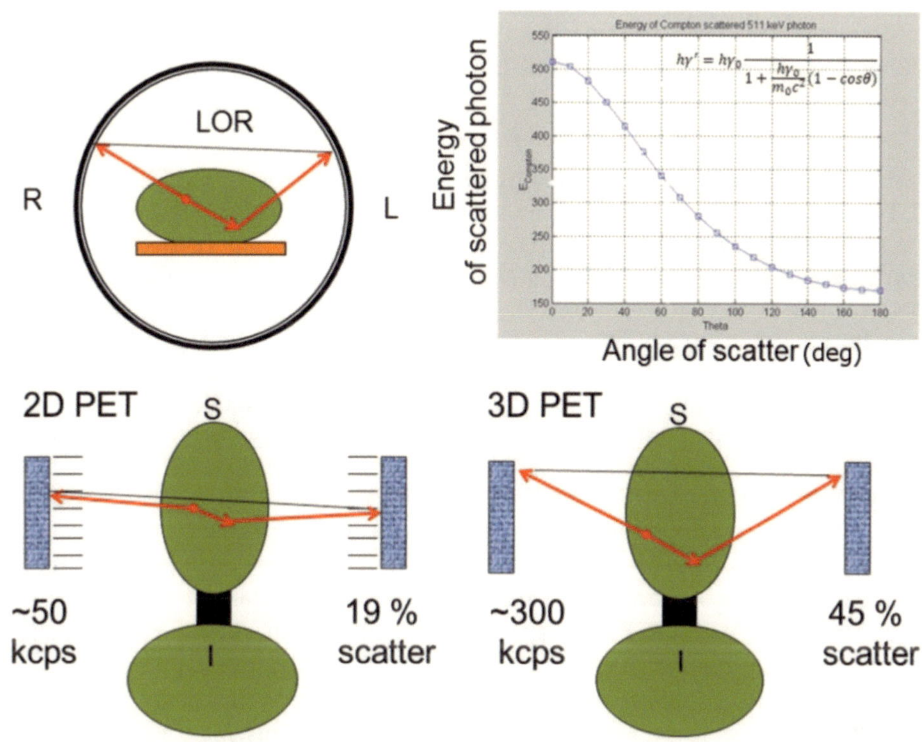

Fig. 8. An illustration of the perturbing role of scatter: erroneous LORs (top left and bottom); dependence of the energy of the Compton scattered annihilation photons on angle of scatter in degrees (top right); illustrations and example count rates in kilo-counts per second (kcps) and scatter fractions for 2D and 3D PET modes, respectively, for a water phantom with a 20-cm diameter filled with 1 mCi ^{18}F-FDG and placed in a Monte Carlo model of a clinical PET scanner (bottom).

In practice, the largest contribution to the errors seen in scatter correction is due to an inaccurate estimate of the scatter fraction. The reason is that the scatter fraction is often obtained by using a tail fit of the projection data outside the patient, which can be affected by patient motion, pulse pileup, or spilled activity. This causes the entire distribution of the scatter counts to be over- or under- corrected. This uniform over- or under- correction in the projection data, can however be re-distributed unevenly by the attenuation and normalization corrections.

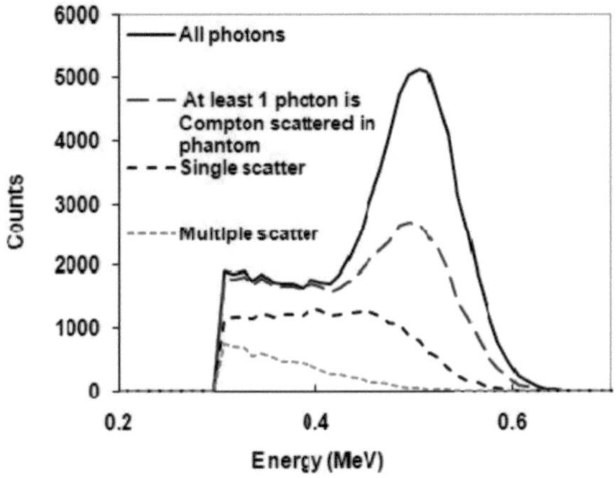

Fig. 9. Photon spectra of coincident photons reaching the detectors of the GE Discovery LS PET/CT scanner, after being emitted from a digital model of the NEMA-2 2001 scatter fraction phantom (20.3 mm diameter) ('NEMA NU 2-2001, Performance Measurements of Positron Emission Tomographs,' 2001), as simulated by the GATE Monte Carlo code. (Jan et al., 2004). Photons with energies below 300 keV are discarded since the coincidence energy windows typically range from 350 or 375 keV to 650 keV. The different spectra correspond to photons from all coincidences (solid line), photons from coincidence of which at least one photon was scattered in the phantom (long dash), spectra of only single-scattered photons (short dash), and spectra of only multiple-scattered photons (dotted line).

In the case of extreme over correction the edges of the images will show zero counts and the resulting images have a "bleached out" appearance. This is most often seen when activity outside the patient's body as determined from the CT mask is present. This alters the tail fit from which the scatter fraction is estimated. An example of this occurs when a patient begins a scan with arms up (CT arms up) and then part way through the scan lowers their arms. Alternatively, this can happen at high activities when pulse pile-up can lead to compounding the true counts so that they produce pulses above the energy window and to compounding scattered counts to fall inside that window. This may increase the tail of scattered events in the sinogram and lead to scatter overcorrection. This is most often seen near the bladder or heart in normal scans and sometimes with short half-life tracers due to their high initial activity. In either case, resulting images have a dramatic loss of contrast and appear bleached out. In the case of severe over correction, because of the loss of contrast and quantitative accuracy, the affects on segmentation can be dramatic. However, these images are often poor enough that no usable diagnostic information remains, and it is obvious that they are not useful for segmentation.

Poor modeling of the scatter distribution can cause local regions of the projection data to be over or under-corrected. Discrepancies in the modeled scatter distribution are further scaled by the system sensitivity and attenuation corrections during image reconstruction. The net result is that the over-corrected regions will show reduced uptake and the under-corrected regions will show increased uptake. However, because the scatter distribution, even after being scaled is smoothly varying in projection space, poor modeling of the shape of the distribution is generally difficult to identify and likely a small effect. The exception to this is when the entire distribution is improperly scaled due to a poor estimate of the scatter fraction.

Although, the scatter distribution is a slowly varying function of position in projection space, the application of the attenuation correction scales these counts so that they concentrate in the more highly attenuated regions in the images (Fig.10). Because of this, in some regions of the thorax the apparent number of scattered photons in the images may approach the number of true coincidences (Kang et al., 2009). Therefore, an inaccuracy of the

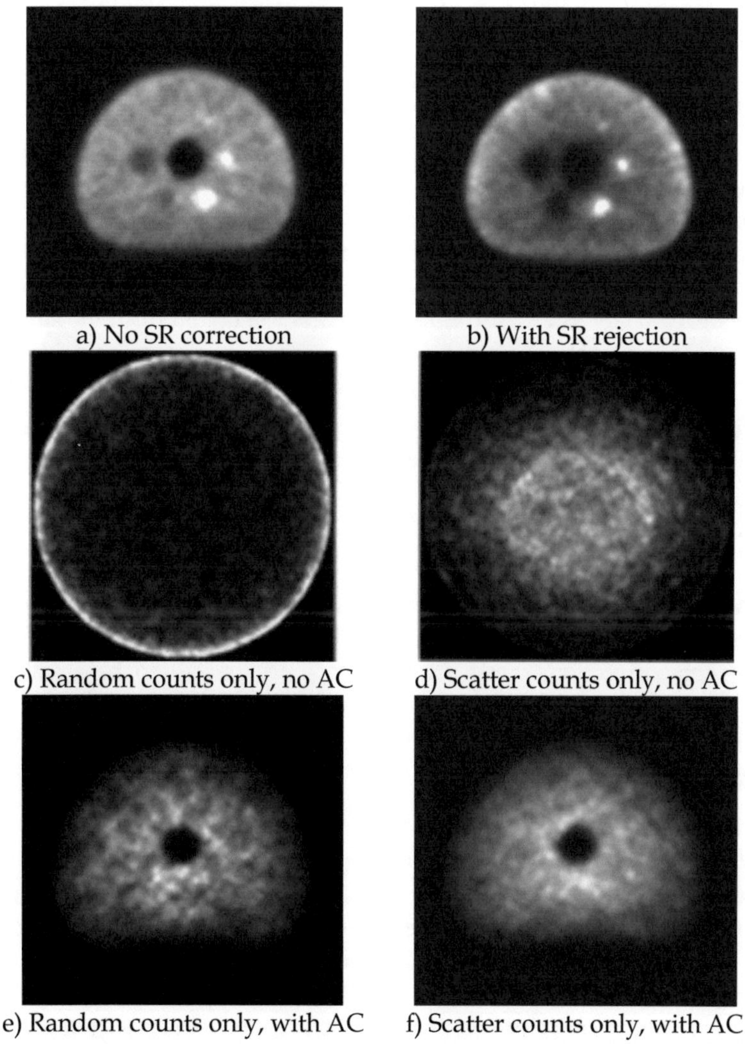

Fig. 10. (a-f) Effect and distribution of scattered and random (SR) coincidences for the NEMA-2 Image Quality phantom, as obtained from a Monte Carlo simulated scan (Jan et al., 2004; Schmidtlein et al., 2006), which allows exact separation of these events.

scatter correction of about 15% (Chang et al., 2009), can result in a similar quantification error in the PET signal for these regions. This can alter the tumor to background ratio, which can affect most segmentation methods.

Finally, the scattered events can affect segmentation accuracy if the AC map is shifted with respect to the PET image due to patient movement between the CT and the subsequent PET scan. In addition to shifting the true counts image as was shown in Section 5.2 (Fig 7), this will cause a similar shift of the scatter counts image (Fig.10f). The under- and over-corrections will be most pronounced at the extreme edges of the patient along the axis of the shift. However, unless the shift is substantial, the overall effect may be small if the attenuation correction is smoothed. In general, this is a second order effect when compared to the effect of the attenuation correction misregistration on the true coincidences.

5.4 Random corrections

The number of random events increases with increasing the injected activity and may exceed the number of true events by few times. However, the random correction is very accurate. Usually it is obtained in one of the following three ways: (i) real time subtraction of the count rate from a delayed timing window for which no true coincidences are possible, (ii) off-line correction using a low-noise estimate of the random events rate obtained by smoothing the delayed sinogram; or (iii) random rates calculated from the single events rate in each detector. Direct subtraction of real time measured random coincidences increases noise in the corrected image. Brasse et al (Brasse et al., 2005) have shown that while smoothed delayed random estimates provide the lowest noise images, singles-based random estimates perform only marginally worse, but without the dead-time penalty and increased data bandwidth of the delayed counts approach.

In analogy with the discussion in Section 5.3, although random counts are quite smooth and uniform, because of the attenuation correction, any uncorrected random counts will be pushed in the regions with high attenuation (Fig.10) and they may cause inaccuracies similar to these described for scattered photons. However due to much higher accuracy of the random events correction, these inaccuracies are expected to be smaller than those introduced by the inaccuracy of the scattered events correction.

5.5 Normalization correction

The normalization correction corrects for the "non-uniformity of detector response related to the geometry of the scanner" and for the difference in sensitivity between the different detector channels (Bailey, 1998). It is performed during routine re-calibration of the scanner by using a uniform activity cylinder or by a scanning rod source. The vendor of the scanner specifies the source and the correction procedures. For more information on different approaches for normalization correction see (Bailey, 1998) and (Badawi, 1999). Improper or out of date normalization files can add some artifacts to the reconstructed image. The most common artifacts are caused by unaccounted for change in the efficiency of some detectors. They can be seen in transverse slices as ring-like light and dark intensity patterns centered on the transverse axis. The effect on automated segmentation schemes is likely to be similar to that of CT streak artifacts but less intense.

5.6 Dead time

Corrections are needed to account for count loses due to the electronics dead time. Since the losses are larger at high count rates, this can be done by repetitive scans of a decaying source. High count rates can also lead to mis-positioning and misclassifying events due to pulse pile-up in block detector systems (Badawi, 1999). Mis-positioning may cause loss of imaging accuracy if normalization is performed at count rates very different from these in clinical scans. Additionally, at high activities, pulse pile-up can cause true counts to be pushed out and scattered events pushed in the coincidence energy window (event misclassification). As discussed in Section 5.3, this may lead to an overestimation of the scatter correction and therefore can affect segmentation as described in section 5.3.

5.7 Image reconstruction and noise

PET image reconstruction is inherently noisy due to the Poisson processes that govern the detection and the interpretation of the emitted photons (e.g. decay, detection, energy spectrum). While all modern PET scanners are supplied with and clinics use statistically based (iterative) image reconstruction, it is useful to discuss the resolution and noise properties of images generated with older, deterministic, image reconstruction methods first. In deterministic image reconstruction methods, such as filtered back-projection, the back-projection process mixes the Poisson distributed projection data via the projection operator (often a uniformly spaced Radon transform) to generate images whose voxels have a Gaussian noise distribution (Alpert et al., 1982; Schmidtlein et al., 2010). The resulting images have better signal-to-noise ratios for high contrast objects than for low contrast objects (this is not true for OSEM, as explained below). Additionally, the projection operator and related post-filtering tend to smooth the noise and create covariance between neighboring voxels. Post filtering greatly increases the ability to interpret the images.

The most popular iterative image reconstruction algorithm is Ordered Subsets Expectation Maximization (OSEM), which is a form of Maximum Likelihood Expectation Maximization (MLEM) with accelerated convergence achieved by iterating over smaller subsets of the data (typically an angular component of the sinogram) (Tarantola et al., 2003). This iterative reconstruction seeks the most likely image given the data and a statistical model of the system. However, like all un-regularized maximum likelihood estimates, these reconstruction methods begin to fit the noise of the data if iterated too many times. Furthermore, the signal-to-noise (SNR) ratio over the image is more uniform, and because of that hot objects will have higher noise compared to colder objects (Schmidtlein et al., 2010). As a result, the ability of iterative statistical reconstruction to produce increased contrast in low uptake regions is one of the primary reasons that these methods are superior to deterministic methods for diagnostic purposes.

Overall, the noise of voxels in OSEM generated images is best described as log-normally or multi-variate normally distributed (Barrett et al., 1994) where the standard deviation is proportional to the voxel intensity. It follows then from the proportionality and the non-uniform sampling that the noise and resolution properties in these images are position dependent (Fessler & Rogers, 1996). In addition, the covariance between neighboring voxels is increased, that adds complexity when evaluating the statistical properties of regions of interest (Buvat 2002; Schmidtlein et al, 2010). Following iterative reconstruction, most data is typically smoothed to reduce the effects of the data over-fitting. To avoid these effects and/or non-uniform spatial resolution, some penalized-likelihood (regularization) schemes have been developed (Fessler & Rogers, 1996), but are rarely used. Li (Li, 2011) most recently analyzed the noise properties of penalized-likelihood algorithms.

Two new features that are now available with the latest generation of PET scanners are point spread function modeling (PSF) and time-of-flight (TOF) reconstruction. Both of these modifications to the reconstruction process alter the noise in the reconstructed images by altering the projection operator. PSF reconstruction uses the measured spatial resolution of the scanner to account for blurring (Table 2). Counter intuitively (deconvolution is usually a noise amplifying process) this process results in smoother images. This behavior can be explained by realizing that, with the addition of the PSF information into the system model, the over fitting normally seen in maximum likelihood models is constrained by the improved system model (mathematically this can also be seen through the propagation of the PSF kernel through the forward and back projectors (Rapisarda et al., 2010; Tong et al., 2010). In TOF reconstruction, the use of the timing information restricts lines-of-response (LOR) in the projection matrix to a smaller portion of the object. In addition this reduces both the amount of random and scattered events in the object. Hence, for TOF reconstruction the contrast can be improved, though the effect is most pronounced in patients with more scatter (Chang et al., 2011).

Therefore resolution, contrast and signal-to-noise ratio are dependent on the reconstruction type and parameters. With few exceptions among the statistical auto-segmentation methods, e.g. (Yu, Caldwell, Mah, & Mozeg, 2009; Hatt et al., 2009), most other auto-segmentation methods are dependent on these characteristics of the images.

5.8 Misregistration and motion

Patient motion (e.g. breathing) can lead to loss of registration between CT and PET images. Due to the much longer PET acquisition time a PET image encompasses lesion positions over different breathing phases. This can affect the accuracy of the contours shown in Fig.1. Breathing motion artefacts in PET/CT images can be corrected for by binning PET data according to the breathing phase (e.g. in 10 bins), and then correct each of those data sets for attenuation using a phase-matched CT image set deduced from 4D-CT images. This method is referred to as 4D PET/CT (Nehmeh et al., 2004). Another technique is the breath hold technique PET/CT acquisition, where both PET and CT images will be acquired at the same breathing amplitude, e.g. deep inspiration (Nehmeh et al., 2011). The basis of this technique as well as a description of the different motion tracking devices are summarized in a review (Nehmeh & Erdi, 2008).

An interesting case of registered PET/CT images is shown in Fig.11. In this case, motion is suspected to be the reason for what seems to be activity in the air cavity. The behavior of the PET signal at tissue-air and tissue-lung interfaces was separately investigated and showed a steep PET signal drop for a cork or air cavity next to ^{18}F activity (Fig.12) (Kirov et al., 2004). Therefore, motion is suspected to be the reason for what seems to be activity in the air cavity.

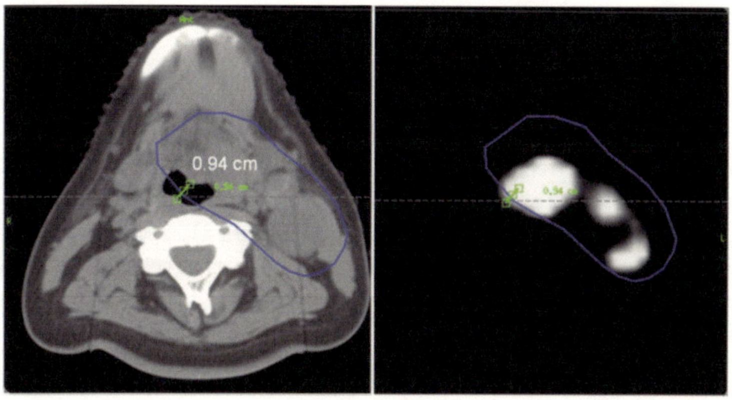

Fig. 11. A RTP contour displayed on registered CT (left) and PET (right) images from a FDG-based PET/CT scan. PET signal appears to originate from ~ 1-cm wide air cavity inside the trachea, as seen with respect to the RTP contour.

At 3 mm and beyond into the cavity the PET signal intensity drops to 30% below the peak value. Increased signal is observed on the opposing wall of the cavity due to positrons crossing the cavity (Fig. 12). The intensity of this peak is ~ 0.2% of that of the main peak. This was confirmed also by a Monte Carlo simulation, which gives the positron annihilation position.

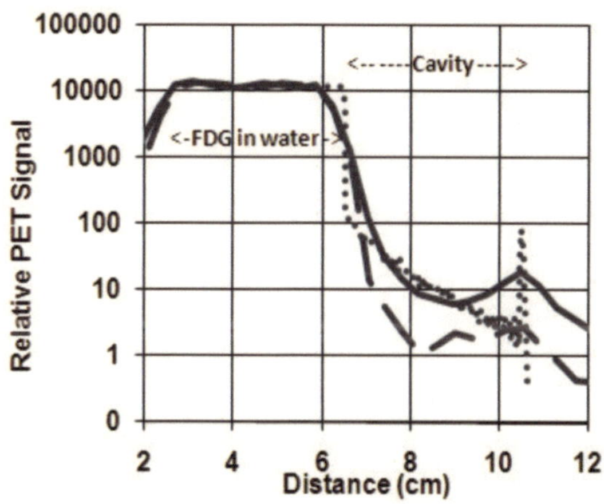

Fig. 12. Effect of the presence of air and lung cavities positioned next to activity on the PET image intensity. Relative PET signal profiles across FDG-air (solid line) and FDG-cork (dashed line) interfaces, as obtained by OSEM reconstruction of a 2D high sensitivity scan on the GE Discovery LS PET scanner. The profiles were summed over three neighboring slices at the center of the image to reduce noise. The positron annihilation position for this geometry, as obtained from a Monte Carlo simulation (Fig.4), is shown with the dotted line.

5.9 Other artifacts

In addition to the physical processes described above, other sources of error in PET images may be due to improper calibration, faulty detector blocks, or another malfunctioning of the scanner hardware as well as spilled activity on the cover of the detector rings, e.g. contamination from urinal splash.

5.10 Overall PET inaccuracy

For simple phantoms, the overall quantification inaccuracy of PET scans has been measured. However, for more realistic cases in which the tracer distribution is a complex superposition of the perturbing effects of the various phenomena discussed above, PET accuracy is both unknown and not yet well investigated. In a Monte Carlo based investigation it was shown how different corrections and reconstruction algorithms can affect accuracy for non-uniform activity and attenuation varying in one direction (Kirov et al., 2007). The development of a new class of physical phantoms, capable of producing realistic activity distributions, similar to those observed in clinical scans (Kirov et al., 2011), will further aid in quantification of the overall PET inaccuracy.

The artifacts discussed in the previous sections and summarized in Table 3, ultimately contribute to the inaccuracy of the segmentation boundary in the form of offsets and global inaccuracies as well as in uncertainty of the boundary location due to the noise of the voxel intensities. Here we present an example of a formalism that allows to explicitly represent the overall uncertainty of the position of the segmentation contour as a function of these inaccuracies and the uncertainty associated with a noise model based on a spherical tumor with constant uptake in an image reconstructed with OSEM. In this case, assuming that the uptake is increasing in a direction perpendicular to the segmentation boundary, the intensity of a given voxel at position r can be approximated as a truncated Taylor series expansion by

$$X(r) \cong X_T(R_T) + \left.\frac{dX}{dr}\right|_T (r - R_T)\,. \tag{1}$$

Here $X(r)$ is image intensity at a voxel at position, r, and, R_T is the position of the segmentation edge. It should be noted that this edge is a function of the segmentation method; however, once the segmentation is performed it is at a fixed position. By using a central difference approximation of the derivative, this can be rearranged to represent an estimate of the distance from the segmentation edge, $\delta_{R_T} = r - R_T$ as,

$$\delta_{R_T} = r - R_T \cong \frac{2\Delta r\,[X - X_T]}{X_{T+} - X_{T-}}, \tag{2}$$

where, $X = X(r)$, $X_T = X(R_T)$, $X_{T+} = X(R_T + \Delta r)$, $X_{T-} = X(R_T - \Delta r)$, and Δr is the distance between voxels. Now by assuming the independence of one voxel to another (i.e. ignoring the covariance), the uncertainty of the boundary at any particular position can be estimated by,

$$\sigma_\delta^2 \cong \left(\frac{2\Delta r}{X_{T+} - X_{T-}}\right)^2 (\sigma_X^2 + \sigma_{X_T}^2) + \left(\frac{2\Delta r[X - X_T]}{[X_{T+} - X_{T-}]^2}\right)^2 (\sigma_{X_{T+}}^2 + \sigma_{X_{T-}}^2), \tag{3}$$

where the first term represents the contribution of uncertainty from the voxel intensities, and the second term represents the contribution due to the uncertainty from the gradient. Here, σ_δ^2 is the variance of the distance from the segmentation contour corresponding to threshold T, and σ_X^2 is the variance of voxel intensity. The above equation can be further simplified by substituting R_{T+} and R_{T-} for r in (2), averaging these two results, and then by using the approximation,

$$\frac{2[X_{T+}-X_T]}{X_{T+}-X_{T-}} \approx \frac{2[X_T-X_{T-}]}{X_{T+}-X_{T-}} \approx 1 .$$

Noting this and using the approximation that, for MLEM reconstructed images, the variances of the data are proportional to the square of the mean , $\sigma_X^2 \cong \alpha^2 X^2$, (Barrett et al., 1994; Schmidtlein et al., 2010), and evaluating X at R_T this can be rewritten to give the effect of noise on segmentation as,

$$\sigma_\delta^2 \cong \left(\frac{2\alpha\,\Delta r}{X_{T+}-X_{T-}}\right)^2 \left(X_T^2 + \frac{3}{4}X_{T+}^2 + \frac{3}{4}X_{T-}^2\right). \quad (4)$$

The parameter, α, can be estimated by finding a region of uniform uptake, such as the liver, through direct measurement. The uncertainties introduced by the physical artifacts (Table 3) and their corrections discussed in this chapter as well as other factors including biological uncertainty can in principle be incorporated into the parameters of Eq.(3) to quantitatively model the overall uncertainty of the segmentation, provided that their covariances are not significant. The above formalism ignores the covariance between neighboring voxels. In practice, the covariance can be included and estimated as shown by Buvat (Buvat, 2002), and the variance can be estimated by using a staggered checkerboard pattern (Schmidtlein et al., 2010).

Factor	Brief Description of Effect on Segmentation
PET Resolution	Tracer distribution blurring and variation of segmentation threshold with object size
Photon Attenuation	AC artifacts can strongly affect relative voxel intensities and therefore, the position of the delineation contour
Photon Scatter	Although slowly varying photon scatter can affect local intensities due to the effect of attenuation correction (Fig.10); the effects of severe over-correction can confound segmentation
Random Coincidences	Generally negligible effects due to accurate corrections
Depth of Interaction	Decreased spatial resolution and increased edge uncertainty
Electronics Dead Time	Can affect voxel intensities and also the scatter fraction estimate
Image Reconstruction	Parameters of iterative reconstruction (e.g., iteration number, post-reconstruction filters) modify the smoothness of an image to which segmentation methods are sensitive
Registration with the Attenuation Image	Attenuation artifacts and scatter artifacts
Motion	In addition to offsetting the lesion position, motion can cause loss of resolution, attenuation artifacts, and scatter artifacts

Table 3. Contribution of the various physical PET artifacts to segmentation inaccuracy.

6. Challenges for PET based tumor segmentation

According to Udupa et al, (Udupa et al., 2006) the image segmentation task is a process consisting of two stages: a high level process to recognize the rough region of interest (ROI) containing the tumor and a lower level process to delineate the tumor within that ROI. Although the delineation stage may be based mostly on low level information (the image intensities), it often requires high level information and interpretation including knowledge from areas which are not present nor reflected in the PET image, namely anatomy, physiology and pathology. This imposes the need for the segmentation to be performed by a physician expert or by a team of such experts (e.g. a nuclear medicine physician and a radiation oncologist) (MacManus & Hicks, 2008). At the same time manual only PET segmentation may lead to large inter- and intra- observer variations, due for example to different intensity windowing during display. This has prompted the development of PET auto-segmentation methods which are based on the intensities of the image voxels or on properties derived from these intensities. It has been shown that the use of such methods lead to reduction of inter-observer variability in delineation (van Baardwijk et al., 2007).

A vast variety of PET auto-segmentation methods with different level of complexity have been developed in the last 15 years. Several recently published reviews present comprehensive list and classifications of these methods (Boudraa & Zaidi, 2006; Lee, 2010; Zaidi & El Naqa, 2010). A simpler classification can be based in part on the numerical simplicity of the approach and in part on the popularity of that approach. In order of increasing complexity (and decreasing popularity) the line-up is as follows: a) methods using a fixed threshold value in terms of intensity or standard uptake value (SUV), e.g. (Erdi et al., 1997; Mah et al., 2002; Paulino & Johnstone, 2004); b) adaptive threshold methodse.g. (Erdi et al., 1997; Black et al., 2004; Nehmeh et al., 2009; Nestle et al., 2005; Seuntjens et al., 2011) and c) advanced segmentation methods, which include a large variety of more complex numerical approaches using gradient (Geets et al., 2007), statistical (Aristophanous et al., 2007; Hatt et al., 2009; Dewalle-Vignion et al., 2011), region growing (Day et al., 2009); deformable models (Li et al., 2008), texture analysis (Yu, et al., 2009) as well as other supervised or unsupervised learning methods (Zaidi, 2006; Zaidi & El Naqa, 2010; Belhassen & Zaidi, 2010). A similar classification is adopted by the educational task group on PET auto-segmentation within the American Association of Physicists in Medicine (AAPM TG211).

The advantage of the fixed threshold methods is their simplicity, ease of implementation and use. Large discrepancies between some of these methods with respect to volumes visually determined by a physician were found for non-small lung cancer (NSLC) (Nestle et al., 2005) and for head and neck cancer (Greco et al., 2008). By design the adaptive threshold methods should provide better accuracy, however it is very important to adapt the parameters in each of these methods to the scanner and protocol used in each institution (Fig. 13) and to pay special attention to the phantom data sets used for this process (Lee, 2010). It is known that the fixed and adaptive threshold methods are challenged by irregularly shaped non-uniform activity distributions (Black et al., 2004; Hatt, Cheze le Rest, van Baardwijk, et al., 2011). Finally, the advanced segmentation tools have been demonstrated to be more accurate and robust to non-uniform activity distributions, (Geets et al., 2007; Montgomery et al., 2007; Li et al., 2008; Hatt, Cheze Le Rest, Albarghach, et al.,

2011), however their implementation, if not part of a commercial software may be significantly more demanding. Although the anatomical, metabolic and functional contours do not necessarily need to match, using images from different imaging imaging modalities (e.g. CT, PET, and MRI) is beneficial for tumor segmentation (El Naqa et al., 2007; Yu, Caldwell, Mah, & Mozeg, 2009; Yu et al., 2009).

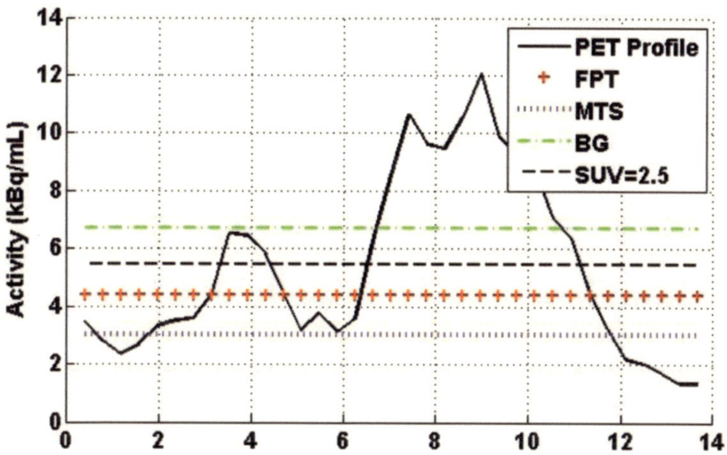

Fig. 13. PET segmentation thresholds obtained with different automatic segmentation algorithms that use a fixed threshold displayed on top of a profile of the activity across a real lesion: FPT – 40 % of peak activity, MTS- mean target SUV (Black et al., 2004) , BG – background-based method (Nestle et al., 2005).

Despite these developments, the segmentation of PET images is still a challenge since the quantitative accuracy of PET with respect to the underlying histopathology is not well known. The quantitative accuracy of the PET image is affected by how well the selected tracer identifies the biological target and by the physical factors summarized in this chapter. In addition to using an accurate auto-segmentation tool by an experienced physician, resolution of each of these two problems for each patient is needed to claim reliable and accurate PET based tumor delineation.

7. Acknowledgements

The authors would like to acknowledge the contributions of Dr. Ellen Yorke, Dr. John Humm, Dr. Heiko Schöder, and Dr. Howard Amols, all of Memorial Sloan-Kettering Cancer Center in New York City, for their helpful discussions of the material presented; of Erin Sculley, of Bucknell University in Lewisburg, PA, for her help in the analysis of some of the data presented; of Dr. Slobodan Devic, of McGill University in Montreal, for providing thoughtful comments, and of Ms. Sandhya George of Memorial Sloan-Kettering Cancer Center for her help in editing and formatting of the text.

8. Disclaimer

The material in this chapter is not to be used as a substitute for medical advice, diagnosis or treatment of any health condition or problem. Radiation therapy and planning and PET/CT imaging should only be undertaken by qualified individuals. Your facility's installation and set-up may differ from our experience and the ideas presented in this chapter are for discussion purposes only. You should not rely on the material presented here without independent evaluation and verification. Follow safety procedures and the instructions of medical equipment manufacturers. Medical physics treatment practices change frequently and therefore information contained in this chapter may be outdated, incomplete, or incorrect.

9. References

Aerts, H. J., Lambin, P., & Ruysscher, D. D. 2010, 'FDG for dose painting: a rational choice', *Radiother Oncol*, vol. 97, no. 2, pp. 163-4.

Alessio, A. & MacDonald, L. 2008, 'Spatially Variant Positron Range Modeling Derived from CT for PET Image Reconstruction', *IEEE Nucl. Sci. Symp. and Med. Imaging Conf., Dresden, pp 3637 - 3640.*

Alessio, A. M. & Kinahan, P. E. 2006, 'Improved quantitation for PET/CT image reconstruction with system modeling and anatomical priors', *Med Phys*, vol. 33, no. 11, pp. 4095-103.

Alpert, N. M., Chesler, D. A., Correia, J. A., Ackerman, R. H., Chang, J. Y., Finklestein, S., Davis, S. M., Brownell, G. L., & Taveras, J. M. 1982, 'Estimation of the local statistical noise in emission computed tomography', *IEEE Trans Med Imaging*, vol. 1, no. 2, pp. 142-6.

Aristophanous, M., Penney, B. C., Martel, M. K., & Pelizzari, C. A. 2007, 'A Gaussian mixture model for definition of lung tumor volumes in positron emission tomography', *Med Phys*, vol. 34, no. 11, pp. 4223-35.

Badawi, R. 1999, *Introduction to PET Physics (web-page tutorial)*, <http://depts.washington.edu/nucmed/IRL/pet_intro/intro_src/section6.html>.

Bailey, D. L. 1998, '*Quantitative procedures in 3D PET', in The Theory and Practice of 3D PET*, Developments in Nuclear Medicine (P H Cox ed.), ed. B. Bendriem and D.W. Townsend, Vol. 32, Kluwer Academic Publishers, Rdrecht / Boston /London.

Barrett, H. H., Wilson, D. W., & Tsui, B. M. 1994, 'Noise properties of the EM algorithm: I. Theory', *Phys Med Biol*, vol. 39, no. 5, pp. 833-46.

Belhassen, S. & Zaidi, H. 2010, 'A novel fuzzy C-means algorithm for unsupervised heterogeneous tumor quantification in PET', *Med Phys*, vol. 37, no. 3, pp. 1309-24.

Bentzen, S. M. & Gregoire, V. 2011, 'Molecular imaging-based dose painting: a novel paradigm for radiation therapy prescription', *Semin Radiat Oncol*, vol. 21, no. 2, pp. 101-10.

Black, Q. C., Grills, I. S., Kestin, L. L., Wong, C. Y., Wong, J. W., Martinez, A. A., & Yan, D. 2004, 'Defining a radiotherapy target with positron emission tomography', *Int J Radiat Oncol Biol Phys*, vol. 60, no. 4, pp. 1272-82.

Boellaard, R. 2009, 'Standards for PET image acquisition and quantitative data analysis', *J Nucl Med*, vol. 50 Suppl 1, pp. 11S-20S.

Boudraa, A. O. & Zaidi, H. 2006, 'Image Segmentation Techniques In Nuclear Medicine Imaging', in H. Zaidi (ed), *Quantitative analysis in Nuclear Medicine Imaging*, Springer, Singapore, pp. 308-57.

Boussion, N., Cheze Le Rest, C., Hatt, M., & Visvikis, D. 2009, 'Incorporation of wavelet-based denoising in iterative deconvolution for partial volume correction in whole-body PET imaging', *Eur J Nucl Med Mol Imaging*, vol. 36, no. 7, pp. 1064-75.

Brasse, D., Kinahan, P. E., Lartizien, C., Comtat, C., Casey, M., & Michel, C. 2005, 'Correction methods for random coincidences in fully 3D whole-body PET: impact on data and image quality', *J Nucl Med*, vol. 46, no. 5, pp. 859-67.

Buvat, I. 2002, 'A non-parametric bootstrap approach for analysing the statistical properties of SPECT and PET images', *Phys Med Biol*, vol. 47, no. 10, pp. 1761-75.

Chang, T., Chang, G., Clark, J., & Mawlawi, O. 2009, ' Accuracy of Scatter and Attenuation Correction in PET imaging.', *Abstract presented at the 2009 AAPM annual meeting, Med. Phys.*, vol. 36, no. 6, p. 2469.

Chang, T., Clark, J., & Mawlawi, O. 2011, 'Evaluation of Image quality on a Time-of-Flight PET/CT scanner', *Abstract presented at the 2011 joint AAPM/COMP meeting, Med. Phys.*, vol. 38, p. 3787.

Cherry, S. R., Sorensen, J. A., & Phelps, M. E. 2003, *Physics in Nuclear Medicine*, Saunders, Elsevier.

Daisne, J. F., Sibomana, M., Bol, A., Doumont, T., Lonneux, M., & Gregoire, V. 2003, 'Tri-dimensional automatic segmentation of PET volumes based on measured source-to-background ratios: influence of reconstruction algorithms', *Radiother Oncol*, vol. 69, no. 3, pp. 247-50.

Day, E., Betler, J., Parda, D., Reitz, B., Kirichenko, A., Mohammadi, S., & Miften, M. 2009, 'A region growing method for tumor volume segmentation on PET images for rectal and anal cancer patients', *Med Phys*, vol. 36, no. 10, pp. 4349-58.

De Bernardi, E., Faggiano, E., Zito, F., Gerundini, P., & Baselli, G. 2009, 'Lesion quantification in oncological positron emission tomography: a maximum likelihood partial volume correction strategy', *Med Phys*, vol. 36, no. 7, pp. 3040-9.

Dewalle-Vignion, A. S., Betrouni, N., Lopes, R., Huglo, D., Stute, S., & Vermandel, M. 2011, 'A new method for volume segmentation of PET images, based on possibility theory', *IEEE Trans Med Imaging*, vol. 30, no. 2, pp. 409-23.

El Naqa, I., Yang, D., Apte, A., Khullar, D., Mutic, S., Zheng, J., Bradley, J. D., Grigsby, P., & Deasy, J. O. 2007, 'Concurrent multimodality image segmentation by active contours for radiotherapy treatment planning', *Med Phys*, vol. 34, no. 12, pp. 4738-49.

Erdi, Y. E., Mawlawi, O., Larson, S. M., Imbriaco, M., Yeung, H., Finn, R., & Humm, J. L. 1997, 'Segmentation of lung lesion volume by adaptive positron emission tomography image thresholding', *Cancer*, vol. 80, no. 12 Suppl, pp. 2505-9.

Erdi, Y. E., Rosenzweig, K., Erdi, A. K., Macapinlac, H. A., Hu, Y. C., Braban, L. E., Humm, J. L., Squire, O. D., Chui, C. S., Larson, S. M., & Yorke, E. D. 2002, 'Radiotherapy treatment planning for patients with non-small cell lung cancer using positron emission tomography (PET)', *Radiother Oncol*, vol. 62, no. 1, pp. 51-60.

Fessler, J. A. & Rogers, W. L. 1996, 'Spatial resolution properties of penalized-likelihood image reconstruction: space-invariant tomographs', *IEEE Trans Image Process*, vol. 5, no. 9, pp. 1346-58.

Ford, E. C., Kinahan, P. E., Hanlon, L., Alessio, A., Rajendran, J., Schwartz, D. L., & Phillips, M. 2006, 'Tumor delineation using PET in head and neck cancers: threshold contouring and lesion volumes', *Med Phys*, vol. 33, no. 11, pp. 4280-8.

Fox, J. L., Rengan, R., O'Meara, W., Yorke, E., Erdi, Y., Nehmeh, S., Leibel, S. A., & Rosenzweig, K. E. 2005, 'Does registration of PET and planning CT images decrease interobserver and intraobserver variation in delineating tumor volumes for non-small-cell lung cancer?', *Int J Radiat Oncol Biol Phys*, vol. 62, no. 1, pp. 70-5.

Gambhir, S. S., Czernin, J., Schwimmer, J., Silverman, D. H., Coleman, R. E., & Phelps, M. E. 2001, 'A tabulated summary of the FDG PET literature', *J Nucl Med*, vol. 42, no. 5 Suppl, pp. 1S-93S.

Geets, X., Lee, J. A., Bol, A., Lonneux, M., & Gregoire, V. 2007, 'A gradient-based method for segmenting FDG-PET images: methodology and validation', *Eur J Nucl Med Mol Im*, vol. 34, no. 9, pp. 1427-38.

Greco, C., Nehmeh, S. A., Schoder, H., Gonen, M., Raphael, B., Stambuk, H. E., Humm, J. L., Larson, S. M., & Lee, N. Y. 2008, 'Evaluation of different methods of 18F-FDG-PET target volume delineation in the radiotherapy of head and neck cancer', *Am J Clin Oncol*, vol. 31, no. 5, pp. 439-45.

Gregoire, V. & Chiti, A. 2011, 'Molecular imaging in radiotherapy planning for head and neck tumors', *J Nucl Med*, vol. 52, no. 3, pp. 331-4.

Gregoire, V., Haustermans, K., Geets, X., Roels, S., & Lonneux, M. 2007, 'PET-based treatment planning in radiotherapy: a new standard?', *J Nucl Med*, vol. 48 Suppl 1, pp. 68S-77S.

Grootoonk S, Spinks T J, Sashin D, Spyrou N M and Jones T 1996 , 'Correction for scatter in 3D brain PET using a dual energy window method' *Phys Med Biol* 41 2757-74

Hatt, M., Cheze Le Rest, C., Albarghach, N., Pradier, O., & Visvikis, D. 2011, 'PET functional volume delineation: a robustness and repeatability study', *Eur J Nucl Med Mol Imaging*, vol. 38, no. 4, pp. 663-72.

Hatt, M., Cheze le Rest, C., Turzo, A., Roux, C., & Visvikis, D. 2009, 'A fuzzy locally adaptive Bayesian segmentation approach for volume determination in PET', *IEEE Trans Med Imaging*, vol. 28, no. 6, pp. 881-93.

Hatt, M., Cheze le Rest, C., van Baardwijk, A., Lambin, P., Pradier, O., & Visvikis, D. 2011, 'Impact of tumor size and tracer uptake heterogeneity in 18F-FDG PET and CT Non-Small Cell Lung Cancer tumor delineation', *Journal of Nuclear Medicine*, vol. 52, no. 11, pp. 1690-7.

Haerle, S. K., Strobel, K., Ahmad, N., Soltermann, A., Schmid, D. T., & Stoeckli, S. J. 2011, 'Contrast-enhanced (1)F-FDG-PET/CT for the assessment of necrotic lymph node metastases', *Head Neck*, vol. 33, no. 3, pp. 324-9.

Jan, S., Santin, G., Strul, D., Staelens, S., Assie, K., Autret, D., Avner, S., Barbier, R., Bardies, M., Bloomfield, P. M., Brasse, D., Breton, V., Bruyndonckx, P., Buvat, I., Chatziioannou, A. F., Choi, Y., Chung, Y. H., Comtat, C., Donnarieix, D., Ferrer, L., Glick, S. J., Groiselle, C. J., Guez, D., Honore, P. F., Kerhoas-Cavata, S., Kirov, A. S.,

Kohli, V., Koole, M., Krieguer, M., van der Laan, D. J., Lamare, F., Largeron, G., Lartizien, C., Lazaro, D., Maas, M. C., Maigne, L., Mayet, F., Melot, F., Merheb, C., Pennacchio, E., Perez, J., Pietrzyk, U., Rannou, F. R., Rey, M., Schaart, D. R., Schmidtlein, C. R., Simon, L., Song, T. Y., Vieira, J. M., Visvikis, D., Van de Walle, R., Wieers, E., & Morel, C. 2004, 'GATE: a simulation toolkit for PET and SPECT', *Phys Med Biol*, vol. 49, no. 19, pp. 4543-61.

Kang, H., Schmidtlein C R, Mitev K , Gerganov G , Madzhunkov Y, Humm J L, Amols H I , & Kirov, A. S. 2009, 'Monte Carlo based evaluation of 3D PET quantification inaccuracy for the lung', *Abstract presented at the 51 Annual Meeting of the AAPM, Anaheim, CA , Med. Phys.*, vol. 36, p. 2426.

Kinahan, P. E., Alessio, A. M., & Fessler, J. A. 2006, 'Dual energy CT attenuation correction methods for quantitative assessment of response to cancer therapy with PET/CT imaging', *Technol Cancer Res Treat*, vol. 5, no. 4, pp. 319-27.

Kirov, A. S., Caravelli, G., Palm Å, Chui C, & LoSasso T 2006, 'Pencil Beam Approach for Correcting the Energy Dependence Artifact in Film Dosimetry for IMRT verification', *Med. Phys.*, vol. 33, no. 10, pp. 3690-9.

Kirov, A. S., Danford, C., Schmidtlein, C. R., Yorke, E., Humm, J. L., & Amols, H. I. 2007, 'PET Quantification Inaccuracy of Non-Uniform Tracer Distributions for Radiation Therapy', *IEEE Nuclear Science Symposium and Medical Imaging Conference Record, Proceedings paper M13-5, p. 2838-2841.*

Kirov, A. S., Piao, J. Z., & Schmidtlein, C. R. 2008, 'Partial volume effect correction in PET using regularized iterative deconvolution with variance control based on local topology', *Phys Med Biol*, vol. 53, no. 10, pp. 2577-91.

Kirov, A. S., Schmidtlein C R, Bidaut L M, Nehmeh S A, Yorke E, Humm J L, Larson S, Ling C C, & Amols, H. I. 2004, 'Experimental and Monte Carlo Characterization of Positron Range Artifacts in PET Near Body Cavities ', *Abstract presented at the 2004 Annual Meeting of the AAPM, Med. Phys.*, vol. 31, p. 179.

Kirov, A. S., Sculley, E., Schmidtlein, C. R., Siman, W., Kandel, B., Zdenek, R., Schwar, R., Ayzenberg, G., Yorke, E., Schöder, H., Humm, J. L., & Amols, H. 2011 'A New Phantom Allowing Realistic Non-Uniform Activity Distributions for PET Quantification', *Abstract presented at the 2011 Joint AAPM/COMP meeting, Med. Phys.*, vol. 38, no. 6, p. 3387.

Lee, J. A. 2010, 'Segmentation of positron emission tomography images: some recommendations for target delineation in radiation oncology', *Radiother Oncol*, vol. 96, no. 3, pp. 302-7.

Lee, N. Y., Mechalakos, J. G., Nehmeh, S., Lin, Z., Squire, O. D., Cai, S., Chan, K., Zanzonico, P. B., Greco, C., Ling, C. C., Humm, J. L., & Schoder, H. 2008, 'Fluorine-18-labeled fluoromisonidazole positron emission and computed tomography-guided intensity-modulated radiotherapy for head and neck cancer: a feasibility study', *Int J Radiat Oncol Biol Phys*, vol. 70, no. 1, pp. 2-13.

Li, H., Thorstad, W. L., Biehl, K. J., Laforest, R., Su, Y., Shoghi, K. I., Donnelly, E. D., Low, D. A., & Lu, W. 2008, 'A novel PET tumor delineation method based on adaptive region-growing and dual-front active contours', *Med Phys*, vol. 35, no. 8, pp. 3711-21.

Li, Y. 2011, 'Noise propagation for iterative penalized-likelihood image reconstruction based on Fisher information', *Phys Med Biol*, vol. 56, no. 4, pp. 1083-103.

Ling, C. C., Humm, J., Larson, S., Amols, H., Fuks, Z., Leibel, S., & Koutcher, J. A. 2000, 'Towards multidimensional radiotherapy (MD-CRT): biological imaging and biological conformality', *Int J Radiat Oncol Biol Phys*, vol. 47, no. 3, pp. 551-60.

LoSasso, T. 2003, 'Quality Assurance of IMRT', *A Practical Guide To Intensity-Modulated Radiation Therapy*, Medical Physics Publishing, Madison, Wisconsin.

Mackie, T. R. & Gregoire, V. 2010, *International Commission on Radiation Units and Measurements (ICRU) Report 83. Prescribing, Recording, and Reporting Photon-Beam Intensity-Modulated Radiation Therapy (IMRT)*, Vol. 10(1), Oxford, UK.

MacManus, M. P. & Hicks, R. J. 2008, 'Where do we draw the line? Contouring tumors on positron emission tomography/computed tomography', *Int J Radiat Oncol Biol Phys*, vol. 71, no. 1, pp. 2-4.

Mah, K., Caldwell, C. B., Ung, Y. C., Danjoux, C. E., Balogh, J. M., Ganguli, S. N., Ehrlich, L. E., & Tirona, R. 2002, 'The impact of (18)FDG-PET on target and critical organs in CT-based treatment planning of patients with poorly defined non-small-cell lung carcinoma: a prospective study', *Int J Radiat Oncol Biol Phys*, vol. 52, no. 2, pp. 339-50.

Mawlawi, O., Pan, T., & Macapinlac, H. A. 2006, 'PET/CT imaging techniques, considerations, and artifacts', *J Thorac Imaging*, vol. 21, no. 2, pp. 99-110.

Montgomery, D. W., Amira, A., & Zaidi, H. 2007, 'Fully automated segmentation of oncological PET volumes using a combined multiscale and statistical model', *Med Phys*, vol. 34, no. 2, pp. 722-36.

Nehmeh, S. A., El-Zeftawy, H., Greco, C., Schwartz, J., Erdi, Y. E., Kirov, A., Schmidtlein, C. R., Gyau, A. B., Larson, S. M., & Humm, J. L. 2009, 'An iterative technique to segment PET lesions using a Monte Carlo based mathematical model', *Med Phys*, vol. 36, no. 10, pp. 4803-9.

Nehmeh, S. A. & Erdi, Y. E. 2008, 'Respiratory motion in positron emission tomography/computed tomography: a review', *Semin Nucl Med*, vol. 38, no. 3, pp. 167-76.

Nehmeh, S. A., Erdi, Y. E., Kalaigian, H., Kolbert, K. S., Pan, T., Yeung, H., Squire, O., Sinha, A., Larson, S. M., & Humm, J. L. 2003, 'Correction for oral contrast artifacts in CT attenuation-corrected PET images obtained by combined PET/CT', *J Nucl Med*, vol. 44, no. 12, pp. 1940-4.

Nehmeh, S. A., Erdi, Y. E., Pan, T., Pevsner, A., Rosenzweig, K. E., Yorke, E., Mageras, G. S., Schoder, H., Vernon, P., Squire, O., Mostafavi, H., Larson, S. M., & Humm, J. L. 2004, 'Four-dimensional (4D) PET/CT imaging of the thorax', *Med Phys*, vol. 31, no. 12, pp. 3179-86.

Nehmeh, S. A., Haj-Ali, A. A., Qing, C., Stearns, C., Kalaigian, H., Kohlmyer, S., Schoder, H., Ho, A. Y., Larson, S. M., & Humm, J. L. 2011, 'A novel respiratory tracking system for smart-gated PET acquisition', *Med Phys*, vol. 38, no. 1, pp. 531-8.

'NEMA NU 2-2001, Performance Measurements of Positron Emission Tomographs' 2001, National Electrical Manufacturers Association, Rosslyn, VA.

Nestle, U., Kremp, S., Schaefer-Schuler, A., Sebastian-Welsch, C., Hellwig, D., Rube, C., & Kirsch, C. M. 2005, 'Comparison of different methods for delineation of 18F-FDG

PET-positive tissue for target volume definition in radiotherapy of patients with non-Small cell lung cancer', *J Nucl Med*, vol. 46, no. 8, pp. 1342-8.

Nestle, U., Weber, W., Hentschel, M., & Grosu, A. L. 2009, 'Biological imaging in radiation therapy: role of positron emission tomography', *Phys Med Biol*, vol. 54, no. 1, pp. R1-25.

Ollinger, J. M. 1996, 'Model-based scatter correction for fully 3D PET', *Phys Med Biol*, vol. 41, no. 1, pp. 153-76.

Palta, J. R. & Mackie, T. R. 2011, 'Uncertainties in External Beam Radiation Therapy', Medical Physics Publishing, Madison, Wisconsin.

Paulino, A. C. & Johnstone, P. A. 2004, 'FDG-PET in radiotherapy treatment planning: Pandora's box?', *Int J Radiat Oncol Biol Phys*, vol. 59, no. 1, pp. 4-5.

Petit, S. F., Dekker, A. L., Seigneuric, R., Murrer, L., van Riel, N. A., Nordsmark, M., Overgaard, J., Lambin, P., & Wouters, B. G. 2009, 'Intra-voxel heterogeneity influences the dose prescription for dose-painting with radiotherapy: a modelling study', *Phys Med Biol*, vol. 54, no. 7, pp. 2179-96.

'A Practical Guide To Intensity-Modulated Radiation Therapy' 2003, Medical Physics Publishing, Madison, Wisconsin.

Rapisarda, E., Bettinardi, V., Thielemans, K., & Gilardi, M. C. 2010, 'Image-based point spread function implementation in a fully 3D OSEM reconstruction algorithm for PET', *Phys Med Biol*, vol. 55, no. 14, pp. 4131-51.

Rehfeld, N. S., Heismann, B. J., Kupferschlager, J., Aschoff, P., Christ, G., Pfannenberg, A. C., & Pichler, B. J. 2008, 'Single and dual energy attenuation correction in PET/CT in the presence of iodine based contrast agents', *Med Phys*, vol. 35, no. 5, pp. 1959-69.

Schmidtlein, C. R., Beattie, B. J., Bailey, D. L., Akhurst, T. J., Wang, W., Gonen, M., Kirov, A. S., & Humm, J. L. 2010, 'Using an external gating signal to estimate noise in PET with an emphasis on tracer avid tumors', *Phys Med Biol*, vol. 55, no. 20, pp. 6299-326.

Schmidtlein, C. R., Kirov, A. S., Nehmeh, S. A., Erdi, Y. E., Humm, J. L., Amols, H. I., Bidaut, L. M., Ganin, A., Stearns, C. W., McDaniel, D. L., & Hamacher, K. A. 2006, 'Validation of GATE Monte Carlo simulations of the GE Advance/Discovery LS PET scanners', *Med Phys*, vol. 33, no. 1, pp. 198-208.

Schöder, H. & Ong, S. C. 2008, 'Fundamentals of molecular imaging: rationale and applications with relevance for radiation oncology', *Semin Nucl Med*, vol. 38, no. 2, pp. 119-28.

Seuntjens, J., Mohammed, H., Devic, S., Tomic, N., Aldelaijan, S., Deblois, F., J. Seuntjens, S. Lehnert, & Faria, S. 2011, 'Uptake Volume Histograms: A Novel Avenue Towards Delineation of Biological Target Volumes (BTV) in Radiotherapy', *Med. Phys.*, vol. 38, no. 6, p. 3786.

Soret, M., Bacharach, S. L., & Buvat, I. 2007, 'Partial-volume effect in PET tumor imaging', *J Nucl Med*, vol. 48, no. 6, pp. 932-45.

Steenbakkers, R. J., Duppen, J. C., Fitton, I., Deurloo, K. E., Zijp, L. J., Comans, E. F., Uitterhoeve, A. L., Rodrigus, P. T., Kramer, G. W., Bussink, J., De Jaeger, K., Belderbos, J. S., Nowak, P. J., van Herk, M., & Rasch, C. R. 2006, 'Reduction of observer variation using matched CT-PET for lung cancer delineation: a three-dimensional analysis', *Int J Radiat Oncol Biol Phys*, vol. 64, no. 2, pp. 435-48.

Surti, S., Karp, J. S., & Kinahan, P. E. 2004, 'PET instrumentation', *Radiol Clin North Am*, vol. 42, no. 6, pp. 1003-16.

Tarantola, G., Zito, F., & Gerundini, P. 2003, 'PET instrumentation and reconstruction algorithms in whole-body applications', *J Nucl Med*, vol. 44, no. 5, pp. 756-69.

Tomic, N., Thompson, C. J., & Casey, M. E. 2005, 'Investigation of the "Block Effect" on spatial resolution in PET detectors', *IEEE Trans. Nucl. Sci.*, vol. 52, no. 3, pp. 599-605.

Tong, S., Alessio, A. M., & Kinahan, P. E. 2010, 'Noise and signal properties in PSF-based fully 3D PET image reconstruction: an experimental evaluation', *Phys Med Biol*, vol. 55, no. 5, pp. 1453-73.

Trebossen R, Bendriem B, Frouin V and Syrota A 1993 Spectral-Analysis of Scatter Distributions in Dual-Energy Acquisition Mode on a Positron Tomograph *Journal of Nuclear Medicine* 34 P186-P

Udupa, J. K., Leblanc, V. R., Zhuge, Y., Imielinska, C., Schmidt, H., Currie, L. M., Hirsch, B. E., & Woodburn, J. 2006, 'A framework for evaluating image segmentation algorithms', *Comput Med Imaging Graph*, vol. 30, no. 2, pp. 75-87.

van Baardwijk, A., Bosmans, G., Boersma, L., Buijsen, J., Wanders, S., Hochstenbag, M., van Suylen, R. J., Dekker, A., Dehing-Oberije, C., Houben, R., Bentzen, S. M., van Kroonenburgh, M., Lambin, P., & De Ruysscher, D. 2007, 'PET-CT-based auto-contouring in non-small-cell lung cancer correlates with pathology and reduces interobserver variability in the delineation of the primary tumor and involved nodal volumes', *Int J Radiat Oncol Biol Phys*, vol. 68, no. 3, pp. 771-8.

Yu, H., Caldwell, C., Mah, K., & Mozeg, D. 2009, 'Coregistered FDG PET/CT-based textural characterization of head and neck cancer for radiation treatment planning', *IEEE Trans Med Imaging*, vol. 28, no. 3, pp. 374-83.

Yu, H., Caldwell, C., Mah, K., Poon, I., Balogh, J., MacKenzie, R., Khaouam, N., & Tirona, R. 2009, 'Automated radiation targeting in head-and-neck cancer using region-based texture analysis of PET and CT images', *Int J Radiat Oncol Biol Phys*, vol. 75, no. 2, pp. 618-25.

Zaidi, H. 2001, 'Scatter modelling and correction strategies in fully 3-D PET', *Nucl Med Commun*, vol. 22, no. 11, pp. 1181-4.

Zaidi, H. & El Naqa, I. 2010, 'PET-guided delineation of radiation therapy treatment volumes: a survey of image segmentation techniques', *Eur J Nucl Med Mol Imaging*, vol. 37, no. 11, pp. 2165-87.

Zaidi, H. & Hasegawa, B. 2003, 'Determination of the attenuation map in emission tomography', *J Nucl Med*, vol. 44, no. 2, pp. 291-315.

Zaidi, H. & Koral, K. F. 2004, 'Scatter modelling and compensation in emission tomography', *Eur J Nucl Med Mol Imaging*, vol. 31, no. 5, pp. 761-82.

Zanzonico, P. 2006, 'PET-based biological imaging for radiation therapy treatment planning', *Crit Rev Eukaryot Gene Expr*, vol. 16, no. 1, pp. 61-101.

3

Kinetic Modelling in Human Brain Imaging

Natalie Nelissen[1], James Warwick[2] and Patrick Dupont[1]
[1]*K.U.Leuven*
[2]*Stellenbosch University*
[1]*Belgium*
[2]*South Africa*

1. Introduction

Kinetic modelling is an important tool in Positron Emission Tomography (PET) which enables us to study the kinetics of tracers. Two important applications of this technique are its use in drug development and in the study of the neurochemistry of the brain. A major issue that we encounter when using kinetic modelling is the selection of the model and understanding its limits and pitfalls. Furthermore, the acquisition, reconstruction and processing of PET data also affects the kinetic modelling thereof. Therefore, we define the following three main objectives for the reader of this chapter:

- To understand how the acquisition, reconstruction and processing of data affects its kinetic modelling.
- To understand the rationale, the limits and the pitfalls of each model.
- To understand how model selection can be performed.

2. Acquisition

The acquisition process can be roughly divided into four different parts:

1. Preparation and monitoring of the patient
2. Injection of the tracer
3. PET measurement
4. Sampling of blood (optional)

2.1 Preparation and monitoring of the patient

Most studies for quantification of tracer kinetics last for a relatively long time (typically 60-90 minutes). Therefore, it is important to pay attention to the comfort of the patient when he or she is positioned in the scanner as well as to use elements which can reduce head movement (e.g. a tape around the head to fixate it). Due to the optimal performance at the centre of the scanner, the head needs to be positioned in the central part of the field of view. If needed, monitoring can be performed during the acquisition (e.g. ECG or blood pressure). When the EEG needs to be monitored, this gives rise to local hot spots at the location of the electrodes and introduces a small positive quantification bias in the reconstructed image in voxels located in the brain (Lemmens et al. (2008)). This is caused by metal artifacts from the CT used for attenuation correction. Algorithms for metal artifact reduction in CT can be used to reduce this problem (De Man et al. (2000)).

It is noteworthy to mention that the position of the patient (typically head first, supine) should be indicated when preparing the PET acquisition. This ensures the correct orientation of the reconstructed images since in most cases, left/right cannot be reliably determined based on the images alone (in contrast to cranial/caudal and anterior/posterior orientations).

2.2 Injection of the tracer

When injecting the subject with the tracer, a cannula has to be in place (typically in an arm vein). Most often a bolus injection is given, sometimes in combination with a constant infusion of the tracer over the time period of the study to obtain a faster equilibrium (Carson (2000)).

In most human PET (or SPECT) imaging studies, only a very small amount of ligand is injected, often in the range of pico to nanograms. This usually requires a high specific activity, i.e. the amount of radioactively labelled versus unlabelled molecules, at the time of injection. E.g. if the specific activity of a ligand is $4TBq/mmol$ at injection time and if we inject $400MBq$, the total amount of ligand injected is $0.1\mu mol$. When using certain tracers (e.g. $[^{11}C]$-Carfentanil, a highly potent and selective μ opioid receptor agonist) the total amount of compound administered has to be lower than some predefined value (e.g. $0.03\mu g/kg$ body weight in case of $[^{11}C]$-Carfentanil), ensuring sub-pharmacological doses.

To know the exact amount of activity injected, the remaining dose after injection (rest dose) should be measured as well as the exact time of dose measurement, injection time and rest dose measurement. Accurate timing requires the same or cross-calibrated clocks. The effective dose injected can be calculated as:

$$D = D_i * e^{-\frac{ln(2)}{t_{1/2}}(t_0 - t_i)} - D_e * e^{-\frac{ln(2)}{t_{1/2}}(t_e - t_0)} \tag{1}$$

in which D is the effective dose injected at time t_0, D_i is the dose measured before injection at time t_i and D_e is the rest dose after injection as measured at time t_e. The half-life of the tracer is given by $t_{1/2}$.

2.3 PET measurement

Several high resolution PET scanners are available on the market for which the performance is well characterized. New clinical scanners typically operate as a PET-CT scanner in which the CT can be used for attenuation correction. For this purpose, a low dose CT, limiting the radiation exposure, is sufficient. However, there are still high resolution dedicated PET scanners in operation which most often use $^{68}Ga/^{68}Ge$ or ^{137}Cs sources for attenuation correction. The CT or PET scan used to correct for attenuation, sometimes called the transmission scan, is not performed simultaneously and therefore a mismatch between the head position during the transmission scan and the emission scan (i.e. the actual PET measurement) can occur. This will lead to artifacts and can give rise to large errors in the modelling. Therefore it is recommended that the coregistration between the transmission and the emission scans is explicitly evaluated by an expert. This can be done by reconstructing the PET emission image without attenuation correction and simultaneously viewing it with the reconstructed transmission scan.

PET measurements used for kinetic modelling are dynamic measurements. Two strategies are possible depending on the scanner: a list-mode acquisition or a dynamic acquisition in which time frames have to be specified before the start of the acquisition. List-mode acquisition has the major advantage that rebinning in frames can be done afterwards and - if necessary - another rebinning scheme can be used. However, due to the large amount of data (depending on the number of events and the length of the scan), the option of using multiple rebinning schemes is not always feasible in practice. The frame definition actually defines the sampling resolution of the dynamic PET study. Since we need to reconstruct every frame, two properties should be kept in mind: a frame should contain enough events to ensure a reliable reconstruction, and during a frame the distribution of the tracer should be more or less constant. These two requirements are not met in the beginning of the acquisition and a trade-off has to be chosen. Sampling is certainly not uniform with short frames in the beginning and gradually longer frames towards the end. An example of a frame definition used when performing a 60 minutes $[^{11}C]$-Flumazenil (a GABA-A antagonist) acquisition is 4 x 15s, 4 x 60s, 2 x 150s, 10 x 300s.

Since dynamic PET measurements are long, motion correction should be applied. First, by paying attention to patient comfort when positioning them in the scanner, by fixating the head, and by giving adequate instructions beforehand, major movements can be avoided. Second, coregistration of the different frames can be performed to correct for small movements (see later). Some groups are currently investigating how one can use tracking devices (e.g. Montgomery et al. (2006)) or, in case of the new MRI-PET scanners, simultaneous MRI scanning (Catana et al. (2011)) to continuously monitor any movement and to correct the list mode using these measurements. This is still work in progress but the initial results look promising.

Besides the frame definition, which only in case of list mode data can be changed after the acquisition, a number of settings are irreversible, i.e. they cannot be changed after the measurement. These are the time coincidence window, energy window, settings for scatter and random measurements, measurements for attenuation, start and duration of the scan, etc. Corrections for randoms, scatter and attenuation are necessary in brain imaging and are relatively easy to perform. Scatter correction has an impact on the final results but few studies have been done to quantify this. Attenuation correction is typically done when quantification is necessary but when using a PET transmission scan, this might add additional noise from the transmission scan through propagation into the reconstruction of the emission data. Nowadays, this is much less of a problem when using CT for attenuation correction since it is less noisy than a PET transmission scan.

Since often a bolus injection is given, dead time can be significant in the first minute. Adequate dead time correction is necessary in order to correctly measure the high initial activity. Therefore, the dead time correction available on the system should be well characterized.

The start and duration of the scan depend on the tracer and its kinetics as well as on the model that will be applied to determine the physiological parameters. In many applications it is common practice to start the scan at the time of injection although, for simplified methods, the scan can be started at later a time point when equilibrium is approached. The duration of the scan determines the amount of data generated. Furthermore, the duration is also determined by the system under study: we assume that the physiological and metabolic processes which affect our measurement are more or less constant for the duration of the measurement, unless we explicitly want to manipulate these processes in e.g. activation studies.

Importantly, it is necessary to correct for decay of the isotope unless one takes this into account explicitly in the models. In this chapter we assume that decay correction has been performed.

2.4 Sampling of blood

A number of kinetic models that are commonly used in PET require the sampling of arterial blood to determine the arterial blood or plasma concentration which indicates how much tracer is available for uptake in the brain. This can be done by measuring radioactivity of the blood/plasma samples with a well counter and scaling this number by the volume measured. A major problem that arises with some tracers is that radioactive metabolites are formed which are also detected and indistinguishable from intact tracer, since we measure the isotope attached to a molecule and not the molecule itself. Often metabolites are formed outside the brain and do not cross the blood-brain-barrier. In such a case, the input function can easily be corrected by multiplying it with the intact fraction of the tracer at each time point. The intact fraction can be obtained by taking blood samples at different time points and analyzing them with high-performance liquid chromatography (HPLC) which separates intact tracer from metabolites based on different retention times (due to different chemical interactions) in a column .

For this procedure, it is required that the blood samples have a larger volume for accurate processing compared to the samples needed for the determination of the input function. Typically, 5-7 samples are taken and a model describing the intact fraction as function of time is fitted through the data points to obtain the intact fraction for every time within the measurement interval.

The most popular models used for this are:

1. The mono-exponential model given by

$$F(t) = Ae^{-\frac{ln(2)}{\alpha}t} \tag{2}$$

   describing the fraction $F(t)$ of intact tracer over time. The parameter A describes the amplitude, while α describes the biological half live. Sometimes an additional constraint $A = 1$ (i.e. at the time of the injection, we have 100% intact tracer) is imposed.

2. The bi-exponential model given by

$$F(t) = Ae^{-\frac{ln(2)}{\alpha}t} + Be^{-\frac{ln(2)}{\beta}t} \tag{3}$$

   in which A and B are the amplitudes of the two processes each described by a half-life α respectively β. An additional constraint $A + B = 1$ with the same interpretation as above can be imposed. An equivalent model is given by:

$$F(t) = Ae^{-\frac{ln(2)}{\alpha}(t-t_{delay})} + (1-A)e^{-\frac{ln(2)}{\beta}(t-t_{delay})} \tag{4}$$

   in which t_{delay} is a time-constant describing the delay before metabolisation takes place.

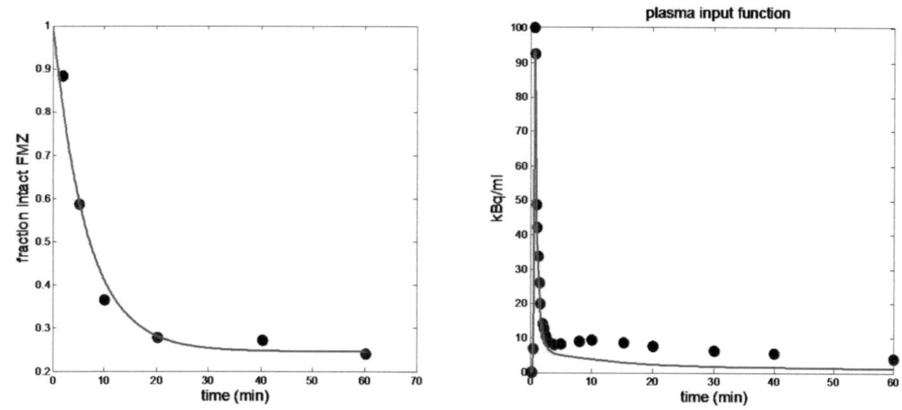

(a) Intact fraction of tracer (b) Plasma input function

Fig. 1. Example of intact fraction and the plasma input function of $[^{11}C]$-Flumazenil

3. A third model is the Hill model described by:

$$F(t) = \frac{b}{1 + (\frac{a}{t})^n} \tag{5}$$

in which a, b and n are parameters that can be interpreted respectively as the time to obtain half of the maximum value, the maximum value obtained at $t = 0$ if $n < 0$ (or the asymptotic value at infinity if $n > 0$) and the steepness of the slope. If $n < 0$ and $b = 1$, the Hill function starts at 1, then gradually decreases followed by a steep decrease and ending with a gradual decrease towards 0.

An example of calculating the intact fraction of $[^{11}C]$-Flumazenil is seen in figure 1 (left). The blue line indicates a fit of the bi-exponential model (equation 3) with the constraint $A + B = 1$ while the black dots represent the individual measurement points. The optimization was performed using multidimensional unconstrained nonlinear minimization (Nelder-Mead) implemented in Matlab. The initial value for the fitting parameters are $A = 0.5$, $\alpha = 10$ min and $\beta = 100$ min. The resulting fitted parameters are $A = 0.75$, $\alpha = 4.6$ min and $\beta = 4.32 * 10^{12}$ min. An example of a plasma input function is given in figure 1 (right). Black dots represent the measurement of each sample (corrected for decay) and the blue line is the input function after taking into account the intact fraction of tracer at each time point (using the fitted function obtained in figure 1 (left).

Unfortunately, this fitting procedure is not described in many publications but can have a major impact on the results. Furthermore, it is important to characterize the metabolites in terms of their effect on the PET measurement in the tissue of interest. If the contribution of the radioactive metabolite to the measured PET signal in the brain cannot be neglected, it should be incorporated into the kinetic model.

Several groups have looked at alternatives to determine the arterial input function. A popular approach is the so-called image-derived input function. Typically, a function which represents the input function is derived from the dynamic images by determining the time-activity curve in a small region including the carotid artery, positioned manually or (semi)automatically.

Due to the limited spatial resolution of the PET image this function has to be corrected for partial volume effects. Furthermore, activity in surrounding structures can affect this function through spill-in effects.

One way of correcting for these effects is to take into account a recovery coefficient (ratio of observed to true activity, estimated based on phantoms and computer simulations) and the spill-in fraction from surrounding tissue (obtained from a nearby ROI) (Chen et al. (1998)). Another option is to use a reconstruction algorithm with resolution recovery in combination with a high-resolution PET (Mourik et al. (2008)). A possible alternative strategy that does not use using any anatomical information, is to extract a time-activity curve by means of an independent component analysis (ICA), which implicitly accounts for spill-over effects (Naganawa et al. (2005)).

Depending on the method (e.g. the amplitude of the independent components is relative), the extracted image-derived input function may need to be scaled using the concentration determined in one or a few blood samples. Sometimes arterial samples can be replaced by venous samples (Chen et al. (1998)), usually at later time points when venous and arterial concentrations of tracer are almost equal. A more desirable alternative is to use so-called blood free methods. For example, Croteau et al. (2010) fitted a tri-exponential function to the extracted carotid time curve, using the carotid diameter as measured on MRI to correct for the partial volume effect. In Backes et al. (2009), the measured time-activity curve C_m was corrected as follows to obtain the image derived input function ($C_{input-ID}$):

$$C_{input-ID}(t) = \frac{C_m(t)}{a_v + (1 - a_v)(1 - e^{-kt})} \tag{6}$$

in which a_v is the fraction of vessel in the ROI and k is the rate constant for the transport to surrounding tissue. The main disadvantage of this method is that both parameters a_v and k have to be estimated empirically.

Recently, in Zanotti-Fregonara et al. (2011) different approaches to determine the image-derived input function were compared. The overall conclusion was threefold: 1) image-derived input functions have to be carefully evaluated for a particular tracer and setting, 2) blood samples are still necessary to obtain a reliable input function and 3) techniques which use the integral of the input function (e.g. the Logan plot) give better results compared to techniques in which the input function is used directly.

Another approach is to use a population based input function (usually in combination with one or a few venous blood samples) (Hunter et al. (1996), Hapdey et al. (2011)). A population based approach can also be used to correct an image derived input function for the intact fraction of tracer.

Importantly, blood/plasma samples are measured in a well counter, dose is determined by a dose calibrator and the activity in the brain is measured with PET. Each of these devices has a different sensitivity and performance (optimal range of activity which can be measured reliably). Since we need to combine the measurements in our modelling, the different machines need to be cross-calibrated.

A summary of the main points to consider for the acquisition is given in table 1.

Subject preparation
- optimal positioning in scanner
- head fixation and comfort of the subject

Tracer injection
- constant infusion or bolus injection
- effective dose injected
- amount of injected ligand / specific activity

Transmission scan
- PET based ($^{68}Ga/^{68}Ge$ or ^{137}Cs) or low-dose CT

Emission scan
- list-mode or dynamic acquisition (frame definition)
- scanning parameters (start and end time, time coincidence window, ...)
- correction for decay, dead-time, scatter, randoms, ...
- cross-calibration with dose calibrator and well counter
- if possible: on-line motion correction

Other measurements
- if input function needed
  - image derived
  - timing of blood samples
  - arterial or venous samples
- if metabolite correction needed
  - timing of arterial samples
  - model to describe intact tracer fraction
- EEG, ECG, blood pressure, ...

Table 1. Main points to consider for the acquisition.

3. Reconstruction

Each frame is reconstructed into a 3D image. There are two major classes of reconstruction: filtered back projection and iterative reconstruction. Filtered back projection has the advantage that it is fast and robust but the disadvantage that in low count measurements streak artifacts occur in the reconstructed images. Iterative reconstruction techniques have the advantage that a-priori information can be taken into account (e.g. the noise model, scatter and attenuation measurements) avoiding precorrection of the raw data before reconstruction which results in superior image quality. The disadvantage is that convergence is not uniform throughout the image making it sensitive to bias due to the limited number of iterations that is often applied. Reconstruction time is also much longer compared to filtered back projection. A very popular and widely used method is OSEM (ordered subsets expectation maximization). This method includes a Poisson-noise model and has a non-negativity constraint. The latter can cause some bias in the parameters estimated when modelling the data. Several studies (Boellaard et al. (2001), Oda et al. (2001), Belanger et al. (2004), Morimoto et al. (2006)) have compared iterative reconstruction methods with filtered back projection. The overall conclusion was that both methods have a similar quantitative accuracy although in some situations, filtered back projection may still be preferable. In a more recent study by Reilhac et al. (2008), using simulations, it was shown that the positivity constraint in maximum likelihood expectation maximization (MLEM)-based algorithms leads to overestimation of the activity in regions with low activity (e.g. in a reference region) which causes a significant bias in binding potential estimates. However, the use of a resolution model reduces low-statistics bias (Walker et al. (2011)).

Usually, the dynamic PET data are reconstructed frame by frame in an independent way without taking into account the temporal relationship between subsequent frames. To overcome this shortcoming, a 4D reconstruction has been developed in which all frames are reconstructed simultaneously (for a recent overview, see Rahmim et al. (2009)). During this 4D reconstruction, different techniques (e.g. iterative temporal smoothing, wavelet based techniques to control noise) can be used to handle temporal information. A particularly interesting approach is to model the data directly from the sinograms. This was first described by Maguire et al. (1996) and is now more widely studied in the context of 4D reconstruction. Because it is rather difficult to model the noise distribution in reconstructed images, the spatially variant noise distribution is neglected when doing kinetic modelling. By calculating sinograms of the physiological parameters directly from the raw data this problem can be circumvented. These sinograms are subsequently reconstructed to form parametric images. The best results with this approach so far have been obtained when using a Gjedde-Patlak model as shown by Wang et al. (2008), and Wang and Qi (2009), but other models are also possible.

Another new development is the use of anatomical knowledge that is available from other imaging modalities (like MRI). One such a technique is the anatomically based maximum a posteriori reconstruction (A-MAP) (Baete et al. (2005)), which corrects the images for partial volume effects, the importance of which is described in the next section.

A summary of the main points to consider for the reconstruction is given in table 2.

Definition of frames (rebinning from list mode)
Pre-corrections if necessary (e.g. random correction)
Reconstruction method: iterative reconstruction or filtered back-projection
reconstruction time
inclusion of additional measurements (scatter, attenuation, . . .)
filtering
effect of reconstruction on final results (bias, variance, resolution)
Optionally, take into account:
temporal relation between frames (4D reconstructions)
anatomical knowledge (partial volume correction)
Data management
Quality assurance of reconstructed images

Table 2. Main points to consider for the reconstruction

4. Processing

Since dynamic PET measurements are long, patient movement is almost inevitable and motion correction should be applied. Implicit in the previous step of reconstruction is that either the transmission scan or the CT scan are in (near) perfect spatial alignment with the PET frames to be attenuation corrected. Also, the different PET frames themselves should be spatially aligned since the next step of kinetic modelling assumes that the time course (in voxels or areas) is derived from the same location.

Motion correction poses two particular difficulties: the first frames are too noisy to use and any movement occurring during a frame is neglected. The first issue can be solved by creating a sum image of the first few minutes reasonably assuming that there was no significant motion during this period and by coregistering all subsequent frames to this sum image. The second issue is more problematic, but as long as movements are small (i.e. less than a few mm in displacement or a few degrees in rotation) this leads to limited additional blurring of the image and will not cause a major problem.

Realigning PET frames to the first frame or a sum image can be done by simply minimising the intensity differences between the images, but in some cases it may be necessary to use more complex measures of similarity between the images based on more general information than simple intensity, such as mutual information or cross correlation. Examples of such situations are when tracer uptake patterns differ drastically over time or when one needs to coregister another imaging modality (e.g. a CT or MRI image) to a PET frame. When realigning within an imaging modality (e.g. PET frames) rigid (6 parameters: 3 translational and 3 rotational parameters) spatial transformations are usually sufficient. Coregistrations between different modalities benefit from affine (12 parameter) transformations allowing additionally 3 directions of zoom and of skew although a rigid body transformation is often acceptable.

Having a high resolution structural scan, usually a T1-weighted MRI, of the same subject coregistered to the PET scan may serve multiple purposes. First, the MRI can be used to draw anatomical volumes of interest (VOIs) for subsequent kinetic modelling with much higher precision than is possible based on PET scans and, importantly, unbiased from the pattern of tracer uptake. Second, the structural scan can be used to calculate a potentially more precise (due to higher resolution of the source image) spatial transformation that takes the subject's brain into a common stereotactic space, such as Montreal Neurological Institute (MNI) space. This allows direct comparisons across subjects in this standard space. Alternatively, the obtained spatial transformation can be inverted and applied to MNI space VOI templates to bring them into the subject's native space if one prefers to avoid interpolation issues and working on distorted images. Third, the structural scan provides high resolution anatomical information needed to perform partial volume correction.

The partial volume effect (PVE) stems from the relatively low spatial resolution of the PET scanner. This can be quantified by means of the system's point spread function (PSF), which describes the degree to which a point source is 'blurred' by the imaging system. More specifically, when imaging a radioactive point source (perfect impulse function), this object appears larger but less intense (bell shaped curve), since the total number of counts is preserved. Applied to brain imaging, this means that for structures that are smaller than the sampling resolution (about 4 mm FWHM for modern scanners), e.g. the cortex, the measured signal is a mix of the true radiotracer concentrations in the multiple tissue types present. As such, the measured activity in grey matter is affected by spill-out onto other tissues (e.g. CSF) and spill-in from adjacent white matter.

This effect poses a particular problem when one wishes to study decreases in tracer binding in patients. A lower measured signal could mean a true decrease in tracer binding, PVE due to tissue atrophy or a mixture of both. In order to disentangle these effects, a formal partial volume correction (PVC) can be applied, based on prior higher resolution knowledge about the underlying tissue types and the point spread function of the scanner.

The basic idea is to view the measured PET signal as a convolution of the true image by the PSF and correct the measured PET signal in a voxel/region by modelling it as a combination of effects in the various tissue types present, taking into account the proportion of those tissue classes in that voxel/region.

The prior anatomical knowledge is derived from a high resolution structural scan, nowadays usually an MRI scan, which is segmented into the tissue types of interest, commonly taken to be grey matter, white matter and cerebrospinal fluid (CSF). The image values in such segmentation maps (e.g. a voxel with a value of 0.8 in a grey matter map) can be interpreted as the tissue fraction (80% of the voxel consists of grey matter) or probability (80% chance that the voxel belongs to grey matter). Importantly, the quality and accuracy of these segmentations will propagate into the partial volume corrected PET images. .

Here, for illustrative purposes, we describe a commonly used method, the Müller-Gärtner partial volume correction (Müller-Gärtner et al. (1992)), to correct the activity in grey matter tissue.

$$I_{GM} = \frac{I_{measured} - (I_{WM}P_{WM}) \otimes PSF - (I_{CSF}P_{CSF}) \otimes PSF}{P_{GM} \otimes PSF} \tag{7}$$

where I_{GM} is the partial volume corrected image, $I_{measured}$ the original PET image, I_{WM} and I_{CSF} the tracer uptake in white matter and CSF, P_{GM}, P_{WM} and P_{CSF} the tissue probabilities, and PSF the system's point spread function.

The corrected image value I_{GM} is obtained by subtracting from the measured value $I_{measured}$ the contributions of white matter and CSF signal. These contributions are given by the tissue's tracer uptake e.g. I_{WM} weighted by the proportion P_{WM} of that particular tissue class in the voxel/area and convolved with the PET system's PSF to match the resolution of the higher-resolution tissue probability maps with the PET image. In order to obtain 'pure' grey matter tracer uptake (i.e. independent of how much grey matter is present in the voxel/area), the result is divided by the proportion of grey matter P_{GM}, again convolved with the PSF.

The PSF of a PET system can be measured and varies spatially, being the most narrow at the centre of the scanner. For brain scans, this spatial variability is thought to be negligible. P_{GM}, P_{WM} and P_{CSF} are derived from the tissue probability maps. Under the assumption that tracer uptake is homogeneous throughout white matter, a representative uptake value for I_{WM} can be obtained by measuring the PET signal within a 'pure' WM area where there is no significant spill-in from other tissues, such as the centrum semiovale. Likewise I_{CSF} can be derived from a pure CSF region or can be assumed to be zero since CSF should not show any tracer uptake.

While the Müller-Gärtner PVC is a postprocessing method performed after image reconstruction, a similar strategy can be applied during iterative reconstruction incorporating anatomical information as a priori knowledge, such as A-MAP (Baete et al. (2005)). The latter approach offers a better spatial resolution, since smoothing (which is done during reconstruction in order to suppress noise) can be restricted to a specific tissue class instead of increasing spill-over between tissue classes, yielding sharper anatomical boundaries.

PVC can be applied on a voxel- or VOI-based level, the advantages and disadvantages of which are discussed in more depth later. Errors in registration of tissue maps to the PET image, misclassifications in the tissue probability maps, and VOI misplacement may all introduce errors that propagate in further analyses on partial volume corrected data.

Theoretically, PVC would preferably be applied prior to kinetic modelling, since there is usually not a simple linear relationship between raw counts and kinetic modelling output measures that are eventually used to describe processes of interest.

Images can be smoothed prior to kinetic modelling (parametric imaging), or are smoothed implicitly by using the VOI approach. Either method will attempt to find the kinetic modelling coefficient that best describe the data, either in each voxel or in each VOI independently of the other voxels/VOIs.

A summary of the main points to consider for the processing is given in table 3.

Motion correction
sum the first frames (e.g. first 5 minutes assuming no movement)
align all images of the remaining frames
method
evaluation of motion parameters
Coregistration with high-resolution anatomical MRI
method (transformation, cost-function)
PET image (e.g. summed image of all frames)
Use high-resolution anatomical MRI
to draw volumes of interest
to correct for partial volume effects
to determine the spatial transformation to a common anatomical space
Smoothing of PET data (noise reduction)

Table 3. Main points to consider for image processing

5. Kinetic models

5.1 Pharmacological terminology

When describing the pharmacokinetics of a tracer, the most commonly used method is a compartmental model (figure 2), where distinct pools of tracer (spatial location or chemical state) are assigned to different compartments. It is assumed that the tracer concentration in a compartment, given by C (e.g. expressed in Bq ml^{-1}), is homogeneous (instantaneous mixing assumption). The rate of exchange of tracer between 2 compartments is given by a rate constant k (in fraction per time, e.g. min^{-1}).

The rate at which the tracer crosses the blood-brain barrier (BBB) to enter the first brain compartment is given by K_1, the only rate constant historically denoted in upper case and having units of ml plasma per cubic cm tissue per min (ml cm^{-3} min^{-1}). This rate constant for blood-brain barrier transport is related to perfusion (blood flow).

In a capillary model, the following relation can be derived

$$K_1 = EF \tag{8}$$

where E is the unidirectional extraction from blood into brain during the tracer's first pass through the capillary bed, and F denotes the blood flow. Regarding the capillary as a rigid tube, the Renkin-Crone model posits that

$$E = 1 - e^{-\frac{PS}{F}} \tag{9}$$

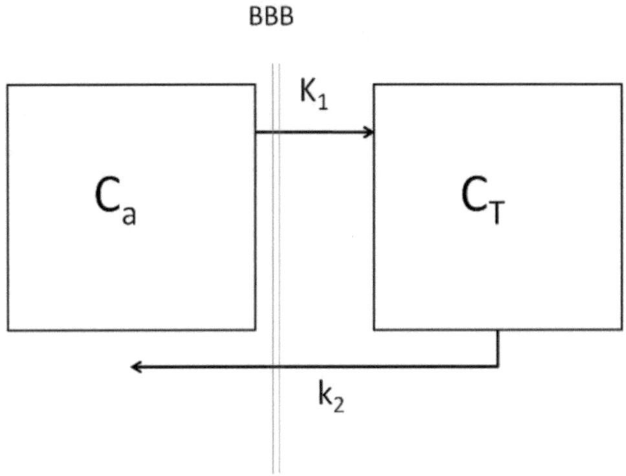

Fig. 2. One-tissue compartement model

with PS the permeability surface product (the tracer's total permeability across the capillary membrane).

On one end of the spectrum, for tracers with a large permeability surface product (freely diffusible tracers e.g. water), extraction is virtually independent of perfusion and approaches 1 (the exponential term is very small). As a result, K_1 approximates blood flow for such tracers. On the other end, for tracers with a permeability surface product much lower than the blood flow, E can be approximated by PS/F and hence K_1 is no longer related to blood flow but is proportional tot the permeability surface product ($K_1 \approx$ PS).

Two interacting compartments commonly found in a model are ligand and receptor. A ligand is a chemical that binds to a receptor. If this binding results in a chemical response i.e. 'activates' the receptor, the ligand is called an agonist. More specifically, the term 'agonist' is used for molecules that induce a pharmacological response mimicking the action of the naturally occurring compound, e.g. the binding of morphine to opioid receptors mimics the action of the endogenous endorphins. An 'inverse agonist' induces the opposite pharmacological response as the agonist. Finally, a ligand is called an antagonist if its binding does not activate the receptor or appears to 'deactivate' it by displacing an agonist.

Receptor occupancy refers to the percentage of receptors that are currently being occupied by ligands. The aim of PET receptor displacement studies is to detect changes in receptor occupancy caused by the experimental action of introducing a nonradioactive ligand. By measuring the difference in binding of the radioactive tracer, which is applied before and after the pharmacological challenge, the occupancy of the nonradioactive ligand can be inferred. For example, if the non-radioactive compound occupies 25% of binding sites, relative tracer binding will decrease by around 25% as well. This is explained in more detail in a later section.

In vitro, ligand-receptor kinetics is described by the well-known Michaelis-Menten relationship for a reversible binding.

$$L + R \underset{k_{\text{off}}}{\overset{k_{\text{on}}}{\rightleftharpoons}} LR \tag{10}$$

where L = ligand, R = receptor, LR = ligand-receptor complex, k_{on} = rate constant of association and k_{off} = rate constant of dissociation. According to the law of mass action, the kinetics of this system are described by

$$\frac{dC_{LR}}{dt}(t) = k_{on}C_L(t)C_R(t) - k_{off}C_{LR}(t) \tag{11}$$

with C_L, C_R and C_{LR} being the concentration of respectively L, R and LR.

When the system reaches a dynamic equilibrium:

$$k_{on}C_LC_R = k_{off}C_{LR} \tag{12}$$

Rearranging the previous equation gives the definition of the dissociation constant, K_D:

$$K_D = \frac{k_{off}}{k_{on}} = \frac{C_LC_R}{C_{LR}} \tag{13}$$

The affinity of a receptor for the ligand is defined as $1/K_D$.

Furthermore, the total concentration of receptors, free and bound, or receptor density is

$$B_{max} = C_{LR} + C_R \tag{14}$$

Here we have assumed that none of the receptors are bound by endogenous ligands.

Rearranging the two previous equations gives

$$C_{LR} = \frac{B_{max}C_L}{K_D + C_L} \tag{15}$$

This relationship is termed a saturation binding curve. B_{max} is the asymptotic value representing the occupation of all available receptors. K_D is the concentration of ligand at which 50% of all receptors have been saturated (if $C_L = K_D$, then $C_{LR} = 0.5B_{max}$). The initial slope of the saturation curve is B_{max}/K_D.

The *in vitro* binding potential is defined as

$$BP = \lim_{C_L \to 0} \frac{C_{LR}}{C_L} \tag{16}$$

Since PET studies employ tracer doses (i.e. occupying a negligible percentage of receptors, often taken to be 5%), the concentration of free ligand is very small compared to K_D and hence may be ignored. Using equation 15, BP can be written as:

$$BP = \frac{B_{max}}{K_d} \tag{17}$$

It is usually assumed that changes in BP are mainly due to changes in total number of receptors (B_{max}) while affinity (=$1/K_D$) of the tracer for the receptor is similar. While *in vitro* ligand binding consists of a single compartment, *in vivo* PET models include plasma and one or more tissue compartments, thus requiring a slightly different definition of BP, as will described in more detail later.

A related concept to BP is the volume of distribution (or distribution volume). Similar to BP, there are also slightly different *in vivo* definitions of the volume of distribution, which will be discussed later. In its original pharmacological definition, the apparent volume of distribution is the virtual plasma volume that the drug would have to occupy in order to adopt the same (uniformly distributed) concentration in the body as in the blood plasma. Put differently, it is the ratio of the total drug amount in the body (administered dose) over the drug's plasma concentration (at equilibrium). For example, if 5 mg of a drug is present in the body, and its plasma concentration is 250 ng per ml, then a virtual volume of 20 l plasma would be needed to contain 5 mg of the drug.

In PET, the volume of distribution V_T is based on a similar conceptual idea but has been adapted slightly: it relates to a specific organ of interest instead of the entire body and uses the tracer's concentration (amount per volume) instead of volume (Innis et al. (2007)).

$$V_T = \frac{C_T}{C_a} \tag{18}$$

where C_T is the tracer's concentration in the tissue and C_a is the tracer's arterial plasma concentration, assuming equilibrium has been reached. Hence, its values are expressed in ml per cm^3 which is in fact unitless since 1 ml = 1 cm^3. For example, if the tracer's concentration is 50 kBq cm^{-3} in the brain and 2.5 kBq ml^{-1} in plasma, then V_T is 20, or, in other words: in order to have the same amount of tracer as in 1 cm^3 of brain, 20 ml of plasma would be needed.

In contrast to the *in vitro* definition of binding potential, the *in vivo* situation is much more complex. A fraction f_p of tracer is bound to plasma proteins and will not pass the blood brain barrier. Usually, a reliable estimate of this fraction is difficult. Another fraction of intact tracer is protein bound in the brain (non-specific binding representing the non-displaceable compartment). The free fraction of tracer available for binding to the receptor is denoted f_{ND} according to the consensus nomenclature (Innis et al. (2007)). Therefore, three different definitions of binding potential in PET exist which can be expressed as a ratio at equilibrium:

1. BP_F: the ratio of the concentration of specifically bound tracer to the concentration of free tracer in tissue. We assume that the concentration of free tracer in tissue equals the concentration of free tracer in plasma.
2. BP_P: the ratio of the concentration of specifically bound tracer in tissue to the concentration of intact tracer in plasma (both free and protein bound).
3. BP_{ND}: the ratio of the concentration of specifically bound tracer in tissue to the concentration of non-displaceable tracer in tissue.

There is a linear relation between these three values: $BP_{ND} = f_{ND}B_F$ and $BP_P = f_pB_F$.

Analogous to the different definitions of binding potential, different definitions exist for the volume of distribution. The total tracer concentration C_T in tissue can be written as the sum of three different parts:

$$C_T = C_{LR} + C_{NS} + C_L \tag{19}$$

in which C_{LR} is the concentration of tracer bound to the receptor, C_{NS} is the concentration of nonspecific bound tracer and C_L is the concentration of free available tracer. The concentration of the non-displaceable part is given by $C_{ND} = C_L + C_{NS}$. Besides V_T, the volume of distribution of all radioligand, we also define the distribution volume of the non-displaceable part of the tracer as:

$$V_{ND} = C_{ND}/C_a. \tag{20}$$

Note that in an *in vivo* setting, B_{max} should actually be replaced by B' which is the maximum concentration of available receptors, i.e. not occupied by endogenous ligands or compartmentized in a low affinity state.

The binding potential that we measure with PET is BP_{ND} and the relation with the volume of distribution is:

$$BP_{ND} = \frac{V_T - V_{ND}}{V_{ND}} = \frac{V_T}{V_{ND}} - 1 = DVR - 1 \tag{21}$$

with DVR the volume of distribution ratio.

BP and V_T are combinations of the rate constants introduced in the compartmental models as will be shown in a later section.

A common assumption in compartmental modelling is that the underlying physiological processes are not influenced by the presence of the tracer and are in a steady-state, i.e. the rate constants do not change over time. In this case, linear differential equations can be used to describe how changes in concentration in one compartment influence concentration in another one. The tissue compartments can refer to physical locations (e.g. outside vs. inside the cell) or chemical states (e.g. free vs. bound ligand).

The general aim is to estimate one or more of the rate constants, either individually or in some combination such as BP and V_T. The parameter estimation is based on the measured PET signal in the brain and the concentration in arterial blood measured by the arterial input function.

5.2 Model simplification

Accurate models describing the full behaviour of a tracer are too complex to be used in practice. Therefore, model simplifications are used. We show here the example of the well-known tracer $[^{18}F]$-FDG used when measuring the metabolic rate of glucose consumption. In figure 3, a model for the PET tracer $[^{18}F]$-FDG, consisting of both physical spaces (vascular, interstitial and cellular) and chemical compartments (FDG and FDG-6-PO_4) is shown. Constants K_1, k_2, k_5 and k_6 describe the rate of transport of FDG between the physical compartments, while rate constants k_3 and k_4 give the phosphorylation and dephosphorylation rates respectively. The blood-brain-barrier is indicated by BBB.

The transport of glucose or FDG across the cell membrane in cerebral tissue is very fast as compared with the transport across the capillary wall and the phosphorylation reaction catalyzed by hexokinase. The concentration ratio between the interstitial space and the cellular space is nearly in equilibrium at all times. Therefore, the interstitial and the cellular space can be approximated as a single compartment. This leads to the well-known two-tissue compartment of $[^{18}F]$-FDG (figure 4). In addition in the brain almost no dephosphorylation of FDG-6-PO_4 takes place within the first hour which leads to a further simplification in which $k_4 = 0$.

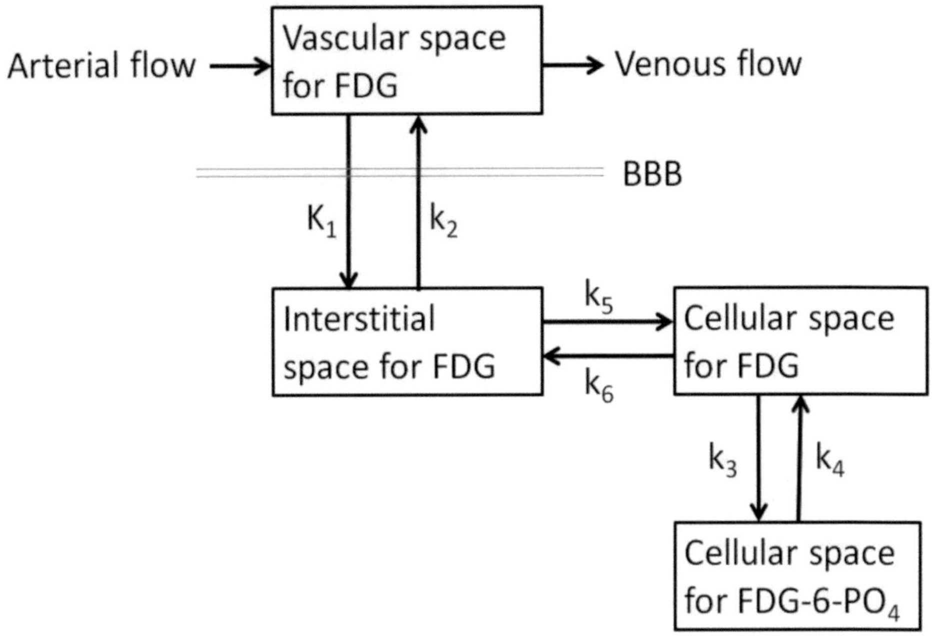

Fig. 3. Extended FDG model

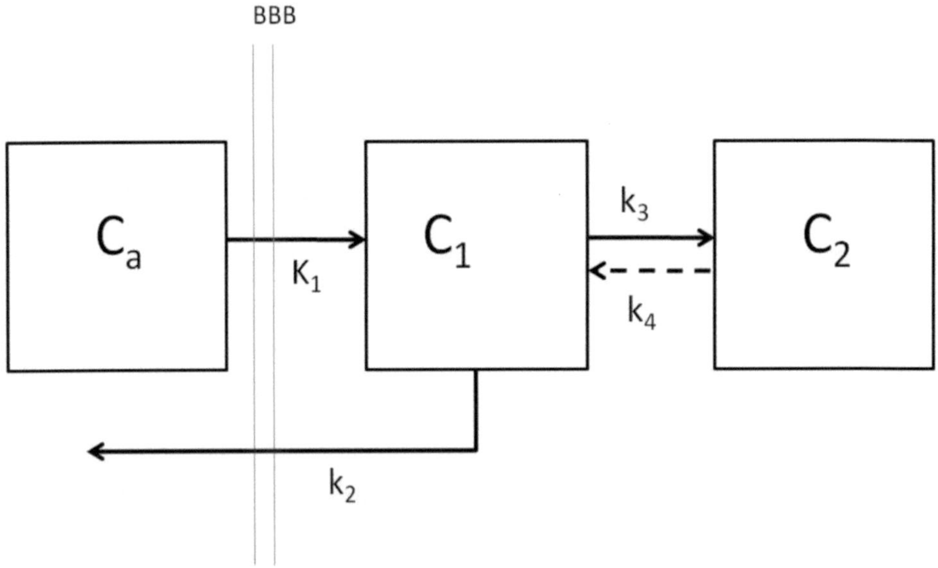

Fig. 4. simplified FDG model

FDG and glucose behave differently because FDG becomes trapped after phosphorylation. Influx/uptake of FDG is only proportional to the influx/uptake of glucose. The constant of proportionality is called the lumped constant LC.

5.3 Compartmental models

5.3.1 One-tissue compartment model

In the one-tissue compartment model, we have two rate constants K_1 and k_2 describing the model (see figure 2). The differential equation is given by:

$$\frac{dC_T}{dt}(t) = K_1 C_a(t) - k_2 C_T(t), \tag{22}$$

where C_a is the arterial plasma concentration of intact tracer and C_T is the concentration of tracer in tissue. This model is also called the Kety-Schmidt model originally developed to model tracers measuring regional cerebral blood flow.

The solution of this equation is given by:

$$C_T(t) = K_1 \int_0^t e^{-k_2(t-s)} C_a(s)ds = K_1 e^{-k_2 t} \otimes C_a \tag{23}$$

Using this expression, the rate constants can be estimated based upon the measurement of C_a and C_T at different time points. This estimation is a nonlinear operation.

A linear alternative can be formulated by integrating both sides of the differential equation 22:

$$C_T(t) - C_T(0) = K_1 \int_0^t C_a(s)ds - k_2 \int_0^t C_T(s)ds. \tag{24}$$

Assuming $C_T(0) = 0$, we find the following linear relation:

$$\frac{C_T(t)}{\int_0^t C_a(s)ds} = K_1 - k_2 \frac{\int_0^t C_T(s)ds}{\int_0^t C_a(s)ds}. \tag{25}$$

From this equation, K_1 and k_2 can be estimated using linear regression. The distribution volume can then be calculated as:

$$V_T = \frac{K_1}{k_2}. \tag{26}$$

5.3.2 Two-tissue reversible compartment model

In the two-tissue compartment model, K_1 and k_2 again describe the exchange of tracer with the blood pool similar as in the one-tissue compartment model. Two additional rate constants, k_3 and k_4, model the interactions between the 2 tissue compartments.

Tracer behaviour in this model (5) is described by the following set of differential equations:

$$C_T(t) = \frac{dC_{f+ns}}{dt}(t) = K_1 C_a(t) - (k_2 + k_3)C_{f+ns}(t) + k_4 C_b(t)$$

$$\frac{dC_b}{dt}(t) = k_3 C_{f+ns}(t) - k_4 C_b(t)$$

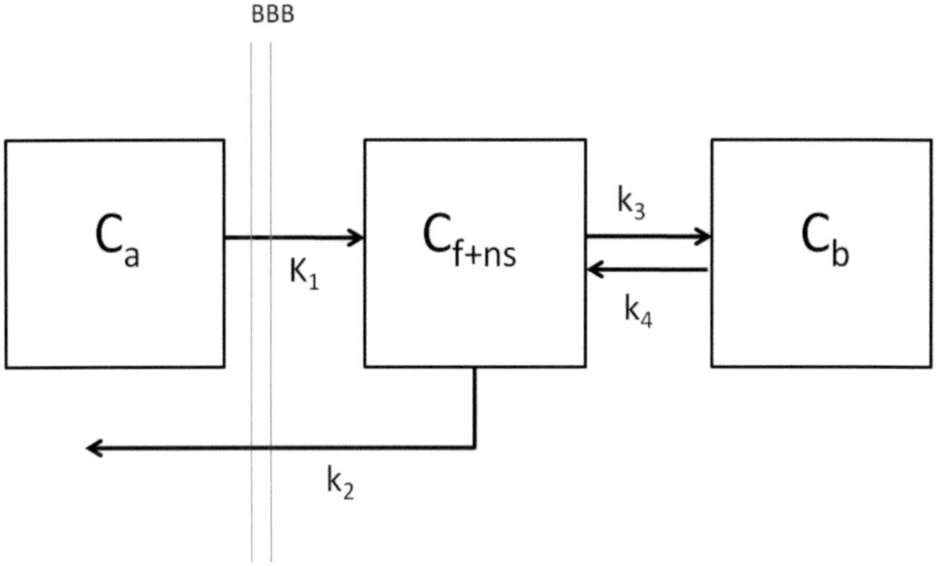

Fig. 5. Two-tissue reversible compartment model

where C_{f+ns} denotes the concentration of free and non-specifically bound tracer and C_b is the concentration of specifically bound tracer. Reworking these equations gives

$$C_{f+ns}(t) + C_b(t) = (\phi_1 e^{-\theta_1 t} + \phi_2 e^{-\theta_2 t}) \otimes C_a(t) \tag{27}$$

$$\phi_1 = \frac{K_1(\theta_1 - k_3 - k_4)}{\Delta}$$

$$\phi_2 = \frac{K_1(\theta_2 - k_3 - k_4)}{-\Delta}$$

$$\theta_1 = \frac{k_2 + k_3 + k_4 + \Delta}{2} \tag{28}$$

$$\theta_2 = \frac{k_2 + k_3 + k_4 - \Delta}{2} \tag{29}$$

$$\Delta = \sqrt{(k_2 + k_3 + k_4)^2 - 4k_2k_4} \tag{30}$$

The distribution volume is given by:

$$V_T = \frac{K_1}{k_2}(1 + \frac{k_3}{k_4}) \tag{31}$$

An example of a time-activity curve in a right frontal region in a normal subject injected with [^{11}C]-FMZ and the corresponding fit obtained using the two-tissue compartment model, is given in figure 6. The initial values for the rate constants were: $K_1 = 0.300$ ml cm^{-3} min^{-1}; $k_2 = 0.100$ min^{-1}; $k_3 = 0.050$ min^{-1}; $k_4 = 0.030$ min^{-1} and the fitted values were $K_1 = 0.302$ ml cm^{-3} min^{-1}; $k_2 = 0.076$ min^{-1}; $k_3 = 0.010$ min^{-1} ; $k_4 = 0.041$ min^{-1}. We also fitted the fraction of blood in the VOI (see below): the initial value was $V_b = 0.05$ and the fitted value was $V_b = 0.08$.

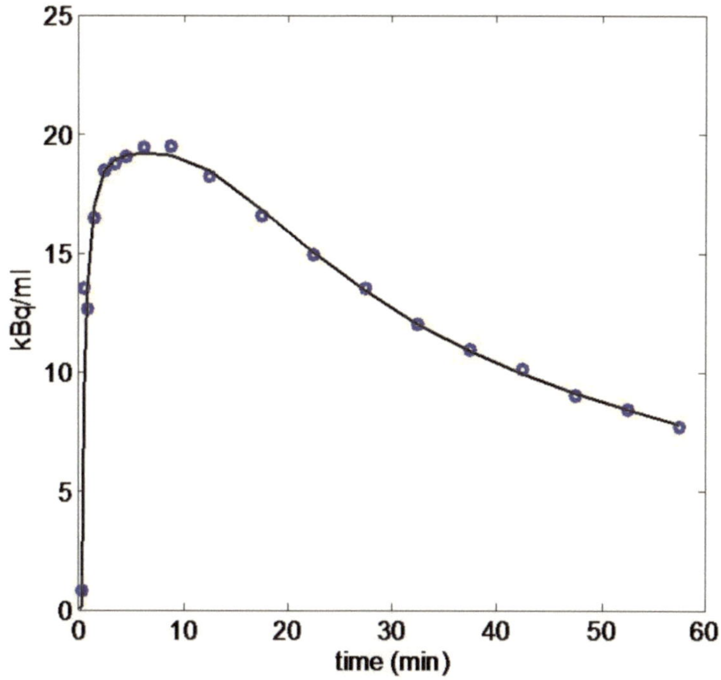

Fig. 6. Measured time activity curve (dots) and the corresponding fit (full line) using a two-tissue compartment model

5.3.3 Two-tissue irreversible compartment model

In case of irreversible binding, e.g. FDG, k_4 can be assumed to be 0 and the compartmental model equations simplify to:

$$\frac{dC_{f+ns}}{dt}(t) = K_1 C_a(t) - (k_2 + k_3) C_{f+ns}(t)$$

$$\frac{dC_b}{dt}(t) = k_3 C_f(t)$$

$$C_T(t) = C_{f+ns}(t) + C_b(t) = \{\frac{K_1 k_2}{k_2 + k_3} e^{-(k_2+k_3)t} + \frac{K_1 k_3}{k_2 + k_3}\} \otimes C_a(t) \quad (32)$$

$$K_I = \frac{K_1 k_3}{k2 + k3} \quad (33)$$

K_I is the net influx constant, the overall net rate of tracer uptake into tissue.

5.4 Graphical models

5.4.1 Gjedde-Patlak approach

This is an example of a graphical method which is derived using the assumption that $k_4 = 0$ (irreversible tracer) and that there is a steady state between the tissue concentration in the reversible compartment and the blood or plasma concentration. Under these conditions we find:

$$\frac{C_T(t)}{C_a(t)} = K_I \frac{\int_0^t C_a(s)ds}{C_a(t)} - \frac{K_1 k_2}{(k_2 + k_3)^2} \tag{34}$$

with C_T being the tissue concentration, C_a the arterial blood or plasma concentration, K_I is given by equation (33) and K_1, k_2 and k_3 the time independent rate-constants. Equation (34) is an asymptotic relation but in practice the steady state is reached within 20-30 minutes for tracers like $[^{18}F]$-FDG. The time after which we *assume* steady state is denoted by t^*.

5.4.2 Logan approach

For tracers with reversible binding kinetics, the following linear regression can be performed, assuming the relationship becomes linear (steady-state) after $t = t^*$:

$$\frac{\int_0^t C_T(s)ds}{C_T(t)} = A + V_T \frac{\int_0^t C_a(s)ds}{C_T(t)} \tag{35}$$

The slope V_T is the distribution volume given by equation (31) and the intercept is given by $A = -\frac{k_2 k_4}{k_2+k_3+k_4}$.

Figure 7 shows an example of a time-activity curve of $[^{11}C]$flumazenil (FMZ) transformed according to the above formula in which $X = \frac{\int_0^t C_a(s)ds}{C_T(t)}$ and $Y = \frac{\int_0^t C_T(s)ds}{C_T(t)}$. The estimated value for $V_T = 4.89$ and t^* was chosen as $t^* = 20min$.

5.5 Reference models

5.5.1 Reference Tissue Model (RTM)

Sometimes, the arterial input function can be replaced by a reference region providing an indirect input function. More specifically, in this reference region there should be no specific tracer binding, hence making it possible to estimate the contribution of non-specific tracer binding to the signal in the tissue of interest (Lammertsma et al. (1996)).

Figure 8 depicts a reference tissue model, described by the following differential equations:

$$\frac{dC_r}{dt}(t) = K_1' C_a(t) - k_2' C_r(t)$$

$$\frac{dC_{f+ns}}{dt}(t) = K_1 C_a(t) - (k_2 + k_3) C_{f+ns}(t) + k_4 C_b(t)$$

$$\frac{dC_b}{dt}(t) = k_3 C_{f+ns}(t) - k_4 C_b(t)$$

where C_r is the nonspecific tracer concentration (and the measured PET signal) in the reference region, and K_1' and k_2' are the rate constant describing resp. tracer influx into and outflow from the reference tissue. The two lower equations are those of the standard 2-tissue compartment model described higher, with $C_T(t) = C_{f+ns}(t) + C_b(t)$.

It is assumed that the volume of distribution of the non-specifically bound tracer is similar in both the tissue of interest and the reference region, i.e. $K_1/k_2 = K_1'/k_2'$. Hence, C_T can be

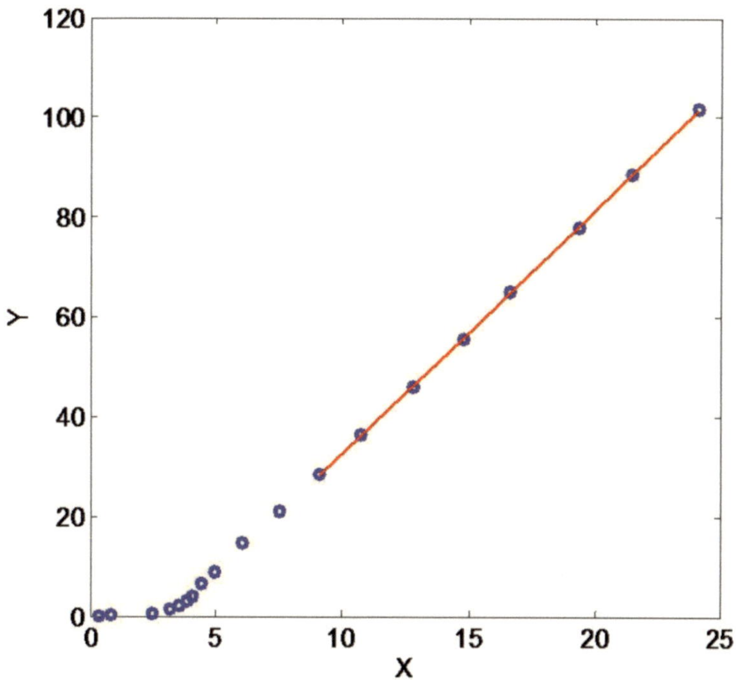

Fig. 7. Logan plot

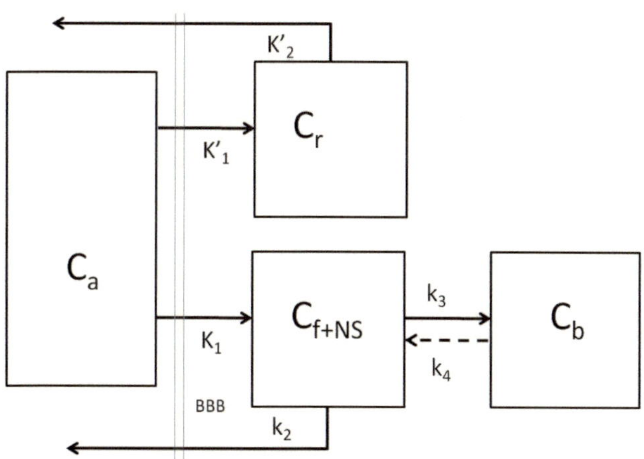

Fig. 8. Reference tissue model

described as a function of C_r omitting the need for the arterial input function C_a. The solution is given by:

$$C_T(t) = R_1[C_r(t) + A_1 e^{-\theta_1 t} + A_2 E^{-\theta_2 t}] \otimes C_r \tag{36}$$

with

$$\begin{aligned} A_1 &= \frac{\theta_1 - k_3 - k_4}{\Delta}(\frac{k_2}{R_1} - \theta_1) \\ A_2 &= \frac{k_3 + k_4 - \theta_2}{\Delta}(\frac{k_2}{R_1} - \theta_2) \\ R_1 &= \frac{K1}{K_1'} \end{aligned} \tag{37}$$

and the parameters θ_1, θ_2 and Δ are given by equations (28-30). The parameters R_1, k_2, k_3 and k_4 have to be estimated.

5.5.2 Simplified Reference Tissue Model (SRTM)

The reference tissue model can be further simplified if it can be assumed that the free and bound compartments of the tissue of interest are not readily distinguishable, i.e. can be described by one compartment. This reduces the number of parameters to be estimated from four to three, reducing standard errors on the estimates and speeding up convergence. The solution in this case is given by (Lammertsma & Hume (1996)):

$$C_T(t) = R_1 C_r(t) + k_2(1 - \frac{R_1}{1 + BP_{ND}})C_r \otimes e^{-\frac{k_2 t}{1+BP_{ND}}} \tag{38}$$

with R_1 given by equation (37). The parameters $R_1, k_2,$ and B_{ND} have to be estimated.

5.5.3 Reference logan

The Logan approach described above can also be applied when using a reference region instead of the arterial input function. In that case the operational equation becomes (Logan et al. (1996)):

$$\frac{\int_0^t C_T(\tau)d\tau}{C_T(t)} = DVR\frac{\int_0^t C_r(\tau)d\tau}{C_T(t)} + B \tag{39}$$

in which $DVR = B_{ND} + 1$ and B is assumed to be constant (when C_T/C_r is constant after some time t*).

5.5.4 Multilinear reference tissue model (MRTM)

In the reference Logan model, it is assumed that C_T/C_r becomes constant after some time. If this is not the case, the Ichise model MRTM_0 can be used (Ichise et al. (2003)):

$$\frac{\int_0^t C_T(\tau)d\tau}{C_T(t)} = DVR\frac{\int_0^t C_r(\tau)d\tau}{C_T(t)} + A'\frac{C_r(t)}{C_T(t)} + b \tag{40}$$

in which $DVR = B_{ND} + 1$, $A' = -DVR/k_2'$ and b is assumed to be constant.

This equation can be rearranged in the following form (MRTM):

$$C_T(t) = -\frac{DVR}{b}\int_0^t C_r(s)ds + \frac{1}{b}\int_0^t C_T(s)ds - \frac{DVR}{k_2'b}C_r(t). \tag{41}$$

The advantage of this expression is that C_T is not present in the independent variables because C_T can be noisy.

Other variants of these models exist in which k_2' is assumed to be known. The difference between these models is mainly based on the strategy to determine k_2'.

5.6 Displacement studies

Displacement studies are important in the validation process of a new tracer. Based on *in vitro* experiments, the affinity for a receptor system can be determined but this doesn't guarantee that the tracer will behave *in vivo* exactly as predicted. By performing an *in vivo* displacement study, the binding to a certain receptor system can be proven. The underlying assumption is that the drug used for the displacement study has a well-characterized affinity for the receptor system under investigation which is higher than the affinity of the tracer itself. If this is not the case, the displacement will be more subtle and may not be detectable.

A displacement study starts with the injected tracer (either as bolus or constant infusion) having reached an equilibrium state. This is disturbed by introducing a nonradioactive competitor which can be either endogenous (e.g. subject performs a cognitive task resulting in neurotransmitter release) or exogenous (e.g. infusion of a drug). The nonradioactive ligand 'displaces' the radioactive one by occupying available receptors hence promoting tracer wash-out (assuming the tracer is not bound irreversibly). The decrease in tracer binding can be detected either by comparing two scans, one with and one without nonradioactive competitor, or by modelling the competition (e.g. Morris and Yoder (2007)).

5.7 Occupancy studies

Occupancy studies are important to test new drugs. Too little occupancy of specific target receptors will not lead to a drug effect while a dose that is much higher than needed to occupy almost all receptors of the target, will not show additional benefits and may cause more negative side-effects than necessary.

Occupancy O of a target receptor system by a drug is defined as:

$$O(t) = 100.\frac{V_T(0) - V_T(t)}{V_T(0) - V_{ND}} \tag{42}$$

in which $V_T(0)$ is the volume of distribution at baseline (i.e. no drug is given), $V_T(t)$ is the volume of distribution at time t after drug intake and V_{ND} is the volume of distribution of the non-displaceable part of the tracer, i.e. the free and non-specifically bound tracer (e.g. as measured in a reference region where the target receptor is absent). Note that the occupancy is expressed in % and that it is time-dependent. It can also vary across different parts of the brain.

Unlike displacement studies, occupancy studies start with a certain equilibrium level of cold ligand (the drug of interest) present, followed by injection of the tracer to estimate the remaining fraction of available receptors not bound by the drug. In addition to one baseline scan in the absence of the drug, this typically requires multiple scans at different time points. These time points depend on the kinetics of the drug under investigation. The number of time points is limited by constraints on the amount of blood that can be sampled (if applicable) and on the radiation exposure to the subject. Therefore, occupancy studies are often first performed in monkeys in which at least the constraint on the radiation exposure is weaker compared to humans. In such a case, the occupancy is expressed as function of the plasma concentration of the drug and this relationship is usually modelled with a Hill function. Based on these animal data and on plasma kinetics data in humans, a few time points can be selected to determine the occupancy in-vivo in humans.

5.8 Optimization procedures

The model estimate $\hat{y}_i$ of the PET measurement y_i of frame i is given by:

$$\hat{y}_i = \frac{\int_{t_i^b}^{t_i^e} \{(1 - V_b)C_T(s) + V_b C_a(s)\} ds}{t_i^e - t_i^b} \tag{43}$$

in which t_i^b and t_i^e are the begin time respectively end time of frame i. V_b is the fraction of blood in the volume of interest which can be fitted or fixed to some value. If we have an appropriate sampling scheme, we can approximate M_i by

$$\hat{y}_i = (1 - V_b)C_T(t_i) + V_b C_a(t_i) \tag{44}$$

where the midscan time of frame i is given by $t_i = (t_i^e - t_i^b)/2$.

The cost function O that is used very often, is then defined as:

$$O = \sum_{i=1}^{N} w_i (y_i - \hat{y}_i)^2 \tag{45}$$

in which N is the number of frames, w_i is the weigth of frame i, and $\hat{y}_i$ is the model estimate of observation y_i. The weight is typically inversely proportional to the variance σ_i^2 in frame i:

$$w_i = \frac{1}{\sigma_i^2}. \tag{46}$$

Several models for the variance can be used: e.g. a uniform variance model, a model taking into account the decay correction factors or a model based on the length of the frame, the number of trues and the decay factor that is used. Each of these models will introduce some bias compared to the true variance which is very difficult to determine (Yaqub et al. (2006)). Weights are normalized so that they sum to 1. A priori it is not easy to determine which weighting scheme is the most appropriate but often a uniform weighting scheme is used.

In some models (e.g. reference Logan), we assume that $\hat{y}_i = C_T(t_i)$.

Every model contains one or more parameters which have to be estimated. In some cases parameters can be calculated based on a linear regression but often it is necessary to use non-linear estimation methods. Furthermore, many parameters of interest are by definition positive and it can be useful to constrain the solution to a physiologically acceptable range.

A major problem when using non-linear estimation methods, is that they are time consuming and depend on the initial values that have to be set. In a high-dimensional space (in which each dimension represents a parameter that has to be fitted) with noisy data, the cost function has many local minima. Depending on the initial condition and on the mathematical algorithm that is used, the result of the optimization problem is a local minimum that unfortunately need not to be the global minimum. If we use global optimization algorithms like simulated annealing, we will in theory find the global minimum but the time to find the solution is much longer compared to the other optimization algorithms.

In addition to the presence of local minima, other factors affecting the accuracy of the solution are the initial values if needed, the noise in the data, and the correlation that may be present among different variables.

A summary of the main points to consider for kinetic modelling is given in table 4.

Models
- compartmental models
  - number of compartments
  - interpretation of compartments
  - reversible or irreversible binding
  - parameters of interest
- graphical models (linearization)
  - choice of model
  - assumptions
  - if needed, start time for linearization (t^*)
- reference models
  - compartmental or graphical model
  - choice of reference region
  - assumptions regarding reference region tracer kinetics

Displacement studies
- assumptions about competitor drug's kinetics and affinity
- compare 2 scans or model competition

Occupancy studies
- assumptions about inital cold ligand's kinetics and affinity
- selected time points for scans (e.g. based on animal studies)

Optimization
- cost function
- initial values
- constrain solution to physiologically acceptable range
- mathematical algorithm for optimization

Volume of interest or voxel-based approach
- size of the smoothing kernel reflecting expected effect size (voxel-based)
- processing time
- VOI definition
- error estimates (voxel-based)

Table 4. Main points to consider for kinetic modelling

6. Model selection

When comparing models or when looking for the best model, the problem of a gold standard arises. Often, a two-tissue compartment model with a measured input function is considered the "best" model. Although this might theoretically be one of the best models, in practice this model is sensitive to all kinds of errors (movement of the patient, errors in timing, errors in determining the input function, etc). This is of course true for other methods as well but simplified models tend to be more robust. One way to solve this, is to use more realistic simulations to study the sensitivity of models to this type of error. Furthermore, when real measurements are used, a strict quality assurance protocol should be in place to evaluate the quality of all data and to minimize errors.

Despite this, comparing different models is complex. Models with more parameters tend to more accurately describe the data. Let P be the number of parameters in the model, N the number of observations and SS the residual sum of squares given by:

$$SS = \sum_{i=1}^{N} w_i (y_i - \hat{y}_i)^2 \tag{47}$$

in which w_i is the weight of observation i, y_i is the i-th observation and $\hat{y}_i$ is the model estimate of observation i.

Several measures exist to help in model selection, the two most popular ones being the Akaiki and the Schwarz criteria:

1. The Akaike information criterion AIC is defined as in Turkheimer et al. (2003):

$$AIC = N \ln(\frac{SS}{N}) + 2P. \tag{48}$$

   Usually, N is not large enough compared to P (i.e. $\frac{N}{P} < 40$) and in such a case we have to use an expression with a correction term (Turkheimer et al. (2003)):

$$AIC_{cor} = N \ln(\frac{SS}{N}) + 2P + \frac{2P(P+1)}{N-P-1}. \tag{49}$$

2. Another criterion that is used sometimes, is the Schwarz criterion given by:

$$SC = N \ln(\frac{SS}{N}) + P \ln(N). \tag{50}$$

In both cases, the model with the lowest value is the most appropriate.

To study the agreement between two different models (or a model and the gold standard), a Bland-Altman plot can be used. This is a plot in which the difference between two model parameters is plotted as function of the average value. It offers a better way of assessing the agreement between two different methods than plotting a correlation between the two different methods since a correlation can simply be high when there is a lot of variability within each method.

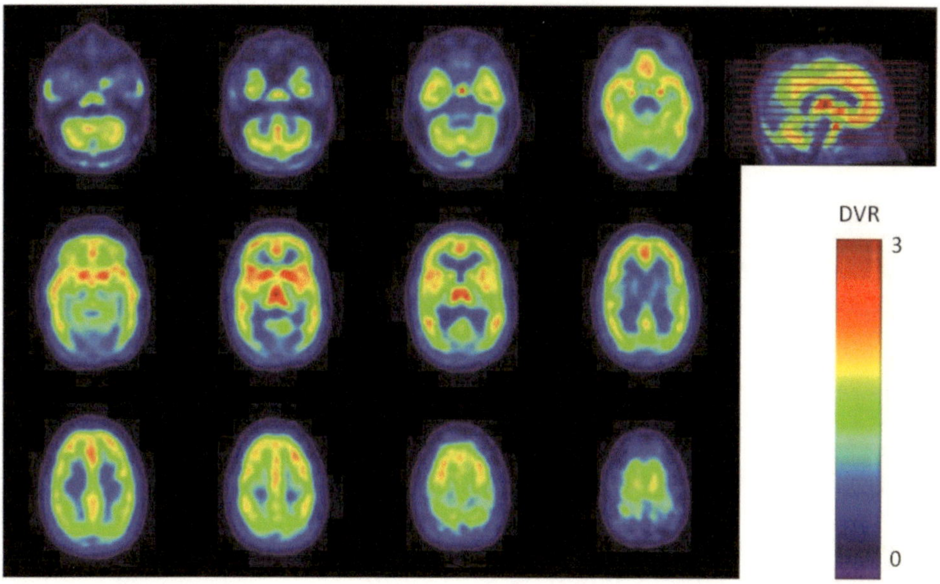

Fig. 9. Parametric image of DVR when using the tracer [^{11}C]-Carfentanil to measure opioid receptors

7. Parametric imaging

In traditional parametric image analysis, a kinetic model is performed in each (brain) voxel independently. In contrast, VOI based analysis is spatially biased due to the observer drawing VOIs or at least selecting usually anatomical areas to include in each VOI. Since there is no averaging of the signal over multiple voxels (and potentially large areas), voxel-based analysis is more sensitive than VOI based approaches to pick up small localised changes, but also to noise that will propagate throughout the analysis. As a trade-off, some spatial sensitivity is sacrificed to reduce the effect of noise in the input data (frames of raw counts) by smoothing the data prior to kinetic modelling, e.g. with a Gaussian kernel with a small full width at half maximum (FWHM) such as 6 mm.

Partial volume correction can be performed in a voxel-wise manner as well, by segmenting a coregistered anatomical MRI image into grey matter, white matter and cerebrospinal fluid. The effects of misregistrations and inaccurate segmentations are more likely to impact voxel-wise analyses whereas they may average out in VOI-based analyses.

The resulting output will be parametric images of the kinetic modelling parameters, such as k3 or DVR (figure 9), which can then be entered into voxel-wise statistical analyses after being spatially warped into a common stereotactic (e.g. MNI) space and another smoothing operation is performed. This pre-analysis smoothing serves to correct for remaining inaccuracies in spatial normalisation and normal intersubject variability, but also to ensure assumptions are met for voxel-wise parametric statistics (more specifically, its correction for multiple comparisons by means of Gaussian random field theory). In general, the size of the smoothing kernel determines the size of the effects the analysis is most sensitive to. Smoothing kernels around 10 mm FWHM are commonly used.

8. Future developments

A great challenge is to apply kinetic modelling in small animal brain imaging. Small animal imaging using dedicated PET systems has its own problems and limitations and although theoretically most of what is described in this chapter could be used, in practice it is generally not possible. For a review on kinetic modelling in small animal imaging with PET, the reader is referred to Dupont and Warwick (2009).

A new development is the use of PET to detect endogenous releases of neurotransmitters using a stimulation paradigm. This is a great challenge since the signal changes are very weak. Therefore, simulations are needed first to quantify the effect of different stimulus paradigms and to estimate signal changes (Muylle et al. (2008)).

In this chapter we have looked at relatively simple models described by first order differential equations in which the rate constants were time-independent. More complex models are developed however models with too many parameters are not suitable for use in PET imaging. On the other hand, simple measures like standard uptake value (SUV) or a simple ratio can be investigated in different pathological conditions and compared with parameters derived from kinetic modelling as described in this chapter. These very simple measures clearly have several drawbacks and should be used with care, but they are easy to determine, which is important when using them in a clinical setting.

9. References

Backes, H.; Ullrich, R.; Neumaier, B.; Kracht, L.; Wienhard, K. & Jacobs, A.H. (2009). Noninvasive quantification of 18F-FLT human brain PET for the assessment of tumour proliferation in patients with high-grade glioma, *European Journal of Nuclear Medicine and Molecular Imaging* Vol. 36: 1960-7.

Baete, K.; Nuyts, J.; Van Laere, K.; Van Paesschen, W.; Ceyssens, S.; De Ceuninck, L.; Gheysens, O.; Kelles, A.; Van den Eynden, J.; Suetens, P. & Dupont, P. (2004). Evaluation of Anatomy Based Reconstruction for Partial Volume Correction in Brain FDG-PET, *NeuroImage* Vol. 23: 305-317.

Belanger, M.J.; Mann, J.J. & Parsey, R.V. (2004). OS-EM and FBP reconstructions at low count rates: effect on 3D PET studies of [11C] WAY-100635, *NeuroImage* Vol. 21: 244-50.

Boellaard, R.; van Lingen, A. & Lammertsma, A.A. (2001). Experimental and clinical evaluation of iterative reconstruction (OSEM) in dynamic PET: quantitative characteristics and effects on kinetic modeling, *Journal of Nuclear Medicine* Vol. 42: 808-17.

Catana, C.; Benner, T.; van der Kouwe, A.; Byars, L.; Hamm, M.; Chonde, D.B.; Michel, C.J.; El Fakhri, G.; Schmand, M. & Sorensen, A.G. (2011). MRI-assisted PET motion correction for neurologic studies in an integrated MR-PET scanner, *Journal of Nuclear Medicine* Vol. 52: 154-61.

Carson, R.E. (2000). PET physiological measurements using constant infusion, *Nuclear Medicine and Biology* Vol. 27: 657-60.

Chen, K.; Bandy, D.; Reiman, E.; Huang, S.C.; Lawson, M.; Feng, D.; Yun, L.S. & Palant, A.J. (1998). Noninvasive quantification of the cerebral metabolic rate for glucose using positron emission tomography, 18F-fluoro-2-deoxyglucose, the Patlak method, and an image-derived input function, *Journal of Cerebral Blood Flow & Metabolism* Vol. 18: 716-23.

Croteau, E.; Lavallée, E.; Labbe, S.M.; Hubert, L.; Pifferi, F.; Rousseau, J.A.; Cunnane, S.C.; Carpentier, A.C.; Lecomte, R. & Bénard, F. (2010). Image-derived input function in dynamic human PET/CT: methodology and validation with 11C-acetate and 18F-fluorothioheptadecanoic acid in muscle and 18F-fluorodeoxyglucose in brain, *European Journal of Nuclear Medicine and Molecular Imaging* Vol. 37: 1539-50.

De Man, B.; Nuyts, J.; Dupont, P.; Marchal, G. & Suetens, P. (2000). Reduction of metal streak artifacts in x-ray computed tomography using a transmission maximum a posteriori algorithm, *IEEE Transactions on Nuclear Science* Vol. 47: 977-981

Dupont, P. & Warwick, J. (2009). Kinetic modeling in small animal imaging with PET, *Methods* Vol. 48: 98-103.

Hapdey, S.; Buvat, I.; Carson, J.M.; Carrasquillo, J.A.; Whatley, M. & Bacharach, S.L. (2011). Searching for alternatives to full kinetic analysis in 18F-FDG PET: an extension of the simplified kinetic analysis method, *Journal of Nuclear Medicine* Vol. 52: 634-41.

Hunter, G.J.; Hamberg, L.M.; Alpert, N.M.; Choi, N.C. & Fischman, A.J. (1996). Simplified measurement of deoxyglucose utilization rate, *Journal of Nuclear Medicine* Vol. 37: 950-5.

Ichise, M.; Liow, J.S.; Lu, J.Q.; Takano, A.; Model, K.; Toyama, H.; Suhara, T.; Suzuki, K.; Innis, R.B. & Carson, R.E. (2003). Linearized reference tissue parametric imaging methods: application to [11C]DASB positron emission tomography studies of the serotonin transporter in human brain, *Journal of Cerebral Blood Flow & Metabolism* Vol. 23: 1096-112.

Innis, R.B.; Cunningham, V.J.; Delforge, J.; Fujita, M.; Gjedde, A.; Gunn, R.N.; Holden, J.; Houle, S.; Huang, S.C.; Ichise, M.; Iida, H.; Ito, H.; Kimura, Y.; Koeppe, R.A.; Knudsen, G.M.; Knuuti, J.; Lammertsma, A.A.; Laruelle, M.; Logan, J.; Maguire, R.P.; Mintun, M.A.; Morris, E.D.; Parsey, R.; Price, J.C.; Slifstein, M.; Sossi, V.; Suhara, T.; Votaw, J.R.; Wong, D.F. & Carson, R.E. (2007). Consensus nomenclature for in vivo imaging of reversibly binding radioligands, *Journal of Cerebral Blood Flow & Metabolism* Vol. 27: 1533-9.

Lammertsma, A.A. & Hume, S.P. (1996). Simplified reference tissue model for PET receptor studies, *NeuroImage* Vol. 4: 153-8.

Lammertsma, A.A.; Bench, C.J.; Hume, S.P.; Osman, S.; Gunn, K.; Brooks, D.J. & Frackowiak, R.S. (1996). Comparison of methods for analysis of clinical [11C]raclopride studies, *Journal of Cerebral Blood Flow & Metabolism* Vol. 16: 42-52.

Lemmens, C.; Montandon, ML.; Nuyts, J.; Ratib, O.; Dupont, P. & Zaidi, H. (2008). Impact of metal artifacts due to EEG electrodes in brain PET/CT Imaging, *Physics in Medicine and Biology*, Vol. 53: 4417-4429.

Logan, J.; Fowler, J.S.; Volkow, N.D.; Wang, G.J.; Ding, Y.S.& Alexoff, D.L. (1996). Distribution volume ratios without blood sampling from graphical analysis of PET data, *Journal of Cerebral Blood Flow & Metabolism* Vol. 16: 834-40.

Maguire, R.P.; Calonder, C. & Leenders, K.L. (1996). Patlak Analysis applied to Sinogram Data in Myers, R.; Cunningham, V.; Bailey, D. & Jones T. (Eds.), *Quantification of Brain Function Using PET*, Academic Press, New York, pp. 307-311.

Montgomery, A.J.; Thielemans, K.; Mehta, M.A.; Turkheimer, F.; Mustafovic, S. & Grasby, P.M. (2006). Correction of head movement on PET studies: comparison of methods, *Journal of Nuclear Medicine* Vol. 47: 1936-44.

Morimoto, T.; Ito, H.; Takano, A.; Ikoma, Y.; Seki, C.; Okauchi, T.; Tanimoto, K.; Ando, A.; Shiraishi, T.; Yamaya, T. & Suhara, T. (2006). Effects of image reconstruction algorithm on neurotransmission PET studies in humans: comparison between filtered backprojection and ordered subsets expectation maximization, *Annals of Nuclear Medicine* Vol. 20: 237-43.

Morris, E.D. & Yoder, K.K. (2007). Positron emission tomography displacement sensitivity: predicting binding potential change for positron emission tomography tracers based on their kinetic characteristics, *Journal of Cerebral Blood Flow & Metabolism* Vol. 27: 606-17.

Mourik, J.E.; van Velden, F.H.; Lubberink, M.; Kloet, R.W.; van Berckel, B.N.; Lammertsma, A.A. & Boellaard, R. (2008). Image derived input functions for dynamic High Resolution Research Tomograph PET brain studies, *NeuroImage* Vol. 43: 676-86.

Müller-Gärtner, H.W.; Links, J.M.; Prince, J.L.; Bryan, R.N.; McVeigh, E.; Leal, J.P.; Davatzikos, C. & Frost, J.J. (1992). Measurement of radiotracer concentration in brain gray matter using positron emission tomography: MRI-based correction for partial volume effects, *Journal of Cerebral Blood Flow & Metabolism* Vol. 12: 571-83.

Muylle, T.; Dupont, P. & Van Laere, K. (2008). On the detection of endogenous ligand release with PET: A simulation study, *NeuroImage* Vol. 41: T75.

Naganawa, M.; Kimura, Y.; Ishii, K.; Oda, K.; Ishiwata, K. & Matani, A. (2005). Extraction of a plasma time-activity curve from dynamic brain PET images based on independent component analysis, *IEEE Transactions on Biomedical Engineering* Vol. 52: 201-210.

Oda, K.; Toyama, H.; Uemura, K.; Ikoma, Y.; Kimura, Y. & Senda, M. (2001). Comparison of parametric FBP and OS-EM reconstruction algorithm images for PET dynamic study, *Annals of Nuclear Medicine* Vol. 15: 417-23.

Rahmim, A.; Tang, J. & Zaidi, H. (2009). Four-dimensional (4D) image reconstruction strategies in dynamic PET: beyond conventional independent frame reconstruction, *Medical Physics* Vol. 36: 3654-70.

Reilhac, A.; Tomei, S.; Buvat, I.; Michel, C.; Keheren, F. & Costes, N. (2008). Simulation-based evaluation of OSEM iterative reconstruction methods in dynamic brain PET studies, *NeuroImage* Vol. 39: 359-68.

Turkheimer, F.E.; Hinz, R. & Cunningham, V.J. (2003). On the Undecidability Among Kinetic Models: From Model Selection to Model Averaging, *Journal of Cerebral Blood Flow & Metabolism*, Vol. 23: 490-498.

Walker, M.D.; Asselin, M.C.; Julyan, P.J.; Feldmann, M.; Talbot, P.S.; Jones, T. & Matthews, J.C. (2011). Bias in iterative reconstruction of low-statistics PET data: benefits of a resolution model, *Physics in Medicine and Biology* Vol. 56: 931-49.

Wang, G.; Fu, L. & Qi, J. (2008). Maximum a posteriori reconstruction of the Patlak parametric image from sinograms in dynamic PET, *Physics in Medicine and Biology* Vol. 53: 593-604.

Wang, G. & Qi, J. (2009). Generalized algorithms for direct reconstruction of parametric images from dynamic PET data, *IEEE Transactions on Medical Imaging* Vol. 28: 1717-26.

Yaqub, M.; Boellaard, R.; Kropholler, M.A. & Lammertsma, A.A. (2006). Optimization algorithms and weighting factors for analysis of dynamic PET studies, *Physics in Medicine and Biology* Vol. 51: 4217-32.

Zanotti-Fregonara, P.; Liow, J.S.; Fujita, M.; Dusch, E.; Zoghbi, S.S.; Luong, E.; Boellaard, R.; Pike, V.W.; Comtat, C. & Innis, R.B. (2011). Image-derived input function for human brain using high resolution PET imaging with [C](R)-rolipram and [C]PBR28, *PLoS ONE* Vol. 25: e17056.

4

Free Software for PET Imaging

Roberto de la Prieta
Universidad Rey Juan Carlos
Spain

1. Introduction

In recent years, there has been a large influx of image analysis software made freely available to the public. *Free software* or *libre software* is any software that can be used, studied, modified, copied and redistributed in modified or unmodified form either without or with minimal restrictions (see Stallman (2002) and Free Software Foundation (2011) for licenses, copylefts and further details). In practice, and in particular for the software reviewed here, straightforward availability at no cost as well as open code source are also granted. Multiplatform availability is also very common, i.e. the product is available for different operating systems and architectures. Additionally, free software users –be them clinicians or software engineers– can take advantage of other nice features such as on-line documentation, user forums and email lists that are also provided with some applications.

Free software is advantageous to the community in several ways. First, by providing a platform on which to perform analysis without having to re-implement and re-program the details of the algorithms themselves. Second, it also promotes *open research*, the dissemination of source code, data, and publication, with the goals of research reproducibility, method validation and advancement (see OpenScience Project (2011)). Thus, in this spirit, free software is the main focus of this chapter's software compilation.

It is worth saying that although any imaging processing software makes the analytical technicalities less complicated, a free software user must ensure that the implementation of the method is sufficiently understood in order to interpret the results accurately. It is the user's responsibility to verify that the software be well documented, validated, and kept up to date in order to ensure that the quality requirements of the particular task are met. Likewise, another caveat of free software is that any specific license restrictions for software use (i.e. some free software packages are restricted to academic research and not available for commercial applications) are left to the user.

Due to the above mentioned advantageous features, free software has become an appealing choice for many technical and non technical applications. Specifically, PET imaging practitioners –researchers and eventually clinicians– may benefit from a number of advantages by incorporating some pieces of free software to their set of tools. The main focus of this chapter is a practical one. It is intended as a, possibly incomplete, free software guide to available packages that help to accomplish daily or less usual tasks related to this medical imaging field. We will review a variety of free packages ranging from plain image viewers, to the more complex or demanding system modeling and image reconstruction applications.

Other tasks such as image manipulation/post-processing and quality evaluation are also addressed. The chapter is divided in sections according to the above mentioned key tasks.

A thorough discussion of the theory and methodologies underlying the applications is outside the scope of this chapter, although some guidelines will be given. The reader should instead refer to the given bibliography for suggested material covering these topics. Finally, the listings of freely available PET imaging software included in this chapter are not intended to be exhaustive. The software reviewed here was included because the author was familiar with it.

2. Image viewers

A wide variety of (free) image viewers are available for medical imaging allowing the user visualization of images in either a raw format, a proprietary format or a standardized format (such as DICOM, Analyze, PACS). Additionally, these packages usually include some or many preprocessing and postprocessing capabilities. Here we will briefly review the following (see table 1 and fig,1): AMIDE (Loening & Gambhir (2003)), MRIcro (Rorden (2011)), OsiriX (Rosset et al. (2004)), GpetView (Watabe (2011)). The reader may also consult Tamburo (2010) for a more detailed list including 3DSlicer, ImageJ and VTK among others.

2.1 AMIDE

AMIDE is a completely free tool for viewing, analyzing, and registering volumetric medical imaging data sets. It has been written on top of the Gtk+ libraries, and runs on any system that supports this toolkit (Linux, Windows, Mac OS X, etc. AMIDE is available at `http://amide.sourceforge.net/` and some of it features include:

- Arbitrary orientation, thickness, and time period slice viewing of a data set
- Multiple data sets can be loaded and viewed at once, with either linked or fused views. Each data set can be viewed from any orientation. Fusing can be done by blending or overlay
- Nearest neighbor and trilinear interpolation functions
- Zooming
- The following color maps are supported: Black/White,White/Black,Red/Green/Blue Temperature, Hot Metal/Blue/Green, Spectrum, NIH/UCLA
- Threshold: data sets are thresholded independently. Data sets can be thresholded over the entire data set or over each slice.
- Three-dimensional regions of interest (ROIs) can be drawn directly on the images and statistics can be generated for these ROIs. Currently supported ROIs are ellipsoids, elliptic cylinder's, boxes, and isocontours
- Imports raw data files (8bit,16bit,32bit,float,etc). Also imports Acr/Nema 2.0, Analyze (SPM), DICOM 3.0, InterFile3.3, ECAT 6/7, and Gif87a/89a (using the (X)medcon/libmdc)
- Imports most clinical DICOM files (using the DCMTK library)
- Allows cropping and clearing regions of data sets
- Anisotropic filtering wizard. Current filters: Gaussian, 1D Median, and 3D Median
- Saves studies (ROI and Data Set data) as XML data
- Series of slices can be viewed

- Fly through movies can be generated as MPEG1 files
- True volume rendering support with the capability of rendering multiple data sets at a time. Series of renderings can be saved as MPEG1 movies. Data sets can also be rendered as stereoscopic image pairs
- Alignment of data sets is supported using fiducial markers. This is done by placing fiducial reference points on the data sets to be aligned, and then running an alignment wizard to perform a rigid body transformation (Procrustes method)
- A profile tool is included that can calculate Gaussian fits and FWHM's of the generated line profiles. Profiles can also be saved for external use.

2.2 MRIcro

MRIcro allows Windows and Linux users to view medical images. It is a standalone program, but includes tools to complement SPM (software that allows neuroimagers to analyze Magnetic Resonance Imaging (MRI), functional MRI (fMRI) and PET images, see 5.4.1). MRIcro allows efficient viewing and exporting of brain images. In addition, it allows neuropsychologists to identify regions of interest (ROIs, e.g. lesions). MRIcro can create Analyze format headers for exporting brain images to other platforms. Users familiar with other Windows programs will find that this software is fairly straightforward to use. MRIcro is available at `http://www.cabiatl.com/mricro/`.

2.3 OsiriX

OsiriX is an image processing software dedicated to DICOM images produced by imaging equipment such as (MRI, CT, PET, PET-CT, SPECT-CT or Ultrasounds. It can also read many other file formats: TIFF (8,16, 32 bits), JPEG, PDF, AVI, MPEG and Quicktime. It is fully compliant with the DICOM standard for image communication and image file formats. OsiriX is able to receive images transferred by DICOM communication protocol from any PACS or imaging modality (C-STORE SCP/SCU, and Query/Retrieve: C-MOVE SCU/SCP, C-FIND SCU/SCP, C-GET SCU/SCP). A drawback of this tool comes from the fact that it is only available for Mac OS and iPhone platforms (`http://www.osirix-viewer.com/`).

2.4 GpetView

GpetView is a light-weight image viewer based on Gtk+ library. The supported image format is ANALYZE(TM) format (Mayo Foundation). GpetView can run on Unix-systems, such as Linux, Solaris, IRIX, Mac OS-X etc. From Version 2.0, GpetView can also run on Win32 system, if you have installed Glib and Gtk+(2.x). Glib andGtk+ can be found at `http://www.gtk.org`. For Windows users, you can find Gtk+ libraries at `http://gladewin32.sourceforge.net/modules/news/`

GpetView has the following features;

- Very light-weight
- View images as transverse, coronal, or sagittal
- Change color-map (support Analyze lkup file)
- Zoom images
- ROIs include shapes of circle, ellipse, rectangle, polygon and automatic edge detection
- Image histogram and profile

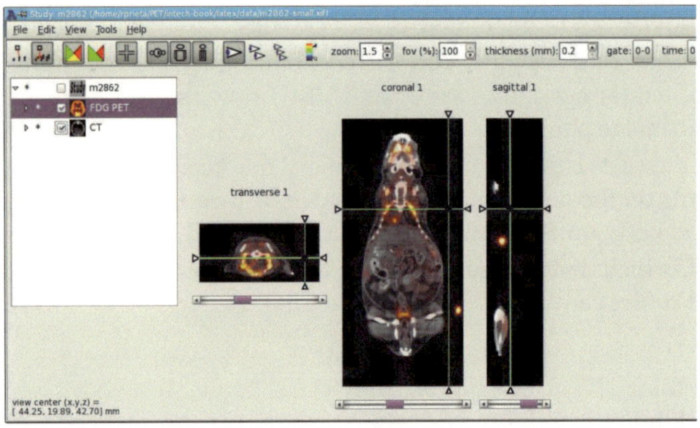

(a) AMIDE

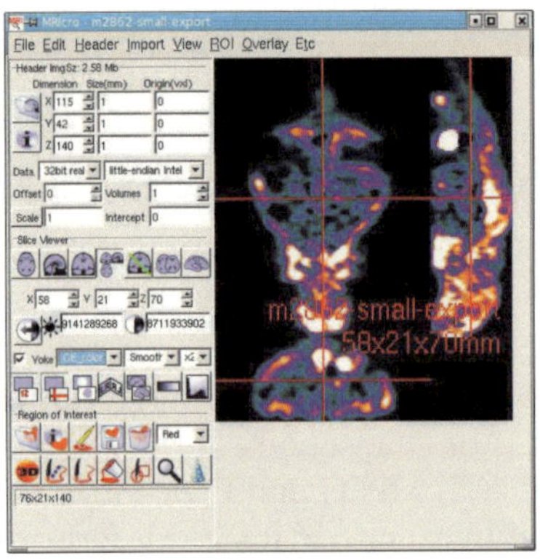

(b) MRIcro

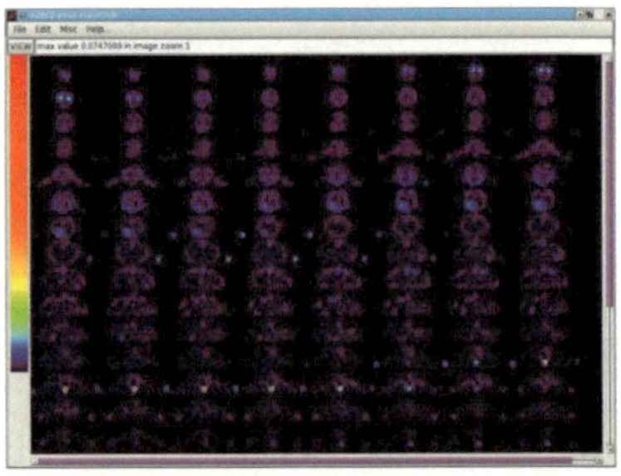

(c) GpetView

Fig. 1. Some screenshots of image viewers

	AMIDE	MRIcro	OsiriX	GpetView
Programming language	C language	?	Objective C/Various	C language
Open source	yes	no	yes	yes
License	GPL	BSD	LGPL	GPL
64-bit support	yes	yes	yes	yes
Multiplatform	♣♣♣	♣♣♣	♣	♣♣♣
Easy to install	♣	♣♣♣	♣♣♣	♣
Easy to use	♣♣	♣♣	♣♣♣	♣♣♣
Fast	♣♣	♣	♣♣♣	♣♣♣
Disk space	♣♣	♣♣♣	♣♣	♣♣♣
Rendering	♣♣	–	♣♣♣	–
Color maps	♣♣♣	♣♣	♣♣♣	♣
Image formats	♣♣♣	♣♣	♣♣♣	♣

Table 1. Comparison of viewers features

3. Image reconstruction

Because the process of data acquisition is random in nature there always exists an unavoidable resolution/noise (or equivalently, bias/variance) trade-off in all the nuclear medicine imaging modalities. Any reconstruction algorithm is somehow intended to solve this compromise in some optimal way. Before going into the software package specific features, we will take a bird's-eye view of some important issues concerning PET reconstruction.

3.1 Algorithms

Algorithms for image reconstruction from projections (in particular, PET and SPECT image reconstruction) fall into two broad categories: *direct* and *indirect* methods.

3.1.1 Analytic methods

Algorithm of this first group, a.k.a. direct methods, represent a closed formula obtained by discretization of different expressions of the inverse Radon transform. Thus, for 2D reconstruction we find the well known Filtered Backprojection (FBP) or Convolution Backprojection (CBP) algorithms (see, for instance Kak & Slaney (1988)). For 3D acquisition, the situation is more involved and many options are at hand. However, the 3D Re-Projection (3DRP) algorithm, a.k.a PROMIS (Kinahan & Rogers (1989)), has become an option of choice.

At this point, it is worth mentioning two approaches in order to enhance the performance of direct methods. First of all, the use of the standard Ram-Lak or *ramp* filter in the convolution or filtering step give rise to the striking artifacts characteristic of this methods. To alleviate those undesirable effects various windowing filters have been proposed in the literature (Hamming, Shepp-Logan, Parzen, etc.) in order to de-emphasize the high frequencies of the ramp filter. Unfortunately the introduction of a window filter to reduce noise will produce an unavoidable image *blurring* effect. In practice, by the selection of the cut-off filter parameter the user choose the resolution/noise trade-off desired for a particular reconstruction. Secondly, another important part of the direct method is the backprojection step in which the projection profiles are smeared back to the image domain. Because of the finite sampling data, the process needs an interpolation step. In this sense, one can use nearest-neighbor, linear, bi-linear, cubic, or spline interpolation among other choices.

3.1.2 Rebinning methods

Approximate direct methods, a.k.a. *rebinning* methods, manipulate the 3D projection data in order to obtain a richer 2D set that can be reconstructed using some 2D direct method. This reduces the amount of data and speeds-up the reconstruction process. Popular rebinning algorithms include, from less to more sophisticated approaches, Single Slice Rebinning (SSRB), Multiple Slice Rebinning (MSRB), Fourier Rebinning (FORE), and variations such as FOREX and FOREJ (see Daube-Witherspoon & Muehllehner (1987); Defrise et al. (1997); Lewitt et al. (1994)).

3.1.3 Iterative methods

On the other hand, indirect methods, i.e. *iterative* algorithms take a different approach. Starting from an initial guess for the image to reconstruct (for example a constant image or a 2D FBP reconstruction) they make successive improved guesses by projecting and backprojecting the data between image and sinogram spaces. Iterative methods in ET, though leading to a much higher computational burden, have shown better performance than direct methods because (i) they take into account the discrete nature of the measured data, and (ii) due to their ability to incorporate a measurement or *system model*. This is achieved by means of the so-called *transition* or *system matrix* (SM). Algorithms in this category include the Algebraic Reconstruction Technique (ART) (see Kak & Slaney (1988)) and variations such as SART, MART, the Least Squares (LS), and generalizations such as Weighted Least Squares fit (WLS), and the penalized version (PWLS) (see Fessler (1994); Kaufman (1993)). In addition to the above mentioned features (i) and (ii) a special class of iterative algorithms called *statistical iterative algorithms* are able to incorporate (iii) a statistical model for the process of data acquisition (or *noise model*). The well known Maximum Likelihood Expectation Maximization (ML-EM) algorithm of Shepp & Vardi (1982) and its accelerated version Ordered Subsets EM (OSEM) of Hudson & Larkin (1994) belong to this class. Finally, the class of penalized or regularized algorithms incorporate (iv) constraints (positivity, anatomical tissue boundaries information) or *a priori* regularization/penalization. Bayesian Maximum a Posteriori (MAP) algorithms belong to this category. The reader may consult Lewitt & Matej (2003) Defrise et al. (2005) and Qi & Leahy (2006) for a review on reconstruction algorithms in ET.

All in all, and according to Fessler (1994) a statistical iterative reconstruction algorithm can be regarded as made of five components: (i) a finite parametrization of the positron-annihilation distribution, *e.g.* its representation as a discretized image, (ii) a system model that relates the unknown image to the expectation of each detector measurement, (iii) a Statistical model for how the detector measurements vary around their expectations, (iv) an objective function that is to be maximized to find the image estimate, (v) a numerical algorithm, typically iterative, for maximizing the objective function, including specification of the initial estimate and a stopping criterion.

3.2 System matrix

The quality of an iterative reconstruction algorithm heavily relies on the above-mentioned system matrix (SM) (Rafecas, Boning, Pichler, Lorenz, Schwaiger & Ziegler (2004), Qi & Huesman (2005)). The introduction of system modeling techniques (i.e. detailed descriptions of the physical phenomena underlying the data acquisition process) in the generation of the SM improves the reconstruction both in terms of resolution and quantitative accuracy. The SM may be generated from measurements taken in the real system where the reconstruction is to be performed (Frese et al. (2003), Panin et al. (2006), Tohme & Qi (2009)). This approach has been succesfully incorporated within the clinical setting. However, while this method results in demonstrated improvements in image quality, it requires extensive and very accurate point source measurements (e.g. using a positioning robot).

A widely used approach to calculate the SM is to perform a Monte Carlo simulation. Monte Carlo integration can incorporate complex but interesting effects of the physics underlying PET data acquisition (see next section). However, Monte Carlo codes are complex and often quite time consuming, and they may produce noisy results if not monitored adequately. Thus, MC based integration might be impractical if the number of tubes of response (TORs) is too big, not enough computation is available or the setup of the scanner has to be changed often.

On the other hand, a number of analytical approaches have been proposed in the literature in order to compute the system matrix since the seminal work of Shepp & Vardi (1982). There, two-dimensional *(2D) angle of view* and *area of intersection* models were used to approximate the geometric sensitivity of a PET scanner and also a more elaborated model including positron range effects was proposed.

The *length of intersection* model, a.k.a. *ray-tracing*, has efficient implementations such as the Siddon algorithm (Siddon (1985)) that has been applied to PET in Herman & Meyer (1993) and Zhao & Reader (2003) or the orthogonal distance-based ray-tracer of Aguiar et al. (2010). The ray-tracing technique allows for *on the fly* calculation of the matrix elements thus avoiding SM storage problems. However, while ray-tracing is fast, the length of intersection is not a physically meaningful quantity representing the probability of detection and it is known to yield artifacts (i.e. missmatched projector/backprojector pairs). Similarly, the *3D volume of intersection* (Ollinger & Goggin (1996), Scheins et al. (2006)) should be corrected somehow if one desires a reasonably accurate model incorporating the effects of radial distance to the center of the field of view.

The natural 3D generalization of the 2D angle of view model, the *solid angle of view* model has also been used to compute the geometric sensitivity of a scanner, either by approximate (Terstegge et al. (1996), Qi et al. (1998), Huesman et al. (2000), Soares et al. (2003), Markiewicz et al. (2005)) or exact calculations (de la Prieta et al. (2006), Iriarte et al. (2009)) or by a combination of several contributions (geometry, positron range, photon non-colinearity, inter-crystal scatter and penetration) in a factorized matrix (see Mumcuoglu et al. (1996), Qi et al. (1998), Rahmim et al. (2008) and the references therein)

Interesting analytic 2D models taking into account the linear attenuation of a beam of gamma-rays impinging on a crystal scintillator have been proposed in Lecomte et al. (1984), Schmitt et al. (1988), Karuta & Lecomte (1992) and Selivanov et al. (2000). These models have been further developed and adapted for multilayer small-diameter PET scanners in Strul et al. (2003).

In spite of being sparse in nature, the calculation and efficient storage of the SM remains an extremely challenging task for currently available clinical tomographs, due to the large number of matrix elements (between 10^{13} in small animal PET systems to 10^{16} for a standard clinical human PET scanner) and storage requirements (on the orther of TeraBytes), so it needs especial manipulation techniques in real systems (Johnson et al. (1995), de la Prieta (2004), Rehfeld & Alber (2007), Ortuño et al. (2010)). This is the reason why prototyping languages, such as MATLAB, have not yet offered a solution for 3D realistic sized PET reconstruction (though some freely available MATLAB add-ons for 2D PET reconstruction can be found at `http://www.eecs.umich.edu/~fessler/code/` and in the MATLAB Central web page) In this sense, some researchers have shown renewed interest in high performance computing solutions such as PC clusters (Jones et al. (2006), Beisel et al. (2008)) and Graphic Processing Units (GPUs) (Herraiz et al. (2009), Zhou & Qi (2011)).

Different solutions to the various problems posed by the incorporation of such a matrix in the projection/backprojection steps of the iterative reconstruction algorithm are scattered throughout the literature. In practice, scanner manufacturers implement those algorithms in proprietary software packages that come with the workstation of the scanner equipment. Although tremendous effort has been devoted to the development of strategies and code to generate the SM and incorporate it in the reconstruction procedures –see for instance ASPIRE (Fessler (1997)), FIRST (Herraiz et al. (2006)) and PRESTO (Scheins & Herzog (2008))–, to the best of our knowledge, not many truly free software packages are available to this end (see also section 5.6).

3.3 Software for Tomographic Image Reconstruction (STIR)

In this section we will review the STIR library (Thielemans et al. (2006)) This library evolved from the European Union funded PARAPET project, and was later extended by Hammersmith Immanet and made into an Open Source project. The software is licensed under the GPL, LGPL and PARAPET licenses (see the STIR Sourceforge site for details, Thielemans & al. (2011)). STIR is an object oriented library for reconstruction of 2D/3D PET data written in C++ language. Let's see some of its features and practical considerations in further detail.

3.3.1 Installation

The installation of STIR should be straightforward for most Unix flavors: it is well known to work in AIX, Solaris and Linux. It can also be used in Windows versions using Cygwin (Cygwin (2011)). STIR requires a version of the *C++ boost libraries* (The boost libraries (2011))) to be downloaded and installed in the system. Once this requirement is met one can download the STIR sources in a .zip compressed file and then use the *GNU make* utility to compile the program to be run. The recommended compiler is *GNU gcc* but the use of other ones is also possible such as the free version of the Visual C++ Compiler.

Some extra features are possible at compile time:

- Parallel code with Open MPI (Open MPI (2011)) for the most relevant iterative algorithms and preliminary threaded code for some algorithms
- Enabling ECAT 7 file format support requires the Louvain la Neuve Ecat (LLN) library (`ftp://ftp.topo.ucl.ac.be/pub/ecat`)
- Enabling AVW support for data I/O, processing, analysis, visualization with the AVW Analyze library (`http://mayoresearch.mayo.edu/mayo/research/robb_lab/avw.cfm`)

Further details guiding the user in the process of installation in specific architectures are provided in the User's Manual.

3.3.2 Running STIR programs

Most STIR programs accept a single parameter in the command line, which is usually optional:

```
> executable_name [parameter filename]
```

The parameter file is a text file which uses an Interfile-like syntax. It is composed of keywords, corresponding to the names of the various parameters, with the values entered next to them. Spaces and tabs are normally irrelevant. Parameters omitted from the parameter file are assigned a default value. If a parameter file is not passed to the executable, the user is prompted for the required information.

3.3.3 File formats

The STIR utility and reconstruction programs frequently need to read and write files of image and projection data. Files formats are encountered in which data and header information are maintained in separate files (e.g. interfile). In other formats, data files carry header information (e.g. the native GE Advance sinogram format).

Currently STIR supports the following formats: (a native version of) Interfile, GE VOLPET sinogram , ECAT6 and ECAT7 data. First steps have been taken to be able to use the AVW library as well as SimSET file formats.

Some scanners produce list mode data, which is essentially a list of events. STIR provides utilities to use the list mode files, for example to convert them to sinograms. It is also possible to reconstruct images directly from list mode data, although this has not been tested very well as of yet STIR 2.1. Currently supported list mode formats are specific to the ECAT HR+ and ECAT EXACT 3D scanners. There are some unfinished classes available on the STIR web-site to read LMF format files, in conjunction with the LMF library. However, these are obsolete as the OpenGATE project distributes scripts to enable STIR to read LMF format files.

3.3.4 STIR reconstruction algorithms

The library implements the following algorithm list:

- Analytical: 2DFBP, 3DRP
- Rebinning methods: SSRB
- Statistical algorithms: OSMAPOSL, OSSPS

OSMAPOSL is an ordered subset (OS) implementation of the One Step Late (OSL) algorithm of Green (1990), with various additional refinements (i.e Metz filter) and capabilities (see Jacobson et al. (2000) for a description of many details of the implementation. OSSPS is an OS implementation of the Paraboloidal Surrogate algorithm described in Ahn & Fessler (2003).

Although the OSMAPOSL can be regarded as a generalization of ML-EM, OSEM and MRP algorithms [1] the list is of STIR available algorithms is somehow expandable (see next section) The 'situation' is summarized in Table 2.

The STIR library offers the user some (limited) choices in the projector/backprojector pairs (such as linear or B-Spline interpolation in the backprojector) and also in the image filters (separable convolution median or separable cartesian Metz filter) and statistical Priors (quadratic, median root) of the iterative algorithms.

3.3.5 STIR utilities

The library includes a number of valuable and independent utilities allowing to display results (X Windows, PGM, MathLink) perform operations with images and sinograms, convert between data formats, filter and compare data, precorrection or uncorrection, scatter correction, kinetic modeling, add noise and perform different tests.

3.3.6 STIR: future developments

The future improvements of the library will presumably pursue the following lines

- Add more automatic testing programs

[1] i.e. those algorithms can be obtained by adjusting the regularization parameter λ and the number HS subsets N_s. In short, $\lambda = 0$, $N_s = 0$ for ML-EM, $\lambda = 0$, $N_s > 0$ for OSEM, and $\lambda > 0$, $N_s = 0$ for MRP

Direct methods (ANALYTICAL)	Approximate	SSR √ MSR FORE
	Exact	FBP2D √ 3DRP √ ..
Indirect methods (ITERATIVE)	No model	ART, MART, SIRT ..
	Noise model (STATISTICAL)	.. LS, WLS, PWLS RAMLA ML-EM √ OSEM √ OSMAP-OSL √ PML ..

Table 2. Reconstruction algorithms implemented by STIR

- Add more algorithms: potentially ART, FORE and OSCB (the latter, based on the conjugate barrier method of Ben-Tal & Nemirovski (1999))
- Add more projectors/backprojector pairs and more priors
- Extend the parallelization of OSMAPOSL and OSSPS to FBP3DRP, or use Open MPI (Open MPI (2011))
- Add compatibility of the interpolating backprojector with recent data processors of the library
- Add more kinetic models: Spectral Analysis, Logan Plot

3.4 PET Reconstruction & Utilities Software (PETRUS)

PETRUS is a library that the author of this chapter is developing and will hopefully be released soon. PETRUS is intended to be efficient, versatile and portable and features both commercial and research multi-ring multi-block scanner modeling. It also incorporates original strategies for the management of the transition matrix at three different levels: compression, symmetries (de la Prieta (2004) and sensitivity modeling (de la Prieta et al. (2006)).

4. System modeling and simulation

In order to obtain the best performance of an imaging system it is desirable to have an accurate description of the physical phenomena underlying the process of data acquisition. Thus in PET, relevant models include –among others– geometric sensitivity, positron range, photon pair non-colinearity, Compton scatter in tissues, detector sensitivity, inter-crystal scatter and penetration and detector dead-times. Additionally, one may have some statistical models

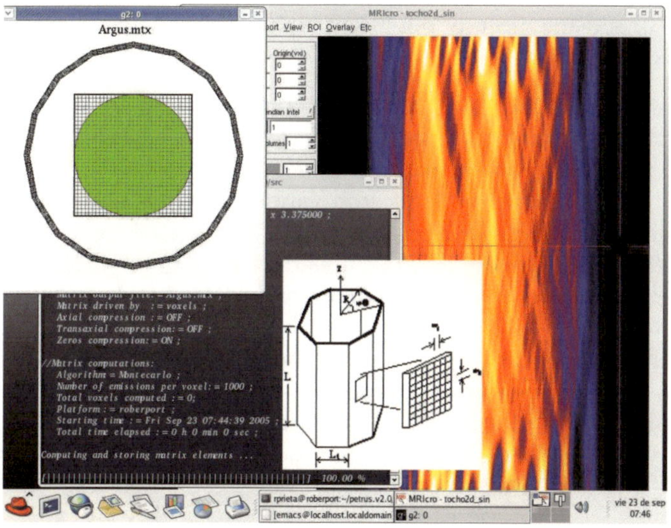

Fig. 2. Screenshot of PETRUS library at work

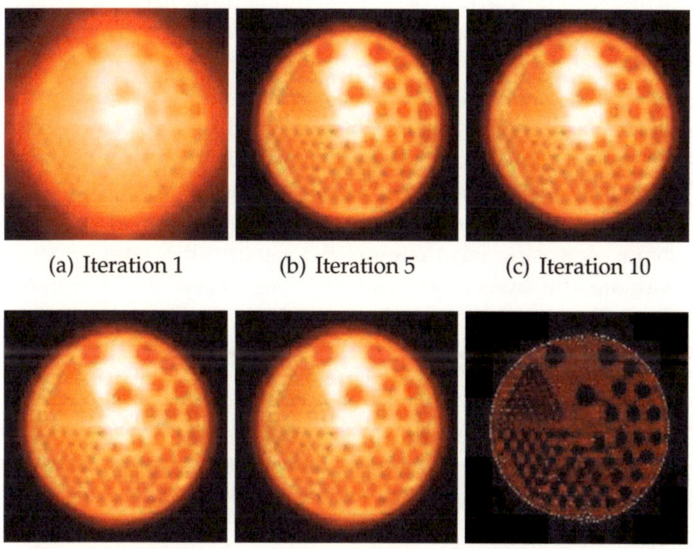

(a) Iteration 1 (b) Iteration 5 (c) Iteration 10

(d) Iteration 50 (e) Iteration 100 (f) Iteration 500

Fig. 3. Simulated acquisition of a Derenzo/Jaszczak digital phantom with 5×10^5 counts, reconstructed using the ML-EM algorithm implementation of the PETRUS library

for sinogram data, including compensation for the effect of randoms substraction and the presence of scatter.

The reader may consult Charlton & Humberston (2000) Cherry et al. (2003) for background on the physics of PET data acquisition. Concerning PET technology, instrumentation and state-of-the-art machinery, the reader may want to consult Bendriem & Townsend (1998),

Bailey et al. (2005), and the recently published monograph Phelps (2006) for further details and overview of clinical uses.

Interestingly, system modeling plays a very important role in ET for optimizing detector design, configuration and materials (see Levin & Zaidi (2007) and Stickel & Cherry (2005))[2] and for assesing acquisition and processing protocols, for example to study differences in image quality when using radionuclides with various positron ranges (Bai et al. (2005)) or properties that are not possible to measure directly like the behavior of scattered photons (Dewaraja et al. (2000)). Likewise, it is also a valuable tool in the design and assessment of correction and reconstruction methods (Zaidi & Koral (2004), Holdsworth et al. (2002)) and in the study of an imaging system response (Alessio et al. (2006)). System modeling, may also be used in the generation of the system matrix either by means of analytical calculations (see previous section) or by Monte Carlo computations (Rafecas, Mosler, Dietz, Pogl, Stamatakis, McElroy & Ziegler (2004), Alessio et al. (2006),Vandenberghe et al. (2006), Rahmim et al. (2008)). Finally, system modeling helps data production for evaluation purposes, for instance by using a digital phantom (see section 5.1) and in the description and validation of recently issued code.

In addition to the computationally more advantageous but perhaps more heterogeneous analytical approaches, Monte Carlo (MC) simulations have become a standard tool in ET (Zaidi (1999), Buvat & Castiglioni (2002), Buvat et al. (2005)) because of their ability to simultaneously model many complex processes and phenomena by statistical methods using random numbers. In a MC analysis of PET, a computer model is created with characteristics as similar as possible to the real imaging system. In this model the photon and charged particle interactions are simulated based on known probabilities of occurrence, with sampling of the probability density functions (PDFs) using uniformly distributed random numbers. The simulation is similar to a real measurement in that the statistical uncertainty decreases as the number of events increases, and therefore the quality of the reported average behavior improves. To evaluate the trajectories and energies deposited at different locations the radiation transport is simulated by sampling the PDFs for the interactions of the charged particles or photons.

General purpose MC software such as EGS4 (Nelson et al. (1985)), ITS (Jordan (1993)), MCNP (Briesmeister & Los Alamos National Laboratory (1986)) and Geant4 (Agostinelli et al. (2003)) have mainly been developed for high energy physics and include a complete set of particle and cross-section data up to several GeV. On the other hand, a number of libraries for MC simulation dedicated to SPECT and PET have been released in the last decade. These packages have been designed to solve problems for a specific type of imaging system and have improved its performance by using large optimization strategies such as the variance reduction methods. The major drawbacks may be the long computing times required for some applications and the limited flexibility when simulating different types of geometries. Examples of this software packages are SIMIND (Ljungberg & Strand (1989)), PETSIM (Thompson et al. (1992)), PET-SORTEO (Reilhac et al. (2004)) and PeneloPET (España et al. (2009)). However, two packages have become very popular among the PET community: SimSET (Lewellen et al. (1998), University of Washington, Division of Nuclear Medicine (2006)) and in recent years GATE (Jan et al. (2004),OpenGATE Collaboration (2011)). We will briefly review the main features of them and make some comparisons.

[2] See also: *Virtual PET scanner. From simulation in GATE to a final multiring Albira PET/CT camera*, in this same monograph

4.1 Geant4 Application for Tomography Emission and Radiotherapy (GATE)

In 2001, a workshop was organized in Paris about the future of MC simulations in nuclear medicine. From the discussions about the disadvantages of available software, it became clear that a new dedicated toolkit for tomographic emission was needed which could handle issues such as decay kinetics, detector dead times and patient movements. An object-oriented solution was preferred. The coding began with the Lausanne PET instrumentation group with help from several other physics and signal processing groups. A workshop was organized the year after to define the development strategy. In 2002, the first OpenGATE meeting took place in Lausanne, with the first live demonstration of the first version of GATE. Since then a number of new versions has been released and a user email list with currently more than 1200 subscribers is available.

GATE is based on the Geant4 Monte Carlo code (Agostinelli et al. (2003)) and uses its libraries to simulate particle transport. The basic idea with GATE is that the user should not need to carry out any programming, but instead employ an extended version of Geant4 script language. The program has a layered architecture with a core layer that defines the main tools and features of GATE in C++, an application layer with C++ base classes and at the top, a user layer where the simulations are set up using command based scripts. One feature of GATE is the possibility of simulating time-dependent phenomena such as source kinetics and movements of geometries, for example patient motion, respiratory and cardiac motion, changes of activity distribution over time and scanner rotation. Geant4 does however require static geometries during a simulation. Because of the relatively short duration of a single event compared to a typical movement, this problem can be solved by dividing the simulation into short time steps and updating the geometries at every step.

4.1.1 Simulation architecture

GATE simulations are based on the execution of scripted commands gathered in macros. A simulation is generally divided into seven steps as follows:

1. The verbosity level is set for each simulation module. This means that it is possible to decide the amount of information about the simulation returned by the program. In the first step, the visualization options are also chosen.
2. The geometries are defined. In this step, the geometry, denoted 'world', in which the simulation is going to take place is initially defined. After that the scanner and phantom geometries are defined.
3. This step defines the detection parameters in the so called digitizer module. Here the characteristics of the system are prescribed such as energy and timing resolution. It is also possible to include dead time and other features related to the creation of the image.
4. The physical processes are chosen for the simulation. This includes the choice of interactions library, enabling or disabling interaction effects and setting cut-off energy or range for secondary particle production.
5. The radioactive source is defined. This includes particle type, activity and half-life, source geometry, emission angle and source movement.
6. Output format is chosen. Different output formats are available for different imaging systems.
7. The experiment is initialized and started.

Scanner type	Studied FoM	Agreement	References
ECAT EXACT HR+, CPS	Spatial resolution Sensitivity Count rates Scatter fraction	∼ 3% < 7% good at activity < 20 kBq/ml ∼ 3%	Jan & al. (2005a)
ECAT HRRT, Siemens	Spatial resolution Scatter fraction Scattered coinc. profiles Count rates	excellent (<0.2 mm) < 1% very good (visual) good (about 10%)	Bataille & al. (2004)
Hi-Rez, Siemens	Scatter fraction Count rates NEC curves	∼ 1% good at activity < 40 Bq/ml good at activity < 40 Bq/ml	Michel & al. (2006)
Allegro, Philips	Count rate Scatter fraction	< 8% 8%	Lamare & al. (2006)
GE Advance, GEMS	Energy spectra Scatter fraction	not reported < 1%	Schmidtlein & al. (2006)
MicroPET P_4, Concorde	Spatial resolution Sensitivity Miniature Derenzo phantom	about 7% < 4% visual assessment	Jan et al. (2003)
MicroPET Focus 220, Siemens	Spatial resolution Sensitivity Count rates (mouse phantom)	∼ 5% ∼ 3% prompt coinc: < 5.5% delayed coinc: < 13%	Jan & al. (2005b)
Mosaic, Philips	Scatter fraction Count rates	∼ 5% 4 − 15%	Merheb & al. (2006)

Table 3. Commercial PET systems modeled in GATE

4.1.2 Imaging systems in GATE

A number of different imaging systems are available in GATE: (for example 'scanner', 'SPECThead', 'cylindricalPET', 'ECAT', 'CPET' and 'OPET'). A system is defined as a family of geometries compatible with different data output formats. For cylindrical PET the available output formats are: ASCII, ROOT, RAW and list-mode (LMF). Other systems have different options. The purpose of system definition is to make the particle-in-detector interaction histories be processed realistically.

4.1.3 Source and physics

The radioactive source in a GATE simulation is defined by the radionuclide, particle type and position, direction of emitted radiation, energy and activity. The radioactive decay is performed by the Geant4 Radioactive Decay Module. There are two packages available to simulate electromagnetic processes: the standard energy package and the low energy package. The low energy package models photon and electron interaction down to 250 eV and includes Rayleigh scatter and provides more accurate models for medical application. To speed up the simulation, it is possible to set a threshold for secondary particle production.

4.1.4 The digitizer module

The digitizer chain simulates the electronics response of a sensitive detector, which are used to store information about particle interaction within a volume. The digitizer chain consists of some processing modules: the 'hit adder' that calculates the energy deposited in

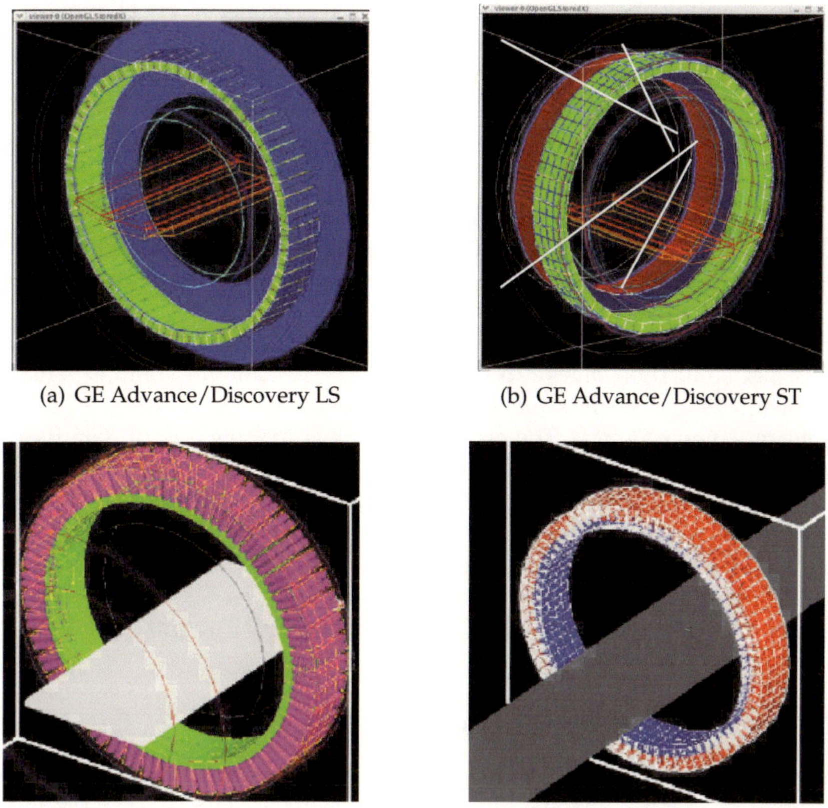

(a) GE Advance/Discovery LS

(b) GE Advance/Discovery ST

(c) Siemens Biograph

(d) HR+ ECAT EXACT

Fig. 4. Screenshots of some PET systems modeled in GATE

a sensitive detector by a given photon, the 'pulse reader' that adds pulses from a group of sensitive detectors yielding a pulse containing the total energy deposited in these detectors and assigned to the position of the largest pulse. There are also some modules wherein the user can define parameters such as energy resolution (the ability to sort photons of different energies), energy window (the energy span within which the photons will be registered), spatial resolution, time resolution (the ability to separate two events with regard to time), dead time and coincidence window (the time interval within which two detected photons will cause an event).

4.1.5 Output formats

Different output formats are available for different systems. The ASCII format is the simplest. It gives all information about the detected photons in a large text file. Each row corresponds to one event and includes information about event number, time of annihilation, positions of annihilation, scatter, energy deposition, detecting crystals and position. This output needs to be further processed to be useful, but GATE can automatically sort out coincidence events from single photon events. The ROOT format is also a very powerful output that can be analyzed by using special software. With this output it is easy to get histograms over distributions of the angles between the two annihilation photons, the energies of the positrons, the time stamps of the decays and the ranges of the positrons. For an 'ECAT' system a sinogram output is available. This output automatically stores the events in 2D sinograms. For a 'cylindricalPET' system, the list mode format (LMF), can be used with other software for image reconstruction. However, only singles can be stored by GATE, which means that coincidence events have to be paired together afterwards. The RAW output gives access to raw images of source position for singles or coincidences. This output should be used in addition to other formats.

GATE is a software for which it is easy to create complicated models of different tomographic systems, making it possible to build a realistic model if one has the correct and detailed manufacturer specifications of a scanner. A major drawback with GATE, as with other MC packages, is that simulation times can be very long, especially for complex situations with voxelized phantoms and sources (on the order of one week on a cluster of 60 computers for realistic simulation of a SM). The other drawback is that the output data files are large, on the order of GB. Compared to other existing dedicated MC software, such as SimSET, GATE seems to be able to handle more complex situations and therefore it is possible to do more realistic simulations. Although in the latest release of GATE (version 6.0.0) a couple of variance reduction methods are available, presumably more efforts will be made be to enhance the computational speed of the simulations. Finally, when using GATE it is also interesting to make use of enhanced data output formats, such as the ROOT output, in order to save disc storage space.

4.2 Simulation System for Emission Tomography (SimSET)

The SimSET package uses MC techniques to model the physical processes and instrumentation used in ET imaging. First released in 1993, SimSET has become a primary resource for many nuclear medicine imaging research groups around the world. The University of Washington Imaging Research Laboratory is continuing to develop SimSET, adding new functionality and utilities.

SimSET consists of different modules. The Photon History Generator (PHG) tracks the photons through the tomograph FOV and creates a photon history list with information about the photons reaching the camera. An object editor is used for definition of the activity and attenuation objects for the PHG. The collimator routine in SimSET is based on the 2D PET collimator that originally was implemented in the MC program PETSIM (Thompson et al. (1992)). The detector and binning modules are used to define Gaussian blurring of energy, and the photon events are then binned by combinations of number of scatters, axial position, angles and photon energy. The data are binned during the simulation run, but they can be reprocessed afterwards by the use of the photon history list.

The main advantages of GATE compared to SimSET are that GATE in contrast to SimSET can handle system dead time, random events, block detector geometries with distances between each crystal (SimSET can only handle continuous detector rings) and dynamic studies with time dependent processes. Unlike GATE, SimSET does not allow for MC simulation of the photon transport within the collimator and only includes an analytical model of the collimator response.

5. Additional tasks

Once the PET data has been collected and reconstructed some common postprocessing tasks or additional analysis may be necessary. On the other hand, one might need to generate simulated data in order to test or compare different reconstruction algorithms. For the sake of completeness, we have compiled here information on several areas of potential interest for the PET imaging practice. Thus, in this section we include a little background and useful links to freely available resources on digital phantoms, postprocessing tasks such as segmentation, registration and statistical analysis of data and quality assessment.

5.1 Digital phantoms

Computer simulated phantoms, a.k.a. digital phantoms (as opposed to physical phantoms) offer a convenient way to examine different imaging protocols in medical and small-animal imaging research. Used in combination with accurate system models of the data acquisition process, phantoms can yield realistic imaging data to serve as a 'ground truth' from which molecular imaging devices and techniques can be evaluated and improved.

5.1.1 Evolution and types of digital phantoms

Existing phantoms can be divided into two general classes: voxel-based and geometry-based phantoms. Voxel-based phantoms, such as the Hoffman phantom (Hoffman et al. (1990)) and the Zubal phantom (Zubal et al. (1994)) are generally build on patient data. They may include anatomical and functional information from different medical imaging modalities. However, they are fixed to a particular anatomy, so that study of the effects of anatomical variations is limited. Also, they are fixed to a specific resolution so the generation of the phantom at other resolutions requires interpolation.

Geometry-based phantoms, a.k.a. mathematical phantoms, such as the Shepp-Logan phantom (Shepp & Logan (1974)), the NEMA phantom (National Electrical Manufacturers Association (NEMA) (2007)), or the Derenzo/Jaszczak phantom (Budinger et al. (1977)) permit, on the other hand, variations and data generation at multiple resolutions (see fig. 5). Although they are based in fairly simple geometric primitives such as spheres and ellipsoids they have found a widespread use to research new instrumentation, image acquisition strategies, and image processing and reconstruction methods during more than three decades. A slightly more realistic description of anatomical details was achieved with the ellipsoid-based (four-dimensional) 4-D Mathematical Cardiac-Torso (MCAT) phantom. In order to study the effects of patient involuntary motion in ET imaging, models for the beating heart and respiration were developed for the MCAT. These models extended the phantom to a fourth dimension: time. This phantom was made reasonably realistic but was not as realistic as voxel-based phantoms.

A new generation of hybrid phantoms focused on the creation of ideal models that sought to combine the realism of a patient-based voxelized phantom with the flexibility of a mathematical or stylized phantom. The use of rational B-splines (NURBS) as a new flexible mathematical basis allowed to move far beyond simple geometrically based phantoms toward a more ideal phantom combining the advantages of voxelized and mathematical models. Thus, the 4-D NURBS-based Cardiac-Torso (NCAT) phantom, was able to accurately model motion and anatomical variations as well as a mathematical phantom. It was created by including information of different imaging modalities (MRI and CT data) The data slices were

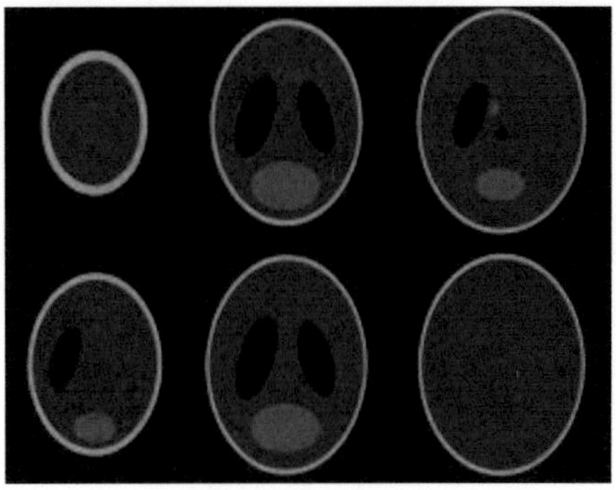

(a) Shepp-Logan phantom

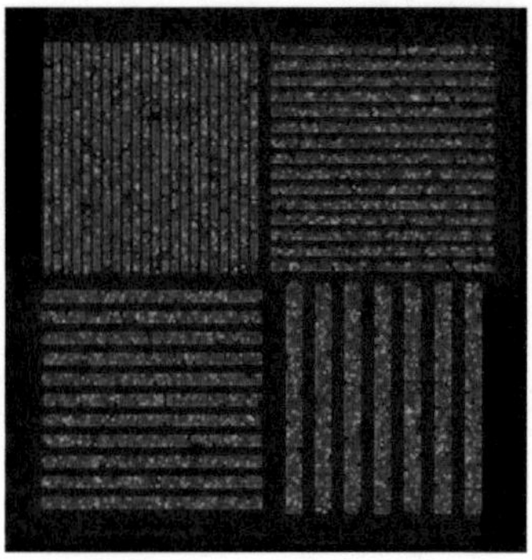

(b) Noisy bar phantom

Fig. 5. Examples of geometry-based or mathematical phantoms: (a) Trans-axial slices trough a 3D version of the Shepp-Logan phantom (b) Bar phantom with added Poisson noise

manually segmented and co-registered and 3-D NURBS surfaces were fit to each segmented structure using NURBS modeling software to generate an anatomical atlas. Each surface shape can be altered easily via affine and other transformations. The shape is defined by a set of control points which form a convex hull around the surface. To alter the surface, one only has to apply transformations to these control points. With this flexibility, NURBS have the same ability to model anatomical variations and patient motion as a mathematical phantom. Since it was based on actual imaging data, the anatomy of the NCAT is much more realistic than that of the MCAT.

In recent years and following the same guidelines, i.e. the combination of segmented patient data from actual imaging studies data with state-of-the-art computer graphics techniques, more precisely NURBS and subdivision surfaces (SDs), yet more realistic phantoms such as the 4-D extended Cardiac-Torso (XCAT) phantom and the Mouse Whole-Body (MOBY) phantom (Segars et al. (2004), figure 6) have been developed providing a level of realism comparable to that of a voxelized phantom. SDs are capable of modeling smooth surfaces of arbitrary topological type more efficiently, as is the case with complex anatomical structures of the body found in the brain and the interior of the breast. NURBS surfaces can only model such structures by partitioning the model into a collection of individual NURBS surfaces, which introduces a large number of parameters to define the model. SDs, on the contrary, initially represent an object as a coarse polygon mesh. This mesh can be iteratively subdivided and smoothed using a refinement scheme to produce a smooth surface.

With the improved anatomical detail and the extension to new areas, not only torso, the XCAT (with more than nine thousands of anatomical objects modeled over the entire human body) and MOBY phantoms are suitable for other medical imaging applications using nuclear medicine or high-resolution techniques such as CT or MRI. Additionally, these phantoms have the potential to open the door to the rapid development of hundreds of realistic patient-specific 4-D computational models. Such a library of computational models will presumably have widespread use in imaging research to develop, evaluate, and improve imaging devices and techniques and to investigate the effects of anatomy and motion. They will also provide vital tools in radiation dosimetry to estimate patient-specific dose and radiation risk and optimize dose-reduction strategies. For more detailed information on the

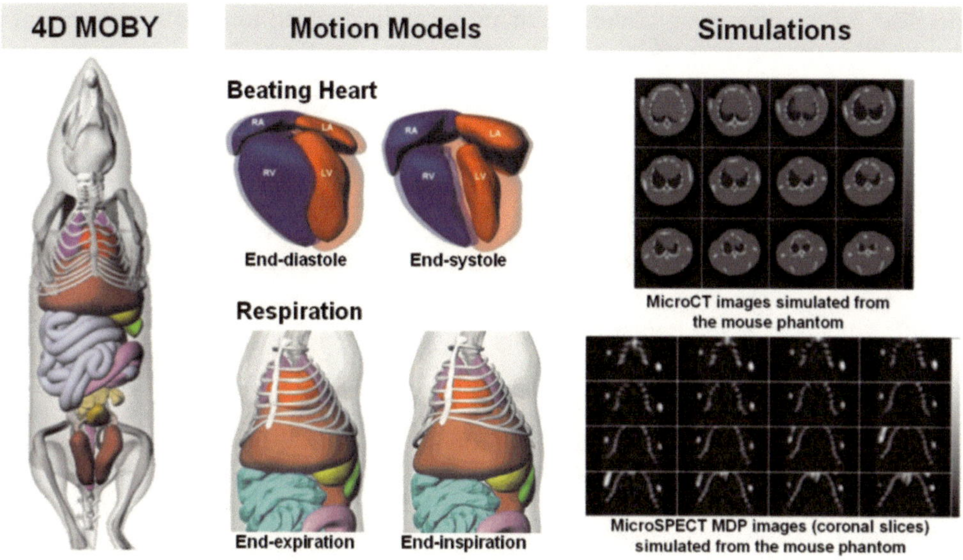

Fig. 6. The 4D MOBY hybrid phantom: (Left) Anterior view of the 4D MOBY phantom. (Middle) Cardiac and respiratory motions of the MOBY phantom. (Right) MicroCT and MicroSPECT images simulated using the phantom

MCAT, NCAT, XCAT and MOBY phantoms the reader may consult Segars & Tsui (2009) and the references therein.

5.1.2 Digital phantom resources

Some useful links to freely available digital phantom resources are the following:

The MC-ET database (Castiglioni et al. (2005)) is an interactive open to the public Internet-published database of MC simulated data for ET. Data can be easily downloaded directly from the web site `http://www.ibfm.cnr.it/mcet/`, after registering as an MC-ET user. Data sets for PET and SPECT include simulated MC data from simple mathematical phantoms, anthropomorphic phantoms as well as some data obtained from real patients where cerebral, thoracic and abdominal regions were considered.

Different versions (CT-based torso, CT-based head, MRI-based high-resolution head phantom) of the Zubal phantom data sets can be downloaded at `http://noodle.med.yale.edu/zubal/`.

The NCAT, XCAT and MOBY phantoms are distributed free-of-charge to academic institutions by emailing the authors. Companies are also welcome to use them, but authors do charge a small licensing fee. Visit the Division of Medical Imaging at Johns Hopkins Medical Institutions web page `http://dmip1.rad.jhmi.edu/xcat/` for more information on how to obtain the phantoms.

The Digimouse phantom (Dogdas et al. (2007)) is available at `http://neuroimage.usc.edu/Digimouse.html`

A detailed list of some computational human phantoms created to date is available in the website `http://www.virtualphantoms.org/phantoms.htm`

5.2 Registration

Registration is the task of aligning or developing correspondences between data. For example, in the medical environment, a CT scan may be aligned with an MRI scan in order to combine the information contained in both. Up to now, this task has renewed importance due to the active research that is taking place in PET/CT and PET/MRI systems.

5.2.1 AIR: Automatic Image Registration

This package (see `http://www.loni.ucla.edu/Software/AIR`) was developed by Robert P. Woods at UCLA as a tool for automated registration of 3D and 2D images within and across subjects and across imaging modalities. The AIR library can easily incorporate automated image registration into site specific programs adapted to any particular need. AIR source code written in C is available to the research community free of charge. The code can be compiled for UNIX, PC or Macintosh platforms. Only source code is available at the website `http://bishopw.loni.ucla.edu/AIR5/` (no executables). The software features:

- Linear spatial transformation models: rigid-body models, global rescaling models, affine models and perspective models. It supports within-modality, across-modality and linear inter-subject registration
- Nonlinear polynomial spatial transformation models ranging from first (linear) to twelfth order

It also includes utilities for re-slicing, re-orienting, re-uniting, resizing and averaging and related and similar tasks.

5.3 Segmentation

Segmentation refers to the process of partitioning a digital image into multiple sets of voxels (segments). More precisely, image segmentation is the process of assigning a label to every voxel in an image such that voxels with the same label share certain visual characteristics. In Medical Imaging, segmentation is typically used to extract organs or body structures of interest from an initial image. Relevant applications include the location of tumors and other pathologies, measuring tissue volumes, computer-guided surgery, diagnosis, treatment planning and study of anatomical structure.

5.3.1 Insight Segmentation and Registration Toolkit (ITK)

ITK (`http://www.itk.org`) is an open-source, cross-platform system that provides developers with an extensive suite of software tools for image analysis. Developed through extreme programming methodologies, ITK employs cutting-edge algorithms for registering and segmenting multidimensional data. ITK uses the CMake build environment to manage the configuration process. The software is implemented in C++ and it is wrapped for Tcl, Python (using CableSwig) and Java. This enables developers to create software using a variety of programming languages. ITK's C++ implementation style is referred to as generic programming (i.e., using templated code). Such C++ templating means that the code is highly efficient, and that many software problems are discovered at compile-time, rather than at run-time during program execution.

Some technical features of the package include:

- Data representation and algorithms to perform segmentation and registration. The focus is on medical applications; although the toolkit is capable of processing other data types
- Data representations in general form for images and meshes
- The toolkit does not address visualization or graphical user interface. These are left to other toolkits (such as VTK, VisPack, 3DViewnix, MetaImage, etc.)
- The toolkit provides minimal tools for file interface. Again, this is left to other toolkits/libraries to provide
- Multi-threaded (shared memory) parallel processing is supported

The development of the toolkit is based on principles of extreme programming. That is, design, implementation, and testing is performed in a rapid, iterative process.

5.4 Statistical analysis

Statistical analysis on image data has been a rapidly growing field in PET and in other functional imaging modalities such as fMRI with interesting applications to kinetic modeling and activation studies.

5.4.1 Statistical Parametric Mapping (SPM)

Statistical Parametric Mapping refers to the construction and assessment of spatially extended statistical processes used to test hypotheses about functional imaging data. These ideas have been instantiated in software that is called SPM. The SPM software package has been designed for the analysis of brain imaging data sequences. The sequences can be a series of images from different cohorts, or time-series from the same subject. The current release is designed for the analysis of fMRI, PET, SPECT, EEG and MEG.

SPM is made freely available to the neuro-imaging community (`http://www.fil.ion.ucl.ac.uk/spm`), to promote collaboration and a common analysis scheme across laboratories. The software represents the implementation of the theoretical concepts of Statistical Parametric Mapping in a complete analysis package. The SPM software is a suite of MATLAB (The MathWorks, Inc) functions and subroutines with some externally compiled C routines. SPM was written to organize and interpret functional neuroimaging data. SPM is an academic software toolkit for the analysis of functional imaging data, for users familiar with the underlying statistical, mathematical and image processing concepts. It is essential to understand these underlying concepts in order to use the software effectively.

5.4.2 SnPM

The Statistical nonParametric Mapping toolbox, available at `http://www.sph.umich.edu/ni-stat/SnPM`, provides an extensible framework for voxel level non-parametric permutation/randomization tests of functional Neuroimaging experiments with independent observations. The SnPM toolbox provides an alternative to the Statistics section of SPM. SnPM uses the General Linear Model to construct pseudo t-statistic images, which are then assessed for significance using a standard non-parametric multiple comparisons procedure based on randomization/permutation testing. It is most suitable for single subject PET/SPECT analysis, or designs with low degrees of freedom available for variance estimation. In these situations the freedom to use weighted locally pooled variance estimates, or variance smoothing, makes the non-parametric approach considerably more powerful than conventional parametric approaches, as are implemented in SPM. Further, the non-parametric approach is always valid, given only minimal assumptions.

5.5 Quality assessment

In the area of image reconstruction, researchers often desire to compare two or more reconstruction techniques and asses their relative merits. SNARK09 provides a uniform framework in which to implement algorithms and evaluate their performance. This software is basically a programming system for the reconstruction of 2D images from 1D projections. It is designed to help researchers interested in developing and evaluating reconstruction algorithms. SNARK09 has been designed to treat both parallel and divergent projection geometries and can create test data for use by reconstruction algorithms. A number of frequently used reconstruction algorithms are incorporated. The software can be downloaded at Gabor T. Herman website (`http://www.dig.cs.gc.cuny.edu/software/`)

5.6 Miscellaneous

Some very interesting pieces of free and open source code can be found in the following locations:

- Prof. Jeff Fessler's web page (`http://www.eecs.umich.edu/~fessler/`) at University of Michigan
- Prof. Charles A. Bouman's web page (`https://engineering.purdue.edu/~bouman/`) at Purdue University
- Turku PET Center's web (`http://www.turkupetcentre.net/software/list.php`)
- Louvain La Neuve University web pages (`ftp://ftp.topo.ucl.ac.be/pub/ecat`)

6. Conclusions

A number of relevant free software applications for PET imaging (viewing, reconstruction, system modeling and postprocessing) as well as key references have been reviewed in this chapter suggesting that free software is a highly valuable option in PET imaging clinics and research practice. We also have provided useful links to specific free software packages and data that the reader might consider useful.

7. Acknowledgments

The author wishes to thank UCLA graduate Nichole Marie LaPeer for her contribution in proof reading and editing this chapter's manuscript.

8. References

Agostinelli, S., Allison, J., Amako, K., Apostolakis, J., Araujo, H., Arce, P., Asai, M., Axen, D., Banerjee, S., Barrand, G. et al. (2003). Geant4-a simulation toolkit, *Nuclear Instruments and Methods in Physics Research-Section A Only* 506(3): 250–303.

Aguiar, P., Rafecas, M., Ortuño, J., Kontaxakis, G., Santos, A., Pavía, J. & Ros, D. (2010). Geometrical and Monte Carlo projectors in 3D PET reconstruction, *Medical physics* 37: 5691.

Ahn, S. & Fessler, J. A. (2003). A Globally Convergent Image Reconstruction for Emission Tomography Using Relaxed Ordered Subsets Algorithms, *IEEE Transactions on Medical Imaging* pp. 623–626.

Alessio, A., Kinahan, P. & Lewellen, T. (2006). Modeling and incorporation of system response functions in 3-D whole body PET, *IEEE Transactions on Medical Imaging* 25(7): 828–837.

Bai, B., Laforest, R., Smith, A. & Leahy, R. (2005). Evaluation of MAP image reconstruction with positron range modeling for 3D PET, *IEEE Nuclear Science Symposium Conference Record*, Vol. 5, IEEE, pp. 2686–2689.

Bailey, D. L., Townsend, D. W., Valk, P. E. & Maisey, M. N. (eds) (2005). *Positron Emission Tomography*, Springer.

Bataille, F. & al. (2004). Monte Carlo simulation for the ECAT HRRT using GATE, *IEEE MIC Conf Records*, Vol. 4, pp. 2570–2574.

Beisel, T., Lietsch, S. & Thielemans, K. (2008). A method for OSEM PET reconstruction on parallel architectures using STIR, *Nuclear Science Symposium Conference Record, 2008. NSS'08. IEEE*, IEEE, pp. 4161–4168.

Ben-Tal, A. & Nemirovski, A. (1999). The conjugate barrier method for non-smooth, convex optimization, *Technical Report Research report #5/99*, MINERVA Optimization Center, Faculty of Industrial Engineering and Management,Technion Israel Institute of Technology.

Bendriem, B. & Townsend, D. W. (eds) (1998). *The Theory and Practice of 3D PET*, Kluwer Academic Publisher, The Netherlands.

Briesmeister, J. & Los Alamos National Laboratory (1986). *MCNP–A general Monte Carlo code for neutron and photon transport*, Los Alamos National Laboratory.

Budinger, T., Derenzo, S., Gullberg, G., Greenberg, W. & Huesman, R. (1977). Emission computer assisted tomography with single-photon and positron annihilation photon emitters, *Journal of Computer Assisted Tomography* 1(1): 131.

Buvat, I. & Castiglioni, I. (2002). Monte Carlo simulations in SPET and PET, *Quarterly Journal of Nuclear Medicine* 46(1): 48–61.

Buvat, I., Castiglioni, I., Feuardent, J. & Gilardi, M. (2005). Unified description and validation of Monte Carlo simulators in PET, *Physics in Medicine and Biology* 50: 329.

Castiglioni, I., Buvat, I., Rizzo, G., Gilardi, M., Feuardent, J. & Fazio, F. (2005). A publicly accessible Monte Carlo database for validation purposes in emission tomography, *European Journal of Nuclear Medicine and Molecular Imaging* 32(10): 1234–1239.

Charlton, M. & Humberston, J. (2000). *Positron physics*, Cambridge Monographs on Atomic, Molecular and Chemical Physics, Cambridge University Press.

Cherry, S. R., Sorenson, J. A. & Phelps, M. E. (2003). *Physics in Nuclear Medicine*, 3rd edition edn, W. B. Saunders Co.

Cygwin (2011). Cygwin web, `http://www.cygwin.com/`.

Daube-Witherspoon, M. E. & Muehllehner, G. (1987). Treatment of axial data in three-dimensional PET, *Journal of Nuclear Medicine* 28: 1717–1724.

de la Prieta, R. (2004). *Biological and Medical Data Analysis*, Vol. 3337 of *Lecture Notes in Computer Science*, Springer, chapter An accurate and parallelizable geometric projector/backprojector for 3D PET image reconstruction.

de la Prieta, R., Hernandez, J., Schiavi, E. & Malpica, N. (2006). Analytical Geometric Model for Photon Coincidence Detection in 3D PET, *IEEE Nuclear Science Symposium Conference Record*, pp. 2229–2232.

Defrise, M., Kinahan, P. E. & Michel, C. J. (2005). *Positron Emission Tomography*, Springer, chapter Image Reconstruction Algorithms in PET.

Defrise, M., Kinahan, P., Townsend, D., Michel, C., Sibomana, M. & Newport, D. (1997). Exact and approximate rebinning algorithms for 3-D PET data, *IEEE Transactions on Medical Imaging* 16(2): 145–158.

Dewaraja, Y., Ljungberg, M. & Koral, K. (2000). Characterization of scatter and penetration using Monte Carlo simulation in ^{131}I imaging, *Journal of Nuclear Medicine: official publication, Society of Nuclear Medicine* 41(1): 123.

Dogdas, B., Stout, D., Chatziioannou, A. & Leahy, R. (2007). Digimouse: a 3D whole body mouse atlas from CT and cryosection data, *Physics in Medicine and Biology* 52: 577.

España, S., Herraiz, J., Vicente, E., Vaquero, J., Desco, M. & Udias, J. (2009). PeneloPET, a Monte Carlo PET simulation tool based on PENELOPE: features and validation, *Physics in Medicine and Biology* 54: 1723.

Fessler, J. (1994). Penalized wighted least-squares image reconstruction for positron emission tomography, *IEEE Transactions on Medical Imaging* .

Fessler, J. (1997). Users guide for aspire 3d image reconstruction software, *Comm. and Sign. Proc. Lab., Dept. of EECS, Univ. of Michigan, Ann Arbor, MI, Tech. Rep* 310.

Free Software Foundation (2011). Free Software Foundation Web, `http://www.fsf.org`.

Frese, T., Rouze, N., Bouman, C., Sauer, K. & Hutchins, G. (2003). Quantitative comparison of FBP, EM, and bayesian reconstruction algorithms, including the impact of accurate system modeling, for the IndyPET scanner, *IEEE Transactions on Medical Imaging* 22(2): 258–276.

Green, P. J. (1990). Bayesian reconstructions from emission tomography data using a modified EM algorithm, *IEEE Transactions on Medical Imaging* pp. 84–93.

Herman, G. & Meyer, L. (1993). Algebraic reconstruction techniques can be made computationally efficient [positron emission tomography application], *IEEE Transactions on Medical Imaging* 12(3): 600–609.

Herraiz, J., Espaa, S., García, S., Cabido, R., Montemayor, A., Desco, M., Vaquero, J. & Udias, J. (2009). GPU acceleration of a fully 3D iterative reconstruction software for PET using CUDA, *Nuclear Science Symposium Conference Record (NSS/MIC), 2009 IEEE*, IEEE, pp. 4064–4067.

Herraiz, J., Espana, S., Vaquero, J., Desco, M. & Udias, J. (2006). FIRST: Fast iterative reconstruction software for (PET) tomography, *Physics in medicine and biology* 51: 4547.

Hoffman, E., Cutler, P., Digby, W. & Mazziotta, J. (1990). 3-D phantom to simulate cerebral blood flow and metabolic images for PET, *IEEE Transactions on Nuclear Science* 37(2): 616–620.

Holdsworth, C., Levin, C., Janecek, M., Dahlbom, M. & Hoffman, E. (2002). Performance analysis of an improved 3-D PET Monte Carlo simulation and scatter correction, *Nuclear Science, IEEE Transactions on* 49(1): 83–89.

Hudson, M. & Larkin, R. (1994). Accelerated Image Reconstruction using Ordered Subsets of Projection Data, *IEEE Transactions on Medical Imaging* 13: 601–609.

Huesman, R., Klein, G., Moses, W., Qi, J., Reutter, B. & Virador, P. (2000). List-mode maximum-likelihood reconstruction applied to positron emission mammography (pem) with irregular sampling, *Medical Imaging, IEEE Transactions on* 19(5): 532–537.

Iriarte, A., Sorzano, C., Carazo, J., Rubio, J. & Marabini, R. (2009). A theoretical model for em-ml reconstruction algorithms applied to rotating pet scanners, *Physics in medicine and biology* 54: 1909.

Jacobson, M., Levkovitz, R., Ben-Tal, A., Thielemans, K., Spinks, T., Belluzzo, . D., Pagani, E., Bettinardi, V., Gilardi, M. C., Zverovich, A. & Mitra, G. (2000). Enhanced 3D PET OSEM reconstruction using inter-update Metz filtering, *Physics in Medicine and Biology* 45(8): 2417–2439.

Jan, S. & al. (2005a). Monte Carlo simulation for the ECAT EXACT HR+ system using GATE, *IEEE Transactions on Nuclear Imaging* 52: 627–633.

Jan, S. & al. (2005b). Monte Carlo simulation of the microPET FOCUS system for small rodents imaging applications, *IEEE Nuclear Science Symposium Conference Record*, Vol. 3, pp. 1653–1657.

Jan, S., Chatziioannou, A., Comtat, C., Strul, D., Santin, G. & Trébossen, R. (2003). Monte Carlo simulation for the microPET P4 system using GATE, *Molecular Imaging and Biology* 5: 138.

Jan, S., Morel, C. & al. (2004). GATE: a simulation toolkit for PET and SPECT, *Physics in Medicine and Biology* 49: 4543–4561.

Johnson, C., Yan, Yan, Y., Carson, R., Martino, R. & Daube-Witherspoon, M. (1995). A system for the 3D reconstruction of retracted-septa PET data using the EM algorithm, *IEEE Transactions on Nuclear Science* 42(4): 1223–1227.

Jones, M., Yao, R. & Bhole, C. (2006). Hybrid MPI-OpenMP programming for parallel OSEM PET reconstruction, *Nuclear Science, IEEE Transactions on* 53(5): 2752–2758.

Jordan, T. (1993). Comments on ITS: 'The integrated TIGER series of electron/photon transport codes-Version 3.0' by J.A. Halbleib et al., *Nuclear Science, IEEE Transactions on* 40(1): 71–72.

Kak, A. & Slaney, M. (1988). *Principles of Computerized Tomographic Imaging*, IEEE Engineering in Medicine and Biology Society, IEEE Press.

Karuta, B. & Lecomte, R. (1992). Effect of detector weighting functions on the point spread function of high resolution PET tomographs: a simulation study, *IEEE Transactions on Medical Imaging* 11(3): 379–385.

Kaufman, L. (1993). Maximum likelihood, least squares, and penalized least squares for PET, *IEEE Transactions on Medical Imaging* 12(2): 200–214.

Kinahan, P. E. & Rogers, J. G. (1989). Analytic 3D Image Reconstruction Using All Detected Events, *IEEE Transactions on Nuclear Science* 36(1): 964–968.

Lamare, F. & al. (2006). Validation of a Monte Carlo simulation of the Philips Allegro/GEMINI PET systems using GATE, *Phys. Med. Biol.* 51: 943–962.

Lecomte, R., Schmitt, D. & Lamoureux, G. (1984). Geometry study of a high resolution PET detection system using small detectors, *IEEE Transactions on Nuclear Science* 31(1): 556–561.

Levin, C. & Zaidi, H. (2007). Current trends in preclinical PET system design, *PET Clinics* 2(2): 125–160.

Lewellen, T., Harrison, R. & Vannoy, S. (1998). The sSimSET program, *Monte Carlo calculations in nuclear medicine: applications in diagnostic imaging, M. Ljungberg; SE. Strand, and M. A. King, Eds. Philadelphia: Institute of Physics* pp. 77–92.

Lewitt, R. M., Muehllehner, G. & Karp, J. S. (1994). Three-dimensional reconstruction for PET by multi-slice rebinning and axial image filtering, *Phys. Med. Biol* 39(3): 321–340.

Lewitt, R. & Matej, S. (2003). Overview of methods for image reconstruction from projections in emission computed tomography, *Proceedings of the IEEE* 91(10): 1588–1611.

Ljungberg, M. & Strand, S. (1989). A Monte Carlo program for the simulation of scintillation camera characteristics, *Computer methods and programs in biomedicine* 29(4): 257–272.

Loening, A. & Gambhir, S. (2003). AMIDE: A free software tool for multimodality medical image analysis, *Mol. Imaging* 2(3): 131–137.

Markiewicz, P., Reader, A., Tamal, M., Julyan, J. & Hastings, D. (2005). An advanced analytic method incorporating the geometrical properties of scanner and radiation emissions into the system model for the true component of 3d pet data, *Nuclear Science Symposium Conference Record, 2005 IEEE*, Vol. 4, IEEE, pp. 2310–2314.

Merheb, C. & al. (2006). Assessment of the Mosaic animal PET system response using list-mode data for validation of GATE Monte Carlo modelling, *Nuclear Instruments and Methods in Physics Research Section A* 569: 220–224.

Michel, C. & al. (2006). Influence of crystal material on the performance of the HiRez 3D PET scanner: A Monte-Carlo study, *IEEE Nuclear Science Symposium Conference Record*, Vol. 4, pp. 1528–1531.

Mumcuoglu, E., Leahy, R., Cherry, S. & Hoffman, E. (1996). Accurate geometric and physical response modelling for statistical image reconstruction in high resolution PET, *IEEE Nuclear Science Symposium, Conference Record*, Vol. 3, IEEE, pp. 1569–1573.

National Electrical Manufacturers Association (NEMA) (2007). NEMA NU 2-2007 Performance Measurements of Small Animal Positron Emission Tomographs (PETs), available at `http://www.nema.org/stds/nu4.cfmg`.

Nelson, W., Hirayama, H. & Rogers, D. (1985). Egs4 code system, *Technical report*, Stanford Linear Accelerator Center, Menlo Park, CA (USA).

Ollinger, J. & Goggin, A. (1996). Maximum likelihood reconstruction in fully 3D PET via the SAGE algorithm, *Nuclear Science Symposium, 1996. Conference Record., 1996 IEEE*, Vol. 3, IEEE, pp. 1594–1598.

Open MPI (2011). Open Source High Performance Computing web, `http://www.open-mpi.org/`.

OpenGATE Collaboration (2011). OpenGATE Collaboration Webpage, `http://www.opengatecollaboration.org`.

OpenScience Project (2011). OpenScience Project Web, `http://www.openscience.org/`.

Ortuño, J., Kontaxakis, G., Rubio, J., Guerra, P. & Santos, A. (2010). Efficient methodologies for system matrix modelling in iterative image reconstruction for rotating high-resolution PET, *Physics in Medicine and Biology* 55: 1833.

Panin, V., Kehren, F., Michel, C. & Casey, M. (2006). Fully 3-D PET reconstruction with system matrix derived from point source measurements, *IEEE Transactions on Medical Imaging* 25(7): 907–921.

Phelps, M. E. (ed.) (2006). *PET: Physics, Instrumentation and Scanners*, 1st edn, Springer, Orlando.

Qi, J. & Huesman, R. (2005). Effect of errors in the system matrix on maximum a posteriori image reconstruction, *Physics in medicine and biology* 50: 3297.

Qi, J. & Leahy, R. (2006). Iterative reconstruction techniques in emission computed tomography, *Physics in Medicine and Biology* 51(15): R541–R578.

Qi, J., Leahy, R., Cherry, S., Chatziioannou, A. & Farquhar, T. (1998). High-resolution 3D Bayesian image reconstruction using the microPET small-animal scanner, *Physics in Medicine and Biology* 43: 1001.

Rafecas, M., Boning, G., Pichler, B., Lorenz, E., Schwaiger, M. & Ziegler, S. (2004). Effect of noise in the probability matrix used for statistical reconstruction of pet data, *Nuclear Science, IEEE Transactions on* 51(1): 149–156.

Rafecas, M., Mosler, B., Dietz, M., Pogl, M., Stamatakis, A., McElroy, D. & Ziegler, S. (2004). Use of a Monte Carlo-based probability matrix for 3-D iterative reconstruction of MADPET-II data, *IEEE Transactions on Nuclear Science* 51(5): 2597–2605.

Rahmim, A., Tang, J., Lodge, M., Lashkari, S., Ay, M., Lautamäki, R., Tsui, B. & Bengel, F. (2008). Analytic system matrix resolution modeling in PET: an application to Rb-82 cardiac imaging, *Physics in Medicine and Biology* 53: 5947.

Rehfeld, N. & Alber, M. (2007). A parallelizable compression scheme for Monte Carlo scatter system matrices in PET image reconstruction, *Physics in Medicine and Biology* 52: 3421.

Reilhac, A., Lartizien, C., Costes, N., Sans, S., Comtat, C., Gunn, R. & Evans, A. (2004). PET-SORTEO: A Monte Carlo-based simulator with high count rate capabilities, *IEEE Transactions on Nuclear Science* 51(1): 46–52.

Rorden, C. (2011). MRIcro web pages, `http://www.cabiatl.com/mricro/`.

Rosset, A., Spadola, L. & Ratib, O. (2004). OsiriX: an open-source software for navigating in multidimensional DICOM images, *Journal of Digital Imaging* 17(3): 205–216.

Scheins, J., Boschen, F. & Herzog, H. (2006). Analytical calculation of volumes-of-intersection for iterative, fully 3-D PET reconstruction, *IEEE Transactions on Medical Imaging* 25(10): 1363–1369.

Scheins, J. & Herzog, H. (2008). PET Reconstruction Software Toolkit-PRESTO a novel, universal C++ library for fast, iterative, fully 3D PET image reconstruction using highly compressed, memory-resident system matrices, *Nuclear Science Symposium Conference Record. NSS'08*, IEEE, pp. 4147–4150.

Schmidtlein, C. & al. (2006). Validation of GATE Monte Carlo simulations of the GE Advance/Discovery LS PET scanners, *Med Phys.* 33(1): 198–208.

Schmitt, D., Karuta, B., Carrier., C. & Lecomte, R. (1988). Fast point spread function computation from aperture functions in high resolution PET, *IEEE Transactions on Medical Imaging* 7(1): 2–12.

Segars, W. & Tsui, B. (2009). MCAT to XCAT: The Evolution of 4-D Computerized Phantoms for Imaging Research, *Proceedings of the IEEE* 97(12): 1954–1968.

Segars, W., Tsui, B., Frey, E., Johnson, G. & Berr, S. (2004). Development of a 4-D digital mouse phantom for molecular imaging research, *Molecular Imaging and Biology* 6(3): 149–159.

Selivanov, V. V., Picard, Y., Cadorette, J., Rodrigue, S. & Lecomte, R. (2000). Detector response models for statistical iterative image reconstruction in high resolution PET, *IEEE Transactions on Nuclear Science* 47(3): 1168–1175.

Shepp, L. A. & Vardi, Y. (1982). Maximum likelihood reconstruction for emission tomography, *IEEE Transactions on Medical Imaging* MI–1(2): 113–122.

Shepp, L. & Logan, B. (1974). The Fourier reconstruction of a head section, *IEEE Trans. Nucl. Sci* 21(3): 21–43.

Siddon, R. (1985). Fast calculation of the exact radiological path for a three-dimensional ct array, *Medical Physics* 12: 252.

Soares, E., Germino, K., Glick, S. & Stodilka, R. (2003). Determination of three-dimensional voxel sensitivity for two-and three-headed coincidence imaging, *Nuclear Science, IEEE Transactions on* 50(3): 405–412.

Stallman, R. (2002). *Free Software, Free Society: Selected Essays of Richard M. Stallman*, Joshua Gay.

Stickel, J. & Cherry, S. (2005). High-resolution PET detector design: modelling components of intrinsic spatial resolution, *Physics in Medicine and Biology* 50: 179.

Strul, D., Slates, R. B., Dahlbom, M., Cherry, S. & Marsden, P. (2003). An improved analytical detector response function model for multilayer small-diameter PET scanners, *Physics in Medicine and Biology* 48: 979–994.

Tamburo, R. J. (2010). Software packages for neuroimage processing, *in* P. Laughlin (ed.), *Neuroimaging research in geriatric mental health*, Springer Publishing Company, LLC, pp. 85–100.

Terstegge, A., Weber, S., Herzog, H., Muller-Gartner, H. & Halling, H. (1996). High resolution and better quantification by tube of response modelling in 3d pet reconstruction, *Nuclear Science Symposium, 1996. Conference Record., 1996 IEEE*, Vol. 3, IEEE, pp. 1603–1607.

The boost libraries (2011). The boost libraries web, `http://www.boost.org`.

Thielemans, K. & al. (2011). STIR: Software for Tomographic Image Reconstruction, `http://stir.sourceforge.net/`.

Thielemans, K., Mustafovic, S. & Tsoumpas, C. (2006). STIR: Software for Tomographic Image Reconstruction Release 2, *Proc. IEEE Medical Imaging Conference Medical Imaging Conf., San Diego, CA*, pp. 1603–1607.

Thompson, C., Moreno-Cantu, J. & Picard, Y. (1992). PETSIM: Monte Carlo simulation of all sensitivity and resolution parameters of cylindrical positron imaging systems, *Physics in Medicine and Biology* 37: 731.

Tohme, M. & Qi, J. (2009). Iterative image reconstruction for positron emission tomography based on a detector response function estimated from point source measurements, *Physics in medicine and biology* 54: 3709.

University of Washington, Division of Nuclear Medicine (2006). SimSET: Simulation System for Emission Tomography, `http://depts.washington.edu/simset/html/simset_home.html`.

Vandenberghe, S., Staelens, S., Byrne, C., Soares, E., Lemahieu, I. & Glick, S. (2006). Reconstruction of 2D PET data with Monte Carlo generated system matrix for generalized natural pixels, *Physics in Medicine and Biology* 51: 3105.

Watabe, H. (2011). GpetView website, `http://www.mi.med.osaka-u.ac.jp/gpetview/gpetview.html`.

Zaidi, H. (1999). Relevance of accurate Monte Carlo modeling in nuclear medical imaging, *Medical Physics* 26: 574–608.

Zaidi, H. & Koral, K. (2004). Scatter modelling and compensation in emission tomography, *European Journal of Nuclear Medicine and Molecular Imaging* 31(5): 761–782.

Zhao, H. & Reader, A. (2003). Fast ray-tracing technique to calculate line integral paths in voxel arrays, *Nuclear Science Symposium Conference Record, 2003 IEEE*, Vol. 4, IEEE, pp. 2808–2812.

Zhou, J. & Qi, J. (2011). Fast and efficient fully 3D PET image reconstruction using sparse system matrix factorization with GPU acceleration, *Physics in Medicine and Biology* 56: 6739.

Zubal, I., Harrell, C., Smith, E., Rattner, Z., Gindi, G. & Hoffer, P. (1994). Computerized three-dimensional segmented human anatomy, *Medical Physics-Lancaster PA-* 21: 299–299.

Part 2

Radiopharmaceuticals

5

Pd^0–Mediated Rapid *C*–[^{11}C]Methylation and *C*–[^{18}F]Fluoromethylation: Revolutionary Advanced Methods for General Incorporation of Short–Lived Positron–Emitting ^{11}C and ^{18}F Radionuclides in an Organic Framework

Masaaki Suzuki[1], Hiroko Koyama[2],
Misato Takashima-Hirano[1] and Hisashi Doi[1]
[1]RIKEN Center for Molecular Imaging Science (CMIS) and
[2]Gifu University Graduate School of Medicine
Japan

1. Introduction

The study of *in vivo* bioscience and medical treatment from molecular point of view requires the precise evaluation of molecule behavior in living systems, especially involving the human body. Positron emission tomography (PET) is a non–invasive imaging technology with a good resolution, high sensitivity, and accurate quantification, which makes it possible to timely and spatially analyze the dynamic behavior of molecules in *in vivo* systems using a specific molecular probe labeled with positron–emitting radionuclides such as ^{11}C, ^{13}N, ^{18}F, and ^{76}Br (Phelps, 2004). PET has been extensively used for the diagnosis of diseases such as cancers, cerebral dysfunction, and etc., and recently, in medical checkups as an early detection approach. In the current paradigm shift to drug discovery, PET molecular imaging will provide an important new scientific platform to execute human microdosing trials during the early stage of drug development, especially from the viewpoint of promoting evidence–based medicine (Lappin & Garner, 2003; Bergström et al., 2003). A core concept and the driving force of molecular imaging would truly be "Seeing is Believing". It is of significant value to unveil the vital functions and phenomena of living systems by molecular imaging the *in vivo* behavior of a ligand and the localization of a biologically significant target molecule. The potential of PET molecular imaging in an interdisciplinary scientific area strongly depends on the availability of suitable radioactive molecular probes with specific biological functions. The development of biologically significant novel PET probes will be accomplished by the combination of an efficient synthetic strategy for designed molecules and new advances in the field of labeling chemistry (Schubiger et al., 2007).

Among the short–lived positron–emitting radionuclides, ^{11}C and ^{18}F with a half–life of 20.4 and 109.8 min, respectively, have often been used for radiolabeling as the most significant radionuclides from both a chemical and biological perspective as well as from the viewpoint of radiation exposure safety. With respect to the ^{11}C-incorporation on organic carbon frameworks, we have been developing multiple-type Pd^0-mediated rapid [^{11}C]methylations onto an arene including a heteroaromatic compound, and alkene, alkyne and alkane structures by [^{11}C]carbon-carbon bond forming reactions (rapid *C*-[^{11}C]methylations) using [^{11}C]methyl iodide and an excess amount of an organostannane or organoboron within a very short time span (5 min) (Suzuki et al., 1997; Hosoya et al., 2004; Hosoya et al., 2006; Doi et al., 2009; Suzuki et al., 2009). These labeling reactions provide a high generality and practicability as groundbreaking methods for introducing the [^{11}C]methyl group into almost any organic framework. Regarding the ^{18}F radionuclide, a rather longer half-lived positron emitter than ^{11}C, the ^{18}F-labeling can be mainly accomplished by ordinary methods involving nucleophile substitution with the ^{18}F anion, as exemplified by the synthesis of 2-[^{18}F]fluoro-2-deoxy-D-glucose ([^{18}F]FDG) (Ido et al., 1978) and 3′-[^{18}F]fluoro-3′-deoxythymidine ([^{18}F]FLT) (Grierson et al, 1997, as cited in Bading & Shields, 2008). In this chapter, newly advanced methodologies for introducing the short-lived ^{11}C radionuclide into various carbon frameworks (rapid *C*-[^{11}C]methylations) and the rather longer half-lived ^{18}F radionuclide into a benzene framework (*C*-[^{18}F]fluoromethylation) are described in detail in addition to their applications for radiolabeling biologically and clinically significant organic molecules.

2. PET molecular imaging technology–principle, properties, and benefits

The short-lived positron emitting radionuclide ^{11}C was first produced by Crane and Lauritsen in 1934 (Lauritsen et al., 1934, as cited in Allard et al., 2008). They investigated the physical properties of this radionuclide and demonstrated that ^{11}C undergoes β^+ decay with a half-life of 20.4 min, yielding ^{11}B as the stable nuclide (Figure 1). A positron (positively charged electron, e^+) ejected by this process collides with a nearby electron within a few millimeters in tissue to produce two high-energy γ-ray photons of 511 keV each. These photons travel in opposite directions at 180 degrees, penetrating the body, and can be detected by a pair of opposing scintillation detectors. If the two opposite detectors are simultaneously hit, it is assumed that the photons come from the same decay event. The data are fed to a computer system that can reconstruct the three-dimensional tomographic imaging and provide a highly accurate quantitative analysis of a radiolabeled drug in a body over time, measured as becquerel (Bq) per pixel. Because of the really high specific radioactivity of positron-emitter labeled compounds, PET enables *in vivo* imaging using an extremely small mass of the compound (sub-femtomole), namely, at extremely low concentrations (sub-picomolar) far below the critical concentration of pharmacological effects. The other typical positron-emitting radionuclides for PET studies, along with their half-lives ($t_{1/2}$) are: ^{15}O ($t_{1/2}$ = 2.07 min); ^{13}N ($t_{1/2}$ = 9.96 min); ^{68}Ga ($t_{1/2}$ = 67.6 min); ^{18}F ($t_{1/2}$ = 109.7 min); ^{64}Cu ($t_{1/2}$ = 12.7 h). The benefits of the use of PET technology in scientific research areas are as follows: (1) O, N, and C are included as ubiquitous elements constituting a biologically active compound in nature, providing the diversity of the labeled compounds without modifying the properties (or functions) of the molecule; (2) the molecule including the positron emitting radionuclide can be externally and quantitatively measured using a PET camera with a high resolution and sensitivity; (3) a short half-life is very relevant to human PET studies in terms of the high required safety for radiation exposure.

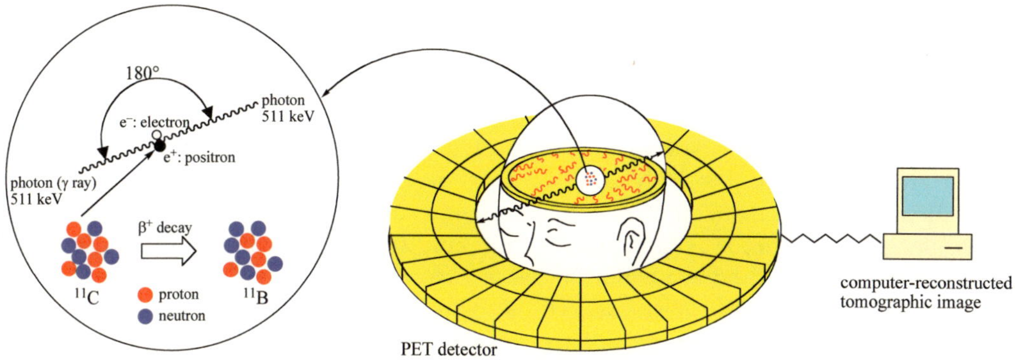

Fig. 1. Principle of the brain imaging by PET as shown by ^{11}C to ^{11}B decay.

3. Rapid chemistry needed for ^{11}C–labeling–working against time

The special aspects of PET radiochemistry such as short half-lives, extremely small amounts of available radionuclides, and relatively high-energy radiation impose severe restrictions on the synthesis of PET probes. In general, the synthesis of a pure, injectable ^{11}C-labeled probe must be accomplished within 2-half lives of ca. 40 min due to the quick decay of the radioactivity. The synthesis process for the pharmaceutical formulation includes the following steps: (1) derivatives of a ^{11}C isotope produced by a cyclotoron to an appropriate labeling precursor such as $^{11}CH_4$, $^{11}CH_3I$, $^{11}CH_3OTf$, ^{11}CO, and $^{11}CO_2$; (2) evaluation of the reaction efficiency (radiochemical yield) by analytical high performance liquid chromatography (HPLC) after the ^{11}C-labeling of the target probe; (3) work-up and chromatographic purification of the desired ^{11}C-labeled probe; and (4) preparation of an injectable solution for an animal/human PET study (pharmaceutical formulation). Therefore, the time allowed for a ^{11}C-labeling reaction should be less than 5 min, inevitably necessitating a rapid chemical reaction. Another difficulty encountered in the synthesis of a ^{11}C-labeled PET probe is the availability of an extremely small amount (nano-mol level) of the ^{11}C-labeling precursor such as [^{11}C]CH_3I. Therefore, the labeling reaction is usually carried out with a large amount (milli-gram level) of the reacting substrate to promote the reaction. In addition, the efficient and secure purification of a small amount of the synthesized ^{11}C-labeled probe from a large amount of the remaining substrate must be considered since a PET probe is usually intravenously injected into both living animals and humans.

4. Attractive features of rapid *C*–[^{11}C]methylation–four kinds of rapid *C*–[^{11}C]methylations

Thus far, in the field of PET chemistry, the [^{11}C]methylation of the hetero atoms of *N*, *O*, and *S* has mainly been explored and utilized because of its simple reaction conditions namely, only by mixing $^{11}CH_3I$ and a large amount of the substrate (Allard et al., 2008). However, a carbon-hetero atom bond tends to be readily metabolized to produce $^{11}CH_3OH$, $^{11}CH_2O$ and $H^{11}COOH$, which are dispersed in whole organs, thus decreasing the credibility of a PET image. It could be said that "the facts are the enemy of the truth." We here considered that the [^{11}C]methylation by [^{11}C]C-C bond formation (referred to as *C*-[^{11}C]methylation)

(Suzuki et al., 1997) will have a number of benefits because of the following reasons: (1) The [^{11}C]methyl group introduced into a carbon will be metabolically stable, and therefore, such a ^{11}C-labeled probe will provide a highly credible PET image; (2) the methyl group is the smallest nonpolar functional group, and therefore, the introduction of a methyl group has the least influence on the biological activity of the parent compound; furthermore, the methyl group is rather positively used in drug design as magic methyl to control the lipophilicity as well as the fixation of the conformation of a molecule; (3) a short half-life of the ^{11}C-incorporated probe is favorable for the rapid screening involving optimization of reaction conditions and the evaluation of the *in vivo* behavior, thus allowing several trials per day. Accordingly, we have devised a plan to realize four types of rapid C-[^{11}C]methylations for arene, alkene, alkyne, and alkane frameworks (Figure 2), which allow the ^{11}C-labeling of almost any organic compound. The following pharmacokinetic (PK)/pharmacodynamic (PD) studies in *in vivo* systems by PET provide a key methodology to eventually promote "evidence-based medicine" at the molecular level. With regard to such a [^{11}C]C-C bond forming reaction, organometallic compounds comprised of the group IA and IIA metals were previously used. For example, [methyl-^{11}C]thymidine was prepared in a radiochemical yield of 20% with radiochemical purities >99% by the reaction of [^{11}C]CH_3I with the lithiated derivative obtained from the bromo precursor (Sundoro-Wu et al., 1984). In such a reaction, however, the use of a moisture-sensitive organolithium compound is difficult to justify the stoichiometry for an extremely small amount of [^{11}C]CH_3I, resulting in the inevitable production of a large amount of an undesired demethylated derivative due to the use of an excess amount of the lithiated substrate. Furthermore, the undesired side reaction such as the rearrangement of the lithiation position occurs under such drastic conditions. Consequently, the tedious separation of demethylated side products and regioisomers is inevitably needed to purify the desired compound. Thus, the reaction based on the use of "soft metalloids" as nucleophilic substrates was ideal for this requirement, if realized, as described in detail in section 5.

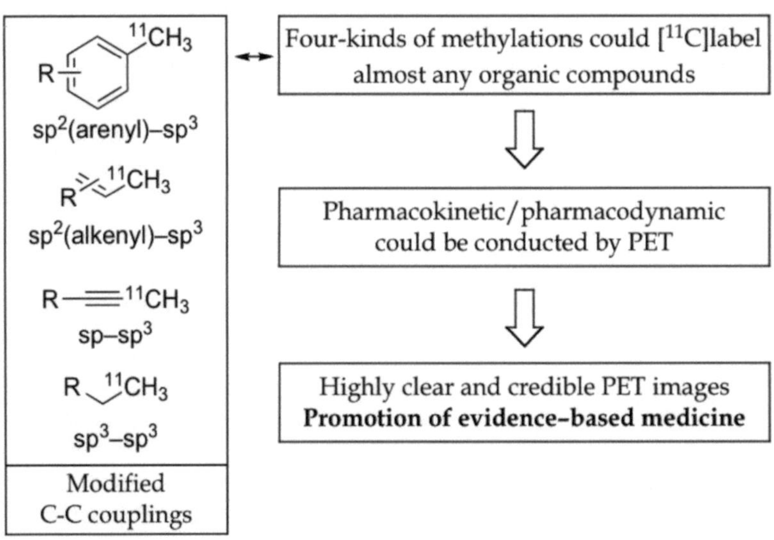

Fig. 2. Attractive features of rapid C-[^{11}C]methylations.

5. Benefits of using of an organostannane as a trapping substrate for [^{11}C]methyl Iodide

A general protocol for the rapid *C*-methylation was established for the first time based on a Stille-type reaction using phenyltributylstannane and CH_3I, then [^{11}C]CH_3I, a frequently-used ^{11}C-labeling precursor (Suzuki et al., 1997). The Stille reaction is among the most generally used C-C bond forming reactions in organic synthesis as a reaction of an organometallic (-metaloid) reagent with an organic electrophile (Stille, 1986). The organotin compounds can be prepared by a number of routes even if containing a variety of reactive functional groups. Moreover, the reagent is not particularly oxygen or moisture sensitive. In the palladium(0)-catalyzed coupling of an organic electrophile with an organotin reagent, essentially only one of the groups on the tin atom selectively enters into the coupling reaction, namely an unsymmetrical organotin reagent comprised of three simple alkyl (except methyl) groups, and the fourth group, such as the arenyl, alkenyl, or alkynyl group. The latter fourth group can selectively transfer. The Stille reaction was thought to be useful for our purpose because of its favorable properties of the triorganostannane compounds, such as (1) their high tolerance to various chemical reactions and chromatographic purification conditions, enabling the incorporation of a radioisotope as the final step of the PET-probe synthesis; and (2) the extremely low polarity of a trialkyltin(IV) derivative, enabling an easy separation of the desired product from a large amount of the remaining tin substrate. However, to the best of our knowledge, at that time, there was little information on the Stille reaction using methyl iodide as an sp^3-hybridized carbon partner in comparison to its wide applicability to sp^2-hybridized arenyl or sp^3-hybridized allylic halides; it seemed rather difficult to realize the methylation in high yield due to the unavoidable scrambling between the methyl group in methyl iodide and phenyl groups in the triphenylphosphine ligand, $P(C_6H_5)_3$, by the reaction of methyl iodide with the less reactive phenyltributylstannane in the presence of $Pd\{P(C_6H_5)_3\}_4$ (Morita et al., 1995). The use of the higher reactive phenyltrimethylsytannane as a substrate also induces the competition between $^{11}CH_3$ in $^{11}CH_3I$ and CH_3 groups in the stannane to produce [^{11}C]ethane as a byproduct (Suzuki et al., 1997, also see section 6). Furthermore, the labeled-compound obtained from the trimethyltin derivative resulted in a much lower specific activity than the tributyltin derivative (Samuelsson & Långström, 2003; Madsen et al., 2003). It should be added that tributyltin derivative is practically non-toxic, while the trimethyl- and triethyltins have a significant acute toxicity (Smith, 1998; Buck et al., 2003). Consequently, we have been obliged to devise new reaction conditions capable of promoting a rapid cross-coupling reaction using the less reactive tributyltin derivative as a substrate for trapping [^{11}C]CH_3I.

6. Realization of Pd^0–mediated rapid *C*–methylations by the reaction of methyl iodide with an excess amount of arenyltributylstannanes (rapid coupling between sp^2(arenyl)– and sp^3–hybridized carbons)

Keeping the ^{11}C radiolabeling conditions of a PET-probe synthesis in mind, we set up a model reaction using methyl iodide and an excess amount of phenyltributylstannane (**1**) (CH_3I/**1** = 1:40 in molar ratio) to possibly restrict the reaction time to less than 5 min (Table 1) (Suzuki et al., 1997). The yield of the methylated product, toluene (**2**), was determined on the basis of the CH_3I consumption. As anticipated, the conventional Stille-reaction conditions with a reaction time of 30 min did not give the desired product at all (Table 1, Entry 1), leading us to introduce the concept of coordinative unsaturation to activate the palladium catalyst. Thus, we found that the use of a coordinatively unsaturated Pd^0 complex, $Pd\{P(o\text{-}CH_3C_6H_4)_3\}_2$ (Paul et al., 1995), generated in situ by mixing $Pd_2(dba)_3$ (dba: dibenzylideneacetone) and the sterically bulky tri-*o*-tolylphosphine ($P(o\text{-}CH_3C_6H_4)_3$; cone angle, 194°) (Tolman, 1977) instead of triphenylphosphine ($P(C_6H_5)_3$; cone angle 145°) (Tolman, 1977), significantly increased the coupling efficiency (76%, Table 1, Entry 2). Next, we introduced an additional concept to shorten the reaction time (from 30 min to 5 min); the simple heating (80 °C) was less effective for lowering the yield, but the stabilization of the transiently formed palladium catalyst, strongly solvated by *N,N*-dimethylformamide (DMF), effectively suppressed the decrease in the yield to a considerable extent. Furthermore, we intended to enhance the reactivity by adding a Cu^I salt with the expectation of Sn to Cu transmetallation, and K_2CO_3 in order to react with the $(n\text{-}C_4H_9)_3SnX$ (X = I and/or Cl) generated during the reaction to neutralize the reaction system. Thus, the reaction using the CH_3I/**1**/$Pd_2(dba)_3$/$P(o\text{-}CH_3C_6H_4)_3$/CuCl/K_2CO_3 system (1:40:0.5:2:2:2) in DMF at 60 °C for 5 min gave the desired product in 91% yield (Table 1, Entry 6) (Suzuki et al., 1997). It should be noted that when phenyltrimethylstannane was used instead of phenyltributylstannane, the reaction produced toluene (**2**) in >100% yield (122–129%) together with ethane, indicating the unexpected cross-coupling reactions (scrambling) between the methyl in methyl iodide and the methyl on the tin atom. The reaction between the phenyl and methyl on the tin atom was also contaminated to yield toluene (undesired product in actual PET probe synthesis) to a significant extent (Suzuki et al., 1997), thereby decreasing the yield of the desired [^{11}C]toluene. The specific radioactivity of desired [^{11}C]toluene would also be deduced by the contamination of [^{12}C]toluene formed by the reaction between the methyl

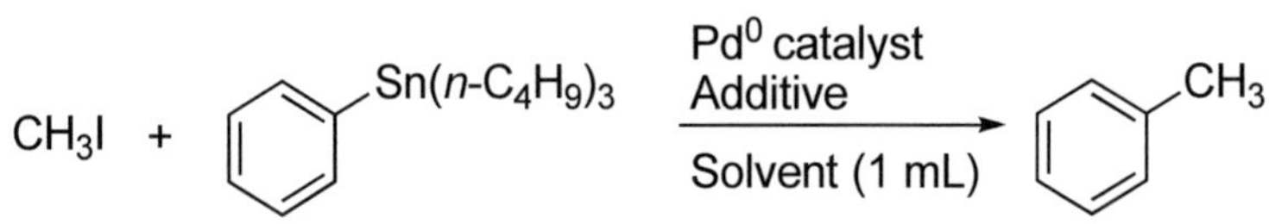

1 2

Entry[a]	Pd^0 comlex (μmol)	Ligand (L) and/or additive (μmol)	Pd^0:L (mol ratio)	Solvent	Temp. (°C)	Time (min)	Yield of **2** (%)[a]
1	$Pd\{P(C_6H_5)_3\}_4$ (10)	–	–	DMSO	40	30	0
2	$Pd_2(dba)_3$ (5)	$P(o\text{-}CH_3C_6H_4)_3$ (20)	1:2	DME	40	30	76
3	$Pd_2(dba)_3$ (5)	$P(o\text{-}CH_3C_6H_4)_3$ (20)	1:2	DME	80	5	41
4	$Pd_2(dba)_3$ (5)	$P(o\text{-}CH_3C_6H_4)_3$ (20)	1:2	DMF	80	5	63
5	$Pd_2(dba)_3$ (5)	$P(o\text{-}CH_3C_6H_4)_3$ (20), CuI (20)	1:2	DMF	60	5	3
6	$Pd_2(dba)_3$ (5)	$P(o\text{-}CH_3C_6H_4)_3$ (20), CuCl (20), K_2CO_3 (20)	1:2	DMF	60	5	91

[a]Reaction was carried out with CH_3I (10 μmol), stannane **1** (400 μmol), and Pd^0 (10 μmol). [b]Yield was determied by GLC analysis based on CH_3I consumption. dba: dibenzylideneacetone; DMSO: dimethyl sulfoxide; DME: 1,2-dimethoxyethane; DMF: *N,N*-dimethylformamide.

Table 1. Rapid cross-coupling of methyl iodide and phenyltributylstannane (**1**).

groups and phenyl groups on the tin atom (Madsen et al., 2003). It was assumed from these results that the reaction of [^{11}C]CH_3I and phenyltrimethylstannane under PET radiolabeling conditions would produce the undesired radioactive and volatile [^{11}C]ethane. As described later (see the section 8.2), these phenomena were observed during the palladium–mediated reaction of 1-(2′-Deoxy-2′-fluoro-β-D-arabinofuranosyl)-5-(trimethylstannyl)uracil to synthesize 1-(2′-Deoxy-2′-fluoro-β-D-arabinofuranosyl)-[methyl-^{11}C]thymidine (Samuelsson & Långström, 2003). Therefore, we concluded that the arenyltributylstannane, though less reactive, would be a much more suitable coupling partner than the arenyltrimethylstannane in view of the increased efficiency of the reaction, relatively low toxicity, and the safety of the radiation exposure.

The conditions of the reaction are significantly different from those of the originally reported Stille coupling reaction. Thus, the coupling of methyl iodide and phenyltributylstannane probably proceeds by the mechanism proposed in Equations 1-5 (Suzuki et al., 1997). In the first step, methyl iodide undergoes oxidative addition with

$$CH_3I + [Pd\{P(o\text{-}CH_3C_6H_4)_3\}_2] \longrightarrow \underset{\mathbf{3}}{[Pd(CH_3)I\{P(o\text{-}CH_3C_6H_4)_3\}]} + P(o\text{-}CH_3C_6H_4)_3 \quad (1)$$

$$\underset{\mathbf{1}}{C_6H_5Sn(n\text{-}C_4H_9)_3} + CuX + P(o\text{-}CH_3C_6H_4)_3 \rightleftharpoons \underset{\mathbf{4}}{[Cu(C_6H_5)\{P(o\text{-}CH_3C_6H_4)_3\}]} + (n\text{-}C_4H_9)_3SnX \quad (2)$$

$$2\,(n\text{-}C_4H_9)_3SnX + K_2CO_3 \longrightarrow \underset{\mathbf{5}}{[(n\text{-}C_4H_9)_3SnO]_2C{=}O} + 2\,KX \quad (3)$$

$$\mathbf{3} + C_6H_5M \longrightarrow \underset{\mathbf{6}}{[Pd(CH_3)(C_6H_5)\{P(o\text{-}CH_3C_6H_4)_3\}]} + MI \quad (4)$$

$$\mathbf{6} \longrightarrow \underset{\text{toluene }(\mathbf{2})}{CH_3\text{-}C_6H_5} + [Pd\{P(o\text{-}CH_3C_6H_4)_3\}] \quad (5)$$

X = Cl or Br; M = $(n\text{-}C_4H_9)_3Sn$ or $Cu\{P(o\text{-}CH_3C_6H_4)_3\}_n$.

a Pd^0 species to generate methyl–Pd^{II} iodide **3** (oxidative addition, Eq. (1)). The Pd^{II} complex **3** may directly react with the phenylstannane **1** to afford the (methyl)(phenyl)Pd^{II} complex **6** (substitution, Eq. (4)); however, the formation of the latter would be facilitated by the phenyl–copper compound **4** formed by the preceding Sn/Cu transmetallation (Eq. (2)). The effect of K_2CO_3 would be explained by the neutralization of $(n\text{-}C_4H_9)_3SnX$ to form the stable bis(tributylstannyl)carbonate **5** (Eq. (3)). At the same time, K_2CO_3 serves to synergically work with a Cu^I salt to promote the Sn/Cu transmetallation (Eqs. (2) and (3)) (Hosoya et al., 2006). Finally, toluene is formed by reductive elimination from the Pd^{II} complex **6** (reductive elimination, Eq. (5)). The significant ligand effect of tri-*o*-tolylphosphine is attributed to its considerable bulkiness (cone angle = 194°, which is greater than that in tri-*tert*-butylphosphine (182°)) (Tolman, 1997), which facilitates the generation of the coordinatively unsaturated Pd^0 and Pd^{II} intermediates (Louie & Hartwig, 1995). Transmetallation to give **6** and/or the reductive elimination of toluene requires the formation of the tricoordinate Pd^{II} complex. DMF may stabilize such Pd intermediates even at high temperatures. It should be noted that J. K. Stille *et al.* previously reported the reaction of methyl iodide and *p*-methoxyphenyltributylstannane in the presence of $Pd\{P(C_6H_5)_3\}_4$ at 50 °C for 24 h, in which the scrambling reaction between the methyl and the phenyl groups in the methyl iodide and triphenylphosphines, respectively, preferably occurred to give the desired *p*-methoxytoluene in only 3% together with 1-methoxy-4-phenylbenzene as the major byproduct in 8% yield, suggesting that the promotion of the Stille reaction using methyl iodide as an sp^3–carbon partner could be difficult (Morita et al., 1995) until our successful result was demonstrated (Suzuki et al., 1997).

7. Application for the synthesis of 15*R*-[^{11}C]TIC methyl ester as specific probe for prostaglandin receptor (IP_2) in the central nervous system

In a preceding study of prostaglangin (PG), we succeeded in developing (15*R*)-16-*m*-tolyl-17,18,19,20-tetranorisocarbacyclin (15*R*-TIC, **7**), which was selectively responsive to a novel prostacyclin receptor (IP_2) in the central nervous system (Suzuki et al., 1996; Suzuki et al., 2000b). The tolyl group in **7** was intended as a trigger component to create a PET molecular probe. Therefore, we planned to apply the rapid C–methylation conditions to the synthesis of a PET molecular probe, the 15*R*-[^{11}C]TIC methyl ester using [^{11}C]CH_3I, prepared from [^{11}C]CO_2 according to an established method (Fowler & Wolf, 1997), and the stannane **8** (Suzuki et al., 2000a). However, we found that the C–[^{11}C]methylation under radiolabeling conditions, even after using an excess amount of a Cu^I salt, lacked reproducibility for some unknown reasons. During the course to overcome this difficulty along with the actual PET–probe synthesis, we encountered some valuable information that led to a solution of the problem by using CuI instead of CuCl that severely retarded the methylation of the phenyltributylstannane (Table 1, Entry 5). In order to minimize this inhibitory effect of CuI, we changed the one–pot operation to a two–pot stepwise procedure during the actual PET–probe synthesis (Figure 3) (Suzuki et al., 2004). This procedure consists of independent syntheses of a methylpalladium complex and a phenyl copper complex at room temperature (25 °C), and then the mixing of these species in one portion at a higher temperature (65 °C, 5 min). As expected, the highly qualified PET probe, the 15*R*-TIC methyl ester ([^{11}C]**9**), was obtained by thus C–[^{11}C]methylation procedure from **8** in an 85% isolated yield (decay-corrected, based on the radioactivity of [^{11}C]CH_3I trapped in the Pd solution; it indicates the production efficiency) with a purity of greater than 98%, which was applicable for a human PET study with a sufficient radioactivity of 2–3 GBq and high reproducibility (Figure 3). The specific radioactivity was 37–100 GBq μmol^{-1}. The total synthesis time was 35–40 min.

After the ethical committee gave its official approval for a human PET study, the principal author, M. Suzuki, was nominated to be the first volunteer. Thus, the 15*R*-[^{11}C]TIC methyl ester ([^{11}C]**9**) was injected into his right arm and it passed through the blood–brain barrier. It was then hydrolyzed in the brain to a free carboxylic acid, which was eventually bound to the IP_2 receptor. PET images of horizontal slices indicated that a new receptor, IP_2, was distributed throughout various structures in the human brain (Figure 4) (Suzuki et al., 2004). A PET study of the middle cerebral artery occlusion using a monkey model demonstrated that 15*R*-TIC revealed a potent neuroprotective effect against focal cerebral ischemia as judged by the [^{15}O]O_2 consumption and the uptake of [^{18}F]FDG (Cui et al., 2006). Recently, rat PET studies using the 15*R*-[^{11}C]TIC methyl ester ([^{11}C]**9**) showed that [^{11}C]**9** could be useful for the *in vivo* analyses of the mrp2–mediated hepatobiliary transport (Takashima et al., 2010). Furthermore, the PK/PD studies of [^{11}C]**9** in humans (submitted for publication) as well as a translational study of Alzheimer's disease patients to evaluate the progress of such neurodegenerative diseases are now in progress. A PET probe of the 17-(3-[^{11}C]methylphenyl)-18,19,20-trinor-prostaglandin $F_{2\alpha}$ isopropyl ester ([^{11}C]**10**) (Björkman et al., 2000) targeting the receptor of prostaglandin $F_{2\alpha}$ ($PGF_{2\alpha}$) was also synthesized using a procedure similar to [^{11}C]**9**.

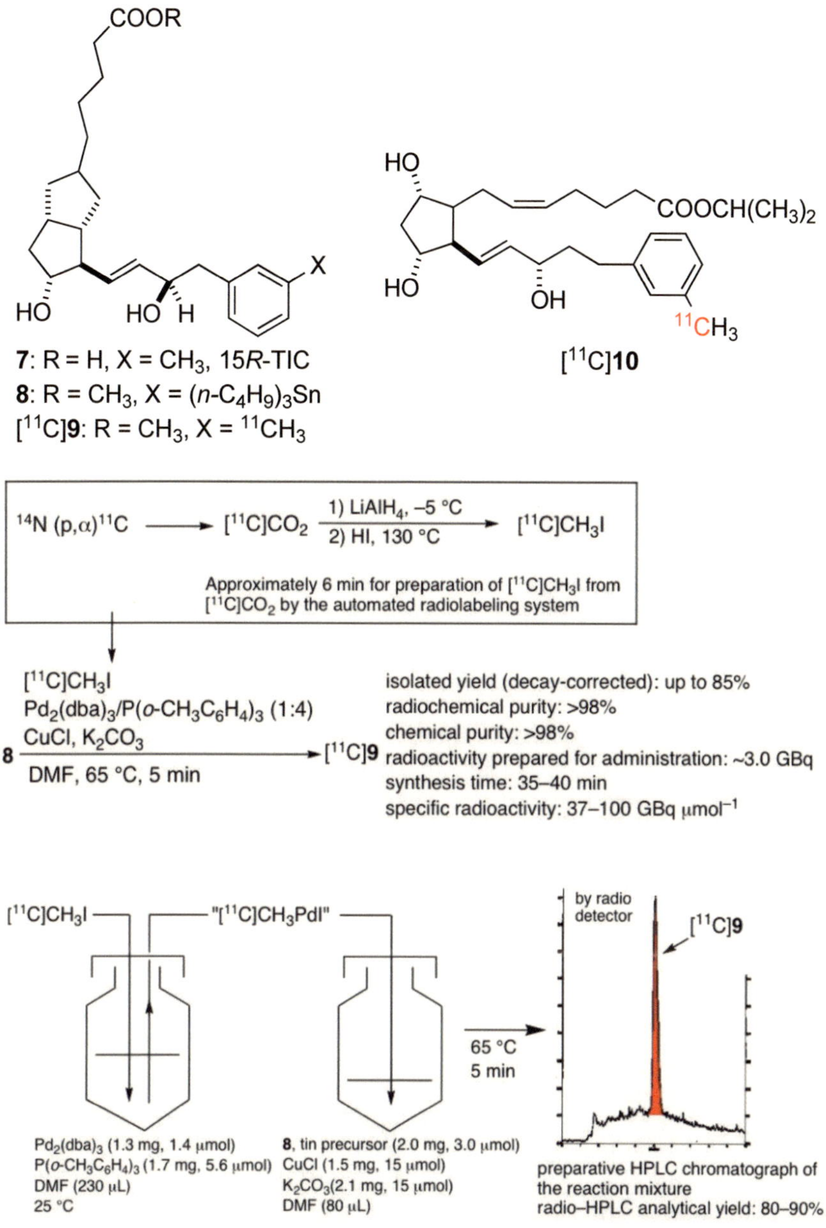

[11C]CH3I, formed from [11C]CO2 according to the established method, was trapped in a solution of $Pd_2(dba)_3$ (1.3 mg, 1.4 μmol) and $P(o\text{-}CH_3C_6H_4)_3$ (1.7 mg, 5.6 μmol) in DMF (230 μL) at room temperature. The solution was transferred to a vial containing stannyl precursor **8** (2.0 mg, 3.0 μmol), CuCl (1.5 mg, 15μmol), and K_2CO_3 (2.1 mg, 15 μmol) in DMF (80 μL), and the resulting mixture was heated at 65 °C for 5 min. Prior to the preparative HPLC, a solid phase extraction column was used to remove the salts and palladium residue from the reaction mixture. The desired product, 15*R*-[11C]TIC methyl ester [11C]**9**, after HPLC separation and intravenous formulation usually had a isolated radioactivity of approximately 2.5 GBq, sufficient for an *in vivo* human PET study.

Fig. 3. Synthesis of 15*R*–[11C]TIC methyl ester ([11C]**9**) under PET radiolabeling conditions.

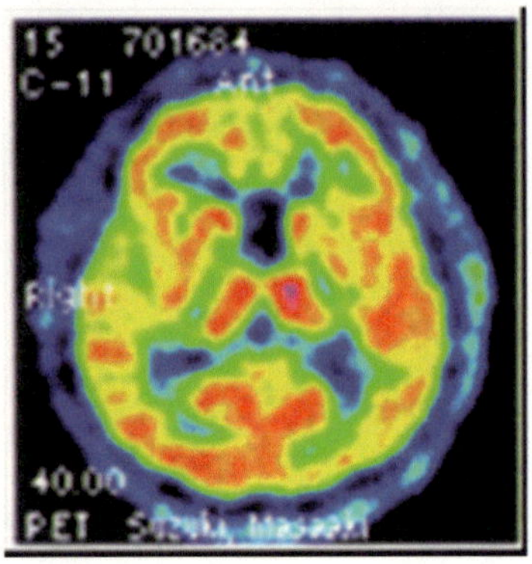

Fig. 4. PET imaging in human brain using [^{11}C]**9**.

8. Rapid *C*–[^{11}C]methylation of heteroaromatic compounds: importance of using a large amount of bulky arenylphosphine, Cu^I/F^- or Cu^I/K_2CO_3 synergic effect, and the selection of an amide solvent

8.1 Pd^0–mediated rapid coupling of methyl iodide and heteroarenylstannanes applicable to 2- and 3-[^{11}C]methylpyridines

There is a strong demand for the incorporation of a short-lived ^{11}C-labeled methyl group into the heteroaromatic carbon frameworks, because such structures often appear in major drugs and their promising candidates. The Pd^0–mediated rapid trapping of methyl iodide with an excess amount of a hetero-aromatic ring-substituted tributylstannane **11a–i** was done (Suzuki et al., 2009) by first using our previously developed CH_3I/**11a–i**/$Pd_2(dba)_3$/$P(o\text{-}CH_3C_6H_4)_3$/CuCl/K_2CO_3 (1:40:0.5:2:2:2) combination system in DMF at 60 °C for 5 min (conditions A; Suzuki et al., 1997), but the reaction produced low yields of the various kinds of heteroaromatic compounds (Table 2, Entries 1-9). An increase in the phosphine ligand (conditions B) significantly improved the yield for the heteroarenyl stannanes, **11b**, **11c**, and **11i**, but the conditions were still insufficient in terms of the range of adaptable heteroaromatic structures. Another CuBr/CsF combination system (conditions C) also provided a result similar to conditions B using an increased amount of the phosphine. Thus, pyridine and the related heteroaromatic compounds still remained as less reactive substrates. Consequently, the problem was overcome by replacing the DMF solvent with *N*-methyl-2-pyrolidinone (NMP). It is of interest that such a solvent effect was not observed for the CuCl/K_2CO_3 combination system, but appeared for the CuBr/CsF reaction system (Table 3, Entry 2), giving 2-methylpyridine (2-picoline, **12d**) in 81% yield. The other solvents, except for the amide-type solvent and amine additives, were not effective (Table 3, Entries 4–11). Thus, the reaction in NMP at 60–100°C for 5 min using the CH_3I/**11a–i**/$Pd_2(dba)_3$/$P(o\text{-}CH_3C_6H_4)_3$/CuBr/CsF (1:40:0.5:16:2:5) combination (conditions D) gave the methylated products **12a–i** in >80% yields (based on the reaction of CH_3I) for all of the heteroaromatic compounds listed in this study (Table 2, Entries 1–9). Thus the combined use of NMP and increased amount of the bulky arenylphosphine is important to efficiently promote the reaction. The conditions using a $Pd\{P(\textit{tert}\text{-}C_4H_9)_3\}_2$/CsF system in NMP reported by G. C. Fu *et al.* (Littke et al., 2002) were not effective by producing only a poor yield (21%, Table 3, Entry 2) as judged by the methylation of 2-pyridyltributylstannane (**11d**). The addition of CuBr to this system improved the yield to only a small extent (39%).

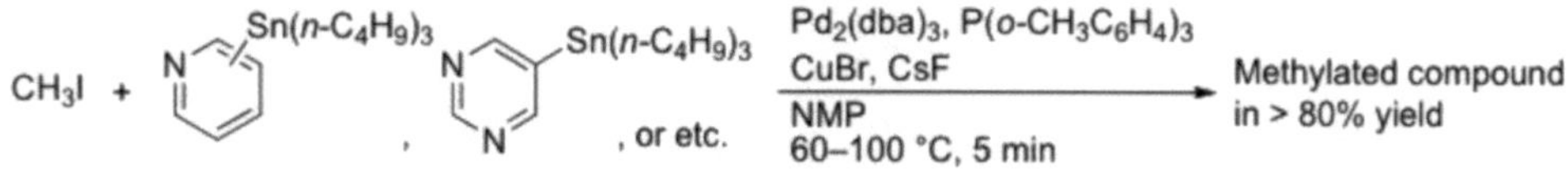

Entry[a]	Heteroarenyl stannane	Methylated product	Yield (%)[b]			
			A[c]	B[c]	C[c]	D[c]
1	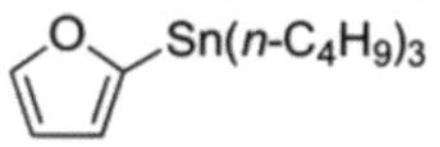 **11a**	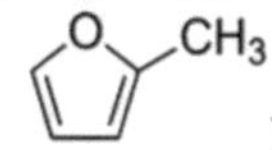 **12a**	28	75	73	80
2	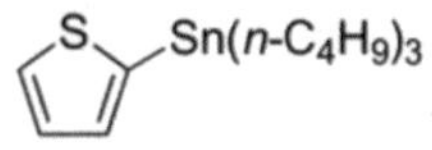 **11b**	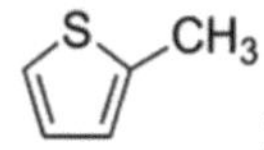 **12b**	57	87	91	94
3	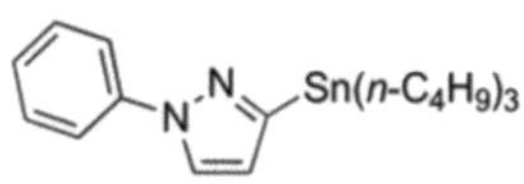 **11c**	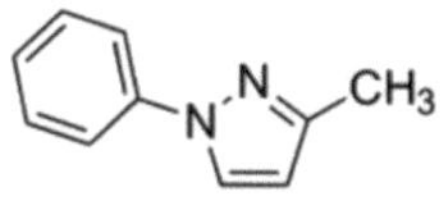 **12c**	52	88	90	94
4	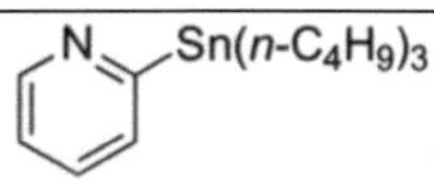 **11d**	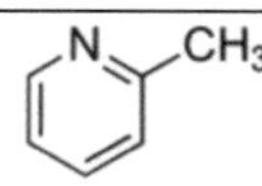 **12d**	16 (14)[d]	67	63	81
5	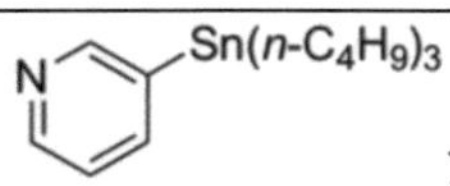 **11e**	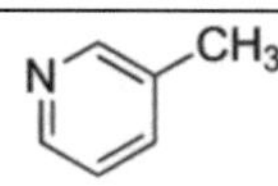 **12e**	25 (53)[e]	61	66	80
6	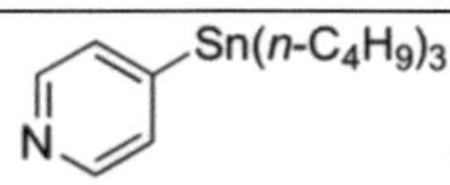 **11f**	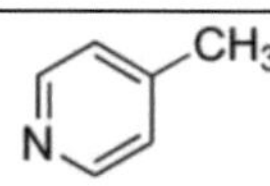 **12f**	79	60	68	87
7	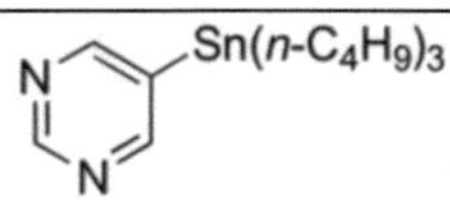 **11g**	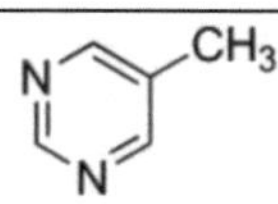 **12g**	3	50	48	62 (87)[f]
8	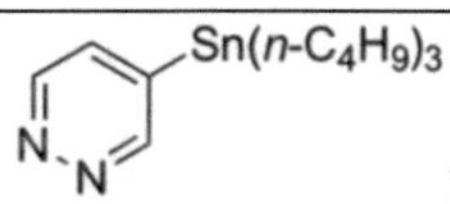 **11h**	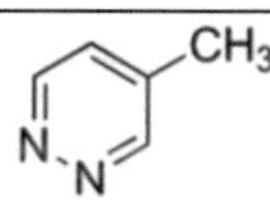 **12h**	25	72	70	90
9	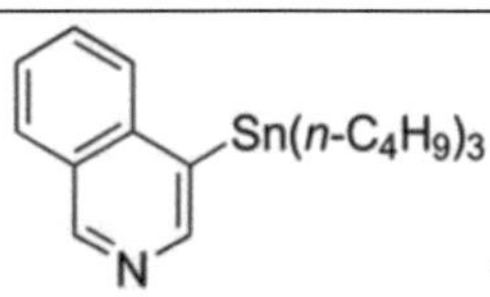 **11i**	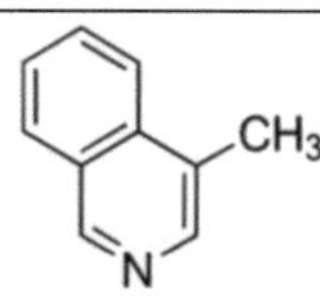 **12i**	12	83	75	83

[a]Reaction was carried out with CH_3I (10 μmol), stannane **11** (400 μmol), and Pd^0 (10 μmol). [b]The products were identified by GLC analyses and comparison with authentic samples. Yields were determined by GLC based on CH_3I consumption using *n*-nonane and *n*-heptane as internal standards, and are the average of 2 or 3 runs. [c]Reaction conditions (molar ratio): A: CH_3I/**11**/$Pd_2(dba)_3$/P(*o*-$CH_3C_6H_4)_3$/CuCl/K_2CO_3 (1:40:0.5:2:2:2) in DMF at 60 °C for 5 min; B: CH_3I/**11**/$Pd_2(dba)_3$/P(*o*-$CH_3C_6H_4)_3$/CuCl/K_2CO_3 (1:40:0.5:16:2:5) in DMF at 60°C for 5 min; C: CH_3I/**11**/$Pd_2(dba)_3$/P(*o*-$CH_3C_6H_4)_3$/CuBr/CsF (1:40:0.5:16:2:5) in DMF at 60 °C for 5 min; D: CH_3I/**11**/$Pd_2(dba)_3$/P(*o*-$CH_3C_6H_4)_3$/CuBr/CsF (1:40:0.5:16:2:5) in NMP at 60 °C for 5 min. [d]CH_3I/**11d**/$Pd_2(dba)_3$/P(*o*-$CH_3C_6H_4)_3$ (1:40:0.5:2) in DMF at 120 °C for 5 min (stepwise procedure) (Iida et al, 2004). [e]CH_3I/**11e**/$Pd_2(dba)_3$/P(*o*-$CH_3C_6H_4)_3$/CuCl/K_2CO_3 (1:40:0.5:2:2:2) in DMF at 80 °C for 3 min (Prabhakaran et al, 2005). [f]The reaction was conducted at 100 °C.

Table 2. General rapid *C*–methylation on various neutral and basic heteroaromatic rings.

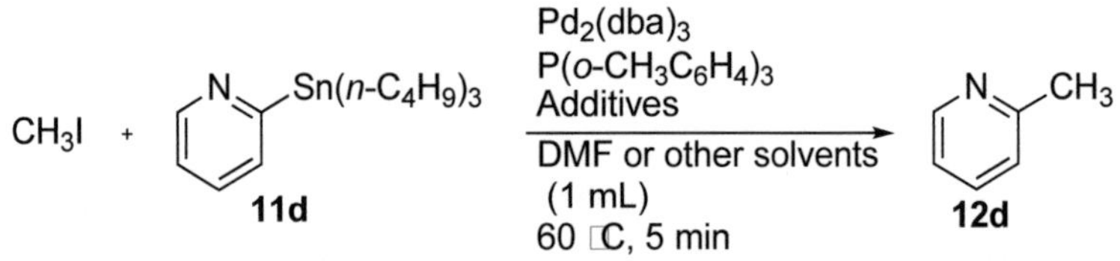

Entry[a]	Solvent	Additive (equiv)	Yield (%)[b]	
			CuCl/K_2CO_3 synergic system	CuBr/CsF synergic system
1	DMF	–	67	65
2	NMP	–	66	81 (21)[c] (39)[d]
3	DMA	–	–	69
4	DMI	–	–	18
5	toluene	–	–	20
6	THF	–	–	38
7	DMSO	–	–	23
8	HMPA	–	–	34
9	DMF	2,6-lutidine (17)	–	19
10	DMF	Triethylamine (14)	–	20
11	DMF	DABCO (18)	–	6

[a]Reaction was carried out with CH_3I (10 μmol), stannane **11d** (400 μmol), and Pd^0 (10 μmol). Reaction conditions (molar ratio): CH_3I/**11d**/$Pd_2(dba)_3$/$P(o\text{-}CH_3C_6H_4)_3$/CuCl/K_2CO_3 (1:40:0.5:16:2:2) or CH_3I/**11d**/$Pd_2(dba)_3$/$P(o\text{-}CH_3C_6H_4)_3$/CuBr/CsF (1:40:0.5:16:2:5) at 60°C for 5 min. [b]Yield (%) of **12d** was determined by GLC analyses based on CH_3I consumption using *n*-heptane as the internal standard. [c]Fu's original conditions (Littke et al., 2002) (molar ratio): CH_3I/**11d**/Pd{P(*tert*-$C_4H_9)_3\}_2$/CsF (1:40:1:2). [d]Fu's original conditions + CuBr (molar ratio): CH_3I/**11d**/Pd{P(*tert*-$C_4H_9)_3\}_2$/CuBr/CsF (1:40:1:2:5). NMP: *N*-methyl-2-pyrrolidinone; DMA: *N,N*-dimethylacetamide; DMI: 1,3-dimethylimidazolidin-2-one; THF: tetrahydrofuran; HMPA: hexamethylphosphoric triamide; DABCO: 1,4-diazabicyclo[2.2.2]octane.

Table 3. Effect of a solvent and additives in increased phosphine and synergic systems on the rapid trapping of methyl iodide with 2-pyridyltributylstannane (**11d**) to give 2-methylpyridine (**12d**).

The utility of the general rapid methylation was well demonstrated by the syntheses of the actual PET tracers, the 2- and 3-[^{11}C]methylpyridines ([^{11}C]**12d** and **e**), using $Pd_2(dba)_3$/$P(o\text{-}CH_3C_6H_4)_3$/CuBr/CsF (1:16:2:5) in NMP at 60°C for 5 min, giving the desired products in 88 and 91% radio-HPLC analytical yields (definition: (radioactivity of desired product on HPLC)/(total radioactivity of distributed materials on HPLC) x 100%; it means reaction efficiency), respectively (Figure 5) (Suzuki et al., 2009).

(*S*)-(+)-2-Methyl-1-[(4-methyl-5-isoquinolinyl)sulfonyl]homopiperazine (H-1152, or referred to as H-1152P, **13**) is known as the most potent, specific, and membrane-permeable inhibitor of small G protein Rho-associated kinase (Rho-kinase). A ^{11}C-labeled H-1152 as a novel PET probe for imaging Rho-kinases was efficiently synthesized for the first time based on the Pd^0-mediated rapid *C*-[^{11}C]methylation for trifluoroacetyl (TFA)-protected heteroarenylstannane precursor using [^{11}C]CH_3I followed by rapid deprotection of the TFA group (Suzuki et al., 2011a). Thus, the *C*-[^{11}C]methylation on the isoquinoline derivative was performed using $Pd_2(dba)_3$/P(o-$CH_3C_6H_4)_3$/CuBr/CsF (1:16:2:5 in molar ratio) in NMP at 80 °C for 5 min and the deprotection of TFA proceeded using 2 M NaOH at 25–50 °C for 1 min, giving [^{11}C]H-1152 ([^{11}C]**13**) with 86 ± 4% (n = 3) radio-HPLC analytical yield. The isolated total radioactivity was 3.8 ± 1.2 GBq (n = 3) with the radiochemical yield of 63 ± 14% (n = 3) (decay-corrected, based on [^{11}C]CH_3I). Both chemical and radiochemical purities were >99%. The total synthesis time was 38 min. The specific radioactivity at the end of the formation was 97 ± 10 GBq μmol^{-1} (n = 3). The use of [^{11}C]**13** for molecular imaging studies of cardiovascular diseases is now in progress.

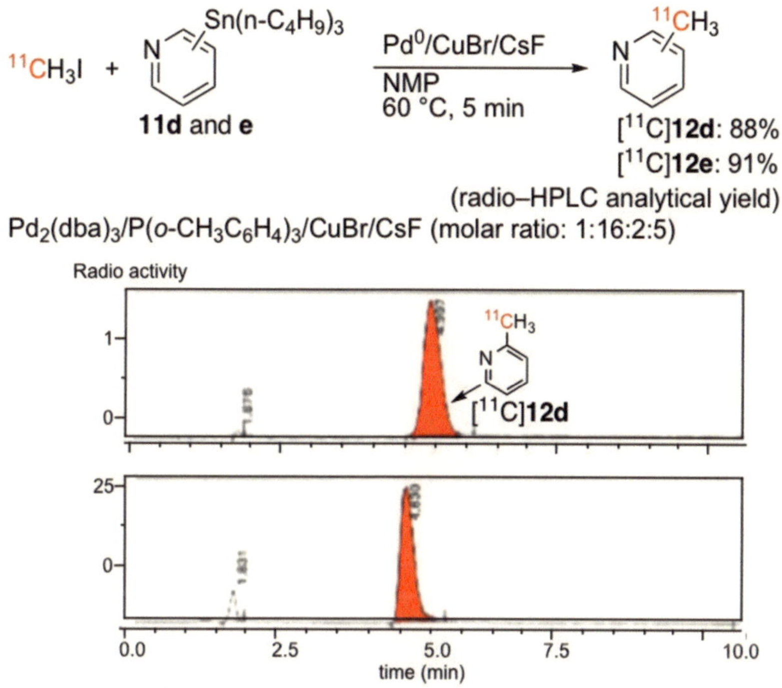

Red carbon in the structure means a radionuclide.

Fig. 5. Syntheses of 2- and 3-[^{11}C]methylpyridines ([^{11}C]**12d, e**).

8.2 Efficient syntheses of [methyl–^{11}C]thymidine and 4'-[methyl–^{11}C]thiothymidine

[^{18}F]FLT has been developed as a more specific tumor imaging agent than [^{18}F]FDG (Grierson et al., 1997, as cited in Bading & Shields, 2008). This pyrimidine analogue lacking a hydroxy group at C-3′ is phosphorylated by thymidine kinase 1 (TK_1) and trapped in cancer cell. The TK_1 activity increases almost 10-fold during the DNA synthesis, and thus, the imaging reflects the cell proliferation differentiating tumor from inflammation (Lee et al., 2009). The first human imaging study was conducted with 1-(2′-deoxy-2′-[^{18}F]fluoro-1-β-D-arabinofuranosyl)thymine ([^{18}F]FMAU) (Sun et al., 2005, as cited in Bading & Shields, 2008), showing that the tumors in the brain, prostate, thorax, and bone could be clearly visualized. However, there is the primary limitation in the use of [^{11}C]- or [^{18}F]FMAU which is being a relatively poor substrate for TK_1 and a relatively good substrate for TK_2, probably accounting for its localization in the mitochondrion–rich human myocardium. On the other hand, 4′-thiothymine (**15b**), which resembles the biological properties of thymidine (**15a**) with a higher stability for the phosphorylase cleavage, underwent the $^{11}CH_3$–labeling for the tumor imaging using a rat, exhibited a higher potential as an attractive PET probe than [^{18}F]FLT (Toyohara et al., 2008). Although the PET imaging studies using various kinds of ^{11}C- and ^{18}F–labeled thymidne analogues have been extensively continued, it is still difficult to synthesize the labeled compounds.

Thus, we applied the rapid C–[^{11}C]methylation of a heteroarenylstannane (see the section 8.1) to the synthesis of the ^{11}C–labeled thymidine and its thio–analogue (Koyama et al., 2011). 1-(2′-Deoxy-2′-fluoro-β-D-arabinofuranosyl)-[methyl–^{11}C]thymine ([^{11}C]FMAU) and 4′-[methyl–^{11}C]thiothymine ([^{11}C]**15b**) have so far been labeled by ^{11}C using 5-trimethyl and/or tributylstannyl precursors via the Stille–type cross–coupling reaction with [^{11}C]methyl iodide (Samuelsson & Långström, 2003; Toyohara et al., 2008). However, as anticipated, the previously reported conditions had fewer effects on the syntheses of 5-tributylstannyl-2′-deoxyuridine (**14a**) and -4′-thio-2′-deoxyuridine (**14b**) using $Pd_2(dba)_3/P(o\text{-}CH_3C_6H_4)_3$ (1:4 in molar ratio) at 130 °C for 5 min in DMF, giving the desired products **15a** and **b** in only 32 and 30% yields, respectively (Table 4, Entries 1 and 4). Therefore, we tried to adapt the current reaction conditions, including the synergic systems developed in our laboratory, for such heteroaromatic compounds. First, the reaction using CH_3I/**14a**/$Pd_2(dba)_3/P(o\text{-}CH_3C_6H_4)_3/CuCl/K_2CO_3$ (1:25:1:32:2:5) at 80 °C gave thymidine (**15a**) in 85% yield (Entry 2). Whereas, CH_3I/**14a**/$Pd_2(dba)_3/P(o\text{-}CH_3C_6H_4)_3$/CuBr/CsF (1:25:1:32:2:5) including another CuBr/CsF system promoted the reaction at a milder temperature (60 °C), giving **15a** in quantitative yield (Entry 3). The chemo–response of the thiothymidine–precursor **14b** was different from the thymidine system **14a**. The optimized conditions obtained for **14a** including the CuBr/CsF system gave 4′-thiothymidine (**15b**) in only 40% yield (Table 4, Entry 5). The reaction using 5–fold amounts of CuBr/CsF at 80 °C gave **15b** in a much higher yield (83%, Entry 6), but unexpectedly, the reaction was accompanied by a large amount of an undesired destannylated product. It was considered that the destannylated product **17** would have been produced by proton transfer to the transmetallated Cu intermediate **16** from $\mathbf{14b}_{\mathbf{Cu2}}$ with the enhanced acidity by Cu^{I} coordination of a sulfur atom in the thiothymidine structure (Figure 6). As expected, such a destannylation was significantly suppressed by changing the medium to a much more basic system, in which the stannyl substrate **14b** would be changed to the deprotonated **18**. Thus, the conditions CH_3I/**14b**/$Pd_2(dba)_3/P(o\text{-}CH_3C_6H_4)_3/CuCl/K_2CO_3$ (1:25:1:32:2:5) at 80 °C gave **15b** in nearly quantitative yield (98%, Table 4, Entry 7).

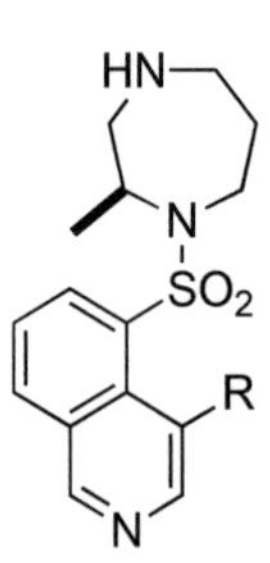

13: R = CH_3, H-1152
[^{11}C]**13**: R = [^{11}C]CH_3, [^{11}C]H-1152

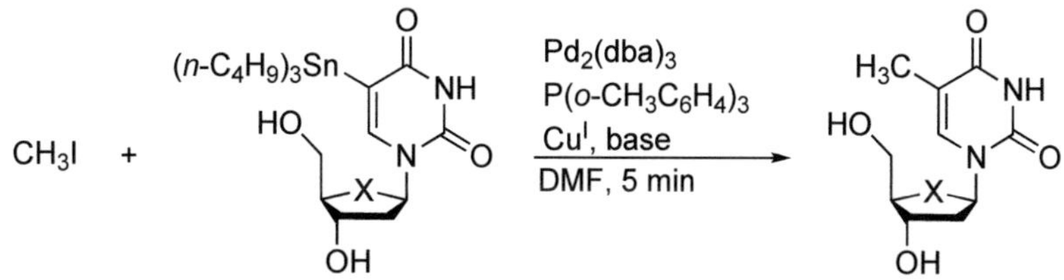

14a: X = O
14b: X = S

15a: X = O
15b: X = S

Entry[a]	X	$P(o\text{-}CH_3C_6H_4)_3$ (equiv)	Cu^I, base (mol ratio)	Yield (%)[b] Temp. (°C)			
				60	80	100	130
1[c]	O	4	none	0	–	–	32
2	O	32	CuCl, K_2CO_3 (2:5)	67	85	–	–
3	O	32	CuBr, CsF (2:5)	100	–	97	–
4	S	4	none	–	–	–	30
5	S	32	CuBr, CsF (2:5)	40	–	–	–
6	S	32	CuBr, CsF (10:25)	64	83	–	–
7	S	32	CuCl, K_2CO_3 (2:5)	83	98	–	–

[a]X = O: reaction was carried out with CH_3I (2.0 μmol), stannane **14a** (50 μmol) and Pd^0 (4.0 μmol). X = S: reaction was carried out with CH_3I (1.0 μmol), stannane **14b** (25 μmol) and Pd^0 (2.0 μmol). [b]The yield was determined by GLC based on CH_3I consumption using acridine as the internal standard. [c]Reaction was carried out with 5 equiv. of **14a** relative to methyl iodide.

Table 4. Synthesis of thymidine (**15a**) and 4′-thiothymidine (**15b**) by the rapid trapping of methyl iodide with 5-tributylstannyl-2′-deoxyuridine (**14a**) and 5-tributylstannyl-4′-thio-2′-deoxyuridine (**14b**).

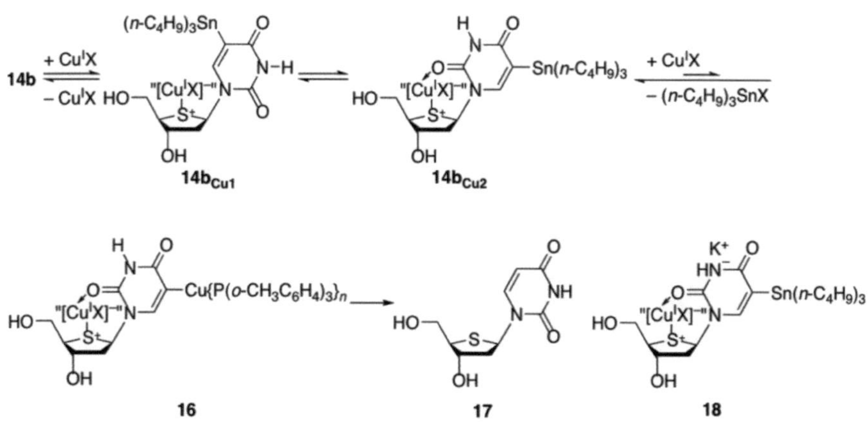

Fig. 6. Assumed equilibration formed in the presence of a Cu^I salt.

Each optimized condition obtained for **14a** and **b** was successfully used for the syntheses of the corresponding PET probes with 87 and 93% radio-HPLC analytical yields (Figure 7) (Koyama et al., 2011). The [^{11}C]compounds were isolated by preparative HPLC after the reaction was conducted under slightly improved conditions using a half-amount of phosphine (16 equiv) to give 45 and 42–59% isolated yields (decay-corrected, based on the radioactivity of $[^{11}C]CH_3I$ trapped in the Pd solution). The total synthesis time was 42 min in each case until the radiopharmaceutical formulation, exhibiting the isolated radioactivity of 3.7–3.8 GBq and the specific radioactivity of 89–200 GBq μmol^{-1} with both a chemical purity of ≥98% and radiochemical purity of ≥99.5% sufficient for both of animal and human PET studies (Koyama et al., 2011). We are currently in the process of applying these synthetic procedures to the PET probe syntheses according to the Guideline of Good Manufacturing Practice (GMP).

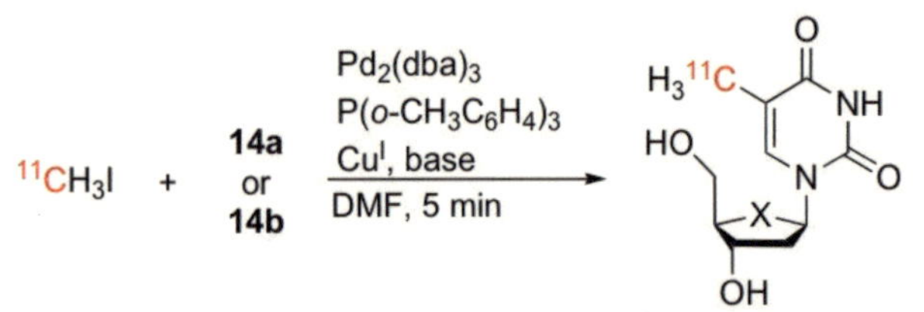

$[^{11}C]$**15a**: X = O: 87%
$[^{11}C]$**15b**: X = S: 93%
(radio–HPLC analytical yield)

X = O: $Pd_2(dba)_3/P(o\text{-}CH_3C_6H_4)_3/CuBr/CsF$ (1:32:2:5)
X = S: $Pd_2(dba)_3/P(o\text{-}CH_3C_6H_4)_3/CuCl/K_2CO_3$ (1:32:2:5)

(A)

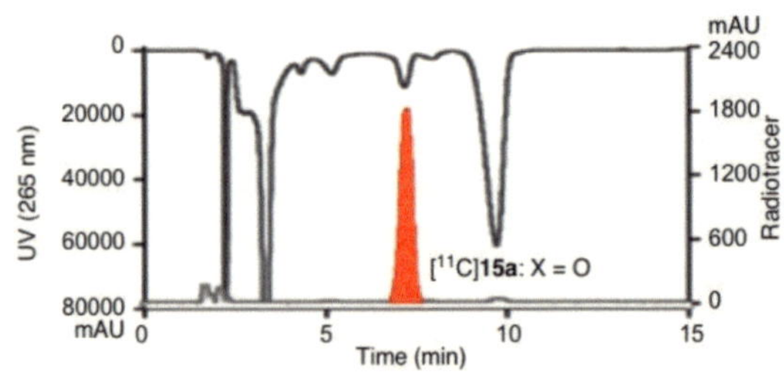

(B)

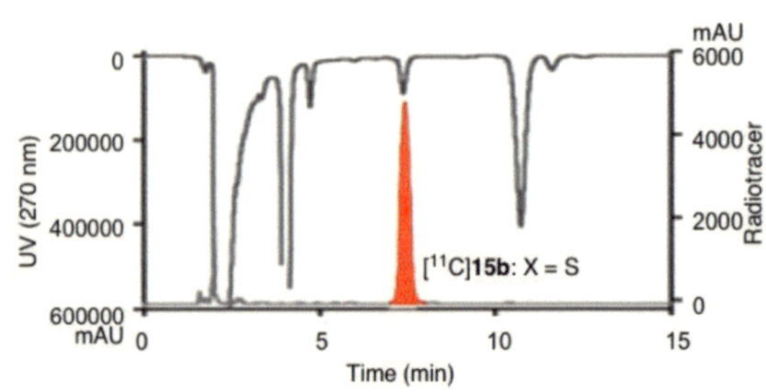

(C)

Fig. 7. Synthetic scheme of [methyl–^{11}C]thymidine ($[^{11}C]$**15a**) and 4'-[methyl–^{11}C]thiothymidine ($[^{11}C]$**15b**) for a PET study (A), and the HPLC chart for the analysis of $[^{11}C]$**15a**, **b** (B and C, respectively, radioactivity and UV vs. time). The peaks at the retention times of 7.6 and 7.4 min labeled B and C are $[^{11}C]$**15a** and **b**, respectively. For the HPLC chart after the isolation of $[^{11}C]$**15a** and **b**, see supporting information in the ref. Koyama et al., 2011.

9. Rapid *C*–[^{11}C]methylation of alkenes: Rapid *C*–methylation of alkenes (rapid coupling between sp^2(alkenyl)–sp^3 hybridized carbons)

The rapid *C*-[^{11}C]methylation of stannyl alkene structures provides methylalkene structures, which are frequently observed in various biologically significant compounds such as retinoids, vitamin K_2, squalene, and other isoprenoids, which are important for cancer chemotherapy. In the process of optimizing the rapid *C*-methylation conditions using twelve types of non-functional and functional 1-alkenyltributylstannanes as model compounds **19a–l** (él), we developed four types of reaction conditions, A–D, that proceeded in DMF at 60 °C for 5 min (Table 5) (Hosoya et al., 2006). Among these, reaction conditions B: CH_3I/**19a–l**/$Pd_2(dba)_3$/$P(o\text{-}CH_3C_6H_4)_3$/CuX (X = Br or Cl)/K_2CO_3 (molar ratio, 1:40:0.5:4:2:5) worked well on various alkenyl stannanes rather than the previously developed conditions A: CH_3I/**19a–l**/$Pd_2(dba)_3$/$P(o\text{-}CH_3C_6H_4)_3$/CuCl/K_2CO_3 (molar ratio, 1:40:0.5:2:2:2). In addition, conditions D consisting of CH_3I/**19a–l**/$Pd_2(dba)_3$/$P(o\text{-}CH_3C_6H_4)_3$/CuX (X = Br, Cl, or I)/CsF (molar ratio, 1:40:0.5:2:2:5) showed the best results from the viewpoint of general applicability, affording the corresponding methylated compounds **20a–l** in 90% or greater yields (for the consumption of methyl iodide) (Hosoya et al., 2006). The high efficiency of the reaction is presumably due to the synergic effect of the Cu^I salt and the fluoride anion to promote the Sn to Cu transmetallation and the formation of coordinatively unsaturated Pd complexes formed by a bulky arenylphosphine. Under conditions C using $P(tert\text{-}C_4H_9)_2(CH_3)$, the yield was lower than that for conditions D using $P(o\text{-}CH_3C_6H_4)_3$, particularly against α,β-unsaturated carbonyl substrates (alkenyltributylstannanes **19i–l** in Table 5, Entries 9–12). In this context, the reactions using the Pd^0 complex, $\{(\pi\text{-allyl})PdCl\}_2/3P(tert\text{-}C_4H_9)_2(CH_3)$, $(CH_3)_4NF$, 3-Å molecular sieves (Menzel & Fu, 2003), $PdCl_2/2P(tert\text{-}C_4H_9)_3$, CuI, and CsF (Mee et al., 2004) gave the desired compound in only the same 2% yields, as judged by the reaction of 1-cyclohexenyltributylstannane (**19e**). Furthermore, the stereo isomerization of a double bond under our conditions did not occur at all under these reaction conditions.

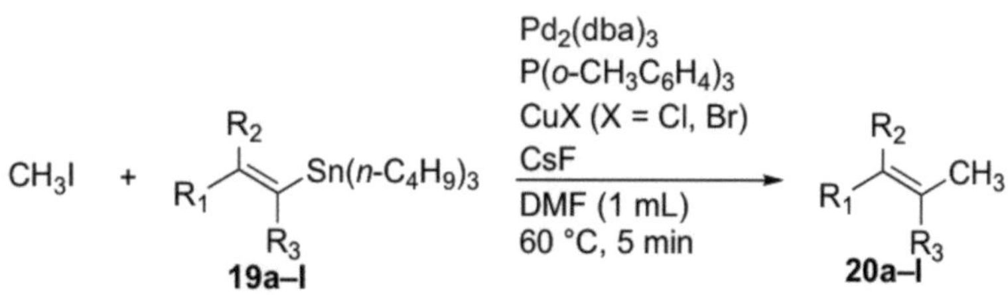

Entry^a	1-Alkenyltributylstannane **19**	Yield of **20**^{b}	Entry^a	1-Alkenyltributylstannane **19**	Yield of **20**^{b}
1	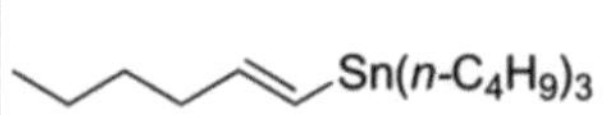 **19a**	98	7	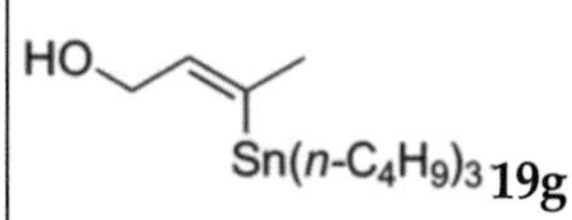 **19g**	99
2	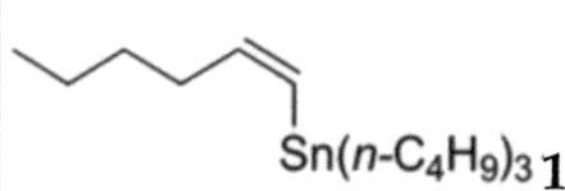 **19b**	99	8	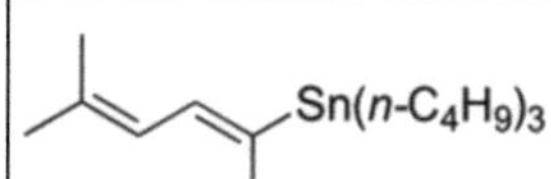 **19h**	89 (91)^c

Entry[a]	1-Alkenyltributylstannane **19**	Yield of **20**[b]	Entry[a]	1-Alkenyltributylstannane **19**	Yield of **20**[b]
3	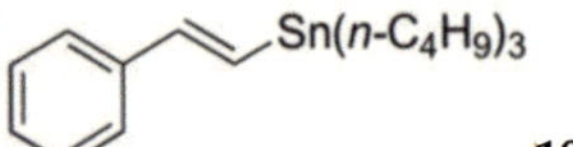 **19c**	83 (88)[c]	9	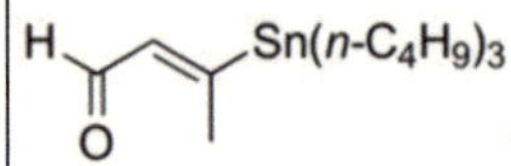 **19i**	85 (96)[c]
4	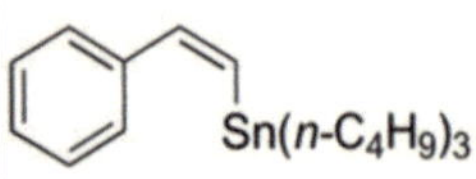 **19d**	84 (89)[c]	10	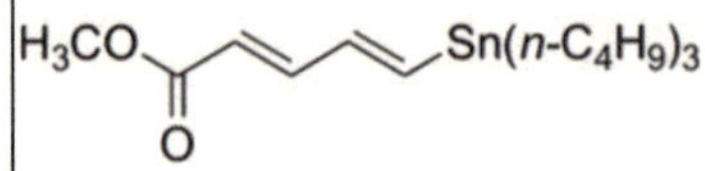 **19j**	86 (93)[c]
5	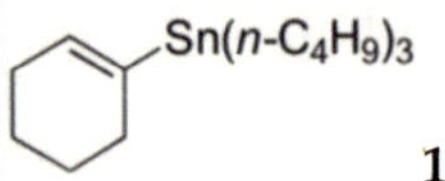 **19e**	99	11	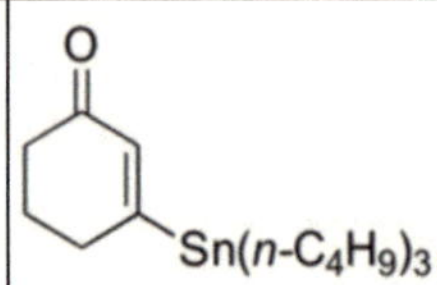 **19k**	95
6	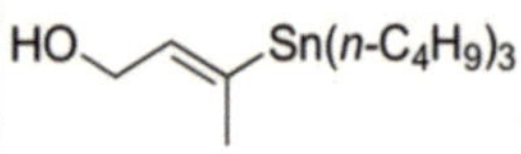 **19f**	99	12[d]	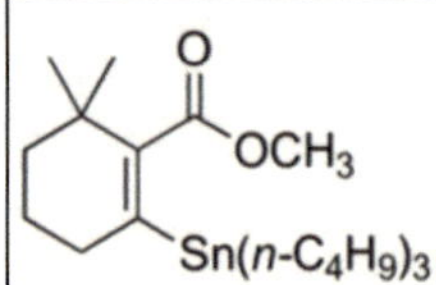 **19l**	84 (91)[c]

[a]Reactions were carried out under conditions D using CH_3I (10 μmol), stannane **19a–l** (400 μmol), $Pd_2(dba)_3$ (5 μmol), $P(o\text{-}CH_3C_6H_4)_3$ (20 μmol), CuBr (20 μmol), and CsF (50 μmol). For the results under conditions A, B, and C, see ref. Hosoya et al., 2006. [b]The products were identified by GLC analyses and comparison to authentic samples. The yields were determined by GLC based on CH_3I. [c]Modified conditions: $Pd_2(dba)_3/P(o\text{-}CH_3C_6H_4)_3$/CuBr/CsF (1:8:4:10 in molar ratio). [d]The reaction using the conditions B: $Pd_2(dba)_3/P(o\text{-}CH_3C_6H_4)_3/CuCl/K_2CO_3$ (1:8:4:10 in molar ratio) gave **20l** in 71% yield.

Table 5. Rapid C–methylation on alkenyl structures.

The utility of the rapid methylation of an alkene was well demonstrated by the synthesis of a ^{11}C–labeled partial retinoid derivative [^{11}C]**20l** using reaction conditions B or D (X = Br), to produce in the high yield of 85% (radio–HPLC analytical yield) for both conditions (Figure 8) (Hosoya et al., 2006, see also section 11.4).

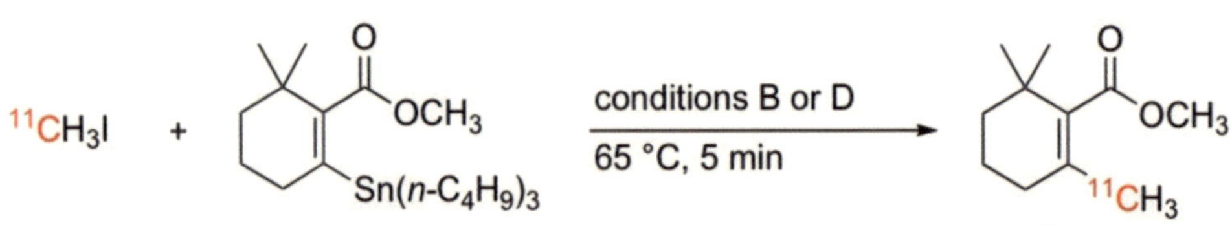

19l [^{11}C]**20l**

B: 85%; D: 85%
(radio–HPLC analytical yield)

(A)

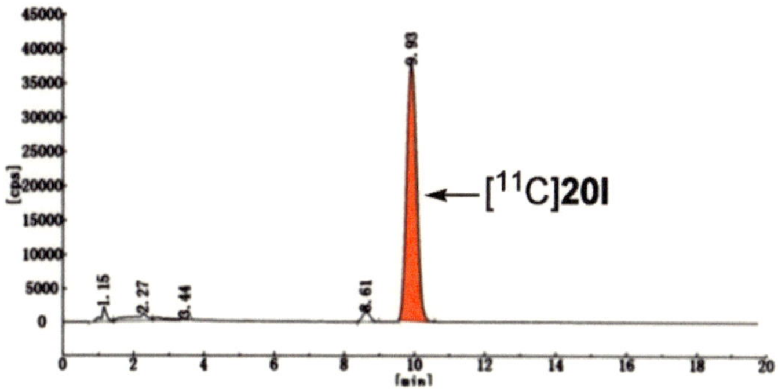

(B)

Fig. 8. Synthetic scheme of ^{11}C-labeled retinoid derivative [^{11}C]**201** (A), and radio-HPLC chart in the analysis of the reaction mixture (B).

10. Rapid *C*–[^{11}C]methylation of alkynes

10.1 Rapid *C*–methylation of alkynes (rapid coupling between sp-sp^3 hybridized carbons)

We set up a model reaction using methyl iodide and an excess amount of 1-hexynyltributylstannane (**21**) (CH_3I/**21** = 1:40) with the reaction time fixed at 5 min (Figure 9) (Hosoya et al., 2004). The reaction with Pd{P(C_6H_5)$_3$}$_4$ gave the desired 2-heptyne (**22**) in a poor yield. The previous conditions, $Pd_2(dba)_3$/P(*o*-$CH_3C_6H_4$)$_3$/CuCl/K_2CO_3, established for the sp^2(arenyl)-sp^3 rapid methylation, were also not applicable for this reaction. Based on the screenings of the phosphine ligand and additives, we found that the bulky and strong σ-electron-donating ligand, P(*tert*-C_4H_9)$_3$, facilitates the methylation (Hosoya et al., 2004). The combinations with fluoride ions, such as CsF or KF, were extremely efficient in promoting the reaction in a high yield. As a consequence, the reaction in the presence of bis(tri-*tert*-butylphosphine)palladium(0) (Pd{P(*tert*-C_4H_9)$_3$}$_2$) and KF in DMF at 60 °C for 5 min resulted in forming **22** in 95% yield (Hosoya et al., 2004).

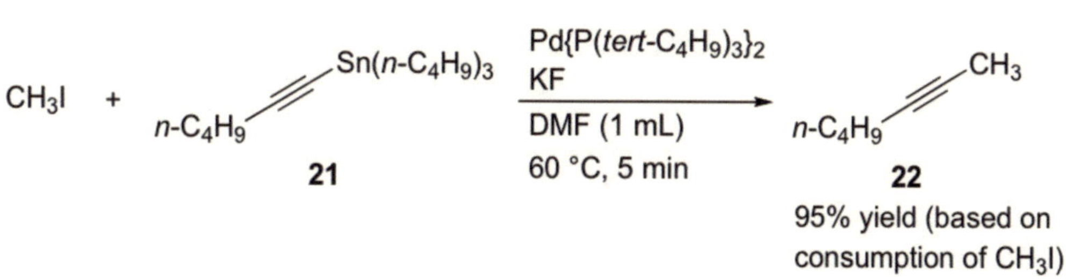

Fig. 9. Rapid coupling of methyl iodide with 1-hexynyltributylstannane (**21**).

The reaction was applicable to various kinds of functionalized alkynylstannanes including the stannyl precursors **23** and **24**, which are the substrates with steroid and deoxyribonucleoside frameworks, giving methylated compounds **25** and **26** in 87 and 74% yields, respectively (Hosoya et al., 2004).

10.2 Synthesis of [^{11}C]iloprost methyl ester

Iloprost (**27**) is a stable prostacyclin (PGI_2) analogue specific for the PGI_2 receptor, IP_1, in peripheral systems used as a potential therapeutic agent (Skuballa & Vorbrüggen, 1981), having the structure of 1-propynyl on the ω-side chain. According to the method established in the previous section, the ^{11}C-labeled iloprost methyl ester ([^{11}C]**29**) was synthesized using [^{11}C]CH_3I and a stannyl precursor **28** in up to 72% radio-HPLC analytical yield. The optimization of the synthesis of [^{11}C]**29** is currently in progress.

11. Rapid *C*–methylations using organoborons as trapping nucleophiles

In general, organoboron compounds are less toxic than organostannanes. Therefore, we intended to elaborate the rapid *C*-methylation based on the Suzuki-Miyaura coupling reaction (Miyaura & Suzuki, 1995) as a complementary method to the Stille-type rapid *C*-methylation. In this context, the Merck group reported the syntheses of [^{11}C]toluene derivatives by the reaction using [^{11}C]methyl iodide and an excess amount of arenylboron in the presence of $PdCl_2$(dppf) (dppf = 1,1'-bis(diphenylphosphino)ferrocene) and K_3PO_4 in DMF under microwave heating at high temperature (Hostetler et al., 2005). In contrast, we intended to establish a more efficient method by moderate thermal conditions based on the use of a Pd^0 complex without using microwaves in view of the careful treatment of a radiolabeled compound, and eventually, succeeded in developing very mild practical reaction conditions thus able to avoid the fear of an accidental radiation exposure (Doi et al., 2009).

11.1 Pd^0–mediated rapid *C*–methylations by coupling reaction of methyl iodide and a large excess arenyl- or alkenyl boronic acid ester

By keeping an actual PET-probe synthesis in mind, we set up the model reaction using methyl iodide and an excess amount of phenylboronic acid pinacol ester (**30**) (CH_3I/**30** = 1:40) with the short reaction time fixed at 5 min (Doi et al., 2009). The results are summarized in Table 6. We first attempted the known conditions frequently used for a

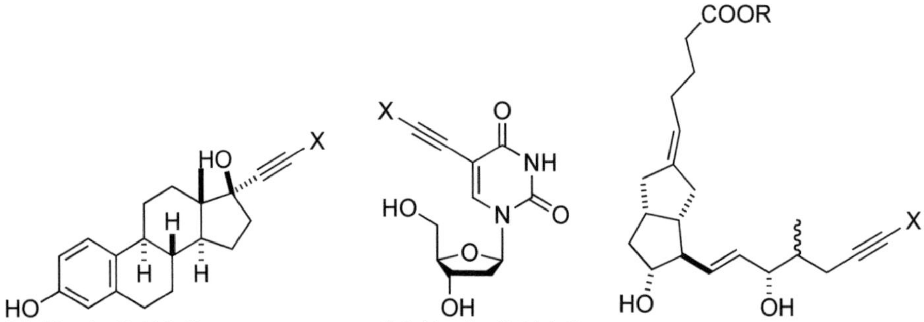

23: X = $(n\text{-}C_4H_9)_3Sn$
25: X = CH_3

24: X = $(n\text{-}C_4H_9)_3Sn$
26: X = CH_3

27: iloprost, R = H, X = CH_3
28: R = CH_3, X = $(n\text{-}C_4H_9)_3Sn$
[^{11}C]**29**: R = CH_3, X = $^{11}CH_3$

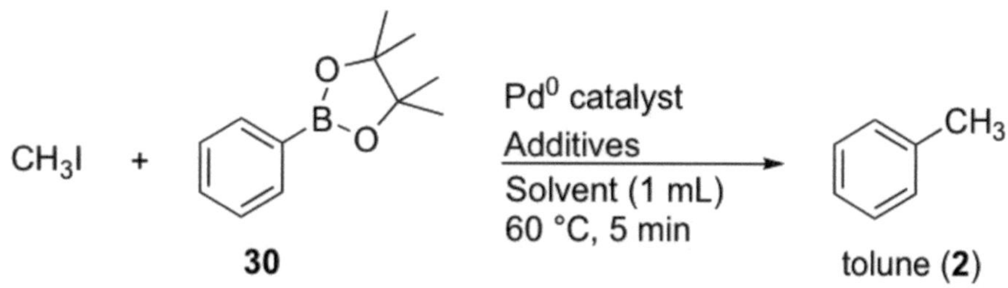

Entry[a]	Pd^0 complex	Ligand (L)	Pd:L (mol ratio)	Additives[b]	Solvent	Yield of **2** (%)[c]
1	Pd{P(C_6H_5)$_3$}$_4$	–	–	K_2CO_3	1,4-dioxane	39
2	$PdCl_2${P(C_6H_5)$_3$}$_2$	–	–	K_3PO_4	DME/H_2O (9:1)	24
3	$PdCl_2$(dppf)·CH_2Cl_2	–	–	K_3PO_4	DME/H_2O (9:1)	28
4	$Pd_2(dba)_3$	P(*o*-$CH_3C_6H_4$)$_3$	1:2	K_2CO_3	DMF	91
5	$Pd_2(dba)_3$	P(*o*-$CH_3C_6H_4$)$_3$	1:2	K_2CO_3	DMF/H_2O (9:1)	94
6	$Pd_2(dba)_3$	P(*o*-$CH_3C_6H_4$)$_3$	1:2	Cs_2CO_3	DMF	92
7	$Pd_2(dba)_3$	P(*o*-$CH_3C_6H_4$)$_3$	1:2	K_3PO_4	DMF	87
8	$Pd_2(dba)_3$	P(*o*-$CH_3C_6H_4$)$_3$	1:2	CuCl/K_2CO_3	DMF	81
9	$Pd_2(dba)_3$	P(*o*-$CH_3C_6H_4$)$_3$	1:2	KF	DMF	81

[a]Reaction was carried out with CH_3I (10 μmol) and **30** (400 μmol), Pd^0 (10 μmol). [b]20 μmol of the additive was used. [c]The yield was determined by GLC based on CH_3I. dppf: 1,1′-bis(diphenylphosphino)ferrocene.

Table 6. Rapid cross-coupling of methyl iodide with phenylboronic acid pinacol ester (**30**).

Suzuki-Miyaura coupling reaction (Miyaura & Suzuki, 1995), but such conditions did not give any satisfactory results (24–39% yields; Table 6, Entries 1-3). Therefore, we attempted the use of a Pd^0 complex coordinated with the bulky phosphine in a non-volatile solvent with a high polarity inspired by our successful studies on the Pd^0-mediated rapid C-[^{11}C]methylations using organostannanes (Suzuki et al., 1997; Hosoya et al., 2004; Hosoya et al., 2006; Suzuki et al., 2009). As expected, the reaction was dramatically accelerated by the use of the tri-*o*-tolylphosphine complex in DMF in the presence of K_2CO_3, K_2CO_3/H_2O, Cs_2CO_3, or K_3PO_4 to give the desired toluene in 87–94% yields (Table 6, Entries 4–7).

The rapid coupling reaction of methyl iodide and **30** probably proceeded via several steps (Eqs. (1)–(5); Doi et al., 2009) as exemplified by the presence of K_2CO_3 or K_2CO_3/H_2O;

$$CH_3I + [Pd\{P(o\text{-}CH_3C_6H_4)_3\}_2] \longrightarrow \underset{\mathbf{3}}{[Pd(CH_3)I\{P(o\text{-}CH_3C_6H_4)_3\}]} + P(o\text{-}CH_3C_6H_4)_3 \quad (1)$$

$$\underset{\mathbf{31}}{C_6H_5Bpin} + K_2CO_3 \text{ (or KOH)} \rightleftharpoons \underset{\mathbf{32}}{K^+[(C_6H_5)B(pin)(OZ)]^-} \quad (2)$$

$$\mathbf{3} + \mathbf{32} \longrightarrow \underset{\mathbf{6}}{[Pd(CH_3)(C_6H_5)\{P(o\text{-}CH_3C_6H_4)_3\}]} + \underset{\mathbf{33}}{K^+[B(pin)(OZ)(I)]^-} \quad (3)$$

$$\mathbf{33} + K_2CO_3 \text{ (or KOH)} \longrightarrow \underset{\mathbf{34}}{K^+[B(pin)(OZ)_2]^-} + KI \quad (4)$$

$$\mathbf{6} \longrightarrow \underset{\text{toluene } (\mathbf{2})}{CH_3\text{-}C_6H_5} + [Pd\{P(o\text{-}CH_3C_6H_4)_3\}] \quad (5)$$

Z = COOK or H

the oxidative addition of methyl iodide to the Pd^0 species to generate the methyl–Pd^{II} iodide **3** (Eq. (1)); the formation of a boronate complex **32** with a high polarity boron–carbon bond by the coordination of a base, such as KCO_3^- or OH^-, in a mixed system of K_2CO_3/H_2O (Eq. (2)); and the substitution of **3** with **32** to afford the [Pd^{II}(methyl)(phenyl)] complex **6** and the unstable borate $K^+[B(pin)(OZ)(I)]^-$ (**33**; Z = COOK or H) (Eq. (3)). The latter would be further converted to the more stable borate, $K^+[B(pin)(OZ)_2]^-$ (**34**), and KI (Eq. (4)). Finally, the reductive elimination from **6** gives the desired toluene (**2**) (Eq. (5)).

The conditions were found to be versatile for various arenyl, alkenyl, and hetero-aromatic ring substituted borons (Doi et al., 2009). Thus, the reactions with of both arenylborons with both electron-donating and electron-withdrawing groups on their aromatic rings and hetero-aromatic, ring-substituted boron compounds smoothly proceeded under the conditions of CH_3I/boron/$Pd_2(dba)_3$/$P(o\text{-}CH_3C_6H_4)_3$/K_2CO_3 (1:40:0.5:2:2) in DMF at 60 °C for 5 min, gave the corresponding methylation products in 80–99% yields. The conditions were also applied to the rapid *C*-methylation of various types of alkenyl compounds, giving the corresponding methylalkenes in 86–99% yields. The *E* and *Z* stereoisomers gave the corresponding methylated products with the retention of stereochemistry, which confirmed that the reaction proceeded in a completely stereocontrolled manner.

Boronic acid and the more lipophilic esters showed the same reactivity as the pinacol boronate, making the labeled probe purification easier (Doi et al., 2009).

The actual [^{11}C]methylation using the above-mentioned conditions (Table 6, Entry 4) was well demonstrated in the synthesis of the [^{11}C]*p*-xylene (Figure 10). Thus, the reaction of the [^{11}C]methyl iodide with pinacol tolylboronate **35** gave the [^{11}C]*p*-xylene ([^{11}C]**36**) in 96% radio-HPLC analytical yield. For the rapid *C*-[^{11}C]methylation, K_2CO_3 was more effective than KF or CsF.

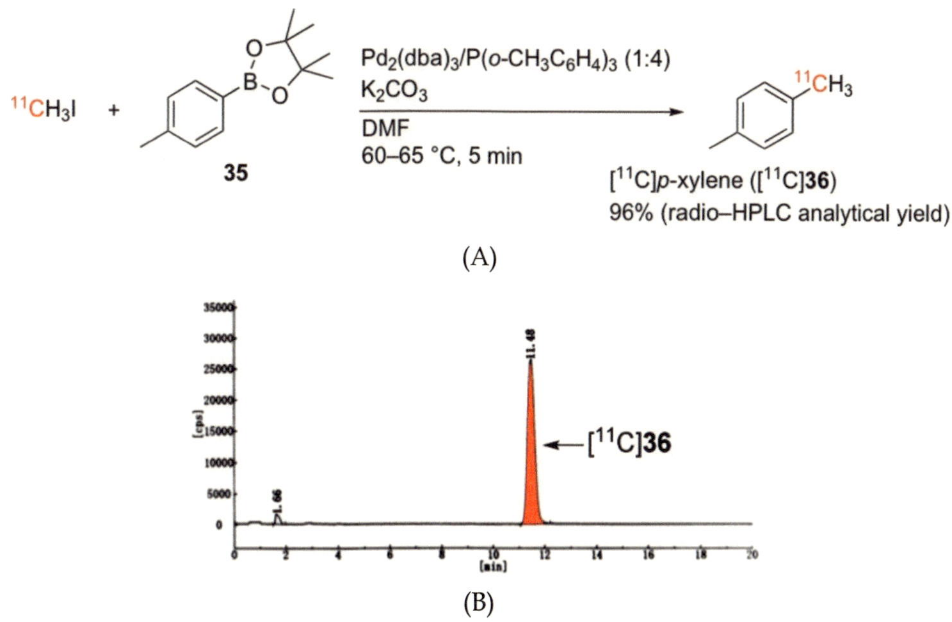

Fig. 10. Synthetic scheme of ^{11}C–labeled *p*-xylene ([^{11}C]**36**) by rapid *C*–[^{11}C]methylation using pinacol tolylboronate (**35**) (A), and radio-HPLC chart in the analysis of the reaction mixture (B).

11.2 Efficient synthesis of [^{11}C]celecoxib and its metabolites, [^{11}C]SC-62807

Celecoxib (4-[5-(4-methylphenyl)-3-(trifluoromethyl)-1*H*-pyrazole-1-yl]benzenesulfonamide, **38**) is a selective cyclooxygenase (COX)-2 inhibitor that has analgesic and anti-inflammatory effects in patients with rheumatoid arthritis, but has no effect on the COX-1 activity at therapeutic plasma concentrations. In humans, celecoxib is extensively metabolized in the liver via sequential two–step oxidative pathways, initially to a hydroxymethyl metabolite (SC-60613), and upon subsequent further oxidation to a carboxylic acid metabolite (SC-62807, **39**). The majority of celecoxib is excreted into the bile as SC-62807. In this context, Wu et al. reported that SC-62807 is a substrate of drug transporters, such as OATP1B1 and BCRP, which presumably mediate its hepatobiliary transport. Therefore, celecoxib or SC-62807 radiolabeled with a short–lived positron–emitting radionuclide could be a potential PET probe for evaluating the function of these drug transporters in hepatobiliary excretion (Takashima-Hirano et al., 2011).

The synthesis of [^{11}C]celecoxib ([^{11}C]**38**) was achieved in one–pot by reacting [^{11}C]methyl iodide with an excess amount of the corresponding pinacol borate precursor **37** using $Pd_2(dba)_3/P(o\text{-}CH_3C_6H_4)_3/K_2CO_3$ (1:4:9 in molar ratio) at 65 °C for 4 min in DMF (Figures 11A and B) according to the method established in a previous section in 55 ± 30% (n = 5) radio–HPLC analytical yield. The isolated radiochemical yield of [^{11}C]**38** was 63 ± 23% (n = 7) (decay-corrected, based on [^{11}C]CH_3I) with a specific radioactivity of 83 ± 23 GBq μmol^{-1} (n = 7) (Takashima-Hirano et al., 2011). The average synthesis time including formulation was 30 min with >99% and >98% radiochemical and chemical purities, respectively. [^{11}C]SC-62807 ([^{11}C]**39**) was also synthesized from the purified [^{11}C]**38** by further rapid oxidation in the presence of an excess amount of $KMnO_4$ under microwave irradiation (Figures 11A and C) with an 87 ± 5% (n = 3) radio–HPLC analytical yield. The isolated radiochemical yield of [^{11}C]**39** was 55 ± 9% (n = 3) (decay-corrected, based on [^{11}C]**38**) and a specific radioactivity of 39 ± 4 GBq μmol^{-1} (n = 3). The average time of synthesis including formulation was 20 min and produced a >99% radiochemically pure product. Now, the synthesis of [^{11}C]**39** was conducted using an automated sequential radiolabeling system equipped with microwave irradiation from the boron precursor **37**. There, nine operations from the [^{11}C]CH_3I production to the formation of [^{11}C]**39** were smoothly done automatically. PET studies in rats and the metabolite analyses of [^{11}C]celecoxib and [^{11}C]SC-62807 showed mostly different excretion processes between these compounds, and consequently, [^{11}C]SC-62807 was rapidly excreted via hepatobiliary excretion without further metabolism (Figure 11D), and therefore evaluated that it has a high potential as a PET probe suitable to investigate the hepatobiliary transport (Takashima-Hirano et al., 2011).

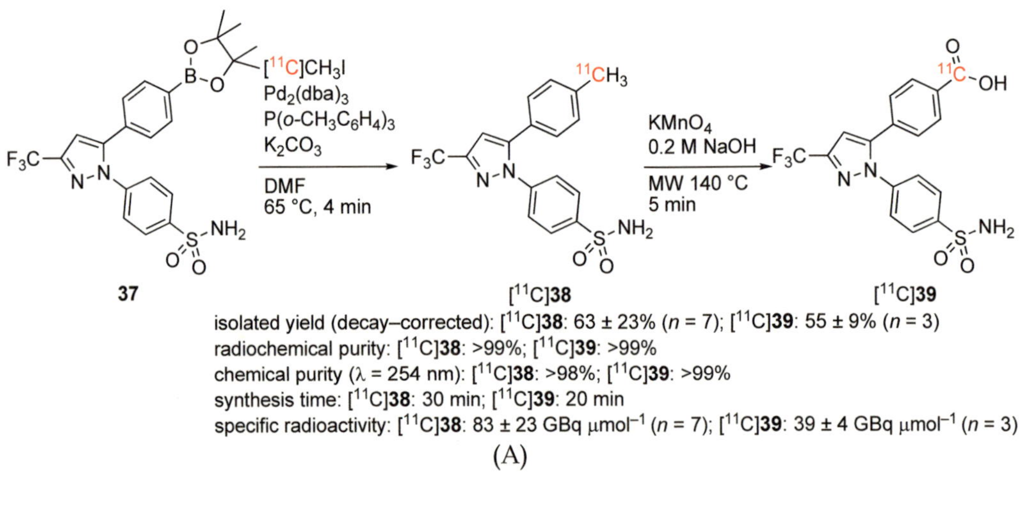

37 [^{11}C]**38** [^{11}C]**39**

isolated yield (decay–corrected): [^{11}C]**38**: 63 ± 23% (n = 7); [^{11}C]**39**: 55 ± 9% (n = 3)
radiochemical purity: [^{11}C]**38**: >99%; [^{11}C]**39**: >99%
chemical purity (λ = 254 nm): [^{11}C]**38**: >98%; [^{11}C]**39**: >99%
synthesis time: [^{11}C]**38**: 30 min; [^{11}C]**39**: 20 min
specific radioactivity: [^{11}C]**38**: 83 ± 23 GBq μmol^{-1} (n = 7); [^{11}C]**39**: 39 ± 4 GBq μmol^{-1} (n = 3)

(A)

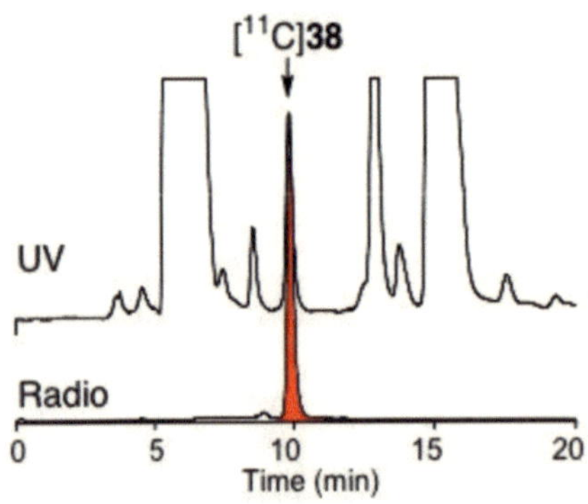

(B)

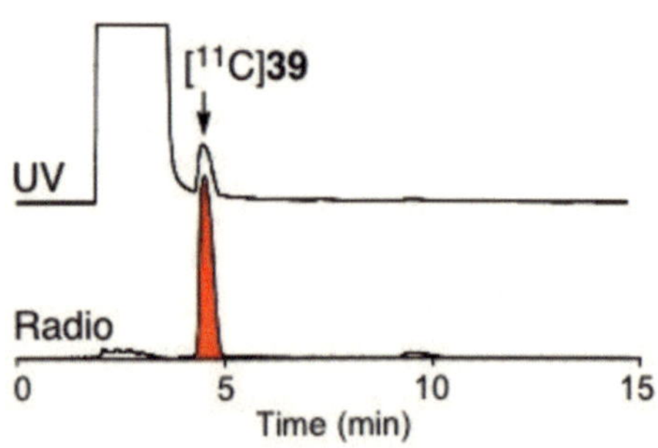

(C)

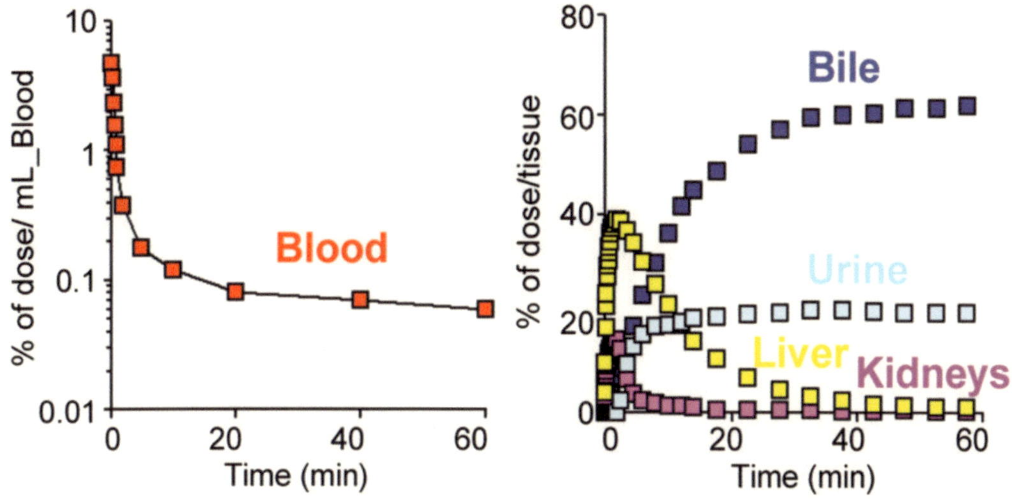

(D)

Fig. 11. Synthetic scheme of [^{11}C]celecoxib ([^{11}C]**38**) and [^{11}C]SC-62807 ([^{11}C]**39**) (A), the HPLC chart for the analysis of [^{11}C]**38** (B) and [^{11}C]**39** (C), and the time profiles of activity in the blood (red point), liver (yellow pont), kidney (pink point), bile (blue point), and urinary bladder (light blue point) determined by PET imaging and blood sampling over 60-min period after administration of [^{11}C]SC-62807 ([^{11}C]**39**) to male Sprague-Dawley rats (D). The peak at a retention time of 9.6 min labeled B is [^{11}C]**38** and the peak at a retention time of 4.4 min labeled C is [^{11}C]**39**. UV absorbance: 254 nm.

11.3 Efficient synthesis of ^{11}C–incorporated acromelic acid analogue

Acromelic acid A (Figure 12), a minor constituent isolated from *Clitocybe acromelalga*, induces allodynia in mice by intrathecal (i.t.) administration. If we can identify the receptor involved in the induction of allodynia, it may provide a trigger to develop novel analgesic drugs for use in the treatment of neuropathic pain. In this context, we have synthesized a novel ^{11}C-labeled PET probe [^{11}C]**41**, which was designed based on the (phenylthio)pyrrolidine derivative **41** that can competitively block the acromelic acid-induced allodynia (Kanazawa et al., 2011). A protocol in which the Pd^0-mediated rapid methylation of the pinacol borate precursor **40** with [^{11}C]CH_3I using $Pd_2(dba)_3$, P(*o*-$CH_3C_6H_4)_3$, and K_2CO_3 in DMF and the following deprotection of the TFA-protected amino acid moiety and hydrolysis of methyl esters were successively performed in one-pot within 5 min (4 and 1 min each) was established for the synthesis of a PET probe [^{11}C]**41** with > 99% of both radiochemical and chemical purities (Kanazawa et al., 2011). The isolated yield was 34–43% (decay-corrected, based on trapped [^{11}C]CH_3I). The obtained radioactivity of [^{11}C]**41** after an injectable formulation under the nomal conditions was 5.0–6.0 GBq and the specific radioactivity was 70–100 GBq μmol^{-1} (Figure 12). The total synthesis time of [^{11}C]**41** was within 30 min (Figure 12).

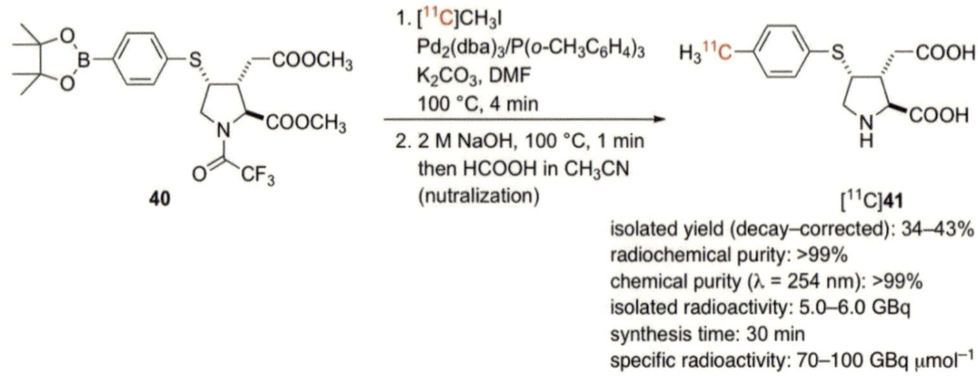

Fig. 12. Efficient synthesis of ^{11}C–labeled acromelic acid analogue [^{11}C]**41**.

11.4 Synthesis of [^{11}C]all-*trans*-retinoic acid

Retinoids are a class of chemical compounds including both naturally dietary vitamin A (retinol) metabolites and active synthetic analogs (Germain et al., 2006). Both experimental and clinical studies have revealed that retinoids regulate a wide variety of essential biological processes, such as vertebrate embryonic morphogenesis and organogenesis, cell growth arrest, differentiation, apoptosis, and homeostasis, as well as their disorders. The all-*trans*-retinoic acid (ATRA), the most potent biologically active metabolite of retinol, has been used in the treatment of acute promyelocytic leukemia. In this context, we focused on the ^{11}C–labeling of ATRA. The Pd^0–mediated rapid C-[^{11}C]methylation using pinacol borate precursor **42** was successfully applied to the synthesis of [^{11}C]ATRA ([^{11}C]**43**) (Suzuki et al., 2011b). The labeling reaction was conducted using [^{11}C]CH_3I in the presence of $Pd_2(dba)_3$, P(*o*-$CH_3C_6H_4)_3$, and Na ascorbate (1:4:9) in DMF–H_2O at 65 °C for 4 min followed by basic hydrolysis of the methyl (at 65 °C) and ethyl ester (at 100 °C) for 2 min, to afford the desired [^{11}C]**43** in 36% radio–HPLC analytical yield (Figure 13). The isolated radioactivity was 1.5 GBq with >99% and 97% radiochemical and chemical purities, respectively. The isolated radiochemical yield was 25% (decay–corrected, based on [^{11}C]CH_3I). Total synthesis time

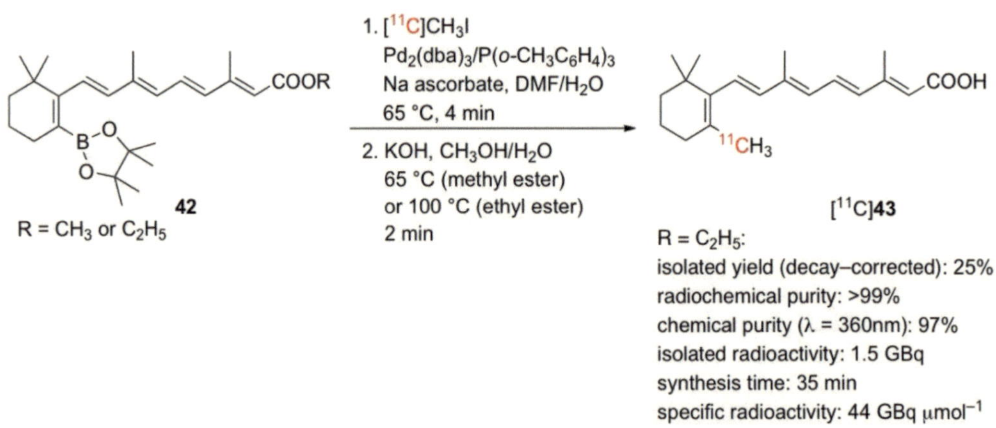

Fig. 13. Synthesis of ^{11}C–labeled all-*trans*-retinoic acid ([^{11}C]ATRA, [^{11}C]**43**).

including HPLC purification and formulation was 35 min. The decomposition of the product has not been observed at 90 min after the end of the synthesis in the presence of sodium ascorbate as judged by the conservation of radiochemical purity >99%.

12. Rapid *C*–[^{11}C]methylation of alkanes

12.1 Rapid *C*–[^{11}C]methylation (rapid coupling sp^3–sp^3 hybridized carbons)

The development of the fourth target of the rapid *C*–[^{11}C]methylations (rapid methylation of an alkane framework) (see Figure 2) by the coupling between sp^3-sp^3 carbons using $^{11}CH_3I$ and organoborons is also currently underway using a similar procedure in our group.

12.2 Another rapid coupling between sp^3–sp^3 hybridized carbons: Efficient synthesis of [^{11}C]NSAIDs and these esters

In order to perform the *in vivo* molecular imaging of cyclooxygenases (COXs), well-known as key enzymes in prostaglandin biosynthesis, we intended to develop a novel method to rapidly incorporate a ^{11}C radionuclide into various 2-arenylpropionic acids that have a common methylated structure, particularly abundant among nonsteroidal anti-inflammatory drugs (NSAIDs). Consequently, we elaborated the rapid ^{11}C-labeling using the reaction of [^{11}C]CH_3I and an enolate intermediate generated from the corresponding ester under basic conditions, followed by the one-pot hydrolysis to convert it into the ^{11}C-incorporated acid as [^{11}C]NSAID (Figure 14A) (Takashima-Hirano et al., 2010b). Methoxy 2-arenylpropionate is much less polar due to the increase in hydrophobicity of an introduced methyl group and the less hyperconjugation between the C-H σ bond of the benzylic position and C=O π^*, which is also possible for the LUMO (π^*) of a phenyl moiety, allowing easy separation of the desired ^{11}C-labeled product from the demethylated compound. This method is quite general and utilized for the syntheses of the following six PET probes of NSAIDs: [^{11}C]ibuprofen ([^{11}C]**50**), [^{11}C]naproxen ([^{11}C]**51**), [^{11}C]flurbiprofen ([^{11}C]**52**), [^{11}C]fenoprofen ([^{11}C]**53**), [^{11}C]ketoprofen ([^{11}C]**54**), [^{11}C]loxoprofen ([^{11}C]**55**), and their corresponding esters as racemates ([^{11}C]**44–49**), with sufficient radioactivity (1.7-5.5 GBq) for animal and human PET studies. The isolated radiochemical yields (decay-corrected) based on [^{11}C]CH_3I of [^{11}C]**44–55** were 26-76%. Notably, we found that methyl esters were particularly useful as pro-radioprobes for the study of neuroinflammation in the brain. The microPET studies of rats with lipopolysaccharide (LPS)-induced brain inflammation clearly showed that the radioactivity of the PET probes, [^{11}C]ketoprofen methyl ester ([^{11}C]**48**) and [^{11}C]ketoprofen ([^{11}C]**54**) specifically accumulated in the inflamed region (Figure 14B), giving the first successful example of the *in vivo* molecular imaging of neuroinflammation by the noninvasive PET technology. A metabolite analysis in the rat brain revealed that the intravenously administrated methyl ester was initially taken up in the brain and then underwent hydrolysis to form a pharmacologically active form of the corresponding acids. Hence, we succeeded in the general ^{11}C-labeling of 2-arenylpropionic acids and their methyl esters as PET probes of NSAIDs to construct a potentially useful PET-probe library for the *in vivo* imaging of inflammation involved in the COX expression (Shukuri et al., 2011). The above racemic NSADs are readily separated by a chiral column to give an optically pure compound. Tetrabutylammonium fluoride (TBAF) was also effective to promote the rapid [^{11}C]methylation of the enolate in THF as found in our (Takashima-Hirano et al., 2010a) and other group (Kato et al., 2010). The [^{11}C]methylation of an analogous enolate has been applied to the synthesis of ^{11}C-labeled α-aminoisobutyric acid as a PET probe for cancer imaging (Kato et al., 2011).

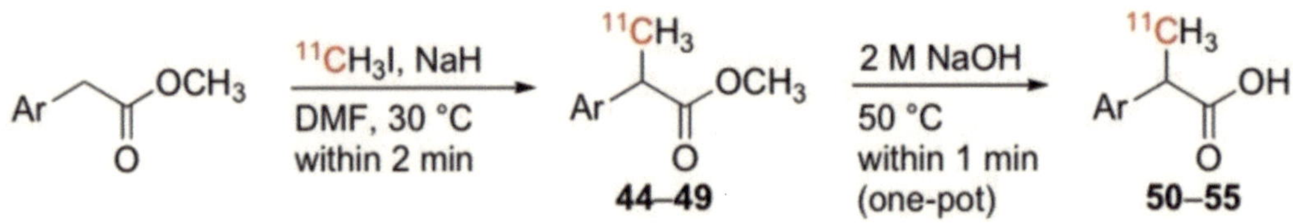

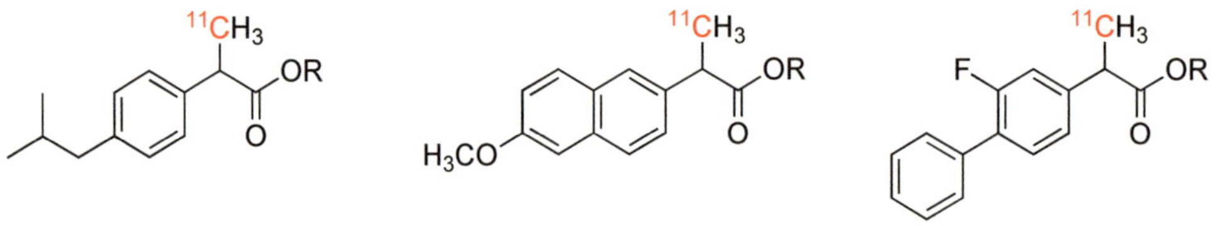

[^{11}C]**44**: R = CH_3,
[^{11}C]ibuprofen methyl ester
[^{11}C]**50**: R = H,
[^{11}C]ibuprofen

[^{11}C]**45**: R = CH_3,
[^{11}C]naproxen methyl ester
[^{11}C]**51**: R = H,
[^{11}C]naproxen

[^{11}C]**46**: R = CH_3,
[^{11}C]flurbiprofen methyl ester
[^{11}C]**52**: R = H,
[^{11}C]flurbiprofen

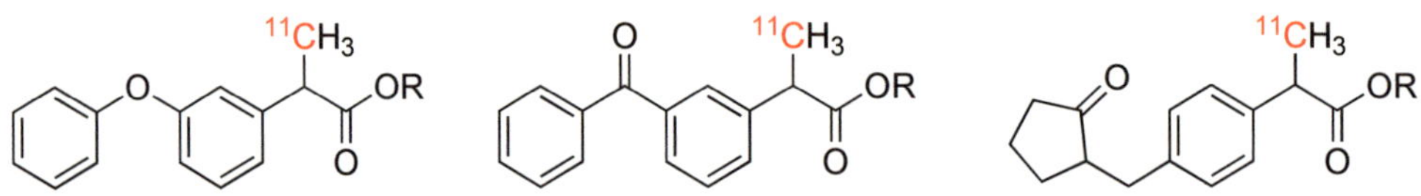

[^{11}C]**47**: R = CH_3,
[^{11}C]fenoprofen methyl ester
[^{11}C]**53**: R = H,
[^{11}C]fenoprofen

[^{11}C]**48**: R = CH_3,
[^{11}C]ketoprofen methyl ester
[^{11}C]**54**: R = H,
[^{11}C]ketoprofen

[^{11}C]**49**: R = CH_3,
[^{11}C]loxoprofen methyl ester
[^{11}C]**55**: R = H,
[^{11}C]loxoprofen

(A)

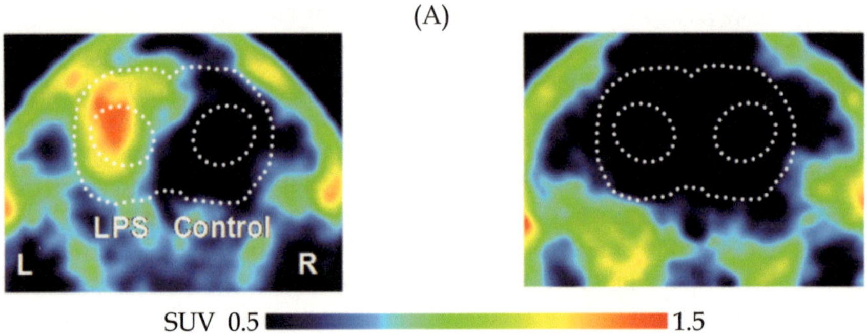

(B)

Fig. 14. Synthesis of ^{11}C-labeled 2-arylpropionoc acids and their esters (A), and PET images of [^{11}C]ketoprofen methyl ester ([^{11}C]**48**, left panel) and [^{11}C]ketoprofen ([^{11}C]**54**, right panel) in rat brain inflammation induced by lipopolysaccharide injection into the left striatum (B). Left PET image showed high accumulation in the area of inflammation, indicating that the methyl ester penetrated the blood-brain barrier and underwent hydrolysis in the brain to produce carboxylic acid as a pharmacologically active form, accumulating the inflammation area.

13. Opportunity for the rapid *C*–[^{18}F]fluoromethylation (rapid ^{18}F–incorporation into an organic framework through the carbon–carbon bond forming reaction)

13.1 Rapid *C*–fluoromethylations

The *C*–[^{11}C]methylation is associated with *C*–[^{18}F]fluoromethylation by a similar coupling methodology using [^{18}F]fluoromethyl bromide ([^{18}F]FCH_2Br) and [^{18}F]fluoromethyl iodide ([^{18}F]FCH_2I) as the available ^{18}F-labeling precursor for the synthesis of various types of PET tracers by *N*- or *O*-[^{18}F]fluoromethylation (Zhang & Suzuki, 2007). There are many benefits based on the success of the ^{18}F-labeling by rapid *C*–[^{18}F]fluoromethylation: (1) capability of a relatively long *in vivo* study complementary to ^{11}C, (2) feasible delivery of ^{18}F-labeled probes to distant PET centers and clinics, (3) insertion of multi-reactions after labeling, and (4) the use as a prosthetic group in click chemistry for the labeling of peptides, nucleic acids, sugars, etc. The application of rapid ^{18}F-labeling to biologically significant organic compounds will be reported in due course.

Initially, we investigated the Pd^0-mediated rapid cross-coupling using non-radioactive fluoromethyl iodide and phenyltributylstannane or a boron compound prior to the actual *C*–[^{18}F]fluoromethylation (Doi et al., 2009). The conditions for rapid *C*-methylation using an organoboron in Table 6, Entry 4, were efficient for the synthesis of the fluoromethyl arene. Furthermore, a slightly improved condition using the 1:3 ratio of $Pd^0/P(o\text{-}CH_3C_6H_4)_3$ was found to be the most effective for promoting the fluoromethylation with pinacol phenylboronate **30**, giving the desired benzyl fluoride in 57% yield (Doi et al., 2009). Thus, the conditions using FCH_2I for the synthesis of an [^{18}F]fluoromethyl-labeled PET probe was established.

13.2 Rapid *C*–[^{18}F]fluoromethylation

We set up the reaction using ca. 0.5 GBq of [^{18}F]FCH_2X (X = Br or I) and a 4-(4,4,5,5-tetramethyl-1,3,2-dioxaborolan-2-yl)benzoic acid methyl ester (**56**) (Figure 15). First, we found that the labeling reaction using [^{18}F]FCH_2I and **56** for 5 min at 65 °C gave the desired *p*-([^{18}F]fluoromethyl)benzoic acid methyl ester ([^{18}F]**57**) using $Pd_2(dba)_3/P(o\text{-}CH_3C_6H_5)_3$ (1:6) and K_2CO_3 in DMF. The radio-HPLC analytical yield of [^{18}F]**57** was 23 %, but a considerable amount of side products with a high polarity appeared, which might be the [^{18}F]fluoride ion derived from the decomposition of [^{18}F]FCH_2I. However, to the best of our knowledge, this result was the first evidence for the Pd^0-mediated rapid *C*–[^{18}F]fluoromethylation. After a broader investigation of not only labeling chemistry, but also the mechanical operations of our radiolabeling system, we concluded that the *C*–[^{18}F]fluoromethylation with [^{18}F]FCH_2Br will be more practical than that with [^{18}F]FCH_2I. Actually, [^{18}F]FCH_2I was essentially more reactive to the Pd^0 complex, but [^{18}F]FCH_2I was not stable and gradually decomposed in the light-exposed solution. For these reasons, we then focused on developing the *C*–[^{18}F]fluoromethylation using [^{18}F]FCH_2Br. The reaction was dramatically promoted under the conditions of 120 °C for 5 and 15 min in DMPU/H_2O (9:1) to give [^{18}F]**57** in 48 and 64% yields, respectively. HPLC analyses showed that the reaction for 5 min resulted in the unreacted [^{18}F]FCH_2Br remaining to a considerable extent, but the reaction for 15 min produced a remarkably sharp peak of [^{18}F]**57** as the main product. The *C*–[^{18}F]fluoromethylation would be completed within 15 min because the reaction for 30 min did not produce a further increase in the yield. The 15-min reaction thus obtained matches well with the ^{18}F-incorporated PET-probe synthesis because of the longer half-life (110 min) of the ^{18}F radionuclide compared to ^{11}C (20.4 min) (Doi et al., 2010).

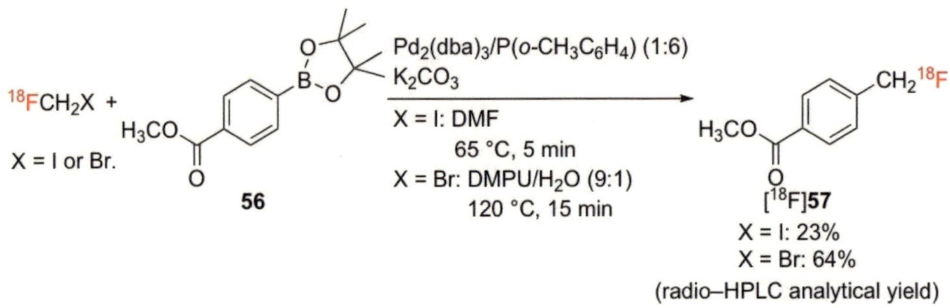

Fig. 15. Rapid C–[^{18}F]fluoromethylation using 4-(4,4,5,5-tetramethyl-1,3,2-dioxaborolan-2-yl)benzoic acid methyl ester (**56**) under PET radiolabeling conditions.

14. Conclusions

In this chapter, a ground-braking methodology based on the use of cutting-edge chemistry was introduced for the synthesis of a short-lived ^{11}C-incorporated PET tracer. First, a general method for the rapid reaction of methyl iodide with an arenyltributylstannane (excess amount) (the Stille-type reaction) was established, producing a methylarene in the presence of the bulky tri-*o*-tolylphosphine-bound coordinatively unsaturated Pd^0 complex, a Cu^I salt, and K_2CO_3 based on a synergic effect to promote the reaction. The reaction was used for the synthesis of the 15*R*-[^{11}C]TIC methyl ester as an actual PET probe. The rapid *C*-methylation was expanded to other types of rapid methylations including the methylation on heteroaromatic frameworks by adding another Cu^I/CsF synergy and choosing the bulky trialkylphosphine for the alkene and alkyne, thus allowing the radio synthesis of various biologically and clinically important molecules. To meet the further demands of an efficient labeling method in PET, we established a rapid methylation using methyl iodide and an organoboron compound (Suzuki-Miyaura type coupling) as a complementary trapping substrate to an organostannane in the presence of Pd^0, tri-*o*-tolylphosphine, and K_2CO_3 or K_2CO_3/H_2O in high yield. The reaction conditions were also applied to the *C*-fluoromethylation, and, after slight modifications, we realized the incorporation of the rather longer half-lived ^{18}F radionuclide into organic frameworks (rapid *C*-[^{18}F]fluoromethylation). Our five original papers (Suzuki et al., 2009; Doi et al., 2009; Hosoya et al., 2006; Koyama et al., 2011; Hosoya et al., 2004, in order for ranking) were ranked Nos. 1-5 among the top 10 articles published in the same domain in BioMedLib (search engine for the 20 million articles of MEDLINE, April 2009-June 2011). Accordingly, a "Bible" on the syntheses of ^{11}C- and ^{18}F-labeled compounds has been continuously updated to provide valuable information required for a PET chemist.

As shown in Figure 16, RIKEN CMIS has utilized three types of remote-controlled synthesizers for ^{11}C- and ^{18}F-labeling, which originally developed with the focus on synthetic organic chemistry.

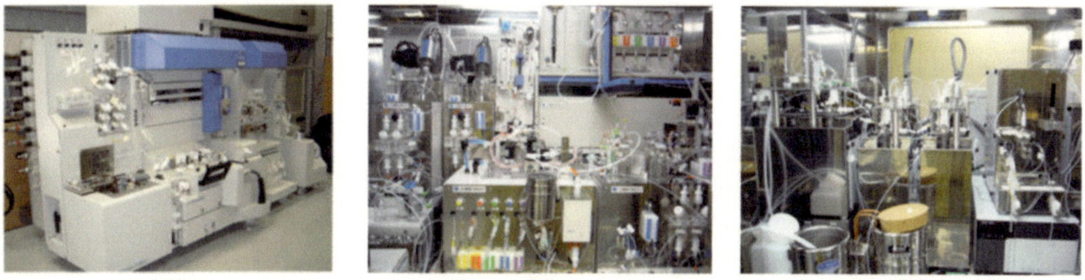

(A) (B) (C)

Fig. 16. Our original remote–controlled synthesizer for ^{11}C– and ^{18}F–labeling; H19D: an early type system hybridized by septum–cannula and robot–arm method for the solution transfer (A), H20S: the improved model for step–wise labeling operations (B), and H20J: standard model focused on the simplicity and operational stability of the remote controlled synthetic procedures (C).

The next step is the application of the descrived synthetic procedure for the synthesis along with the Guidance of Good Manufacturing Practice (GMP) regulation. We also consider that the rapid reactions using a microfluidic system (microreactor) will be important in order to reduce the amount of a substrate (if scarce or very expensive) without lengtheing the reaction time.

The methods thus described have widely been applied by other groups to synthesize ^{11}C-labeled PET probes, such as *N,N*-dimethyl-2-(2-amino-4-[^{11}C]methylphenylthio)benzylamine (MADAM, [^{11}C]**58**, Tarkiainen et al., 2001), the serotonin transporter inhibitor, 5-[^{11}C]methyl-6-nitroquipazine ([^{11}C]**59**, Sandell et al., 2002), [^{11}C]toluene ([^{11}C]**2**, Gerasimov et al., 2002), the central nicotinic acetylcholine inhibitor, 3-[(2S)-azetidin-2-ylmethoxy]-5-[^{11}C]methylpyridine ([^{11}C]**60**, Karimi & Långström, 2002; Iida et al., 2004), [^{11}C]FMAU ([^{11}C]**61**, Samuelsson & Långström, 2003), the serotonin reuptake inhibitor, citalopram analogue, [5-methyl-^{11}C]{3-[1-(4-fluorophenyl)-5-methyl-1,3-dihydroisobenzofuran-1-yl]-propyl}-dimethylamine ([^{11}C]**62**, Madsen et al., 2003), the adrenergic neurotransmitter, 4-[^{11}C]methylmetaraminol ([^{11}C]**63**, Langer et al., 2003), the metabotropic glutamate 1 antagonist, (3-ethyl-2-[^{11}C]methyl-6-quinolinyl)-(*cis*-4-methoxycyclohexyl)methanone ([^{11}C]**64**, Huang et al., 2005), the COX-2 selective inhibitor and prescription drug, [^{11}C]celecoxib ([^{11}C]**38**, Prabhakaran et al., 2005), (+)-*p*-[^{11}C]methylvesamicol for mapping sigma$_1$ receptors ([^{11}C]**65**, Ishiwata et al., 2006), the NK-3 receptor antagonist, [^{11}C]SB 222200 ([^{11}C]**66**, Bennacef et al., 2007), the reboxetin analogues ([^{11}C]**67** and [^{11}C]**68**, Zeng et al., 2009), the derivative of the selective α7 nicotinic acetylcholine receptor partial agonist, 4-[^{11}C]methylphenyl 2,5-diazabicyclo[3.2.2]nonane-2-carboxylate ([^{11}C]CHIBA-1001, [^{11}C]**69**, Toyohara et al., 2009), [^{11}C]α-aminoisobutyric acid for cancer imaging ([^{11}C]**70**), etc.

15. Perspectives

Molecular imaging with PET is the only method for elucidating the whole-body pharmacokinetics of molecules in humans. This technique could be adapted for the efficient screening of drug candidates in humans during the early stage of the drug development process (phase 0 as a pre-clinical trial), and accelerating the path leading to clinical trials, resulting in revolutionizing drug development. The chemistry covering a broad range of designs, syntheses, and labelings is expected to play a central role in this interdisciplinary scientific field.

The objective of the study was to develop a novel chemical methodology for *in vivo* molecular imaging adaptable from animals to humans. As already described, we developed various types of rapid *C*-[^{11}C]methylations and *C*-[^{18}F]fluoromethylations by the Pd^0-mediated cross-coupling reactions between [^{11}C]methyl iodide or [^{18}F]fluoromethyl idodide (or bromide) and organostannanes or organoborons, respectively, for the synthesis of short-lived PET molecular probes. The synthesis method would also be applicable for the incorporation of other carbon isotope units, such as $CH_2{}^{18}F$, $^{13}CH_3$, $^{14}CH_3$, CD_3, and $CH_2{}^{19}F$, allowing the application to accelerator mass spectrometry (AMS) and MRI. In particular, PET and AMS using ^{11}C and ^{14}C (use of 10^{-20} M), respectively, are two methods capable of promoting a human microdose study under political regulations (Europe, 2004; U.S., 2006; Japan, 2008).

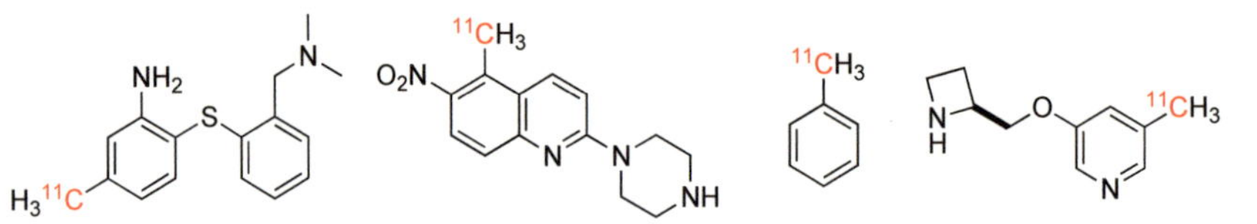

[^{11}C]**58** [^{11}C]**59** [^{11}C]**2** [^{11}C]**60**

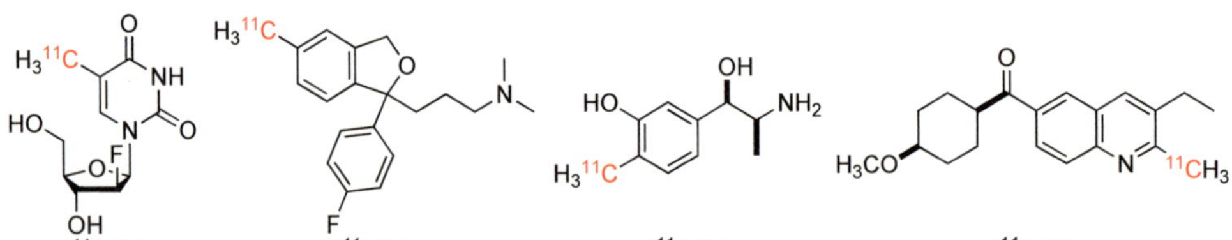

[^{11}C]**61** [^{11}C]**62** [^{11}C]**63** [^{11}C]**64**

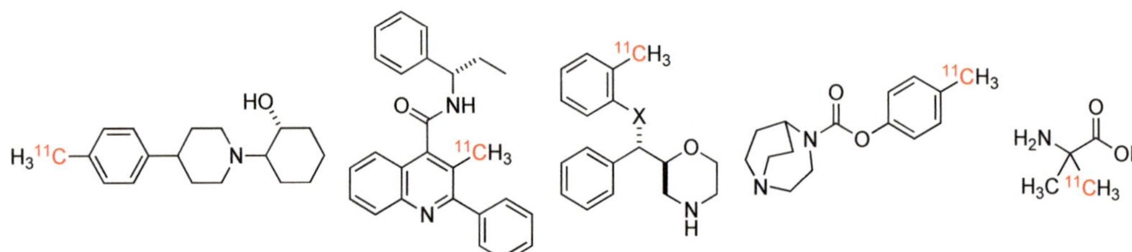

[^{11}C]**65** [^{11}C]**66** [^{11}C]**67**: X = O [^{11}C]**68**: X = S [^{11}C]**69** [^{11}C]**70**

We intend to further expand the rapid *C*-[^{11}C]methylations and [^{18}F]fluoromethylations and their applications in order to construct a library of ^{11}C- and ^{18}F-incorporated biologically significant molecules involved in various diseases important for medical treatment, such as cerebral diseases (Alzheimer's disease (AD), Parkinson's disease (PD), amyotrophic laterals sclerosis (ALS), etc.), cardiovascular diseases (hypertention, stroke, glaucoma, etc.), cancer, diabetes, infection (human immunodeficiency virus (HIV), hepatitis C virus (HCV), influenza, prion, etc.), inflammation, neuropathic pain, and transporter dysfunction, as a frontier research to promote *in vivo* molecular science.

In an advanced medical field, tailor-made medicine, personalized medicine based on single nucleotide polymorphism, and evidence-based medicine based on PK/PD studies in humans are emphasized by the rapid progress of genome science. We believe that the advancement of "*in vivo* molecular science in humans" is strongly required in order to achieve the medical objectives. The progress of *in vivo* human molecular science will serve to overcome the "Death Valley" existing between a preclinical study and the clinical trials in the drug development process in order to revolutionize disease diagnosis and the drug discovery process.

16. Acknowledgement

We would like to express our sincere gratitude to Profs. Ryoji Noyori (President of RIKEN), Bengt Långström (Uppsala University), and Yasuyoshi Watanabe (Director of RIKEN CMIS) for their contribution to the TIC imaging as part of an international collaboration and their valuable advice for the promotion of PET molecular imaging science. We are also grateful to Drs. M. Björkman, T. Hosoya, M. Wakao, K. Sumi, Z. Zhang, Siqin, K. Furuta, M. Kanazawa, H. Tsukada, and other colleagues, whose names are listed in the references, involved in the rapid *C*-[^{11}C]methylation and *C*-[^{18}F]fluoromethylation projects and their application. This study was supported in part by a Grant-in-Aid for Creative Scientific Research (No. 13NP0401), a consignment expense for the Molecular Imaging Program on "Research Base for Exploring New Drugs" (2005–2009), and Japan Advanced Molecular Imaging Program (2010–) from the Ministry of Education, Culture, Sports, Science and Technology (MEXT) of Japan.

17. References

Allard, M.; Fouquet, E.; James, D. & Szlosek-Pinaud, M. (2008). State of art in ^{11}C labelled radiotracers synthesis. *Current Med. Chem.*, Vol. 15, February 2008, pp. 235–277, ISSN: 0929-8673.

Bading, J. R. & Shields, A. F. (2008). Imaging of cell proliferation: status and prospects. *J. Nucl. Med.*, Vol. 49, June 2008, pp. 64S–80S, ISSN: 0161-5505.

Bennacef, I.; Perrio, C.; Lasne, M.-C. & Barré, L. (2007). Functionalization through lithiation of (*S*)-*N*-(1-phenylpropyl)-2-phenylquinoline-4-carboxamide. Application to the labeling with carbon-11 of NK-3 receptor antagonist SB 222200. *J. Org. Chem.*, Vol. 72, March 2007, pp. 2161–2165, ISSN 0022-3263.

Bergström, M.; Grahnén, A. & Långström, B. (2003). Positron emission tomography microdosing: a new concept with application in tracer and early clinical drug development. *Eur. J. Clin. Pharmacol.*, Vol. 59, September 2003, pp. 357–366, print ISSN: 0031-6970, online ISSN: 1432-1041.

Björkman, M.; Doi, H.; Resul, B.; Suzuki, M.; Noyori, R.; Watanabe, Y. & Långström, B. (2000). Synthesis of a ^{11}C-labelled prostaglandin $F_{2\alpha}$ analogue using an improved method for Stille reactions with [^{11}C]methyl iodide. *J. Labelled Compd. Radiopharm.*, Vol. 43, December 2000, pp. 1327–1334, print ISSN: 0362-4803, online ISSN: 1099-1344.

Buck, B.; Mascioni, A.; Que, L. Jr. & Veglia, G. (2003). Dealkylation of organotin compounds by biological dithiols: toward the chemistry of organotin toxicity. *J. Am. Chem. Soc.*, Vol. 125, February 2003, pp. 13316–13317, ISSN: 0002-7863.

Cui, Y.; Takamatsu, H.; Kakiuchi, T.; Ohba, H.; Kataoka, Y.; Yokoyama, C.; Onoe, H.; Watanabe, Yu.; Hosoya, T.; Suzuki, M.; Noyori, R.; Tsukada, H. & Watanabe, Y.

(2006). Neuroprotection by a central nervous system-type prostacyclin receptor ligand demonstrated in monkeys subjected to middle cerebral artery occlusion and reperfusion: a positron emission tomography study. *Stroke*, Vol. 37, November 2006, pp. 2830–2836, ISSN: 0039-2499.

Doi, H.; Ban, I.; Nonoyama, A.; Sumi, K.; Kuang, C.; Hosoya, T.; Tsukada, H. & Suzuki, M. (2009). Palladium(0)-mediated rapid methylation and fluoromethylation on carbon frameworks by reacting methyl and fluoromethyl iodide with aryl and alkenyl boronic acid esters: useful for the synthesis of [^{11}C]CH_3–C- and [^{18}F]FCH_2–C-containing PET tracers (PET = positron emission tomography). *Chem. Eur. J.*, Vol. 15, April 2009, pp. 4165–4171, print ISSN: 0947-6539, online ISSN: 1521-3765.

Doi, H.; Goto, M. & Suzuki, M. (2010). Pd^0-mediated rapid C–[^{18}F]fluoromethylation by the reaction of a [^{18}F]fluoromethyl halide and an organoboron compound. *15th European Symposium on Radiopharmacy and Radiopharmaceuticals*, Edinburgh, Scotland, April 8–11, 2010.

Fowler, J. S. & Wolf, A. P. (1997). Working against time: rapid radiotracer synthesis and imaging the human brain. *Acc. Chem. Res.*, Vol. 30, April 1997, pp. 181–188, ISSN: 1520-4898.

Gerasimov, M. R.; Ferrieri, R. A.; Schiffer, W. K.; Logan, J.; Gatley, S. J.; Gifford, A. N.; Alexoff, D. A.; Marsteller, D. A.; Shea, C.; Garza, V.; Carter, P.; King, P.; Ashby, C. R. Jr.; Vitkun, S. & Dewey, S. L. (2002). Study of brain uptake and biodistribution of [^{11}C]toluene in non-human primates and mice. *Life Sci.*, Vol. 70, April 2002, pp. 2811–2828, ISSN: 0024-3205.

Germain, P.; Chambon, P.; Eichele, G.; Evans, R. M.; Lazar, M. A.; Leid, M.; Lera, A. R. D.; Lotan, R.; Mangelsdorf, D. J. & Gronemeyer, H. (2006). International union of pharmacology. LX. retinoic acid receptors. *Pharmacol. Rev.*, Vol. 58, December 2006, pp. 712–725, print ISSN: 0031-6997, online ISSN: 1521-0081.

Hosoya, T.; Sumi, K.; Doi, H.; Wakao, M. & Suzuki, M. (2006). Rapid methylation on carbon frameworks useful for the synthesis of $^{11}CH_3$-incorporated PET tracers: Pd(0)-mediated rapid coupling of methyl iodide with an alkenyltributylstannane leading to a 1-methylalkene. *Org. Biomol. Chem.*, Vol. 4, pp. 410–415, print ISSN: 1477-0520, online ISSN: 1477-0539.

Hosoya, T.; Wakao, M.; Kondo, Y.; Doi, H. & Suzuki, M. (2004). Rapid methylation of terminal acetylenes by the Stille coupling of methyl iodide with alkynyltributylstannanes: a general protocol potentially useful for the synthesis of short-lived $^{11}CH_3$-labeled PET tracer with a 1-propynyl group. *Org. Biomol. Chem.*, Vol. 2, pp. 24–27, print ISSN: 1477-0520, online ISSN: 1477-0539.

Hostetler, E. D.; Terry, G. E. & Burns, H. D. (2005). An improved synthesis of substituted [^{11}C]toluenes via Suzuki coupling with [^{11}C]methyl iodide. *J. Labelled Compd. Radiopharm.*, Vol. 48, August 2005, pp. 629–634, print ISSN: 0362-4803, online ISSN: 1099-1344.

Huang, Y.; Narendran, R.; Bischoff, F.; Guo, N.; Zhu, Z.; Bae, S.-A.; Lesage, A. S. & Laruelle, M. (2005). A positron emission tomography radioligand for the in vivo labeling of metabotropic glutamate 1 receptor: (3-ethyl-2-[^{11}C]methyl-6-quinolinyl)(*cis*-4-methoxycyclohexyl)methanone. *J. Med. Chem.*, Vol. 48, August 2005, pp. 5096–5099, ISSN: 0022-2623.

Ido, T.; Wan, C.-N.; Casella, V.; Flowler, J. S.; Wolf, A. P.; Reivich, M. & Kuhl, E. E. (1978). Labeled 2-deoxy-D-glucose analogs. ^{18}F-Labeled 2-deoxy-2-fluoro-D-glucose, 2-deoxy-2-fluoro-D-mannose, and ^{14}C-2-deoxy-2-fluoro-D-glucose. *J. Labelled Compd. Radiopharm.*, Vol. 14, pp. 175–183, print ISSN: 0362-4803, online ISSN: 1099-1344..

Iida, Y.; Ogawa, M.; Ueda, M.; Tominaga, A.; Kawashima, H.; Magata, Y.; Nishiyama, S.; Tsukada, H.; Mukai, T. & Saji, H. (2004). Evaluation of 5-^{11}C-methyl-A-85380 as an imaging agent for PET investigations of brain nicotinic acetylcholine receptors. *J. Nucl. Med.*, Vol. 45, May 2004, pp. 878–884, ISSN: 0161-5505.

Ishiwata, K.; Kawamura, K.; Yajima, K.; QingGeLeTu; Mori, H. & Shiba, K. (2006). Evaluation of (+)-*p*-[^{11}C]methylvesamicol for mapping sigma$_1$ receptors: a comparison with [^{11}C]SA4503. *Nucl. Med. Biol.*, Vol. 33, May 2006, pp. 543–548, ISSN: 0969-8051.

Japan's response to microdosing study, Notification No. 0603001, 3 June 2008, Guidance for the Conduct of Microdoing Clinical Trials, Evaluation and Licensing Division, Pharmaceutical and Food Safety Bureau, Ministry of Health, Labour and Walfare, Japan.

Kanazawa, M.; Furuta, K.; Doi, H.; Mori, T.; Minami, T.; Ito, S. & Suzuki, M. (2011). Synthesis of an acromelic acid A analog-based ^{11}C-labeled PET tracer for exploration of the site of action of acromelic acid A in allodynia induction. *Bioorg. Med. Chem. Lett.*, Vol. 21, April 2011, pp. 2017–2020, ISSN: 0960-894X.

Karimi, F. & Långström, B. (2002). Synthesis of 3-[(2S)-azetidin-2-ylmethoxy]-5-[^{11}C]-methylpyridine, an analogue of A-85380, via a Stille coupling. *J. Labelled Compd. Radiopharm.*, Vol. 45, April 2002, pp. 423–434, print ISSN: 0362-4803, online ISSN: 1099-1344.

Kato, K.; Kikuchi, T.; Nengaki, N.; Arai, T. & Zhang, M.-R. (2010). Tetrabutylammonium fluoride-promoted α-[^{11}C]methylation of α-arylesters: a simple and robust method for the preparation of ^{11}C-labeled ibuprofen. *Tetrahedron Lett.*, Vol. 51, November 2010, pp. 5908–5911, ISSN: 0040-4039.

Kato, K.; Tsuji, A. B.; Saga, T. & Zhang, M.-R. (2011). An efficient and expedient method for the synthesis of ^{11}C-labeled α-aminoisobutyric acid: a tumor imaging agent potentially useful for cancer diagnosis. *Bioorg. Med. Chem. Lett.*, Vol. 21, April 2011, pp. 2437–2440, ISSN: 0960-894X.

Koyama, H.; Siqin; Zhang, Z.; Sumi, K.; Hatta, Y.; Nagata, H.; Doi, H. & Suzuki, M. (2011). Highly efficient syntheses of [methyl-^{11}C]thymidine and its analogue 4'-[methyl-^{11}C]thiothymidine as nucleoside PET probes for cancer cell proliferation by Pd^0-mediated rapid C-[^{11}C]methylation. *Org. Biomol. Chem.*, Vol. 9, pp. 4287–4294, print ISSN: 1477-0520, online ISSN: 1477-0539.

Langer, O.; Forngren, T.; Sandell, J.; Dollé, F.; Långström, B.; Någren, K. & Halldin, C. (2003). Preparation of 4-[^{11}C]methylmetaraminol, a potential PET tracer for assessment of myocardial sympathetic innervation. *J. Labelled Compd. Radiopharm.*, Vol. 46, January 2003, pp. 55–65, print ISSN: 0362-4803, online ISSN: 1099-1344.

Lappin, G. & Garner, R. C. (2003). Big physics, small doses: the use of AMS and PET in human microdosing of development drugs. *Nat. Rev. Drug Discov.*, Vol. 2, March 2003, pp. 233–240, ISSN: 1474-1776.

Lee, T. S.; Ahn, S. H.; Moon, B. S.; Chun, K. S.; Kang, J. H.; Cheon, G. J.; Choi, C. W. & Lim, S. M. (2009). Comparison of ^{18}F-FDG, ^{18}F-FET and ^{18}F-FLT for differentiation between tumor and inflammation in rats. *Nucl. Med. Biol.* Vol. 36, August 2009, pp. 681–686, ISSN: 0969-8051.

Littke, A. F.; Schwarz L. & Fu, G. C. (2002). Pd/P(*t*-Bu)$_3$: a mild and general catalyst for Stille reactions of aryl chlorides and aryl bromides. *J. Am. Chem. Soc.*, Vol. 124, June 2002, pp. 6343–6348, ISSN: 0002-7863.

Louie, J. & Hartwig, J. F. (1995). Transmetalation involving organotin aryl, thiolate, and amide compounds. An unusual type of dissociative ligand substitution reaction. *J. Am. Chem. Soc.*, Vol. 117, November 1995, pp. 11598–11599, ISSN: 0002-7863.

Madsen, J.; Merachtsaki, P.; Davoodpour, P.; Bergström, M.; Långström, B.; Andersen, K.; Thomsen, C.; Martiny, L. & Knudsen G. M. (2003). Synthesis and biological evaluation of novel carbon-11-labelled analogues of citalopram as potential radioligands for the serotonin transporter. *Bioorg. Med. Chem.*, Vol. 11, August 2003, pp. 3447–3456, ISSN: 09680896.

Mee, S. P. H.; Lee, V. & Baldwin, J. E. (2004). Stille coupling made easier–the synergic effect of copper(I) salts and the fluoride ion. *Angew. Chem., Int. Ed.*, Vol. 43, February 2004, pp. 1132–1136, print ISSN: 1433-7851, online ISSN: 1521-3773.

Menzel, K. & Fu, G. C. (2003). Room-temperature Stille cross-couplings of alkenyltin reagents and functionalized alkyl bromides that possess β hydrogens. *J. Am. Chem. Soc.*, Vol. 125, April 2003, pp. 3718–3719, ISSN: 0002-7863.

Miyaura, N. & Suzuki, A. (1995). Palladium-catalyzed cross-coupling reactions of organoboron compounds. *Chem. Rev.*, Vol. 95, November 1995, pp. 2457–2483, ISSN: 0009-2665.

Morita, D. K.; Stille, J. K. & Norton, J. R. (1995). Methyl/phenyl exchange between palladium and a phosphine ligand. Consequences for catalytic coupling reactions. *J. Am. Chem. Soc.*, Vol. 117, August 1995, pp. 8576–8581, ISSN: 0002-7863.

Paul, F.; Patt, J. & Hartwig, J. F. (1995). Structural characterization and simple synthesis of {Pd[P(*o*-Tol)$_3$]$_2$}, dimeric palladium(II) complexes obtained by oxidative addition of aryl bromides, and corresponding monometallic amine complexes. *Organometallics*, Vol. 14, June 1995, pp. 3030–3039, pint ISSN: 0276-7333, online ISSN: 1520-6041.

Phelps, M. E. (Ed.) (2004). *PET: Molecular Imaging and Its Biological Applications*, Springer, ISBN-10: 0387403590, ISBN-13: 978-0387403595, New York, Berlin, Heidelberg.

Prabhakaran, J.; Majo, V. J.; Simpson, N. R.; Van Heertum, R. L.; Mann, J. J. & Kumar, J. S. D. (2005). Synthesis of [^{11}C]celecoxib: a potential PET probe for imaging COX-2 expression. *J. Labelled Compd. Radiopharm.*, Vol. 48, October 2005, pp. 887–895, print ISSN: 0362-4803, online ISSN: 1099-1344.

Samuelsson, L. & Långström, B. (2003). Synthesis of 1-(2′-deoxy-2′-fluoro-β-D-arabinofuranosyl)-[*methyl*-^{11}C]thymine ([^{11}C]FMAU) *via* a Stille cross-coupling reaction with [^{11}C]methyl iodide. *J. Labelled Compd. Radiopharm.*, Vol. 46, March 2003, pp. 263–272, print ISSN: 0362-4803, online ISSN: 1099-1344.

Sandell, J.; Yu, M.; Emond, P.; Garreau, L.; Chalon, S.; Någren, K.; Guilloteau, D. & Halldin, C. (2002). Synthesis, radiolabeling and preliminary biological evaluation of radiolabeled 5-methyl-6-nitroquipazine, a potential radioligand for the serotonin transporter. *Bioorg. Med. Chem. Lett.*, Vol. 12, December 2002, pp. 3611–3613, ISSN: 0960-894X.

Schubiger, P. A., Lehmann, L. & Friebe, M. (Eds.) (2007). *PET Chemistry: The Driving Force in Molecular Imaging*, Springer, ISBN-10: 3540326235, ISBN-13: 978-3540326236, New York, Berlin, Heidelberg.

Shukuri, M.; Takashima-Hirano, M.; Tokuda, K.; Takashima, T.; Matsumura, K.; Inoue, O.; Doi, H.; Suzuki, M.; Watanabe, Y. & Onoe, H. (2011). In vivo expression of cyclooxygenase-1 in activated microglia and macrophages during neuroinflammation visualized by PET with ^{11}C-ketoprofen methyl ester. *J. Nucl. Med.*, Vol. 52, July 2011, pp. 1094–1101, print ISSN: 0161-5505, online ISSN: 2159-662X.

Skuballa, W. & Vorbrüggen, H. (1981). A new rout to 6a-carbacyclins—synthesis of a stable, biologically potent prostacyclin analogue. *Angew. Chem., Ent. Ed.*, Vol. 20, pp. 1046–1048, print ISSN: 1433-7851, online ISSN: 1521-3773.

Smith, P. J. (1998). Health and safety aspects of tin chemicals, In: *Chemistry of TIN*, P. J. Smith, (Ed.), pp. 429–441, Blackie Academic & Professional, ISBN: 0-7514-0385-7, UK.

Stille, J. K. (1986). The palladium-catalyzed cross-coupling reactions of organotin reagents with organic electrophiles. *Angew. Chem., Int. Ed.*, Vol. 25, June 1986, pp. 508–524, print ISSN: 1433-7851, online ISSN: 1521-3773.

Sundoro-Wu, B. M.; Schmall, B.; Conti, P. S.; Dahl, J. R.; Drumm, P. & Jacobsen, J. K. (1984). Selective alkylation of pyrimidyldianions: synthesis and purification of ^{11}C labeled thymidine for tumor visualization using positron emission tomography. *Int. J. Appl. Radiat. Isot.*, Vol. 35, pp. 705–708, ISSN: 0020-708X.

Suzuki, M.; Doi, H.; Björkman, M.; Andersson, Y.; Långström, B.; Watanabe Y. & Noyori, R. (1997). Rapid coupling of methyl iodide with aryltributylstannanes mediated by palladium(0) complexes: a general protocol for the synthesis of $^{11}CH_3$-labeled PET tracers. *Chem. Eur. J.*, Vol. 3, December 1997, pp. 2039–2042, print ISSN: 0947-6539, online ISSN: 1521-3765.

Suzuki, M.; Doi, H.; Hosoya, T.; Långström, B. & Watanabe, Y. (2004). Rapid methylation on carbon frameworks leading to the synthesis of a PET tracer capable of imaging a novel CNS-type prostacyclin receptor in living human brain. *Trends Anla. Chem.*, Vol. 23, September 2004, pp. 595–607, ISSN: 0165-9936.

Suzuki, M.; Doi, H.; Kato, K.; Björkman, M.; Långström, B., Watanabe, Y. & Noyori, R. (2000a). Rapid methylation for the synthesis of a ^{11}C-labeled tolylisocarbacyclin imaging the IP_2 receptor in a living human brain. *Tetrahedron*, Vol. 56, Octorber 2000, pp. 8263–8273, ISSN: 0040-4020.

Suzuki, M.; Kato, K.; Noyori, R.; Watanabe, Yu.; Takechi, H.; Matsumura, K.; Långström, B. & Watanabe, Y. (1996). (15*R*)-16-*m*-Tolyl-17,18,19,20-tetranorisocarbacyclin: a stable ligand with high binding affinity and selectivity for a prostacyclin receptor in the central nervous system. *Angew. Chem., Int. Ed.*, Vol. 35, February 1996, pp. 334–336, print ISSN: 1433-7851, online ISSN: 1521-3773.

Suzuki, M.; Noyori, R.; Långström, B. & Watanabe, Y. (2000b). Molecular design of prostaglandin probes in brain research: high, specific binding to a novel prostacyclin receptor in the central nervous system. *Bull. Chem. Soc. Jpn.*, Vol. 73, February 2001, pp. 1053–1070, print ISSN: 1348-0634, online ISSN: 0009-2673.

Suzuki, M.; Sumi, K.; Koyama, H.; Siqin; Hosoya, T.; Takashima-Hirano, M. & Doi, H. (2009). Pd^0-mediated rapid coupling between methyl iodide and heteroarylstannanes: an efficient and general method for the incorporation of a positron-emitting ^{11}C radionuclide into heteroaromatic frameworks. *Chem. Eur. J.*, Vol. 15, November 2009, pp. 12489–12495, print ISSN: 0947-6539, online ISSN: 1521-3765.

Suzuki, M.; Takashima-Hirano, M.; Koyama, H.; Yamaoka, T.; Sumi, K.; Nagata, H.; Hidaka, H. & Doi, H. (2011a). Efficient synthesis of [^{11}C]H-1152, a PET probe specific for Rho-kinases (ROCKs) by Pd(0)-mediated rapid C-[^{11}C]methylation. *2011 World Molecular Imaging Congress*, San Diego, California, September 7-10, 2011, reported by poster presentation.

Suzuki, M.; Takashima-Hirano, M.; Watanabe, C.; Ishii, H.; Sumi, K.; Koyama, H. & Doi, H. (2011b). Synthesis of [^{11}C]all-*trans*-retinoic acid via an alkenylboron precursor by Pd(0)-mediated rapid C-[^{11}C]methylation. *19th International Symposium on Radiopharmaceutical Sciences*, Amsterdam, August 28–September 2, 2011, reported by poster presentation.

Takashima, T.; Nagata, H.; Nakae, T.; Cui, Y.; Wada, Y.; Kitamura, S.; Doi, H.; Suzuki, M.; Maeda, K.; Kusuhara, H.; Sugiyama, S. & Watanabe, Y. (2010). Positron emission tomography studies using (15*R*)-16-*m*-[^{11}C]tolyl-17,18,19,20-tetranorisocarbacyclin methyl ester for the evaluation of hepatobiliary transport. *J. Pharmacol. Exo. Ther.*, Vol. 335, November 2010, pp. 314–323, print ISSN: 0022-3565, online ISSN: 11521-0103.

Takashima-Hirano, M.; Shukuri, M.; Takashima, T.; Cu, Y.-L.; Goto, M.; Tokuda, K.; Wada, Y.; Watanabe, Y.; Onoe, H.; Doi, H. & Suzuki, M. (2010a). ^{11}C-Labeling of nonsteroidal anti-inflammatory drugs and PET imaging. *Molecular Imaging 2010*, Tokyo, Japan, January 21–22, reported by poster presentation.

Takashima-Hirano, M.; Shukuri, M.; Takashima, T.; Goto, M.; Wada, Y.; Watanabe, Y.; Onoe, H.; Doi, H. & Suzuki, M. (2010b). General method for the ^{11}C-labeling of 2-arylpropionic acids and their esters: construction of a PET tracer library for a study of biological events involved in COXs expression. *Chem. Eur. J.*, Vol. 16, April 2010, pp. 4250–4258, print ISSN: 0947-6539, online ISSN: 1521-3765.

Takashima-Hirano, M.; Takashima, T.; Katayama, Y.; Wada, Y.; Sugiyama, Y.; Watanabe, Y.; Doi, H. & Suzuki, M. (2011). Efficient sequential synthesis of PET probes of the COX-2 inhibitor [^{11}C]celecoxib and its major metabolite [^{11}C]SC-62807 and in vivo PET evaluation. *Bioorg. Med. Chem.*, Vol. 19, May 2011, pp. 2997–3004, ISSN: 0960-894X.

Tarkiainen, J.; Vercouillie, J.; Emond, P.; Sandell, J.; Hiltunen, J.; Frangin, Y.; Guilloteau, D. & Halldin, C. (2001). Carbon-11 labelling of MADAM in two different positions: a highly selective PET radioligand for the serotonin transporter. *J. Labelled Compd. Radiopharm.*, Vol. 44, December 2001, pp. 1013–1023, print ISSN: 0362-4803, online ISSN: 1099-1344.

The European Medicines Agency, Evaluation of Medicines for Human Use (EMEA), Position paper on non-clinical safety studies to support clinical trials with a single microdose, CPMP/SWP/2599/02/Rev1, 23 June 2004.

Tolman, C. A. (1977). Steric effects of phosphorus ligands in organometallic chemistry and homogeneous catalysis. *Chem. Rev.*, Vol. 77, June 1977, pp. 313–348, ISSN: 0009-2665.

Toyohara, J.; Sakata, M.; Wu, J.; Ishikawa, M.; Oda, K.; Ishii, K.; Iyo M.; Hashimoto, K. & Ishiwata, K. (2009). Preclinical and the first clinical studies on [^{11}C]CHIBA-1001 for imaging α7 nicotinic receptors by positron emission tomography. *Ann. Nucl. Med.* Vol. 23, May 2009, pp. 301–309, print ISSN: 0914-7187, online ISSN: 1864-6433.

Toyohara, J.; Okada, M.; Toramatsu, C.; Suzuki, K. & Irie, T. (2008). Feasibility studies of 4'-[methyl-^{11}C]thiothymidine as a tumor proliferation imaging agent in mice. *Nucl. Med. Biol.*, Vol. 35, January 2008, pp. 67–74, ISSN: 0969-8051.

U. S. Department of Health and Human Services, Food and Drug Administration, Center for Drug Evaluation and Research, Guidance for Industry, Investigators, and Reviewers, Exploratory IND Studies, January 2006.

Zeng, F.; Mun, J.; Jarkas, N.; Stehouwer, J. S.; Voll, R. J.; Tamagnan, G. D.; Howell, L.; Votaw, J. R.; Kilts, C. D.; Nemeroff, C. B. & Goodman, M. M. (2009). Synthesis, radiosynthesis, and biological evaluation of carbon-11 and fluorine-18 labeled reboxetine analogues: potential positron emission tomography radioligands for in vivo imaging of the norepinephrine transporter. *J. Med. Chem.*, Vol. 52, January 2009, pp. 62–73, ISSN: 0022-2623.

Zhang, M.-R. & Suzuki, K., (2007). [^{18}F]Fluoroalkyl agents: synthesis, reactivity and application for development of PET ligands in molecular imaging. *Curr. Top. Med. Chem.*, Vol. 7, September 2007, pp. 1817–1828, ISSN: 1568-0266.

6

Emerging Technologies for Decentralized Production of PET Tracers

Pei Yuin Keng[1], Melissa Esterby[1,2] and R. Michael van Dam[1]
[1]*Crump Institute for Molecular Imaging, Department of Molecular & Medical Pharmacology, David Geffen School of Medicine, University of California, Los Angeles*
[2]*Sofie Biosciences, Inc.*
USA

1. Introduction

1.1 Increasing diversity of PET

The use of Positron Emission Tomography (PET) to monitor biological processes *in vivo* (Michael E. Phelps 2000) has seen dramatic growth and acceptance in the research, pharmaceutical, and medical communities over the last few decades, with clinical PET growing from ~900,000 scans in 2004 to over 1.74 million in 2010 in the United States alone; growth in foreign markets is comparable (Muschlitz 2011). These scans are conducted in ~2,200 clinical PET centers, all providing molecular imaging diagnostics of the biology of various diseases, including cancer, Alzheimer's, and Parkinson's. Additionally, PET is a powerful tool in the drug discovery and development process, providing *in vivo* pharmacokinetics and pharmacodynamics using radiolabeled versions of new drugs. A portion of clinical PET centers support drug trials carried out by pharmaceutical and biotech companies by synthesizing these molecules. PET biomarkers can also be used to select the best treatment for individual patients. Patient stratification via PET is anticipated to increase the quality of therapeutics available to patients with a concomitant decrease in the cost of bringing these therapeutics to market. (In the current randomized approach to patient selection, ~75% of patients do not have an efficacious response to treatment.) Furthermore, PET has been widely used in preclinical research and its use in cell cultures (Vu et al. 2011) and animal models is growing dramatically due to the recent advent of preclinical PET imaging systems that are easy-to-use, compact, and affordable (Zhang et al. 2010). Coupled with the Critical Path Initiative of the FDA to partner a biomarker with each drug in clinical trials, as well as the ongoing technetium (^{99m}Tc) shortage affecting single photo emission computed tomography (SPECT) imaging, there is an even greater demand for PET, especially so given its superior sensitivity and image quality.

The need to measure and elucidate biological processes in a non-invasive manner in functioning organisms has led researchers to develop more than 1,600 PET probes for metabolism, protein synthesis, receptors, enzymes, DNA replication, gene expression, antibodies, hormones, and therapeutics (Iwata 2004). However, the overwhelming majority of PET for the care of patients utilizes only a single molecular imaging probe, the ^{18}F-labeled glucose analog 2-[^{18}F]fluoro-2-deoxy-D-glucose ([^{18}F]FDG). All cells normally use glucose for a variety of cellular functions, and [^{18}F]FDG PET provides a general assessment of the alterations in glucose metabolism between healthy and diseased states. The primary use of [^{18}F]FDG is to detect, stage, and assess therapeutic responses in cancer (Weber and Figlin 2007). Limitations do exist, however, such as the difficulty in imaging tissues which normally have very high glucose metabolism, and the lack of identification of the specific biochemical pathways through which disease is occurring. [^{18}F]FDG also cannot serve as a companion diagnostic for the discovery, development, and use of new molecular therapeutics. Increasing diversity of tracers beyond [^{18}F]FDG will be needed in the clinic to provide effective diagnostics with more specificity over a greater range of disease and injury (Coenen et al. 2010)(Daniels et al. 2010).

We focus herein on the radioisotope fluorine-18 due to its many desirable chemical and physical properties that lead to excellent stability, resolution, and sensitivity, compared with many other PET radioisotopes (Lasne et al. 2002). Furthermore, the half-life (~110 min) is sufficiently long for transport from production facilities to nearby sites, and [^{18}F]fluoride in [^{18}O]H_2O produced by the $^{18}O(p,n)^{18}F$ nuclear reaction is easy to handle.

1.2 Centralized production of tracers

With existing technology, production of PET probes requires a large capital investment in equipment and infrastructure, and high ongoing personnel and operating costs. Currently, PET probes for clinical PET service are produced in a *centralized* manner by commercial PET radiopharmacies (Fig. 1). A number of universities operate in a similar, centralized manner with a core radiochemistry facility to produce PET probes for an array of basic science and clinical research disciplines. In general, radiopharmacies contain a cyclotron to generate the positron-emitting radioisotope, dedicated probe-specific radiosynthesizers (manual and/or automated) to synthesize and purify radiotracers, and quality control (QC) testing equipment (e.g. gas chromatography (GC), analytical radio-high-performance liquid chromatography (radio-HPLC), dose calibrators, radio-thin layer chromatography (radio-TLC), etc.) to ensure safety of the patient. This workflow requires installation of cumbersome lead-shielded chemistry hoods ("hot cells") to safely contain the radiosynthesis process, specifically allocated workspace for tasks such as QC testing, reagent qualification and storage, etc., and specially trained personnel to operate the entire process, from cyclotron operation to the aseptic dose preparation.

On December 9, 2009, the U.S. Food and Drug Administration (FDA) issued federal regulations (21 CFR Part 212) and an accompanying guidance document to establish current good manufacturing practices (cGMP) for the production, quality control, holding, and distribution of PET probes in routine clinical use. Furthermore, as of December 12, 2011, all manufacturers must register and submit a New Drug Application (NDA) or Abbreviated New Drug Application (ANDA) in order to sell and market PET probes within the U.S. Thus, in addition to the initial and recurring infrastructure and personnel costs, radiopharmacies must spend additional capital to implement and maintain compliance with federal regulations for each tracer produced.

By spreading these significant costs over many customers in the production of one probe, commercial radiopharmacies have made [^{18}F]FDG affordable and readily accessible for clinical and research use. Due to the way tracers are made, there is almost no additional cost in increasing the size of a production run to serve more customers. A batch of [^{18}F]FDG can be increased by simply changing the amount of the radioactive isotope at the beginning of the synthesis, a function of the bombardment time in the cyclotron with no change in the synthesis, purification, and QC steps. This implies a significant financial advantage in producing large batches of a small number of tracers rather than small batches of a large number of tracers. Due to the relatively low demand for a given new tracer, these tracers cannot be provided at a reasonable price in the current centralized model. To obtain the diversity in molecular probes to match the diversity of disciplines and biological problems being studied, research labs must make the significant investments in radiochemistry capability described above (and make their own tracers) or must obtain tracers at high cost from centralized or core production facilities.

1.3 Decentralized production

As technologies advance that simplify the processes involved in making tracers, an alternative, *decentralized,* approach to probe production can be envisioned (Fig. 1). In this paradigm, researchers and clinicians are enabled with the resources to produce on-demand doses of PET probe of interest *themselves*, at low cost, in an automated, user-friendly device. These technologies are aimed at synthesis, purification, and quality control of the PET tracer. Cyclotrons for production of radioisotopes such as fluorine-18 will likely still remain prohibitively expensive for widespread use, even in light of significant reductions in size and cost that have been achieved by ABT's Biomarker Generator dose-on-demand cyclotron (ABT Molecular Imaging, Inc.). Decentralized production, at least for now, will thus still rely on production of radioisotope in centralized facilities. Fortunately, both production and distribution are already well-established, and F-18 can be obtained at very reasonable cost (about $2-4/mCi) in the United States and around the world.

In contrast to the centralized model, where the high costs of equipment, infrastructure, and personnel can be amortized over a large number of customers by producing large batches of PET tracers, decentralized production requires that *each* locally-used batch of a PET tracer to be produced economically. This paradigm shift requires a fundamental change in radiosynthesizer technology such that the following goals are achieved:

- Low capital cost
- Compact size with minimal infrastructure requirements (hot-cell space, etc.)
- User-friendly operation
  - Simple setup and cleanup
  - Fully automated tracer production including synthesis, purification, quality control, and formulation
  - Operation by existing lab technicians
- Multiple runs per day (especially back-to-back production of different tracers)
- cGMP support (e.g. automated batch records, reagents available as kits)
- Integrated quality control
- Ability for end-users to customize/develop syntheses

The last point is important because it will take tremendous effort to develop synthesis protocols for the many currently known and to be discovered tracers. Flexibility in the process enables the entire base of end-users to participate in new method development to ensure a wide diversity of tracers will become available in kit form.

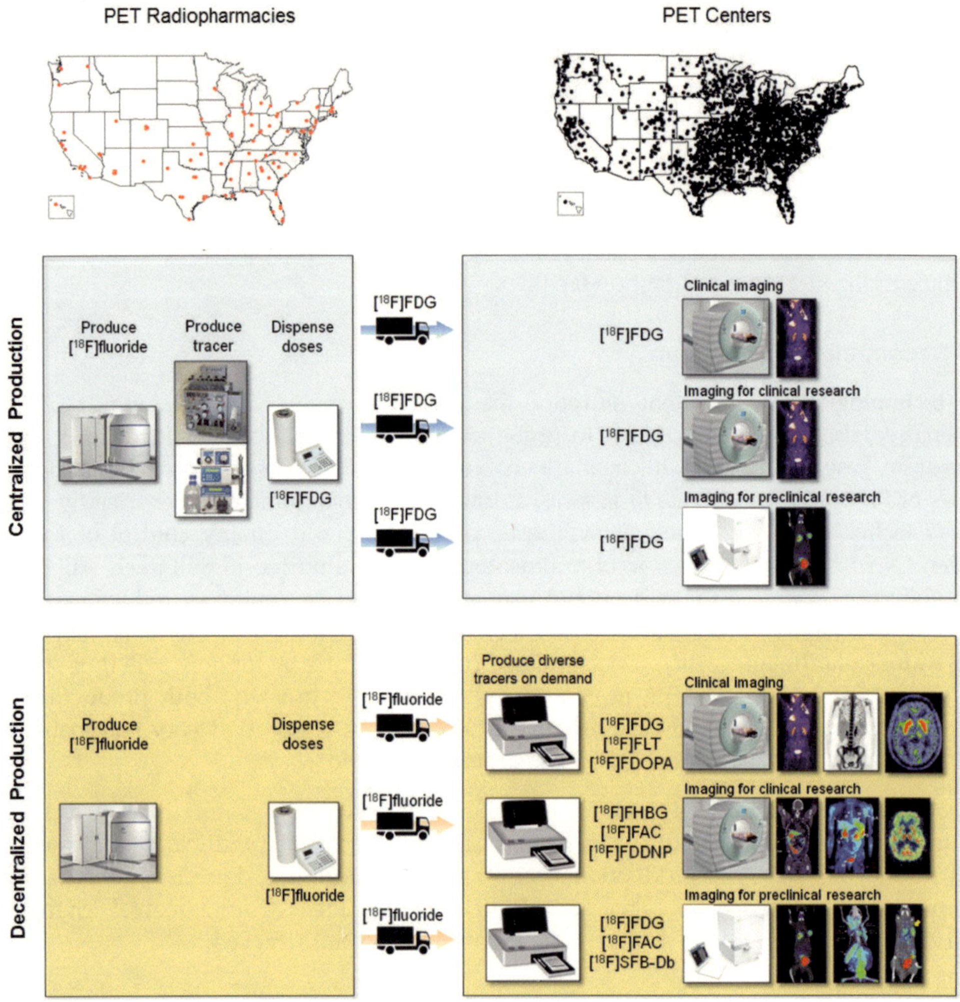

Fig. 1. Centralized and decentralized models of PET tracer production.

A number of research and development efforts in academia and industry are developing technologies that meet many of these needs. Kit-based macroscale radiosynthesizers on the market today are a starting point (Section 3.1), but ultimately microscale systems (Section 3.2) that offer fully integrated radiochemistry solutions on the benchtop will be needed. Several proof-of-concept microfluidic efforts have been described in the scientific literature and several aspects are already beginning to find their way into commercial products. In addition to cassette-based macroscale synthesizers and fully-integrated microscale systems, parallel advances in fundamental radiochemistry (Section 3.3) are resulting in increased yields under milder conditions and simplified purifications. This will increase the diversity of tracers that can be easily adapted into macroscale kit or microfluidic chip format to standardize their production.

2. Emerging technologies

2.1 Kit-based radiochemistry systems

The availability of simple-to-use kits and automated instruments has completely transformed certain areas of biology and biochemistry, putting powerful assays at the fingertips of the masses. For example, polymerase chain reaction (PCR) assays can be performed today on inexpensive equipment by staff with minimal training. In general, kits simplify assays by (i) reducing reagent preparation and setup time, (ii) reducing the possibility of human error or contamination, (iii) facilitating cleanup, and (iv) simplifying operation through automation. Similarly, kits designed for radiotracer production are beginning to put the capability to make PET tracers directly into the hands of the scientists and clinicians who need them.

Once established in kit form and made available to customers, a given synthesis becomes standardized and enables straightforward and reliable production at many different locations. A further advantage of kits is the simplification of reagent handling. Rather than individually managing multiple reagents, the customer need only to manage the kit as a single unit, greatly simplifying compliance with FDA regulations concerning production of tracers for injection into humans.

2.1.1 General approach

Traditional automated radiosynthesizers are built from fixed components, including reaction vial(s), heater(s), tubing, reagent reservoirs, and electronic valves. Reagents are carefully prepared by the operator and loaded into the reagent reservoirs before the start of synthesis. The system performs automated steps to synthesize—and in some cases—purify and formulate a tracer. After production, the system may perform an automated cleaning protocol to eliminate chemical residue from all wetted components and prepare the system for the subsequent production run.

Recently, many commercial groups have made the important technical advance of developing single-use cassette-based synthesizers to dramatically simplify reagent preparation, eliminate cleaning time, and reduce system complexity by eliminating the need for cleaning. The aim of these one-probe, one-cassette synthesizers is to make PET more accessible to laboratory scientists and easy to use by general lab personnel. These systems typically require a new disposable cassette plus a set of reagents (including consumables such as purification cartridges and filters) for each production run. The cassette itself contains most, or all, of the fluid path to accomplish the synthesis. This fluid path consists of valves, a reaction vessel, reagent reservoirs and pumps, and tubing to connect F-18 source, cartridges, and the collection vial. Pinch valves or stopcock valves are generally used for flow control because they allow a clear separation between an inexpensive fluid-contacting component (i.e. the valve itself) and a more expensive valve actuator (e.g. stopcock rotator) that is part of the fixed system onto which the cassettes are installed. Similarly, pumping is often achieved using pressurized inert gas, or by controlling disposable syringes with motion actuators in the fixed system. To reduce complexity and manufacturing costs, in some systems, the fluid path is molded in a manifold structure, such as a bank of stopcock valves.

After a synthesis run, the cassette is discarded and minimal or no cleaning is required. If the scale of the run is high, there can be high level of residual radioactivity remaining in the cassette (e.g. in purification cartridges). In some systems, one must simply wait for the activity to decay to a safe level before removing the cassette and installing a new one for the next run. However, several systems are designed for multiple back-to-back runs, enabling easy and safe cassette replacement with little downtime between syntheses of the same or different tracer. For example, a wash solution may be flushed through the fluid path to a shielded waste container before cassette removal to reduce the radiation dose to the operator. Another approach, taken in the IBA Synthera, is to automatically eject the cassette (while simultaneously cutting the tubing to the collection vial), and drop the cassette into a shielded waste container to isolate the activity and protect the operator. Disposing of cassettes after synthesis also eliminates the possibility of cross-contamination from one tracer to another. It may also enhance reliability, because many components that would otherwise wear or degrade (e.g. seals) in a conventional system would be automatically replaced with fresh components for each run in a cassette-based system.

Mass-produced, probe-specific kits used on a single platform will help standardize radiosynthesis protocols and quality control methods, improving reproducibility and lowering cost. Because the cassettes are intended to be disposed, they are designed to be mass-manufacturable at a low cost relative to the reagent cost. This often implies using inexpensive plastic materials that can easily be formed by molding processes. In many cases, this introduces limitations into the range of reaction conditions (e.g. temperature, pressure, solvents, etc.) that can be implemented in the cassette. New developments in radiochemistry could mitigate this limitation by enabling reactions to be performed under milder conditions (see Section 3.3).

2.1.2 Commercial kit-based systems

There are currently several commercially-available systems that are designed around this concept of reagent kits (Fig. 2).

ABT Molecular Imaging, Inc. "Biomarker Generator". The Biomarker Generator comprises a miniature cyclotron that produces doses of [^{18}F]fluoride (and potentially other isotopes in the future) on demand (e.g. 20 mCi), coupled to a dose-on-demand chemistry module that uses tracer-specific disposable cassettes (ABT Molecular Imaging, Inc.). Unlike other systems, the chemistry module does not require a hot cell but rather includes integrated shielding sufficient to protect operators from the single dose level of radioactivity. Furthermore, it is coupled to an automated QC testing system. A small aliquot of the formulated tracer is diverted to the QC system and the results automatically incorporated into the batch record. The remainder of the tracer is loaded directly into special syringe body that can be used directly for injection into the subject.

Bioscan, Inc. "F18-Plus". This system (Bioscan, Inc.) consists of two compact modules: an FDG-Plus module (for fluorination and deprotection processes) and a ReFORM-Plus module (for formulation) that together provide ten 3-way valves and two reactors. Preassembled sets of tubing, syringes, vials, and a stopcock valve manifold serve as disposable "cassettes." These are installed by the operator, placing components according to a fluid diagram depicted on the front panel of the instrument. Many other systems provide the cassette as essentially a rigid assembly, which may be slightly more straightforward to install.

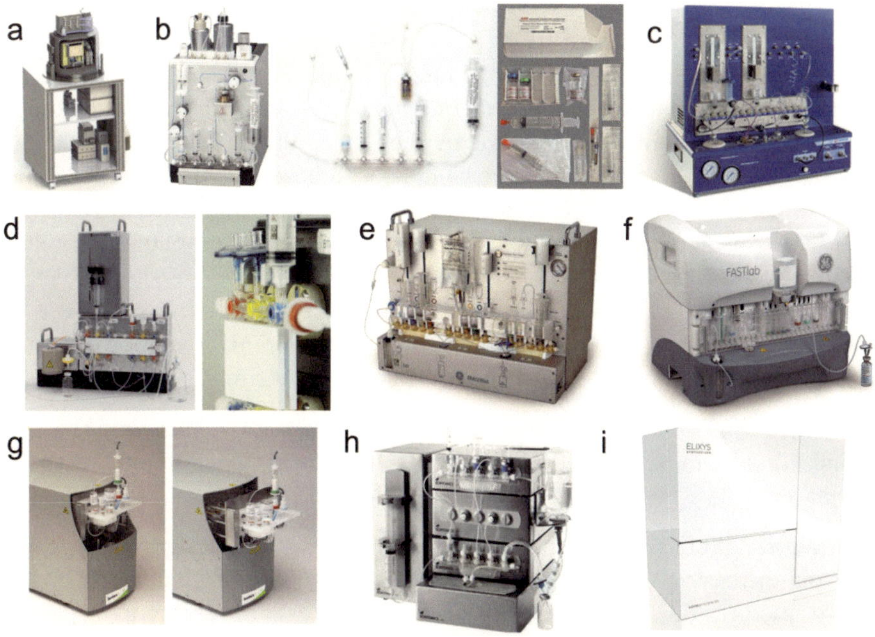

Fig. 2. Commercial cassette-based radiosynthesizers. (a) ABT Biomarker Generator. (b) BIOSCAN F-18 Plus synthesizer (left), disposable cassette (middle), and reagent kit (right). (c) Comecer Taddeo. (d) Eckert & Ziegler PharmTracer. (e) GE TRACERlab MX. (f) GE FASTlab. (g) IBA Synthera in operation (left) and during cassette ejection (right). (h) SCINTOMICS GRP module. (i) Sofie Biosciences ELIXYS.

Comecer "Taddeo". At the time of writing, the Taddeo system (Comecer) is marketed for production of ^{64}Cu-ATSM, but appears to be designed as a more universal synthesis module. Cassettes are based on a stopcock manifold with 15 zero-dead-volume valves, and two reaction vessels are supported.

Eckert & Ziegler "Modular-Lab PharmTracer". The PharmTracer system (Eckert & Ziegler 2011) builds on the strengths (e.g. flexibility and extensibility) of the Eckert & Ziegler Modular-Lab system. Cassettes based on stopcock-manifolds of different sizes (i.e. different numbers of valves) can implement synthesis protocols of varying complexity. The fixed part of the system can be configured to match the desired cassette configuration. The fact that the cassettes use common, off-the-shelf components means they can be reconfigured to develop new protocols.

GE "TRACERlab MX" and "FASTlab". The TRACERlab MX is currently the most widely used synthesis module with disposable cassettes. The FASTlab (GE Healthcare) is a refined version of the TRACERlab, but has highly optimized cassettes and synthesis protocols providing among the highest [^{18}F]FDG yields in the industry. Furthermore, unlike most other cassette-based modules, reagents are pre-loaded, simplifying setup by the operator.

While this simplifies routine production, it hinders development of protocols. Post-synthesis cleaning reduces residual radiation to <0.8% of the starting activity, enabling back-to-back synthesis runs.

IBA "Synthera". The IBA Synthera (IBA) performs one-pot syntheses involving up to four reagents in a compact cassette, the "Integrated Fluidic Processor (IFP)". Tracer-specific cassettes and reagent sets are available for a number of ^{18}F-labeled tracers. Synthera is one of the most compact radiosynthesizers on the market: up to three units fit in a standard mini cell, enabling modular expansion to more complex syntheses. A compact HPLC module is also available containing pump, detectors, and column that can be used for tracers that require HPLC purification. The Synthera system has a mechanism for automatically ejecting the cassette after the synthesis to enable multiple runs. The used cassette (which contains substantial residual activity on purification cartridges, etc.) drops down into a shielded waste container, permitting the hot cell to be opened with minimal radiation exposure to the operator during installation of the cassette for the subsequent run.

SCINTOMICS "GRP (Good Radiopharmaceutical Practice)" Module. This recently commercialized system (SCINTOMICS GmbH) for the production and dispensing of radiopharmaceuticals is based upon stopcock-manifold cassettes.

***Sofie Biosciences** "ELIXYS".* Most of the above systems are designed for "single-pot" syntheses, and increasing the number of synthesis steps to accommodate other tracers either requires user modification of the system, which may obviate the ability to use the cassette, or purchasing additional modules and thereby dramatically increasing the cost of the overall system. The design goal of the ELIXYS system (Sofie Biosciences, Inc.) was to develop a new PET radiosynthesis platform for probe discovery, development, and production that has the flexibility to accommodate a wide range of radiosynthesis conditions, including high temperatures and pressures and multi-pot reactions, to increase diversity in classes of imaging probes. After development and optimization of a tracer, the same system can be used for routine production for research or clinical use.

At the heart of the ELIXYS system is a mechanism to robotically cap the vessel with a "stopper" during sealed reaction steps (Fig. 3), thereby removing all tubing and valves from exposure to high vapor pressures generated during heating of volatile solvents to high temperatures (Herman et al. 2011)(Herman et al. Submitted). Exposure of these components leads to numerous problems that fundamentally limit the capabilities (i.e. range of pressures and temperatures possible) in other systems. Standard vials are loaded into a temperature control fixture with unique spring-loaded design to maintain good thermal contact despite natural variations in vial size. All reactors can be moved to individual positions via computer control to perform unit operations including reagent additions, evaporations, sealed reactions, transfers, and vial removal. Each reactor has an associated disposable cassette that was designed with both probe development, and optimization and routine probe production in mind; each contains up to 10 reagent vials, two cartridge purification positions, three stopcock valves, and two waste vials. By merging easy cassette configurability with an intuitive software platform, the user is able to conduct probe development and optimization and, on the same system, standardize a final protocol for routine use. Additional unique features of the system include a robot to move vials from storage positions to one of two needle ports in each cassette for delivery into to the reaction vessel. The reagent system trades off the complexity of motion by eliminating numerous valves and vastly simplifies the cassette design. A further advantage is that reagent vials remain sealed until delivered to the reaction vessel, thus preventing exposure of sensitive reagents to the atmosphere, which is critical for long multistep radiosynthesis.

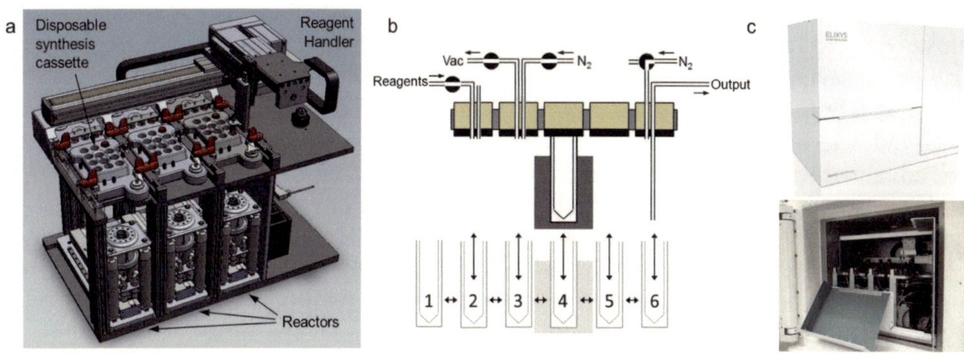

Fig. 3. Sofie Biosciences' universal synthesizer, ELIXYS. (a) 3D schematic of main components. (b) Principle of operation to circumvent issues with high vapor pressures that arise at high temperatures in volatile solvents. This reaction vessel can be moved among 6 different positions and sealed (raised) to a stopper or other interface depending on the desired operation. (c) Photograph of ELIXYS inside a mini-cell.

2.1.3 Millifluidic or minifluidic systems

In addition to the above commercially available systems, there are efforts underway at several companies to develop miniaturized kit-based systems based on the idea of microfluidics. The main distinction from the other, macroscale cassettes previously discussed is that these approaches strive to dramatically reduce manufacturing cost by integrating fluid path, valves, and other components directly into a large "chip", rather than requiring assembly/connection of separate components. Although similar to microfluidics in many ways, the approaches in millifluidics/minifluidics underway generally have larger components (e.g. mm to cm) and volumes (100s of μL) than the true microfluidic efforts described in the next section. Systems are in development at Trasis (Trasis)(Voccia et al. 2009) and GE Healthcare (Christian Rensch et al. 2011). In both platforms, chips are structured in a layered manner to form channels, diaphragm valves (from thin, flexible plastic sheets), inlets and outlets, etc. In the system from GE Healthcare, the diaphragm of the valve is part of the chip, while the solenoid actuator exists in the fixed system. The Trasis system employs pressurized gas delivered by an external system to actuate diaphragm valves. It appears that both systems, while more compact than traditional macroscale modules, would still have to be operated inside a hot cell.

2.2 Microfluidics

Unfortunately, the above macroscale systems still do not address some of the fundamental limitations to PET probe production previously discussed, namely infrastructure requirements, high cost, and need for additional equipment for purification and QC. Another technology that looks promising in its ability to support the decentralized model of PET probe production is microfluidics. Operations for synthesis, purification, and QC can potentially be integrated into a compact, inexpensive device that implements the whole pipeline of PET tracer production beginning with a supply of F-18 from existing commercial radiopharmacies.

The use of micro-reaction technology in many areas of chemistry has grown tremendously over the past several years, due primarily to the highly precise control of reaction conditions that is possible through rapid mixing and heat transport, leading to improved reaction speeds and selectivity compared to macroscale approaches (McMullen and Jensen 2010). These advantages are particularly relevant to the production of radiotracers incorporating short-lived isotopes, leading to a reduction in the amount of required starting material (e.g. radioisotope) and thus the thickness of radiation shielding. A further advantage of microfluidics is the ability to manipulate fluids and perform reactions in extremely small volumes, which are well-matched to the minute mass quantities of radiolabeled tracers needed for PET imaging (e.g. 6 pmol for typical human scan). To exploit numerous advantages of working at small scale, a number of research groups have recently explored microfluidic technology platforms for the production of radiotracers. These efforts have been described in several excellent review articles (Arkadij M. Elizarov 2009)(Miller 2009)(Audrain 2007)(S. Y. Lu and Pike 2007)(Miller et al. 2010).

Microfluidic platforms generally possess a high degree of integration of fluid pathways and active components such as valves, leveraging parallel fabrication techniques such as photolithography from the microelectronics industry and sometimes using expensive materials such as plastics. Such techniques promise to minimize the cost of microfluidic devices produced in high volumes, making them well suited to the disposable one-tracer-one-chip model for decentralized PET tracer production described above.

The myriad of microfluidic platforms that have been explored for chemical reactions can be classified into three basic formats: (i) flow-through (or continuous flow), (ii) droplet or slug, and (iii) batch. In flow-through systems, streams of two or more reagents are mixed and then reacted by flowing through a capillary with a predetermined residence time unit held at a constant temperature. Synthesis of most PET tracers requires multiple reaction steps, often in different solvents. To accommodate this need, liquid-liquid extraction and other processes have been developed in continuous format to enable multi-step reactions (Sahoo et al. 2007). Droplet and slug systems are a variant of flow-through systems, in which individual droplets or slugs (with reaction volumes as low as tens of nanoliters) are separated by an immiscible carrier fluid. Batch microfluidic chip designs use microvalves to isolate small batches of reagents in chambers, providing enhanced control of small volumes including sophisticated operations such as solvent exchange and drying processes (C.-C. Lee et al. 2005)(R. Michael van Dam et al. 2008)(Arkadij M. Elizarov et al. 2010a)(Bejot et al. 2010). These chips enable multi-step organic synthesis in nanoliter to microliter volumes.

2.2.1 Flow-through microfluidics

In a typical flow-through synthesizer, reagents are pumped at constant flow rate (e.g. using syringe pumps) through a fluid path that first induces rapid mixing of the reagents then maintains the mixed fluids under constant conditions (e.g. temperature) for a residence time determined by flow rate and the length/volume of the device. The fluid path may comprise a microfluidic chip or a capillary tube. Both approaches have similar channel dimensions but differ significantly in manufacturing technique. A heater or heat exchanger generally provides energy for the reaction. The large thermal mass of the chip relative to that of the small volume of liquid present within it at any given time ensures the liquid is maintained under very close to ideal isothermal conditions. Providing reaction energy by immersion in a microwave field (Issadore et al. 2009) has also been recently reported.

Flow-through synthesis of [^{18}F]FDG has been reported by a number of groups in glass-based chips (Steel et al. 2007), polymer-based chips (Gillies et al. 2006b), and capillary tubes (Wester et al. 2008)(Ungersboeck et al. 2011). The design of Gillies *et al.* (Gillies et al. 2006b) seeks to maximize mixing and flow-rate and achieved an acceptable yield in only seconds. Commercially available flow-through radiochemistry systems include the Advion Biosciences "NanoTek" (Advion Biosciences, Inc.), and the Scintomics "µ-ICR" (SCINTOMICS GmbH). Several other ^{18}F-labeled tracers have also been synthesized in flow-through systems, including [^{18}F]FMISO (Collier et al. 2010), [^{18}F]fallypride (S. Lu et al. 2009), and part of the synthesis of [^{18}F]FIAU (Anderson et al. 2010). In all cases above, solvent-exchange processes (both for drying of [^{18}F]fluoride, and between reaction steps) were performed off-chip. Typically, this is done via azeotropic evaporation in macroscopic apparatus. The mix of microfluidic and macroscopic elements makes the systems complex and inefficient and is not easily amenable to disposable configuration. Other techniques for drying and activating the fluoride are being developed that could be more readily integrated with flow-through synthesizers. In these approaches, the eluent from the trap-and-release cartridge (C. F. Lemaire et al. 2010)(Wessmann et al. 2011) or electrochemical cell (Saiki et al. 2010)(Alexoff et al. 1989)(C. Rensch et al. 2009)(Sadeghi et al. 2010)(Sadeghi et al. 2011) is directly used in the first reaction step.

Potentially alleviating the above restriction, glass-based and polymer-based chips for continuous solvent-exchange and continuous purification are being developed by investigators involved in the Radiochemistry on Chip (ROC) project (ROC-Project). The concept of this project is to develop a modular set of chips (solvent-exchange chip, reaction chip, purification chip, etc.) that can be assembled to perform different syntheses entirely in continuous-flow format.

2.2.2 Batch microfluidics

In contrast to continuous flow devices, batch devices (Fig. 4) operate on a "finite" batch of reagents all at once to produce a single batch of radiotracer. This batch may be used for a single imaging study, or may be subdivided for multiple studies. Batch microfluidic devices can perform processes that cannot readily be achieved in continuous flow microsystems such as evaporative solvent exchange (including drying of [^{18}F]fluoride, the most critical step in the synthesis of most ^{18}F-labeled tracers) and efficient cartridge purifications.

In general, batch microfluidics can manipulate total volumes much smaller than in continuous flow microfluidics. Performing the radiochemistry in small volume batches in the 40nL - 60µL range (C.-C. Lee et al. 2005)(Arkadij M. Elizarov et al. 2010a)(Bejot et al. 2010) offers numerous additional advantages, including reduced precursor consumption, and accelerated heating and cooling due to reduced mass of liquid. Other potential advantages (not yet established experimentally) include enhanced reaction kinetics by increased concentration of [^{18}F]fluoride, reduced radiolysis, simpler purification and quality control, and increased specific activity (ratio of the radiolabeled to the nonradiolabeled form) due to reduced contact with material surfaces (Berridge et al. 2009) and/or reduced amounts of reagents. Batch devices are therefore the microfluidic platform of choice in building compact radiosynthesizers capable of diverse multi-step syntheses. Beyond the essential functionality for synthesis, it may also be possible to integrate into the chip basic process monitoring and quality control functionality.

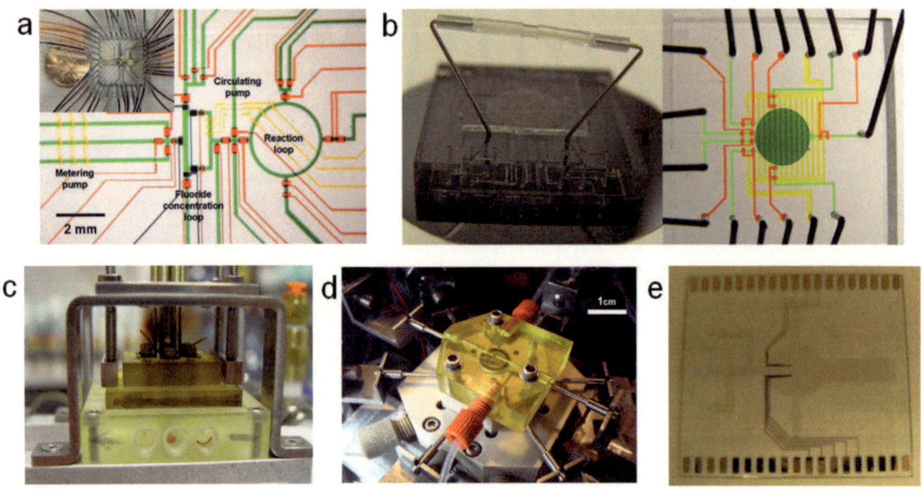

Fig. 4. Batch-format microfluidic platforms for synthesis of PET tracers. (a) Silicone rubber chip (Lee et al. 2005). (b) Scaled-up silicone rubber chip (Elizarov et al. 2010). (c) Chemically-inert pDCPD chip (van Dam et al. 2007) mounted in reagent loading interface and illustrating microvalve actuators. (d) "Open" chip (Bejot et al. 2010) mounted on reagent loading interface and illustrating mechanical actuators for integrated valves.
(e) All-electronic EWOD microfluidic chip (Keng et al. 2011).

Batch Microfluidics with Microvalves

One type of batch microfluidic chips resemble, in many respects, a tiny version of a conventional radiosynthesizer, except with microchannels, microvalves, and micropumps replacing their macroscopic counterparts. The multi-step on-chip synthesis of [^{18}F]FDG, beginning from [^{18}F]fluoride concentration, drying, fluorination, and hydrolysis was first performed as a proof-of-principle study in a microfluidic chip made from poly(dimethylsiloxane) (PDMS) silicone rubber (C.-C. Lee et al. 2005). Since this initial report, additional efforts have demonstrated production of quantities sufficient for preclinical imaging (several mCi) by improvements in chip design and scale-up of reaction volumes from 40nL to 5μL (Arkadij M. Elizarov et al. 2010a). PDMS chips contain tiny microchannels (with width and depth on the order of 100μm) as well as integrated microvalves and micropumps (Melin and Quake 2007) in which small volumes of reagents are manipulated to perform multistep chemical reactions. The underlying technology enables integrated manufacture of chips with tremendous sophistication. Furthermore, the inherent permeability of siliconerubber enables a novel approach to solvent exchange processes. Reagents can be pumped into a reaction chamber, and the chamber sealed by closing valves at all inlets/outlets. As the chip is heated by an external heat source, solvent is removed by pervaporation and permeation.

Despite several publications on these elastomeric chips, device reliability is limited by the inherent incompatibilities of the silicone rubber polymer with many solvents and reagents (Mukhopadhyay 2007), and suspected interaction of the PDMS material with [^{18}F]fluoride ion under certain conditions (W.-Y. Tseng et al. 2010), resulted in up to 95% of [^{18}F]fluoride lost (Arkadij M. Elizarov et al. 2010a). By re-engineering the chip to increase the burst pressure of the micro diaphragm valves and replacing the PDMS with an inert poly-dicyclopentadiene (pDPCD) polymer, the radiosynthesis of [^{18}F]FDG in sufficient quantity for human imaging was demonstrated (R.M. van Dam et al. 2007). The exploration of new materials was enabled by devising a chip architecture that did not require bonding between the device layers.

Rate of solvent evaporation is inherently limited by the gas-permeable membrane present in the above devices, and, for the 5μL volume in the latter reports, becomes a significant fraction of overall process time. Elizarov *et al.* (Bejot et al. 2010) reported the synthesis of N-succinimidyl-4-[^{18}F]fluorobenzoate ([^{18}F]SFB) in a slightly larger (60μL) microreactor in which the membrane is eliminated and evaporation occurs directly from an open liquid-air interface (Arkadij M. Elizarov et al. 2011). A synthesis time of 25 min was achieved, which is substantially faster than that possible on macroscopic modules (60-100 min). The valves were re-engineered in this chip to withstand even higher pressures, but they do not easily lend themselves to a separation between disposable and fixed elements.

Valveless Microfluidics

Recently our group described a novel platform for performing batch synthesis at the microscale, based on a technology known as "electrowetting-on-dielectric" (EWOD). Constructed from inorganic materials coated with a perfluoropolymer layer, these microfluidic chips provide much greater compatibility with diverse reagents and reaction conditions for microscale chemical synthesis. Liquid manipulation is performed electronically, eliminating the need for moving parts such as pumps and valves (inherently increasing reliability), and simplifying the chip and the external control system. Furthermore, it is possible to integrate additional electronically controlled functions into the chip such as sensors to monitor liquid volumes (Gong and Kim 2008) and composition (Schertzer et al. 2010)(Sadeghi et al. Submitted) as well as heaters and temperature sensors for heating liquid droplets or evaporating solvent (Nelson et al. 2010). EWOD devices have the additional advantage of digitally-programmable fluid pathways that could readily be configured for a wide variety of microscale batch organic syntheses, optimization, or screening studies for diverse tracers.

EWOD devices belong to a class of two-dimensional (2-D) droplet-based devices that manipulate droplets using their surface tension (Abdelgawad and Wheeler 2009). A typical EWOD microchip (Fig. 5) consists of two parallel plates: (i) a substrate patterned with electrodes and coated with dielectric and non-wetting layers, and (ii) a cover plate coated with a conductor (to act as a ground electrode), dielectric and non-wetting layers. Droplets are sandwiched into a disc shape between the plates, and electrical potential is applied to individual or multiple electrodes on the patterned substrate to achieve unit operations such as droplet generation, transport, splitting, and merging (S. K. Cho et al. 2003). The open structure of EWOD chips is particularly advantageous in achieving rapid solvent evaporations and solvent exchange. Though generally used for manipulation of aqueous samples and biochemical assays, EWOD chips can manipulate organic solvents (Chatterjee et al. 2006) and ionic liquids (Dubois et al. 2006) critical for performing chemical reactions. With this platform, radiosynthesis of [^{18}F]FDG, and 1-[^{18}F]fluoro-4-nitrobenzene ([^{18}F]FNB) has been demonstrated with high repeatability (S. Chen et al. 2010)(Pei Yuin Keng et al. 2010). So far, mCi quantities of tracer have been produced on chip (Supin Chen et al. 2011)(Pei Yuin Keng et al. Submitted), with further scale-up efforts underway.

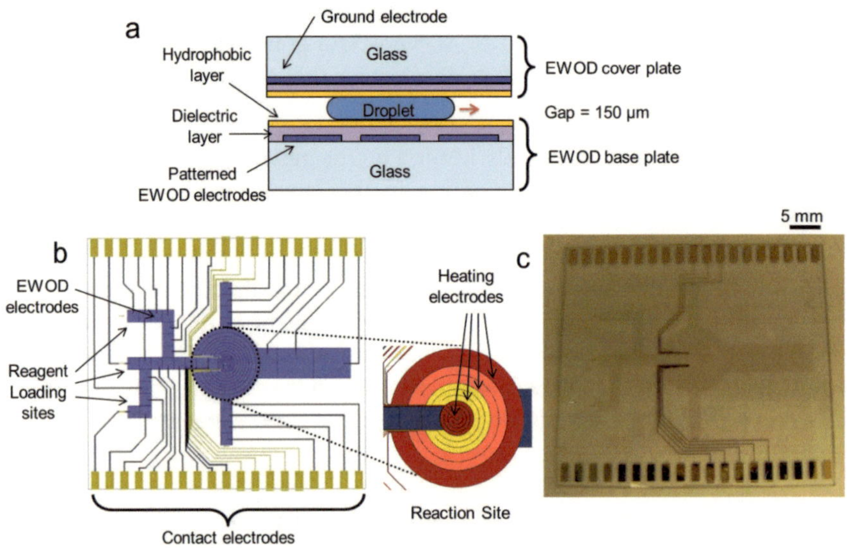

Fig. 5. Electronic microfluidic chip for synthesis of PET tracers. (a) Cross-section of electrowetting-on-dielectric (EWOD) chip illustrating a reagent droplet sandwiched between the base plate and cover plate. (b) Electrode design of a PET tracer synthesis chip. Reagents are moved from the inlet sites to the reaction site in the center of the chip. The reaction site is heated by electrodes to perform reactions or evaporations. During evaporations, vapor can readily escape from the open sides of the chip. (c) Photograph of an EWOD radiosynthesis chip. Adapted from Keng et al. 2011.

2.2.3 Outlook of microfluidic technologies

The main advantages of applying microfluidics to the radiosynthesis of PET tracers thus far have been reduced reaction times, higher synthesis yields, and increased throughput in reaction optimization (Pascali et al. 2010). Microfluidics can also reduce consumption of expensive precursors, increase speed of evaporations and other processes, reduce need for shielding, and potentially increase concentration of [^{18}F]fluoride to normal stoichiometric levels. While these are very important advances, microfluidics also has the potential for tremendous advances in miniaturization and integration that will reduce cost of synthesis, and potentially in the future encompass downstream processes such as purification and quality control testing.

An automated, compact, self-shielded, microscale synthesizer for the on-demand production of individual doses of PET probes in a biological or clinical laboratory setting would overcome many limitations inherent in traditional macroscale systems. First, the need for cost-prohibitive infrastructure associated with developing and bringing novel PET tracers to market will be removed. Second, because of the minute volumes, the amount and expense of cold compounds such as precursors used in radiosynthesis is decreased. Instead of ordering from a limited menu of tracers produced by a centralized radiopharmacy, a scientist or clinician would need only to purchase the benchtop microfluidic synthesizer for their existing laboratory, install their probe-specific "chip" of choice, add the associated radioisotope supplied by the commercial radiopharmacy, and push "START" on the PC control system. The integration of all liquid handling functionality and shielding within a small, self-contained device removes the need of secondary shielding (hot cells) while maintaining the safety of the end user within federal guidelines. Furthermore, a point-of-care device of this kind will address the serious issues facing SPECT by making PET a more practical clinical option and provide a convenient low-cost supply of PET probes for academic and pharmaceutical research.

2.3 Advances in radiochemistry

Recent advancements in microreactor and microfluidic radiosynthesizer technologies have triggered much investigation in modifying conventional radiochemistry approaches to yield PET tracers with higher yield and selectivity, shorter reaction times and milder reaction conditions. Taking advantage of these technology developments and automated high-throughput methods, radiochemists can now perform dozens of parallel optimization experiments in a single day, which was not possible a decade ago. This has catalyzed the discovery of new probes and radiosynthetic approaches. These investigations have also led to the emergence of HPLC-free chemistry, which is critical in realizing the decentralized production of PET tracers because it eliminates the need for expensive HPLC equipment and associated specialized personnel. In addition to fine-tuning reaction parameters, the use of ionic liquid and bulky alcohol as a solvent has also shown increased labeling efficiency, selectivity, and cleaner reaction product, which could facilitate automation, reducing the overall radiosynthesis time and simplifying purification using Sep-pak cartridges. Radiosynthetic strategies utilizing milder reagents and reaction conditions (reduced temperatures and pressure, reduced the use of solvents, etc.) are often more amenable to be performed in reaction systems made from polymeric materials such as disposable kits or microfluidics. These advances represent another avenue for enabling decentralization.

The state-of-the-art [^{18}F]fluoride ion ([^{18}F]F^-) radiolabeling approaches (Scheme 1) involve nucleophilic substitution of a precursor bearing a good leaving group (e.g., triflate and mesylate) in an aprotic organic solvent (usually acetonitrile, dimethyl sulfoxide or dimethylformamide).(Cai et al. 2008) The fluoride anion ($^{18}F^-$) is generated and delivered in [^{18}O]H_2O from the cyclotron, in which the fluoride anion is strongly hydrated by water molecules, hindering its nucleophilicity. To achieve highly reactive fluoride nucleophiles for substitution reactions, the fluoride anion is first transferred from the aqueous phase to the organic phase by complexing with a phase transfer catalyst such as Kryptofix (K_{222}) plus potassium carbonate as a weak base, or tetrabutylammonium hydroxide or tetrabutylammonium bicarbonate. Subsequently, trace amounts of water are removed via repeated cycles of azeotropic distillation with acetonitrile. The activated [^{18}F]KF/K_{222} complex is readily resolubilized in aprotic organic solvent for nucleophilic substitution reactions.

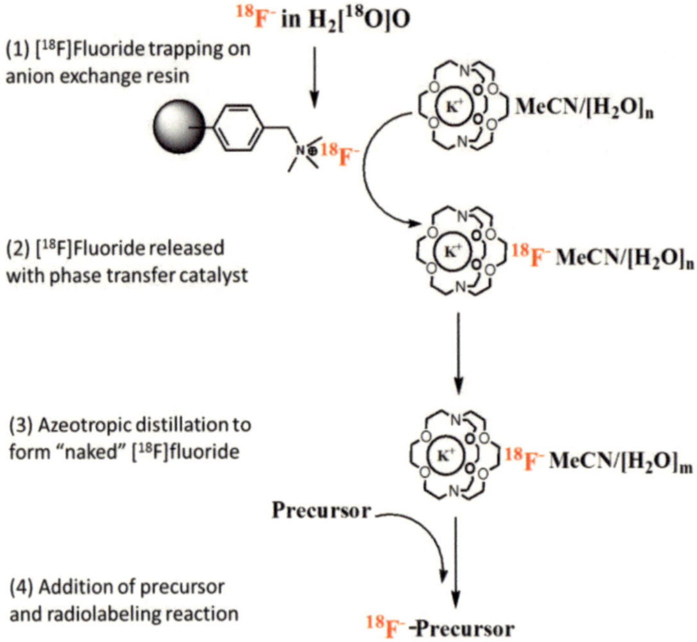

Scheme 1. General radiosynthetic scheme using no-carrier-added [^{18}F]fluoride ion generated from the cyclotron. The first step involves fluoride trapping on an anion exchange resin and release with a phase transfer catalyst. Water is removed via repeated cycles of azeotropic distillation to form the reactive ("naked") fluoride. Then a solution of precursor dissolved in aprotic solvent is added for the radiolabeling reaction.

Traditionally, macroscale radiosyntheses were designed to be performed in inert atmosphere, under anhydrous conditions, or other controlled environments, with evaporations and reactions taking place within a sealed reactor. The majority of fluorine-18 radiolabeling reactions are optimized at high temperature (usually above the boiling point of acetonitrile, which results in high vapor pressure built up in the reaction vessel), excess mass of precursor, and the use of harsh reagents. Along with these stringent reaction conditions, the majority of radiosynthetic strategies require HPLC purification to remove the excess precursors and undesired side products. Hence, radiosyntheses of PET probes have necessitated skilled radiochemists, and specialized, complex, and expensive synthesis modules--factors that have limited the availability of radiotracers. These conventional strategies are not easily implemented onto microfluidic chips (as described in Section 2.2.3) due to the difficulty in performing evaporations at the microscale and other factors.

Due to the increasing demand for PET probes and recent progress of microfluidic synthesis platforms (Miller 2009)(Arkadij M. Elizarov 2009), there is much interest on developing novel, simplified, robust and efficient radiosynthetic strategies to enable facile implementation of radiosyntheses both in the macro- and microscale synthesis modules. In this section, we focus on recent developments in (i) HPLC-free radiosynthesis method, (ii) alcohol and ionic liquid catalyzed radiosynthesis, and (iii) enzymatic fluorination using nucleophilic fluoride ion. The scope of this section is limited to selected (radio)chemistry strategies that have the potential to be implemented with current state-of-the-art automated microreactor and microfluidic platforms.

2.3.1 HPLC free radiochemistry

Current F-18 PET tracer synthesis protocols, with [^{18}F]FDG as the main exception, require HPLC purification due to the formation of radiolabeled or toxic side products that cannot be easily removed via solid phase extraction (SPE) cartridges. Thus, current methods necessitate purification via HPLC to meet the cGMP/FDA regulations before the tracer can be administered into humans (S. Yu 2006). Due to the disadvantages of using HPLC, it is desirable to modify current radiosynthetic strategies to use simpler purification methods, such as SPE. Such modification could potentially reduce the total synthesis time and radiation exposure by eliminating the need for concentrating the purified product before formulation of the PET tracer into injectable doses.

Recent examples have demonstrated the radiosynthesis of 3′-deoxy-3′[^{18}F]fluorothymidine [^{18}F]FLT and 1-α-D-(5′-deoxy-5′fluoro-(1S,2R,3S,4S)arabinofuranosyl)-2-nitroimidazole ([^{18}F]FAZA) followed by cartridge purification to obtain > 99% pure radiotracers (Nandy and Rajan 2009)(Nandy and Rajan 2010). In the simplified radiosynthesis of [^{18}F]FLT, Rajan *et al.* utilized a precursor with minimum-blocking groups, 5′-O-(4,4′-dimethoxytriphenilmethyl)-2,3′-anhydro-thymidine (DMTThy), followed by a single alumina cartridge purification to yield [^{18}F]FLT with >95% radiochemical purity (Nandy and Rajan 2009). The key to eliminating complicated HPLC purification was to reduce the amount of side products such as the leaving group and protecting group that were liberated during the substitution and deprotection reactions. (Nandy et al. 2010) Using the anhydrothymidine precursor (Machulla et al.), the Najan group successfully synthesized and purified [^{18}F]FLT using the custom-made alumina cartridge, which contained 7700 mg of dry alumina (compared with ~600 mg in a typical Sep-Pak alumina cartridge).. Although the anhydrothymidine precursor requires higher synthesis temperature, longer reaction time, and has slightly lower radiochemical yield in comparison to the nosylate-FLT precursor, the ability to purify the crude product using a single alumina cartridge is particularly attractive. Later, the Tang group further optimized the radiosynthesis conditions using the nosylate-FLT precursor to obtain pure [^{18}F]FLT with up to 40% radiochemical yield in 35 minutes using a series of Sep-Pak cartridges; thus eliminating the needs for HPLC purification.(G. Tang et al. 2010)

One of the well-known base catalyzed competing reactions is the bimolecular elimination (E2) reaction, where the leaving group is positioned anti-periplanar to a hydrogen attached to the adjacent carbon. Due to the large excess of base used in a typical radiochemistry reaction in comparison to the [^{18}F]fluoride anion, the majority of the precursor undergoes elimination reaction.(Chirakal et al. 1995) However, the presence of a large amount of side product complicates HPLC purification. Specifically in this version of [^{18}F]FLT synthesis, the elimination by-product, 2′,3′-didehydro-3′-deoxythymidine, an anti-HIV drug (Stauvidin), is permanently incorporated into DNA and results in cytotoxicity.(Grierson and Shields 2000)

By controlling the concentration of base and the precursor-to-base mole ratio, an optimal labeling efficiency could be achieved with minimal side products. In a quantitative investigation by Shuehiro *et al.*, the group showed that 300 ng of impurities is produced under typical [^{18}F]FLT synthesis conditions where the concentration of K_{222} and K_2CO_3 were 74 mmole and 40 mmole, respectively. As the base concentration of the phase transfer catalyst and base were reduced to 10 mM and 7 mM, respectively, the impurities decreased to 1 ng while achieving similar labeling efficiency.(Suehiro et al. 2007) This quantitative report not only showed that higher labeling efficiency could be achieved by reducing the base concentration, but also showed the potential to facilitate automation by enabling purification using SPE cartridges due to the reduced amount of impurities. Applying such methods to other tracers could similarly result in HPLC-free protocols for their production.

2.3.2 Solid phase supported radiosynthesis

The development of solid phase solid supports since 1970 has revolutionized peptide synthesis and combinatorial chemistry of libraries of small molecule analogues.(Ellman 1996) In solid phase organic synthesis, one of the reagents or substrates is bound onto a polymer solid support, while the second reactant (in solution) is flowed through the functionalized solid support. The advantages of solid phase organic synthesis relative to solution phase synthesis include ease of purification, selective product cleavage, recycling of precious catalyst and enabling polymer bound toxic reagents to be handled safely.(Früchtel and Jung 1996) In radiochemistry, large excess of precursor is typically needed to achieve high yield (>60%). To overcome the challenges in isolating the final product from the large excess of precursor, several groups have investigated a new radiosynthetic platform based on nucleophilic cleavage of solid-supported precursor using [^{18}F]fluoride ion (LUTHRA et al. 2003)(Frank Brady et al.)(L. J. Brown et al. 2007) with 70-91% labeling efficiency. In this strategy, a PET probe precursor with a sulfonate linker is attached on a solid phase support, which can be cleaved upon nucleophilic substitution by [^{18}F]F^-. In principle, only the substituted intermediate will be cleaved into the solution phase for the subsequent deprotection reaction, thus minimizing the amount of unreacted starting material in the reaction mixture. However, this solid phase approach has not been widely utilized or commercialized for other PET probes. The limited progress in this area could be due to the multistep synthesis to prepare the solid phase linkers. Additionally, this approach utilizes a perfluorinated linker to activate the nucleophilic substitution reaction, which could arguably decrease the specific activity of PET tracers (Chyng-Yann Shiue et al. 1985).

The Gourveneur group has worked out an alternative strategy to the solid phase approach based on the fluorous detagging of the precursor upon nucleophilic fluorination to simplify purification (Bejot et al. 2009). Taking advantage of the strong partition efficiency of the perfluorinated compound from aqueous and organic phases, fluorous phase extraction has been widely utilized in organic synthesis to facilitate purification and recovery of catalysts. Unlike the solid phase approach, in which the reaction mixture is heterogeneous (i.e., precursor on the solid phase while the nucleophile is in the solution phase), the fluorous detagging strategy is a solution-phase approach with the advantages of rapid reaction kinetics and simplified purification via selective phase separation from liquid. In this strategy, several alkylperfluorosulfonate tags with prosthetic groups such as reactive epoxide, azide, alkyne, and triflate were synthesized and radiolabeled with the

[18F]KF/K2.2.2 complex in acetonitrile. The radiolabeled product was collected via fluorous phase solid extraction (FPSE), in which the unreacted excess precursor tag with the fluorous phase remained on the FPSE cartridge, while the radiolabeled PET probe was eluted with high efficiency (Fig. 6). Additionally, the group has also demonstrated the synthesis of [18F]FMISO, [18F]fluoroethylcholine, and cis-4-[18F]fluoro-L-proline in 53%, 84%, and 42% radiochemical yields, respectively. These results showed that the fluorous detagging strategy could potentially be integrated onto microfluidic device as a universal radiosynthesis platform for the preparation of a wide range of PET probes (Fig. 6).

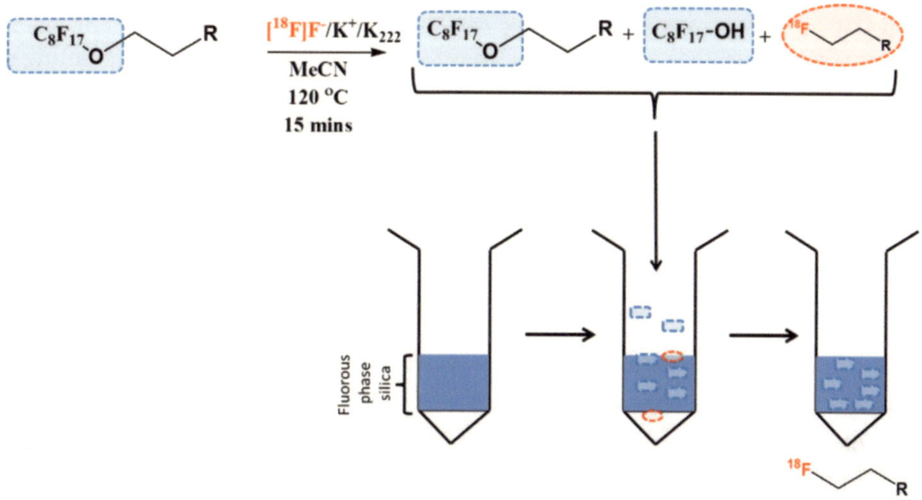

Fig. 6. Fluorous phase synthesis of [18F]F prosthetic groups in acetonitrile followed by fluorous solid phase extraction (FSPE). The reaction mixture is passed through a fluorous silica gel to collect only the fluorinated product.

2.3.3 Alcohol and ionic liquid catalyzed radiosynthesis

The conventional radiolabeling strategies using either quaternary ammonium or Kryptand/K+ as phase transfer catalysts to solubilize the fluoride anion into aprotic organic solvent require vigorous drying steps. This drying, solvent exchange and fluoride activation process is one of the most challenging and time consuming steps in radiosynthesis. In a typical F-18 radiolabeling reaction in an aprotic solvent, multiple cycles of azeotropic distillation are needed to completely remove the hydration shell around the anion to increase the nucleophilicity. To date, only a few types of batch microfluidic chips are capable of performing all the required radiolabeling processes including the drying step on chip, while flow-through microfluidic chips have utilized macroscale drying methods. Since 2002, Chi and his group have successfully demonstrated the (radio)fluorination of alkyl mesylate and [18F]FDG using CsF in the presence of ionic liquid as catalyst (Oh et al. 2011)(D. W. Kim et al. 2002). Ionic liquids are fused salts at room temperature; this class of material has been investigated as an alternative to conventional organic solvents due to their unique characteristics: (1) good solvent for a wide range of reagents, which is ideal in solubilizing different component of reagents into a single phase, (2) polar solvent but non-coordinating, which is very optimal for accelerating nucleophilic substitution reactions, and

(3) non-volatile, which is advantageous to prevent solvent evaporation and pressure build-up during fluorine-18 labeling reactions, the majority of which are performed at high temperature. In radiochemistry, this ionic liquid approach presents a new avenue, which has allowed n.c.a fluoride-18 substitution reactions to be performed in the presence of significant amounts of water (50 μL). As reported by Kim *et al.*, high radiolabeling yield could be attained in shorter time (as rigorous drying steps could be eliminated) at higher temperature with reduced side products. This synthetic strategy could potentially be applicable in current flow-through microfluidic technologies (as discussed in section 3.2.1) integrated with an anion exchange cartridge, in which the trapped fluoride-18 could be released with a mixture of phase transfer catalyst in aprotic solvent containing microliter volume of water to achieve reactive n.c.a. fluoride-18 ion, without additional drying steps. Current limitations of the ionic liquid strategy include high temperature synthesis (120 °C), which may not be applicable for all kinds of precursors, and the need of specialized ionic liquid for a specific reaction.

As mentioned earlier, the nucleophilicity of the fluoride anion decreases in the presence of protic solvents, such as water and alcohol, due to the strong hydrogen bonding interaction. However, recent investigation into bulky, tertiary non-protic alcohols (e.g.: t-butyl alcohol) has shown acceleration of the fluorination reaction rate using a nucleophilic fluoride source (e.g.: CsF, TBAF) while suppressing the formation of elimination by-products, thus have the potential to eliminate the needs of HPLC for the final purification. Furthermore, the resulting nucleophilic TBAF(t-butyl alcohol) complex is easy to handle, which facilitates automation. This strategy has been explored in the radiosynthesis of [^{18}F]FDG, [^{18}F]FLT, [^{18}F]F-FP-CIT, and [^{18}F]FMISO with a 2-3-fold increase in radiochemical yield in comparison to conventional methods reported in the literature.(D. W. Kim et al. 2010)(B. S. Moon et al. 2006) In these studies, the fluorination efficiency increases with the increase of steric hindrance of the bulky alcohol in the order of thexyl alcohol > t-amyl alcohol> t-butyl alcohol. Based on x-ray crystallography, the tertiary alcohol is postulated to enhance substitution efficiency and selectivity by the limited solvation of the fluoride anion, yielding a "flexible fluoride anion."(D. W. Kim et al. 2008) Additionally, the reactivity of the leaving group is enhanced by hydrogen bonding of the tertiary alcohol with the oxygen on the mesylate or triflate group. Under this protic environment, side reactions such as elimination, hydroxylation and intramolecular alkylation reactions, could be suppressed. Both the ionic liquid and the bulky alcohol strategies are particularly attractive for implementation of radiochemistry on microfluidic chips due to the high yield, short reaction time (~5 min), high chemoselectivity, and ease of handling the t-butyl alcohol / fluoride (TBAF) complex in comparison to the anhydrous TBAF in aprotic solvent.

2.3.4 Enzymatic radiofluorination

In nature, enzyme catalysis is highly stereoselective and efficient, lowering the activation barrier and thus enabling milder reaction conditions, shorter reaction times, and simplified purification methods. Recent development and discovery of the fluorinase enzyme (O'Hagan 2006)(Dong et al. 2004) has demonstrated the radiofluorination of (S)-adenosyl-L-methionine (SAM) and [^{18}F]fluoride anion with 95% radiochemical yield and 1 million-fold rate enhancement (Fig. 7a).(H. Deng et al. 2006) Based on the mechanistic studies of the fluorinase enzyme, substrate stabilization appears to be the most critical parameter in this

C-F enzymatic catalysis. Additionally, both crystallographic and theoretical studies suggest that the enzyme dehydrates the solvated fluoride ion through cooperative hydrogen bonding on the serine moieties in the active site (Fig 7b). These hydrogen bonding interactions around the naked fluoride ions decrease the calculated activation energy from 92 kJ/mol to 53 kJ/mole, which can explain the dramatic rate acceleration.(O'Hagan 2006) However, the fluorinase enzyme is extremely specific to the SAM substrate and thus is not applicable to any other substrates. To increase structural diversity of fluorinated biomolecules based on the fluorinase catalytic reaction, a base-swap biotransformation has been demonstrated in a single pot to yield 5′-fluorinated uridine derivatives.(Winkler et al. 2008) Although the fluorinase enzyme has shown potential in accelerating radiolabeling reactions and has the potential to be immobilized into microfluidics (Krenkova and Svec 2009), practical application of enzymatic catalysis is currently limited by their short shelf life, and their intolerance to harsh conditions such as non-aqueous environment and extreme temperatures, which currently hinders application to other fluorination reactions.

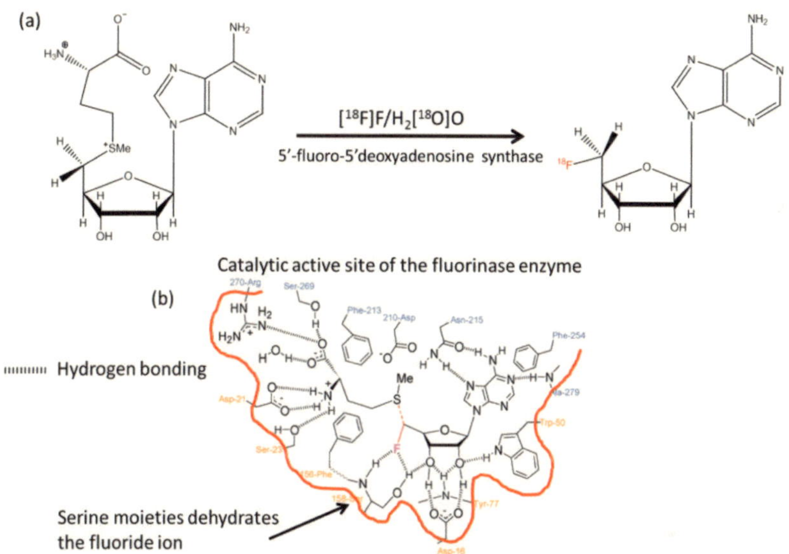

Fig. 7. (a) Enzymatic catalysis of (S)-adenosyl-L-methionine (SAM) and $[^{18}F]F^-$ to 5′-deoxyadenosine (5′-FDA) in using the fluorinase enzyme. (b) Illustration of cooperative hydrogen bonding interactions at the active site of the fluorinase enzyme, [18F]fluoride ion, and the SAM substrate as deduced by x-ray crystallography. Reproduced from O'Hagan 2006.

3. Conclusions

With the number of PET tracers with established research and clinical value increasing, the centralized model of PET tracer production will no longer be able to meet these demands. A paradigm shift to incorporate decentralized production is essential in order to enable imaging scientists to use desired tracers on demand in research or clinical settings. To enable decentralized production, new technologies and automation are needed that simplify tracer production, reduce the cost, size and complexity of equipment required, and eliminate the need for highly skilled radiochemists in routine tracer production. Kit-based radiosynthesizers are a significant step in this direction, with many excellent systems already on the market. Microfluidic technologies under development will further miniaturize and reduce costs of kits, as well as provide fundamental advantages in speed, yield, and perhaps specific activity. In parallel with engineering developments, advances in radiochemistry are making possible syntheses under simpler and milder conditions, thus facilitating their automation. Even with the advances to date, PET tracer production remains expensive and complex and out of reach of most labs. Further developments in miniaturized and automated purification as well as quality-control testing will be instrumental in bringing PET tracer production to the benchtop.

4. Acknowledgments

Financial support was provided in part provided by the Department of Energy Office of Biological and Environmental Research (DE-SC0001249, DE-SC0005056), the National Institutes of Health (R25CA098010) and the UCLA Foundation from a donation made by Ralph & Marjorie Crump for the UCLA Crump Institute for Molecular Imaging. The authors also thank Saman Sadeghi, Michael E. Phelps and Patrick Phelps for valuable feedback on the manuscript.

5. References

Abdelgawad, Mohamed, and Aaron R. Wheeler. (2009). "The Digital Revolution: A New Paradigm for Microfluidics." *Advanced Materials* 21 (8): 920-925.

ABT Molecular Imaging, Inc. Mini-cyclotron. Available from: http://advancedbiomarker.com/product_Mini-Cyclotron.php.

ABT Molecular Imaging, Inc..Micro-chemistry. Available from: http://www.advancedbiomarker.com/product_micro-chemistry.php.

Advion Biosciences, Inc. NanoTek Microfluidic Synthesis System. Available from: http://www.advion.com/biosystems/nanotek/nanotek-positron-emission-tomography.php.

Alexoff, David, David J. Schlyer, and Alfred P. Wolf. (1989). "Recovery of [18F]fluoride from [18O]water in an electrochemical cell." *International Journal of Radiation Applications and Instrumentation. Part A. Applied Radiation and Isotopes* 40 (1): 1-6.

Anderson, Harry, NagaVaraKishore Pillarsetty, Melchor Cantorias, and Jason S. Lewis. (2010). "Improved synthesis of 2′-deoxy-2′-[18F]-fluoro-1-[beta]-d-arabinofuranosyl-5-iodouracil ([18F]-FIAU)." *Nuclear Medicine and Biology* 37 (4): 439-442.

Audrain, Hélène. (2007). "Positron Emission Tomography (PET) and Microfluidic Devices: A Breakthrough on the Microscale?" *Angewandte Chemie International Edition* 46 (11): 1772-1775.

Bejot, Romain, Arkadij M. Elizarov, Ed Ball, Jianzhong Zhang, Reza Miraghaie, Hartmuth C. Kolb, and Véronique Gouverneur. (2011). "Batch-mode microfluidic radiosynthesis of N-succinimidyl-4-[18F]fluorobenzoate for protein labelling." *Journal of Labelled Compounds and Radiopharmaceuticals* 54 (3): 117-122.

Bejot, Romain, Thomas Fowler, Laurence Carroll, Sophie Boldon, Jane E Moore, Jérôme Declerck, and Véronique Gouverneur. (2009). "Fluorous Synthesis of 18F

Radiotracers with the [18F]Fluoride Ion: Nucleophilic Fluorination as the Detagging Process." *Angewandte Chemie International Edition* 48 (3): 586-589.

Berridge, M. S., S. M. Apana, and J. M. Hersh. (2009). "Teflon radiolysis as the major source of carrier in fluorine-18." *Journal of Labelled Compounds and Radiopharmaceuticals* 52 (13): 543-548.

Bioscan, Inc. F18-Plus Nucleophilic Fluorination System. Available from: http://www.bioscan.com/pet-nuclear-medicine/pet-chemistry-synthesizers/f18-plus-nucleophilic-fluorination-system.

Blom, Elisabeth, Farhad Karimi, and Bengt Långström. (2010). "Use of perfluoro groups in nucleophilic 18F-fluorination." *Journal of Labelled Compounds and Radiopharmaceuticals* 53 (1): 24-30.

Brady, Frank, Sajinder Luthra, and Edward, George Robins. (2003). Solid-phase fluorination of uracil and cytosine. International patent WO/2004/056400.

Brown, Lynda J., Denis R. Bouvet, Sue Champion, Alex M. Gibson, Yulai Hu, Alex Jackson, Imtiaz Khan, et al. (2007). "A Solid-Phase Route to 18F-Labeled Tracers, Exemplified by the Synthesis of [18F]2-Fluoro-2-deoxy-D-glucose." *Angewandte Chemie International Edition* 46 (6): 941-944.

Cai, Lisheng, Shuiyu Lu, and Victor W Pike. (2008). "Chemistry with [18F]Fluoride Ion." *European Journal of Organic Chemistry*. 2008 (17): 2853-2873.

Chatterjee, Debalina, Boonta Hetayothin, Aaron R. Wheeler, Daniel J. King, and Robin L. Garrell. (2006). "Droplet-based microfluidics with nonaqueous solvents and solutions." *Lab on a Chip* 6 (2): 199-206.

Chen, S., H. Ding, G.J. Shah, R.M. van Dam, and C-J Kim. (2010). EWOD Microdevices for Synthesis of 18F-Labeled Tracers for Positron Emission Tomography (PET). In *Technical Digest of the Solid-State Sensor, Actuator and Microsystems Workshop*, 37-40. Hilton Head Island, SC, June 6-10.

Chen, Supin, P.Y. Keng, R.M. van Dam, and C-J Kim. (2011). Synthesis of 18F-labeled probes on EWOD for positron emission tomography (PET) preclinical imaging. In *Proceedings of the 24th IEEE International Conference on Micro Electro Mechanical Systems*, 980-983. Cancun, MX, Jan 23-27.

Chirakal, Raman, Brian McCarry, Michael Lonegran, Gunter Firnau, and Stephen Garnett. (1995). "Base-mediated decomposition of a Mannose triflate during the synthesis of 2-deoxy-2-18F-fluoro-D-glucose." *Applied Radiation and Isotopes* 46 (3): 149-155.

Cho, Sung Kwon, Hyejin Moon, and C-J Kim. (2003). "Creating, transporting, cutting, and merging liquid droplets by electrowetting-based actuation for digital microfluidic circuits." *Journal of Microelectromechanical Systems* 12 (1): 70-80.

Churski, Krzysztof, Piotr Korczyk, and Piotr Garstecki. (2010). "High-throughput automated droplet microfluidic system for screening of reaction conditions." *Lab on a Chip* 10 (7): 816-818.

Chyng-Yann Shiue, Joanna S. Fowler, Alfred P. Wolf, Masazumi Watanabe, and Carroll D. Arnett. (1985). "Synthesis and Specific Activity Determinations of No-Carrier-Added Fluorine-18-Labeled Neuroleptic Drugs." *Journal of Nuclear Medicine* 26 (2): 181-186.

Coenen, H.H., P.H. Elsinga, R. Iwata, M.R. Kilbourn, M.R.A. Pillai, M.G.R. Rajan, H.N. Wagner Jr., and J.J. Zaknun. (2010). "Fluorine-18 radiopharmaceuticals beyond

[18F]FDG for use in oncology and neurosciences." *Nuclear Medicine and Biology* 37 (7): 727-740.

Collier, Thomas, Murthy Akula, and George Kabalka. (2010). Microfluidic synthesis of [18F]FMISO. *J Nucl Med.* 51 (Supplement 2): 1462

Comecer. Automatic module for synthesis of therapeutic radiopharmaceuticals model Taddeo. Available from: http://www.comecer.com/nuclear-medicine/radiochemistry/synthesis-modules/radio-pharmaceutical-synthesis-module-model-taddeo/.

van Dam, R. Michael, Carroll Edward Ball, Arkadij M. Elizarov, and Hartmuth C. Kolb. (2007). Fully-automated microfluidic system for the synthesis of radiolabeled biomarkers for positron emission tomography. United States Patent 7,829,032 B2.

van Dam, R.M., A.M. Elizarov, E. Ball, C.K-F Shen, H. Kolb, J. Rolland, L. Diener, et al. (2007). Automated Microfluidic Chip and System for the Synthesis of Radiopharmaceuticals on Human-Dose Scales. In *Technical Proceedings of the 2007 NSTI Nanotechnology Conference and Trade Show*, 3:300-303. Santa Clara, CA, May 20.

Daniels, Stephen, Siti Farah Md Tohid, Winnie Velanguparackel, and Andrew D Westwell. (2010). "The role and future potential of fluorinated biomarkers in positron emission tomography." *Expert Opinion on Drug Discovery* 5: 291-304.

Deng, Hai, Steven L. Cobb, Antony D. Gee, Andrew Lockhart, Laurent Martarello, Ryan P. McGlinchey, David O'Hagan, and Mayca Onega. (2006). "Fluorinase mediated C–18F bond formation, an enzymatic tool for PET labelling." *Chemical Communications* (6): 652-654.

Dong, Changjiang, Fanglu Huang, Hai Deng, Christoph Schaffrath, Jonathan B. Spencer, David O'Hagan, and James H. Naismith. (2004). "Crystal structure and mechanism of a bacterial fluorinating enzyme." *Nature* 427 (6974): 561-565.

Dubois, Philippe, Gilles Marchand, Yves Fouillet, Jean Berthier, Thierry Douki, Fatima Hassine, Said Gmouh, and Michel Vaultier. (2006). "Ionic Liquid Droplet as e-Microreactor." *Analytical Chemistry* 78 (14): 4909-4917.

Eckert & Ziegler. (2011). Modular-Lab PharmTracer. August 4. Available from: http://www.ezag.com/home/business-segments/radiopharma/modular-lab-synthesis-equipment/synthesis-labeling/modular-lab-pharmtracer.html.

Eddings, M.A., S. Olma, M. Wang, Y. Deng, H. Ding, N. Satyamurthy, K. Shen, and R.M. van Dam. (2009). Automated Radiochemistry Platform (ARC-P): Plug-and-play radiochemistry modules for reconfigurable radiosynthesis. Poster presented at the 18th International Symposium on Radiopharmaceutical Sciences (ISRS-18), July 12, Edmonton, AB.

Elizarov, Arkadij M. (2009). "Microreactors for radiopharmaceutical synthesis." *Lab on a Chip* 9 (10): 1326-1333.

Elizarov, Arkadij M., Carroll Edward Ball, Jianzhong Zhang, Hartmuth C. Kolb, Michael R. Van Dam, Lawrence Diener, Sean Ford, and Reza Miraghaie. (2010). Portable Microfluidic Radiosynthesis System for Positron Emission Tomography Biomarkers and Program Code. United States patent application 2011/0097245 A1.

Elizarov, Arkadij M., R. Michael van Dam, Young Shik Shin, Hartmuth C. Kolb, Henry C. Padgett, David Stout, Jenny Shu, Jiang Huang, Antoine Daridon, and James R. Heath. (2010a). "Design and Optimization of Coin-Shaped Microreactor Chips for PET Radiopharmaceutical Synthesis." *J Nucl Med* 51 (2): 282-287.

Elizarov, Arkadij M., Carl Meinhart, Reza Miraghaie, R. Michael Dam, Jiang Huang, Antoine Daridon, James R. Heath, and Hartmuth C. Kolb. (2010b). "Flow optimization study of a batch microfluidics PET tracer synthesizing device." *Biomedical Microdevices* 13 (1): 231-242.

Ellman, Jonathan A. (1996). "Design, Synthesis, and Evaluation of Small-Molecule Libraries." *Accounts of Chemical Research* 29 (3): 132-143.

Früchtel, Jörg S, and Günther Jung. (1996). "Organic Chemistry on Solid Supports." *Angewandte Chemie International Edition in English* 35 (1): 17-42.

GE Healthcare. FASTlab - PET Radiochemistry Solutions. Available from: http://www.gehealthcare.com/euen/fun_img/products/radiopharmacy/products/fastlab-index.html.

Geyer, Karolin, Jeroen D. C. Codée, and Peter H. Seeberger. (2006). "Microreactors as Tools for Synthetic Chemists - The Chemists' Round-Bottomed Flask of the 21st Century?" *Chemistry - A European Journal* 12 (33): 8434-8442.

Gillies, J.M., C. Prenant, G.N. Chimon, G.J. Smethurst, B.A. Dekker, and J. Zweit. (2006a). "Microfluidic technology for PET radiochemistry." *Applied Radiation and Isotopes* 64 (3): 333-336.

Gillies, J.M., C. Prenant, G.N. Chimon, G.J. Smethurst, W. Perrie, I. Hamblett, B. Dekker, and J. Zweit. (2006b). "Microfluidic reactor for the radiosynthesis of PET radiotracers." *Applied Radiation and Isotopes* 64 (3): 325-332.

Gong, Jian, and C-J Kim. (2008). "All-electronic droplet generation on-chip with real-time feedback control for EWOD digital microfluidics." *Lab on a Chip* 8 (6): 898-906.

Grierson, John R., and Anthony F. Shields. (2000). "Radiosynthesis of 3'-deoxy-3'-[18F]fluorothymidine: [18F]FLT for imaging of cellular proliferation in vivo." *Nuclear Medicine and Biology* 27 (2): 143-156.

Herman, Henry, Graciela Flores, Kevin Quinn, Melissa Esterby, Mark Eddings, Sebastian Olma, Huijiang Ding, et al. (Submitted). "Plug-and-play modular radiosynthesizer for multi-pot reactions involving high-pressure conditions."

Herman, Henry, Graciela Flores, Kevin Quinn, Melissa Esterby, Gaurav J. Shah, Michael E. Phelps, Nagichettiar Satyamurthy, and R. Michael van Dam. (2011). Multi-pot radiosynthesizer capable of high-pressure reactions for production of [18F]FAC and analogs. *J Nucl Med.* 52 (Supplement 1): 1440.

IBA. Synthera® for: 18FDG, 18FLT, 18FCH, 18NaF. Available from: http://www.iba-cyclotron-solutions.com/products-cyclo/synthera.

Issadore, David, Katherine J. Humphry, Keith A. Brown, Lori Sandberg, David A. Weitz, and Robert M. Westervelt. (2009). "Microwave dielectric heating of drops in microfluidic devices." *Lab on a Chip* 9 (12): 1701-1706.

Iwata, Ren. (2004). *Reference Book of PET Radiopharmaceuticals*. 2004.10 ed. CYRIC Tohoku University.

Keng, Pei Yuin, Supin Chen, Hui-Jiang Ding, Sam Sadeghi, Michael E. Phelps, N. Satyamurthy, C-J Kim, and R. Michael van Dam. (2010). Optimization of radiosynthesis of molecular tracers in EWOD microfluidic chip. In *Proceedings of the Fourteenth International Conference on Miniaturized Systems for Chemistry and Life Sciences*, 668-670. Groningen, The Netherlands, Oct 3-7.

Keng, Pei Yuin, Supin Chen, Huijiang Ding, Saman Sadeghi, Gaurav J. Shah, Alex Dooraghi, Michael E. Phelps, *et al.* (2011). Micro-chemical synthesis of molecular probes on an electronic microfluidic device. *Proceedings of the National Academy of Sciences of the United States of America*. DOI: 10.1073/pnas.1117566109.

Kim, Dong Wook, Hwan-Jeong Jeong, Seok Tae Lim, and Myung-Hee Sohn. (2010). "Facile nucleophilic fluorination of primary alkyl halides using tetrabutylammonium fluoride in a tert-alcohol medium." *Tetrahedron Letters* 51 (2): 432-434.

Kim, Dong Wook, Choong Eui Song, and Dae Yoon Chi. (2002). "New Method of Fluorination Using Potassium Fluoride in Ionic Liquid: Significantly Enhanced Reactivity of Fluoride and Improved Selectivity." *Journal of the American Chemical Society* 124 (35): 10278-10279.

Kim, Dong Wook, Hwan-Jeong Jeong, Seok Tae Lim, and Myung-Hee Sohn. (2008). "Tetrabutylammonium Tetra(tert-Butyl Alcohol)-Coordinated Fluoride as a Facile Fluoride Source." *Angewandte Chemie International Edition* 47 (44): 8404-8406.

Krenkova, Jana, and Frantisek Svec. (2009). "Less common applications of monoliths: IV. Recent developments in immobilized enzyme reactors for proteomics and biotechnology." *Journal of Separation Science* 32 (5-6): 706-718.

Lasne, Marie-Claire, Cécile Perrio, Jacques Rouden, Louisa Barré, Dirck Roeda, Frédéric Dolle, and Christian Crouzel. (2002). Chemistry of β +-Emitting Compounds Based on Fluorine-18. In *Contrast Agents II*, ed. Werner Krause, 201-258. Berlin: Springer Berlin / Heidelberg.

Lee, C.-C., G. Sui, A. Elizarov, C.J. Shu, Y.-S. Shin, A.N. Dooley, J. Huang, et al. (2005). "Multistep Synthesis of a Radiolabeled Imaging Probe Using Integrated Microfluidics." *Science* 310 (5755): 1793-1796.

Lee, Jessamine Ng, Cheolmin Park, and George M. Whitesides. (2003). "Solvent Compatibility of Poly(dimethylsiloxane)-Based Microfluidic Devices." *Analytical Chemistry* 75 (23): 6544-6554.

Lemaire, Christian F., Joël J. Aerts, Samuel Voccia, Lionel C. Libert, Frédéric Mercier, David Goblet, Alain R. Plenevaux, and André J. Luxen. (2010). "Fast Production of Highly Reactive No-Carrier-Added [18F]Fluoride for the Labeling of Radiopharmaceuticals." *Angewandte Chemie International Edition* 49 (18): 3161-3164.

Lu, S. Y., and V. W. Pike. (2007). Micro-reactors for PET Tracer Labeling. In *PET Chemistry: The Driving Force in Molecular Imaging*, ed. P. Schubinger, 271-287. Berlin: Springer Berlin / Heidelberg.

Lu, Shuiyu, Anthony M. Giamis, and Victor W. Pike. (2009). "Synthesis of [18F]fallypride in a micro-reactor: rapid optimization and multiple-production in small doses for micro-PET studies." *Current radiopharmaceuticals* 2 (1): 1-13.

Luthra, Sajinder, Frank Brady, Harry Wadsworth, Alexander Gibson, and Matthias Glaser. (2002). Solid-phase nucleophilic fluorination. International patent WO/2003/002157.

Machulla, H.-J., A. Blocher, M. Kuntzsch, M. Piert, R. Wei, and J.R. Gierson. "Simplified labeling approach for synthesizing 3'-deoxy-3'[18F]fluorothymidine ([18F]FLT)." *J. Radioanal Nucl Chem* 243 (3): 843-846.

Martarello, Laurent, Christoph Schaffrath, Hai Deng, Antony D Gee, Andrew Lockhart, and David O'Hagan. (2003). "The first enzymatic method for C–18F bond formation: the synthesis of 5'-[18F]-fluoro-5'-deoxyadenosine for imaging with PET." *Journal of Labelled Compounds and Radiopharmaceuticals* 46 (13): 1181-1189.

McMullen, Jonathan P., and Klavs F. Jensen. (2010). "Integrated Microreactors for Reaction Automation: New Approaches to Reaction Development." *Annual Review of Analytical Chemistry* 3 (1): 19-42.

Melin, Jessica, and Stephen R. Quake. (2007). "Microfluidic Large-Scale Integration: The Evolution of Design Rules for Biological Automation." *Annual Review of Biophysics and Biomolecular Structure* 36 (1): 213-231.

Miller, Philip W. (2009). "Radiolabelling with short-lived PET (positron emission tomography) isotopes using microfluidic reactors." *Journal of Chemical Technology & Biotechnology* 84 (3): 309-315.

Miller, Philip W, Hélène Audrain, Dirk Bender, Andrew J deMello, Antony D Gee, Nicholas J Long, and Ramon Vilar. (2011). "Rapid Carbon-11 Radiolabelling for PET Using Microfluidics." *Chemistry - A European Journal* 17 (2): 460-463.

Miller, Philip W., Andrew J. deMello, and Antony D. Gee. (2010). "Application of Microfluidics to the Ultra-Rapid Preparation of Fluorine-18 Labelled Compounds." *Current Radiopharmaceuticals* 3: 254-262.

Moon, Byung Seok, Kyo Chul Lee, Gwang Il An, Dae Yoon Chi, Seung Dae Yang, Chang Woon Choi, Sang Moo Lim, and Kwon Soo Chun. (2006). "Preparation of 3'-deoxy-3'-[18F]fluorothymidine ([18F]FLT) in ionic liquid, [bmim][OTf]." *Journal of Labelled Compounds and Radiopharmaceuticals* 49 (3): 287-293.

Mukhopadhyay, Rajendrani. (2007). "When PDMS isn't the best." *Analytical Chemistry* 79 (9): 3248-3253.

Muschlitz, Lin. (2011). Report finds slowing in PET annual growth rate. July 28. Available from: http://www.auntminnie.com/index.aspx?sec=sup&sub=mol&pag=dis&ItemID=95998.

Nandy, S. K., and M. G. R. Rajan. (2009). "Fully automated and simplified radiosynthesis of [18F]-3'-deoxy-3'-fluorothymidine using anhydro precursor and single neutral alumina column purification." *Journal of Radioanalytical and Nuclear Chemistry* 283 (3): 741-748.

Nandy, S. K., N. V. Krisgnamurthy, and Rajan, M. G. R. (2010). "Evaluation of the Radiochemical Impurities Arising During the Competitive Fluorination of Nosyl Group During the Synthesis of 3'-deoxy-3'fluorothymidine." *J. Radioanal Nucl Chem* 283: 245-251.

Nandy, S.K., and M.G.R. Rajan. (2010). "Simple, column purification technique for the fully automated radiosynthesis of [18F]fluoroazomycinarabinoside ([18F]FAZA)." *Applied Radiation and Isotopes* 68 (10): 1944-1949.

Nelson, Wyatt C., Ivory Peng, Geun-An Lee, Joseph A. Loo, Robin L. Garrell, and Chang-Jin "CJ" Kim. (2010). "Incubated Protein Reduction and Digestion on an Electrowetting-on-Dielectric Digital Microfluidic Chip for MALDI-MS." *Analytical Chemistry* 82 (23): 9932-9937.

O'Hagan, David. (2006). "Recent developments on the fluorinase from Streptomyces cattleya." *Journal of Fluorine Chemistry* 127 (11): 1479-1483.

Oh, Young-Ho, Hyeong Bin Jang, Suk Im, Myoung Jong Song, So-Yeon Kim, Sung-Woo Park, Dae Yoon Chi, Choong Eui Song, and Sungyul Lee. (2011). "SN2 Fluorination reactions in ionic liquids: a mechanistic study towards solvent engineering." *Organic & Biomolecular Chemistry* 9 (2): 418.

Pascali, Giancarlo, Grazia Mazzone, Giuseppe Saccomanni, Clementina Manera, and Piero A. Salvadori. (2010). "Microfluidic approach for fast labeling optimization and dose-on-demand implementation." *Nuclear Medicine and Biology* 37 (5): 547-555.

Phelps, Michael E. (2000). "Positron emission tomography provides molecular imaging of biological processes." *Proceedings of the National Academy of Sciences of the United States of America* 97 (16): 9226-9233.

Rensch, C., C. Boeld, B. Bachmann, S. Riese, G. Reischl, W. Ehrlichmann, N. Heumesser, M. Baller, and V. Samper. (2009). Microfluidic radiosynthesis: electrochemical phase transfer for drying [18F]fluoride. Presented at the International Symposium of Radiopharmaceutical Sciences. Edmonton, AB, Jul 12-17.

Rensch, Christian, Björn Wängler, Christoph Boeld, Marko Baller, Victor Samper, Nicole Heumesser, Walter Ehrlichmann, Stefan Riese, and Gerald Reischl. (2011). [18F]FMISO Synthesis on a chip-based microfluidic research Platform." *J Nucl Med.* 52 (Supplement 1): 288.

ROC-Project. Homepage - Radiochemistry on Chip Project. Available from: http://www.roc-project.eu/site/.

Rolland, Jason P., R. Michael Van Dam, Derek A. Schorzman, Stephen R. Quake, and Joseph M. DeSimone. (2004). "Solvent-Resistant Photocurable Liquid Fluoropolymers for Microfluidic Device Fabrication [corrected]." *Journal of the American Chemical Society* 126 (8): 2322-2323.

Sadeghi, Saman, Huijiang Ding, Gaurav J. Shah, Supin Chen, Chang-Jin Kim, and R. Michael van Dam. (2012). "On-chip droplet characterization: A practical, high-sensitivity measurement of droplet impedance in digital microfluidics." *Analytical Chemistry*, In Press.

Sadeghi, Saman, Jimmy Ly, Yuliang Deng, and R. Michael van Dam. (2010). A robust platinum-based electrochemical micro flow cell for drying of [18F]fluoride for PET tracer synthesis. In *Proceedings of the Fourteenth International Conference on Miniaturized Systems for Chemistry and Life Sciences,* 318-320. Groningen, The Netherlands, Oct 3-7.

Sadeghi, Saman, Jimmy Ly, Yuliang Deng, Nagichettiar Satyamurthy, and R. Michael van Dam. (2011). Electrochemical micro flow cell for rapid PET tracer synthesis." *J Nucl Med.* 52 (Supplement 1): 286.

Sahoo, Hemantkumar R, Jason G Kralj, and Klavs F Jensen. (2007). "Multistep Continuous-Flow Microchemical Synthesis Involving Multiple Reactions and Separations." *Angewandte Chemie International Edition* 46 (30): 5704-5708.

Saiki, Hidekazu, Ren Iwata, Hiroaki Nakanishi, Rebecca Wong, Yoichi Ishikawa, Shozo Furumoto, Ryo Yamahara, Katsumasa Sakamoto, and Eiichi Ozeki. (2010). "Electrochemical concentration of no-carrier-added [18F]fluoride from [18O]water in a disposable microfluidic cell for radiosynthesis of 18F-labeled radiopharmaceuticals." *Applied Radiation and Isotopes* 68: 1703-1708.

Schertzer, M.J., R. Ben-Mrad, and P.E. Sullivan. (2010). "Using capacitance measurements in EWOD devices to identify fluid composition and control droplet mixing." *Sensors and Actuators B: Chemical* 145 (1): 340-347.

SCINTOMICS GmbH. GRP modules. Available from: http://www.scintomics.com/en/production/grp-modules/index.html.

SCINTOMICS GmbH. μ-ICR. Available from:

http://www.scintomics.com/en/production/-mu-icr/index.html.

Sofie Biosciences, Inc. Radiochemistry: Elixys. Available from: http://www.sofiebio.com/elixys.

Steel, C. J., A. T. O'Brien, S. K. Luthra, and F. Brady. (2007). "Automated PET radiosyntheses using microfluidic devices." *Journal of Labelled Compounds and Radiopharmaceuticals* 50 (5-6): 308-311.

Suehiro, Makiko, Shankar Vallabhajosula, Stanley J. Goldsmith, and Douglas J. Ballon. (2007). "Investigation of the role of the base in the synthesis of [18F]FLT." *Applied Radiation and Isotopes* 65 (12): 1350-1358.

Tang, Ganghua, Xiaolan Tang, Fuhua Wen, Mingfang Wang, and Baoyuan Li. (2010). "A facile and rapid automated synthesis of 3′-deoxy-3′-[18F]fluorothymidine." *Applied Radiation and Isotopes* 68 (9): 1734-1739.

Trasis. Miniaturized on-chip-chemistry. Available from: http://www.trasis.com/pages/on_chip_chemistry.html.

Tseng, W-Y, J.S. Cho, X. Ma, A. Kunihiro, A. Chatziioannou, and R.M. van Dam. (2010). Toward reliable synthesis of radiotracers for positron emission tomography in PDMS microfluidic chips: Study and optimization of the [18F] fluoride drying process. In *Technical Proceedings of the 2010 NSTI Nanotechnology Conference and Trade Show*, 2:472-475. Anaheim, CA, June 21.

Unger, Marc A., Hou-Pu Chou, Todd Thorsen, Axel Scherer, and Stephen R. Quake. (2000). "Monolithic Microfabricated Valves and Pumps by Multilayer Soft Lithography." *Science* 288 (5463): 113-116.

Ungersboeck, Johanna, Cécile Philippe, Leonhard-Key Mien, Daniela Haeusler, Karem Shanab, Rupert Lanzenberger, Helmut Spreitzer, et al. (2011). "Microfluidic preparation of [18F]FE@SUPPY and [18F]FE@SUPPY:2 -- comparison with conventional radiosyntheses." *Nuclear Medicine and Biology* 38 (3): 427-434.

Voccia, S., J. Morelle, J. Aerts, C. Lemaire, A. Luxen, and G. Phillipart. (2009). Mini-fluidic chip for the total synthesis of PET tracers. Presented at the 18th International Symposium on Radiopharmaceutical Sciences. Edmonton, AB, Jul 12-17.

Vu, Nam T., Zeta T.F. Yu, Begonya Comin-Anduix, Jonas N. Søndergaard, Robert W. Silverman, Canny Y.N. Chang, Antoni Ribas, Hsian-Rong Tseng, and Arion F. Chatziioannou. (2011). "A β-Camera Integrated with a Microfluidic Chip for Radioassays Based on Real-Time Imaging of Glycolysis in Small Cell Populations." *Journal of Nuclear Medicine* 52 (5): 815 -821.

Weber, Wolfgang A., and Robert Figlin. (2007). "Monitoring Cancer Treatment with PET/CT: Does It Make a Difference?" *J Nucl Med* 48 (1_suppl): 36S-44.

Wessmann, Sarah, Gjermund Henriksen, and Hans-Jürgen Wester. (2011). Preparation of highly reactive [18F]fluoride without any evaporation step. *J Nucl Med.* 52 (Supplement 1): 76.

Wester, Hans-Jürgen, Bent Wilhelm Schoultz, Christina Hultsch, and Gjermund Henriksen. (2008). "Fast and repetitive in-capillary production of [18F]FDG." *European Journal of Nuclear Medicine and Molecular Imaging* 36 (4): 653-658.

Wheeler, Tobias D., Dexing Zeng, Amit V. Desai, Birce Önal, David E. Reichert, and Paul J. A. Kenis. (2010). "Microfluidic labeling of biomolecules with radiometals for use in nuclear medicine." *Lab on a Chip* 10 (24): 3387-3396.

Winkler, Margit, Juozas Domarkas, Lutz F Schweiger, and David O'Hagan. (2008). "Fluorinase-Coupled Base Swaps: Synthesis of [18F]-5'-Deoxy-5'-fluorouridines." *Angewandte Chemie International Edition* 47 (52): 10141-10143.

Yu, S. (2006). "Review of 18F-FDG synthesis and quality control." *Biomedical Imaging and Intervention Journal* 2 (4): e57.

Zhang, Hui, Qinan Bao, Nam T. Vu, Robert W. Silverman, Richard Taschereau, Brittany N. Berry-Pusey, Ali Douraghy, Fernando R. Rannou, David B. Stout, and Arion F. Chatziioannou. (2011). "Performance Evaluation of PETbox: A Low Cost Bench Top Preclinical PET Scanner." *Molecular Imaging and Biology* 13 (5): 949-961.

7

Specific Activity of ^{11}C-Labelled Radiotracers: A Big Challenge for PET Chemists

Vanessa Gómez-Vallejo[1], Vijay Gaja[1], Jacek Koziorowski[2] and Jordi Llop[1]
[1]Molecular Imaging Unit – CIC biomaGUNE
[2]Herlev University Hospital
[1]Spain
[2]Denmark

1. Introduction

Non-invasive *in vivo* molecular imaging using radionuclides is based on the Radiotracer Principle of G. von Hevesy and the magic bullet concept by Ehrlich (1990). Both principles require administration of a radioactive tracer (a molecule labelled with a radioactive isotope which when injected into a living object can be traced by external radiation detection devices) and require that the quantity is in sub-pharmacological amounts, i.e. that minimal mass is injected, which in radiopharmaceutical terms means high specific activity.

1.1 Specific activity: The concept

According to the more updated terminology that is going to be recommended by the IUPAC, the concept of specific activity (A_S) is defined as the activity of a radionuclide divided by the mass (or molar amount) of the sum of all radioactive and stable nuclides (present in the same chemical and physical form) isotopic with the element involved (Bonardi, 2003). Thus, if one thinks of an injectable solution of, for instance, 3,5-dichloro-*N*-[[(2*S*)-1-ethylpyrrolidin-2-yl]methyl]-2-hydroxy-6-([^{11}C]methoxy)benzamide or [^{11}C]Raclopride (a post-synaptic D_2 receptor antagonist which is used for the quantification of D_2-like dopamine receptors (Elsinga et al., 2006) with different clinical applications, e.g. distinction of multiple system atrophy from Parkinson disease (Van Laere et al., 2010)), what one has in solution before administration to the patient is a mixture of different (chemically identical) species (A+B+C+D in Figure 1).

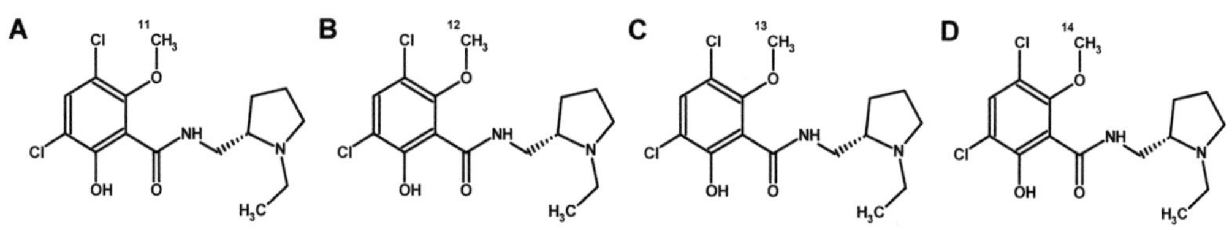

Fig. 1. Chemical structure of [^{11}C]Raclopride and chemically identical species which co-exists with the radioactive specie. All carbon atoms whose mass number is not specified are ^{12}C, ^{13}C or ^{14}C.

The A_S of the radiotracer can thus be expressed as the ratio between the amount of radioactivity (given by the number of molecules containing a Carbon-11 atom, A in Figure 1) and the number of molecules (expressed as mass or molar quantity) containing Carbon-11 or other (stable and unstable) isotopes of Carbon (A+B+C+D in Figure 1).

In the context of radiopharmaceuticals, other definitions have been described for different situations that occur when analyzing the final radioactive product. Thus, the term *effective specific activity* is used to describe the mass or molar quantity of a single species radiotracer relative to the total mass or molar quantity of the radiotracer and non-radioactive compound(s) that have similar biochemical properties. For instance, proteins can be labelled with positron emitters (e.g. ^{68}Ga) by (covalently) attaching a bifunctional chelator to introduce later on the metallic radioactive atom. The chemical structure of the labelled (C in Figure 2) and unlabelled (B in Figure 2) species are very similar (although not identical) and thus it can be anticipated that both compounds will have very similar biochemical properties. Isolation of the labelled compound is not (usually) feasible and *effective specific activity* is defined as the ratio between the amount of radioactivity (given by the number of molecules containing a gallium-68 atom, C in Figure 2) and the number of molecules (expressed as mass or molar quantity) with similar biochemical properties (B and C in the Figure). This concept is mainly applied in the context of macromolecules (e.g. labelled proteins, antibodies, peptides, polymers), nanostructures (nanoparticles, nanotubes) and also when, in smaller molecules, undesired contaminants (which cannot be separated from the labelled structure but have similar biochemical properties) are present in the final solution.

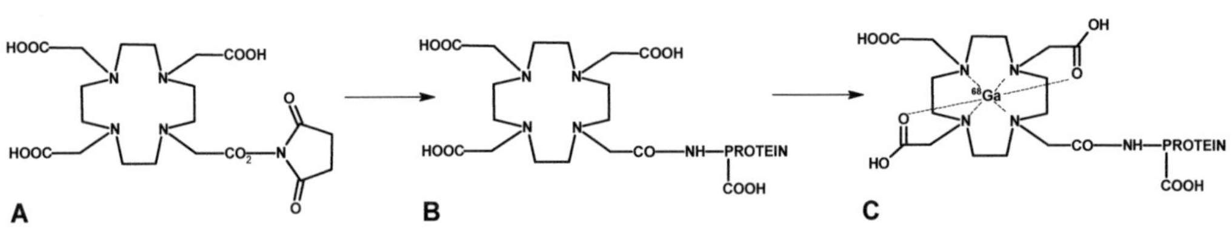

Fig. 2. Schematic reaction pathway for the introduction of a positron emitter (^{68}Ga in the example) in a macromolecule (protein). The labelled and unlabelled structures (B and C) are almost identical and have similar (if not identical) biochemical properties.

When *in vivo* imaging studies are performed, the amount of radioactivity to be administered is somehow fixed within a range: It has to be sufficiently high to allow acquiring good quality images but low enough to prevent saturating of the radio-detectors and, eventually, damage to the organism due to radiation exposure. Thus, the A_S will definitely determine the molar amount of radiotracer. In some applications such as the study of the behaviour of bioactive or toxic molecules, dose exposure studies and the visualization of low density receptors in the brain, the concept of A_S becomes especially relevant, provided that the quantity of injected tracer can definitely produce undesired pharmacodynamic or toxicological effects, as well as target (e.g. receptor) saturation. In some cases, when the injected compound is endogenous and normally found in μM or higher concentrations in the body (e.g. [^{15}O]water, [^{11}C]acetate, [^{11}C]glucose) or that the target or function is not saturated easily (e.g. glucose metabolism - [^{18}F]FDG , hypoxia - [^{18}F]FMISO, enzyme activity; thymidine kinase 1 - [^{18}F]FLT) specific activity is not crucial. For macromolecules it is known that the highest specific activity is not necessary the optimal one. This has been reported for peptides (de Jong et al., 1999; Bernhardt et al., 2003; Schuhmacher et al., 2005; Velikyan et al., 2010) and antibodies (Pandit-Taskar et al., 2008).

Although theoretical A_S values for PET isotopes are very high (e.g. 341.1 TBq/μmol for Carbon-11, 63.3 TBq/μmol for Fluorine-18) these values are usually very far (10-10000 times higher) from those values obtained once the radiotracer has been synthesized. This decrease in A_S is due to a dilution process with the non radioactive isotope, usually occurring during radionuclide production and/or manipulation and preparation of the radiotracer. This fact is well known among the scientific community; however, the number of factors contributing to the introduction of stable isotopes during the production process is very high and usually difficult to be controlled. These potential sources of stable isotopes become relevant when simple calculations are performed. For instance, in 37 GBq of [^{11}C]CO_2 (a radioactive precursor typically used for the preparation of ^{11}C-labelled radiotracers) the number of molecules (when A_S is the theoretical value, 341.1 TBq/μmol) is only 6.53×10^{13} (0.108 nmol). The introduction of (only) 1 or 100 nmol of non radioactive CO_2 will decrease A_S by a factor of 10 or 1000, respectively.

Despite the dramatic consequences of incorporation of minute amounts of non radioactive carbon on A_S, the number of systematic approaches for the study of contamination sources reported in the literature is scarce, and syntheses under (apparently) identical experimental conditions might lead to immense differences in A_S values of the final radiotracer. These facts have led to perpetual discussions among scientists regarding the optimal procedures to be followed to improve A_S, especially in the case of Carbon-11 labelled radiotracers.

1.2 Carbon-11: A challenging isotope

Among all radionuclides, only a few of them have the adequate physical properties to become suitable candidates for the preparation of radiotracers. In the particular case of positron emitters, there are four radionuclides which have been historically used: Carbon-11, Nitrogen-13, Fluorine-18 and Oxygen-15. The wide historical use of these isotopes is due to (i) they can be produced in relatively high yields in commercially available cyclotrons, (ii) they can be easily introduced in biomolecules, (iii) their decay mode is close to 100% positron emission (see table 1) and (iv) their stable isotopes are present in all organic molecules; this last statement is not true in the case of fluorine, but in many cases the substitution of an hydroxyl group (or hydrogen atom) by a fluorine atom does not significantly alter the biological behaviour of the molecule; thus fluorine can be used to prepare analogues of molecules with specific biological characteristics.

Among these four PET isotopes, Fluorine-18 is probably the most widely used, especially for clinical applications. Fluorine-18 forms strong covalent bonds with carbon atoms and can be incorporated into a large variety of organic molecules; on the other hand, substitution of a hydrogen atom by a fluorine atom causes little steric alterations in the molecule; in some particular cases, the biological properties of the radiotracer are even improved with respect to the original molecule. Moreover, Fluorine-18 has a small positron range and its half-life is relatively long (109.8 minutes) allowing the preparation of complex molecules with acceptable radiochemical yields. Finally, the relatively long half-life permits the commercialization of radiotracers as diagnostic tools in the clinical environment.

Radionuclide	Half-life (min)	Decay mode	Max. Energy (MeV)
Fluorine-18	109.8	97% β+ 3% EC*	0.69
Carbon-11	20.4	100 % β+	0.96
Nitrogen-13	9.98	100 % β+	1.19
Oxygen-15	2.05	100 % β+	1.70

Table 1. Physical characteristics of Fluorine-18, Carbon-11, Nitrogen-13 and Oxygen-15. *EC: Electron capture.

Out of the above mentioned clinical environment, Nitrogen-13 and Oxygen-15 can be also potentially used for the synthesis of radiotracers. However, the manufacturing process of radiotracers with these positron emitters presents some difficulties because of their short half-life (9.98 and 2.05 min, respectively) and distribution of radiotracers from one centralized production centre to surrounding centres is not feasible.

Despite the widespread use of these isotopes (which is reflected in a high number of scientific publications in which the preparation and putative applications of ^{18}F-, ^{13}N- and ^{15}O- labelled radiotracers are described) the most challenging and exciting positron emitter is probably Carbon-11, which in general terms cannot be transported from manufacturing centres to surrounding hospitals and thus began to receive increasing attention in the sixties due to the widespread installation of cyclotrons in hospitals and research centres.

There are two main reasons to consider Carbon-11 as the most exciting and challenging PET isotope. First, carbon is present in all organic compounds, and thus a Carbon-11 analog (identical to the unlabelled structure) of any specific organic molecule could be potentially prepared, and second, Carbon-11 can be produced with good yields in two different chemical forms ([^{11}C]CH_4, obtained by irradiating N_2/H_2 mixtures; and [^{11}C]CO_2, obtained by irradiation of N_2/O_2 mixtures (Christman et al., 1975)) which can be easily transformed into other radioactive precursors via well established labelling strategies to perform different types of chemical reactions. Thus, Grignard-type reactions to yield [carbonyl-^{11}C]carboxylates can be carried out by using directly cyclotron generated [^{11}C]CO_2; the latter can be also converted into [^{11}C]CO through the reduction over zinc or molybdenum in an on-line process and further used to produce (e.g. via the palladium-mediated [^{11}C]carbonylation of olefins, alkynes and organic halides) carboxylic acids (Itsenko et al., 2006), amides (Rahman et al., 2003) and imides (Karimi et al., 2001), among others. [^{11}C]CO_2 can be also transformed into [^{11}C]CH_3OH via reduction with $LiAlH_4$; the latter can be further reacted with hydriodic acid to yield [^{11}C]CH_3I which is by far the most commonly used radioactive precursor for introducing Carbon-11 into organic molecules via nucleophilic substitution using amines (Mathis et al., 2003), amides (Hashimoto et al., 1989), phenols (Ehrin et al, 1985) or thiol groups (Langstrom & Lundqvist, 1976). Eventually, [^{11}C]CH_3I can be passed in gas phase through a silver triflate column at high temperature to yield [^{11}C]methyl triflate (Jewett, 1992), which can be used as a highly reactive methylating agent when reactivity of [^{11}C]CH_3I is not sufficient. On the other hand, [^{11}C]CH_4 can be also converted into $[^{11}C]CH_3I$ through a gas-solid iodination reaction at high temperature. In this case, the iodination step is carried out in a quartz tube which contains I_2 vapour at high temperature (Prenant & Crouzel, 1991; Larsen et al., 1997).

This versatility of Carbon-11 as a synthetic tool has led to a immense number of publications in the scientific literature in which the synthetic strategies and optimization steps are described. As a result, nowadays there is a large variety of well established processes that can be followed when the radiosynthesis of a new radiotracer is approached. However, depending on the final application of the tracer, one strategy can be more appropriate than others, and one of the big challenges for radiochemists consists not only of synthesizing the radiotracer with good radiochemical yield and high radiochemical purity but also with a sufficiently high A_S for a particular application.

In this chapter, an exhaustive analysis (based on bibliographic data) of the typical values of A_S obtained for ^{11}C-labelled radiotracers and the main factors affecting this parameter will be performed. Experimental protocols to improve specific activity of ^{11}C-labelled radiotracers will be described and discussed on the basis of bibliographic data and personal experience of the authors.

2. Specific activity in ^{11}C-labelled radiotracers

2.1 Modulation of specific activity

According to IUPAC definition (see above) and in the context of radiopharmaceuticals, specific activity can be expressed using equation (1):

$$A_s = \frac{A_i}{n_i} \qquad (1)$$

Where A_i is the activity (expressed in Bq) of the radiopharmaceutical specie and n_i is the molar amount of the sum of all radioactive and stable forms of the radiopharmaceutical. Usually, A_s is expressed, in the case of ^{11}C-labelled radiopharmaceuticals, in GBq/µmol. From the equation, it is clear that specific activity can be increased either by (i) increasing the amount of radioactivity and/or (ii) decreasing the amount of stable forms.

In the specific case of cyclotron produced ^{11}C, the increase in the amount of radioactivity can be achieved, obviously, by producing higher amounts of radioactive precursor (e.g., $[^{11}C]CO_2$ or $[^{11}C]CH_4$). However, increasing the dose (integrated current) or the beam intensity does not always result in a higher amount of radioactivity and consequently in a higher specific activity of the final radiopharmaceutical. In other occasions, increasing the beam time increases also the incorporation of impurities. For instance, it has been reported that the in-target specific activity of $[^{11}C]CO_2$ peaked at 20-25 minutes of beam time and decreased with longer irradiations, due to incorporation of contamination into the target gas, which was faster that the net production of carbon-11 (Mock, 2006). However, in a certain range and in general terms, increasing irradiation time results in an increase of A_S. In Figure 3, a set of experiments performed by the authors of this chapter (results not published before) are shown. Carbon-11 was produced by irradiation (target current=22 µA, 1-8 µAh) of a gas N_2/H_2 mixture (95/5, filling pressure=16 bar) with high energy (~16 MeV) protons. The resulting [^{11}C]CH_4 was allowed to react with iodine at 720°C to form [^{11}C]methyl iodide in a gas circulating process, to be further reacted with phenol in the presence of a base to yield [^{11}C]anisole. As can be seen, higher specific activity values were obtained with increasing beam time. Although the curve seems to reach a plateau, the presence of a peak as previously reported (Mock, 2006) was not found, probably because no longer irradiation times were investigated.

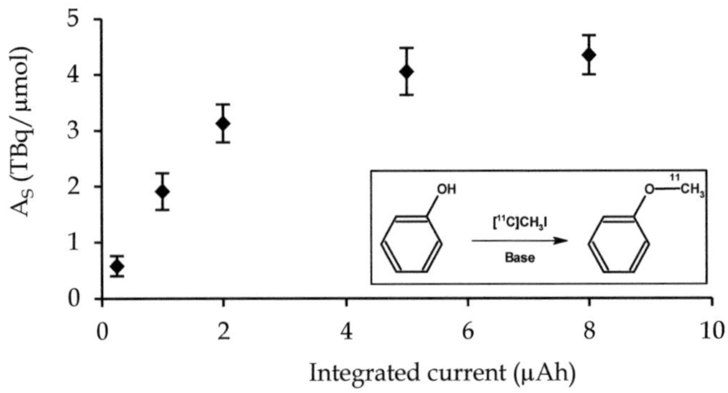

Fig. 3. Specific activity of [^{11}C]anisole (corrected to EOB, end of bombardment) produced using different irradiation times.

Besides increasing the amount of radioactivity, the other possibility to increase specific activity consists of decreasing the amount of stable forms, or in other words, to prevent the introduction of stable isotopes of carbon (mainly ^{12}C) in any of the processes followed for the preparation of the radiopharmaceutical, from the production of ^{11}C in the cyclotron till the final formulation of the radiopharmaceutical. These non radioactive carbon sources might potentially contaminate the reaction environment during radiopharmaceuticals preparation processes, thus decreasing the final specific activity. Actually, some of these sources have been known for a long time. During production of the radioactive precursor (irradiation), impurities in the target gas, impurities coming from the valves, pressure regulators, seals, target body, target windows or even residues from hydrocarbon solvents used to clean metal pieces after manufacturing might affect the final specific activity (Dahl & Schlyer, 1985). During radiotracers synthesis, incorporation of contaminants from the atmosphere, or release of undesired chemicals from tubes, reactors, etc. or even the presence of stable carbon in some of the reagents could also contribute to the decrease of final A_S.

These non radioactive sources will have different effects on the final specific activity depending on the particular configuration of the different equipment at each site. The effects will also vary depending on the synthetic process followed and the chemical structure of such impurities. Thus, every specific scenario should be investigated individually. However, the discussion of all specific scenarios and configurations is beyond the scope of this chapter, and only a few synthetic routes, namely, methylation reactions starting from cyclotron produced [^{11}C]CO_2 and [^{11}C]CH_4 (which are considered by the authors the most frequently used in Carbon-11 radiochemistry) will be discussed. Still, most of the concepts introduced in the following pages can be applied (or extrapolated) to the preparation of ^{11}C-labelled radiotracers by following other routes.

2.2 Interpretation of specific activity: Are reported values always comparable?

If one has a solution of, for instance, [^{11}C]Raclopride, and specific activity is not the theoretical value, species A, B, C and D (Figure 1) are co-existing. The specific activity will be given by equation (2):

$$A_S = \frac{A_A}{n_A + n_B + n_C + n_D} \tag{2}$$

Where A_A is the amount of radioactivity due to the presence of specie A, and n_A, n_B, n_C and n_D are the molar amounts of A, B, C and D, respectively. When the specific activity of a radiotracer is the theoretical value (341.1 TBq/µmol for Carbon-11), n_B, n_C and n_D are zero, and the value of A_S value is not changing over time, because both the amount of radioactivity (A_A) and the molar amount of A (n_A) are decreasing with the same rate.

On the other hand, when the specific activity is far from its theoretical value, then:

$$n_B + n_C + n_D \gg n_A \qquad \text{thus,} \qquad \frac{A_A}{n_A + n_B + n_C + n_D} \sim \frac{A_A}{n_B + n_C + n_D}$$

As ($n_B + n_C + n_D$) is (almost) constant (due to the long half life of ^{14}C) then A_S decreases at the same rate as A_A does. In other words: Every half life, the value of A_S is decreased by a factor of 2. Therefore, in real scenarios the values of A_S have to be reported at a given time point. In the literature, and in the particular case of ^{11}C-labelled radiotracers, authors usually report A_S at the end of synthesis (EOS), end of bombardment (EOB) or end of transfer (of the activity, from the cyclotron to the hot cell where the radiosynthesis takes place). Values at EOB are usually easier to compare, because they do not depend on synthesis time and offer a direct estimation of the amount of stable carbon contributing to the dilution (and consequent decrease in A_S). In some occasions, where systematic studies are performed to search for the sources of contamination, the total amount of carrier (which can be directly compared to previously published values) is reported.

3. Specific activity of ^{11}C-labelled radiotracers produced following methylation

Methylation reactions consist of attaching a CH_3- group (using e.g. CH_3I or CH_3OTf) to a nucleophile (usually an oxygen, nitrogen or sulphur atom) via the S_N2 reaction pathway. When ^{11}C-labelled radiotracers are prepared by following this route, [^{11}C]CH_3I cannot be produced directly in the target in large amounts (Wagner et al., 1981) and has to be synthesized from other synthetic precursors, namely [^{11}C]CO_2 or [^{11}C]CH_4. Both schemes will be discussed separately.

3.1 Methylation reactions starting from cyclotron produced [^{11}C]CO_2

3.1.1 [^{11}C]CO_2 production

The irradiation of nitrogen gas at sufficient beam (proton) energies yields large amounts of [^{11}C]CO_2. During irradiation, ^{14}N is converted into ^{11}C via the ^{14}N(p, α)^{11}C nuclear reaction, with the highest cross-section at 7.5 MeV. According to Christman and co-workers, it is unnecessary to add oxygen to the nitrogen gas, because trace amounts of oxygen already present in the nitrogen (~1 ppm) are sufficient for the oxidation reaction to occur. They reported that, when oxygen was added to the system, copious amounts of nitrogen oxides were produced in addition to the desired $[^{11}C]CO_2$, from the reaction $^{16}O(p, \alpha)^{13}N$ and from radiolysis processes. According to previous reports (Ache & Wolf, 1968) the primary products resulting from the reactions of "hot" carbon atoms with nitrogen-oxygen mixtures at low radiation doses are cyanide and carbon monoxide. The oxidation of these two primary products as a function of the radiation dose by the proton beam are not fully known, but in any case, the final product obtained from this system was shown to be over 90 per cent $^{11}[C]CO_2$, without the incorporation of any chemical oxidation.

Currently, $[^{11}C]CO_2$ is still produced in similar targets to those described by Christman et al., although 0.5-2% oxygen is added to the target gas and some improvements have been incorporated; it was demonstrated (Ferrieri et al., 1993) that the interaction between beam and target walls (independently of the material used for the manufacture of the target) produced the release of non radioactive carbon into the target gas mixture, decreasing thus specific activity. Thus, the use of targets with minimal surface exposure to beam is preferred. Also, and due to multiple scattering suffered by the beam through the foil window and in the gas, a conical-shaped target (a cylindrical target was used in previous experiments conducted by Christman's group) was proposed (Schlyer & Plascjak, 1991). The conical target is still the standard model supplied with some commercial cyclotrons.

3.1.2 $[^{11}C]CH_3I$ production and methylation

The general reaction pathway followed for the preparation of ^{11}C-labelled radiopharmaceuticals via methylation using $[^{11}C]CH_3I$ (or $[^{11}C]CH_3OTf$) produced from $[^{11}C]CO_2$ (historically named the "wet method") can be summarized in 6 steps:[1] (i) $[^{11}C]CO_2$ is generated in a cyclotron via the $^{14}N(p,\alpha)^{11}C$ nuclear reaction by bombarding a N_2/O_2 mixture with high energy protons; (ii) the target content is transferred to a hot cell and trapped in a molecular sieve column (Mock et al., 1995) at room temperature or in a cold trap (liquid nitrogen); (iii) the reactor is prefilled with lithium aluminium hydride solution; (iv) $[^{11}C]CO_2$ is released by increasing the temperature of the trap and bubbled (with the help of an inert gas) in the reactor; (v) After complete trapping, solvent is evaporated to dryness and hydriodic acid (aqueous solution) is added to generate $[^{11}C]CH_3I$ which is distilled by heating under continuous nitrogen flow and (vi) $[^{11}C]CH_3I$ is trapped in a reactor prefilled with the adequate precursor, where methylation takes place. Along this process, the formation of the non-radioactive specie (this is, $[^{x}C]CH_3I$, where ^{x}C is any stable isotope of carbon) is due to the presence, incorporation and/or *in situ* generation of $[^{x}C]CO_2$ before the treatment with hydriodic acid. The specific sources of such ^{x}C in real scenarios and the individual contribution of each one to the decrease of final specific activity have been historically profoundly discussed.

---

1 $[^{11}C]CH_3I$ can be also produced from $[^{11}C]CO_2$ via reduction over a nickel catalyst at high temperature and further reaction with I_2 ("gas phase" method). This reaction pathway will be considered later on.

3.1.3 Search for the sources of ^{12}C in methylation reactions starting from [^{11}C]CO_2 via the wet method

In one of the first reviews in which different sources of carrier carbon were considered (Crouzel et al., 1987) practical recommendations to attain molar activities of 75–175GBq/μmol routinely were suggested. These recommendations included: (i) using (small and properly washed) aluminum targets with Havar, stainless steel or titanium foils, (ii) using high purity target gases with a purification trap installed between the target and the gas supply, (iii) using metal (stainless steel or copper) tubing between the gas supply and target, (iv) performing short irradiations with as high a beam current as possible and (v) using the smallest possible amount of $LiAlH_4$, preferably dissolved in dry (distilled from sodium or potassium) THF. The authors suggested that most of the stable CO_2 was coming from the target under irradiation conditions.

One of the first systematic studies searching for the sources of carrier carbon in ^{11}C-labelled radiotracers produced from [^{11}C]CH_3I synthesized from cyclotron generated [^{11}C]CO_2 was performed 1 year later (Iwata et al., 1988). Although the authors suspected in a first step that $LiAlH_4$ (solution in THF) was the main source of carrier ($LiAlH_4$ can absorb CO_2 from the environment when not stored/prepared under rigorous inert atmosphere), the total carrier amount was not so much reduced as expected with decreasing the concentration of $LiAlH_4$ solution. This fact led them to postulate that a significant amount of carrier might come from the [^{11}C]CO_2 production system (the target), although no significant correlation between the total carrier amount and the volume of the target gas was observed. Finally, they concluded that carrier carbon dioxide was mostly originated in the methanol formed from a trace of THF remaining in the $LiAlH_4$ after the evaporation step, and could be decreased significantly (up to a certain limit) by reducing the amount and concentration of the $LiAlH_4$/THF solution. They concluded that it might be very difficult to overcome this limit, and thus increasing starting ^{11}C-activity and shortening the synthesis time were proposed to be the most adequate solution to achieve higher specific activities.

In a more recent work (Matarrese et al., 2003) another systematic study of the different factors introducing carrier carbon was performed. Although the authors concluded that the critical point to obtain high specific radioactivity was the minimization of lithium aluminum hydride quantity (see table 2 for relation of A_S and quantity of $LiAlH_4$ solutions obtained by Matarrese's group), different modifications were also introduced to the commercial Synthesizer to improve the specific activity. The original reaction vessel design was modified and the tube inlets were accomplished by standard male-luer fittings with disposable needles, while carrier gas flows (the purge gas lines leading to reaction vessels and to dispensing vessels and solid phase extraction unit) were separated, thus allowing the use of different gases for these two purposes. Besides, several routine operations were included before syntheses, mainly: (i) the target was flushed with the target gas mixture (at least 10 target volumes) prior to bombardment; (ii) a leak-test was performed on the liquid nitrogen loop, [^{11}C]CO_2 trapping reaction vessels and connecting tubes; (iii) reaction vessels and liquid nitrogen trap were dried at 150 °C for 30 minutes by a continuous argon flow (100 mL/min); (iv) the PTFE [^{11}C]CO_2 delivery lines connecting the target with the module were continuously flushed with a stream of helium during bombardment and (v) the metallo-organic trapping solution ($LiAlH_4$/THF) was added into the reaction vessel immediately before unloading the [^{11}C]CO_2 target with the sample-lock gas-tight syringe. As can be seen in the table, good specific activity values were reached, especially when the optimal amount of $LiAlH_4$ solution was used, although such values were reported at EOS and synthesis time was not reported; therefore, recalculation at EOB is not possible.

Radioligand	Yield EOB (%)	A_S EOS (GBq/µmol)	$LiAlH_4$ (µmol)
[^{11}C](R)-MDL-100907	55 ± 10	70 ± 30	10
[^{11}C](R)-MDL-100907	60 ± 20	315 ± 89	7
[^{11}C](R)-MDL-100907	54 ± 10	392 ± 166	6
[^{11}C](R)-MDL-100907	53 ± 10	322 ± 181	5

Table 2. Relation between specific radioactivity of [^{11}C](R)-MDL-100907 and quantity of the $LiAlH_4$/THF solutions.

Five years later (Ermert et al, 2008), a different strategy for the preparation of [^{11}C]CH_3I (in which [^{11}C]CO_2 from the target chamber was reduced by a lithium aluminum hydride solution, and the methanol obtained on-line was converted using triphenylphosphine diiodide) was reported. [^{11}C]CH_3I was transformed into [^{11}C]MeOTf via on-line conversion to synthesize [^{11}C]TCH346. Six batches of this radiotracer were prepared within 10 days and specific activity values of 40, 330, 1700, 280, 770 and 5700 GBq/µmol for syntheses 1-6, respectively, were obtained. All syntheses were carried out using the same flask of commercially available lithium aluminum hydride solution repetitively; as the specific activity increased during the course of the synthesis campaign, the authors concluded that essential dilution by stable carbon via the $LiAlH_4$-solution could nearly be excluded, or at least equally important carbon sources appeared to be the target chamber and the penetration of ambient air into the target line and the synthesis unit. In any case, the aforesaid specific activities are higher than those earlier reported and are probably the highest values ever reported for ^{11}C-labelled radiotracers prepared by following this synthetic approach.

Almost simultaneously to the paper reported by Ermert and co-workers, and encouraged by this historical disagreement suggesting that the sources of contamination were extremely dependent on the particular configuration of the systems involved in the production process of each particular site (e.g. quality of the reagents and irradiated gases, target material, synthesis box, etc.) an exhaustive analysis of the potential sources of non radioactive carbon and their individual contribution to the final specific activity was carried out by some of the authors of this chapter (Gómez-Vallejo et al., 2009). In these studies, four synthetic scenarios were defined: (a) syntheses were carried out by executing steps (iii) and (v) of the previous general procedure; (b) syntheses were run by executing steps (iii), (iv) and (v); (c) syntheses were run by executing steps (ii), (iii), (iv) and (v) and (d) syntheses were run by executing all steps included in the general procedure. To assess also the effect of bombarding time on the final amount of [^{x}C]CH_3I, different experiments were carried out at different integrated currents (1, 2, 3 and 10 µAh; scenarios d_1-d_4, respectively).

Under Scenario (a) (where the contribution to the production of stable methyl iodide should come from the presence of CO_2 absorbed in $LiAlH_4$ solution, methanol formed from THF remaining in the $LiAlH_4$ after evaporation step and/or direct CO_2 incorporation from the atmosphere during the synthesis process due to the lack of tightness of the synthesis module) only 15.5 ± 2.7 nmol of non-radioactive CH_3I were generated (Figure 4B). Under scenario (b) conditions (where the contribution of absorbed CO_2 in the molecular sieve was also considered), 45.8 ± 11.7 nmol of CH_3I were generated. Under scenario (c) conditions (where also the contribution from loading and unloading the target was considered, thus CO_2 should come from carbon dioxide absorbed either in the target chamber or in the stainless-steel tubing connecting the target with the synthesis box, and present as an impurity in the target gas), 78.5 ± 12.3 nmol of CH_3I were detected (Figure 4B). Under scenario (d), 537.9 ± 197.5, 832.8 ± 56.3, 907.4 ± 28.2 and 1067.2 ± 59.3 nmol of methyl iodide were obtained for integrated currents of 1, 2, 3 and 10 μAh, respectively (scenarios d_1-d_4, Figure 4B). These results show that the generation of stable methyl iodide under scenarios (a), (b) and (c) is minor when compared to the contribution of bombarding processes during irradiation (see Figure 4A for individual contribution of the sources considered at each scenario). On the other hand, there is a non-linear trend between the increase in the amount of [^{x}C]CO_2 and the increase in integrated current in the target (Figure 4A), suggesting that the decrease in specific activity is probably due to the presence of carbon carrier contamination which undergoes combustion (High temperature, estimated around 260°C and pressure, around 38 bar, are reached into the target chamber during bombardment) mainly during the first minutes of irradiation. This effect of beam integrated current on the amount of stable carbon was also reported by other authors (Mock, 2006).

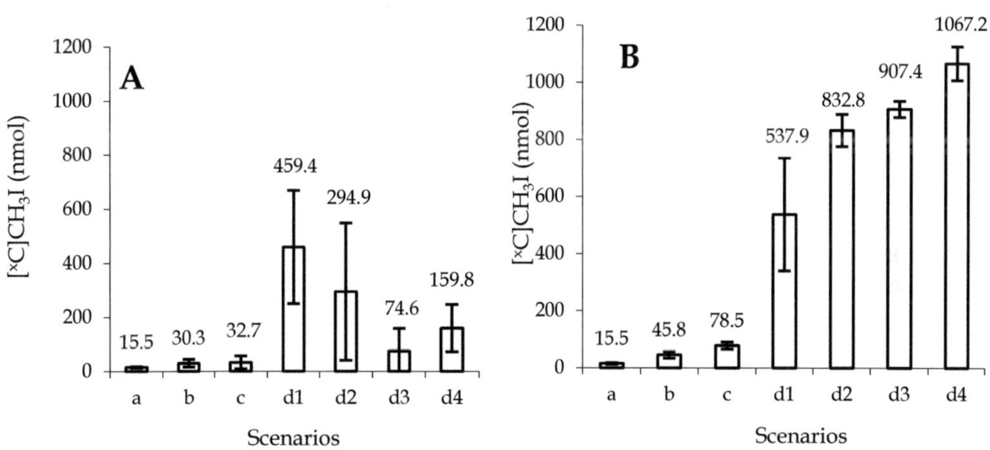

Fig. 4. Amount (in nmol) of [^{x}C]CH_3I generated under scenarios (a), (b), (c) and (d). Individual contribution of the factors considered in each scenario (A) and cumulative contribution (B).

In view of these results, some general procedures (which should help to improve the specific activity of Carbon-11 labelled compounds synthesized by the wet method) were suggested, including: i) loading/unloading (through transfer line into the molecular sieve) the target several times (with the aim of transferring all CO_2 contamination present in the target chamber and/or the transfer line into the molecular sieve); ii) loading/bombarding (integrated current = 1 µAh, target current = 24 µA)/unloading (to waste) the target three times (to "burn" all carbon compounds presumably present in the target chamber); iii) preconditioning (t = 60 minutes, T = 250°C, continuous N_2 flow = 50 mL/min) the molecular sieve column (to eliminate CO_2 from the molecular sieve); iv) cleaning (ethanol/acetone/diethyl ether) and drying (N_2) the synthesis box and keeping the system pressurized after drying to avoid atmospheric contamination; v) using commercially available $LiAlH_4$/THF solution and vi) minimizing the amount of $LiAlH_4$/THF solution used per run; furthermore, keeping the target loaded (P = 21 bar) between two consecutive productions and periodical inspection of general connections and tubing should help in the prevention of external contamination in the target chamber, the transfer line and the synthesis box.

Although by implementing these steps moderate specific activity values could be achieved in the preparation of e.g. [^{11}C]Raclopride (23.2 ± 11.7 GBq/µmol at EOS, 128 ± 64 GBq/µmol at EOB (Catafau et al., 2009)), such values were still far from those reported by Ermert and coworkers in 2008. This is probably due to the fact that the purity of the gases was not considered in the study conducted by Gomez-Vallejo et al., and no purification steps before loading the target were implemented. Also, no specific cleaning of the target chamber was performed before the experiments. In any case, the values obtained by Ermert's group are very far from average specific activities reported in the literature (see table 5); thus, a profound analysis of the specific configuration (and preparation procedures) used by this group could help to get more consistent conclusions related to the sources of non radioactive carbon and the protocols to be followed in order to increase A_S.

One of the lasts works focused in improving specific activities in [^{11}C]CO_2 production was reported recently (Eriksson et al., 2009). Three consecutive test periods were carried out with a standard IBA aluminum target, using 4 different configurations: a) Previously not irradiated target body, using a new window foil with nitrile o-ring; b) used foil with silver o-ring; c) new foil with silver o-ring and d) same basic build as (c) but with nickel plating on the aluminum surface. For configurations (a), (b) and (c) an increase in A_S of 2.4-2.5 GBq/µmol per µAh was observed for second and third production of a series of consecutive runs (results that are consistent with those reported by Gómez-Vallejo et al.), while for (d) the increase was significantly faster (5.4 GBq/µmol per µAh). After several irradiations, a plateau was found for all configurations, but (d) gave better specific activities (2540 ± 190 GBq/µmol) than (a) and (c) (2010 ± 310 GBq/µmol and 1920 ± 220 GBq/µmol, respectively).[2] The specific activity obtained with (d) could be even improved by connecting the helium line (used for activity transfer from cyclotron) only to the ^{11}C target (values up to 5400 ± 1700 GBq/µmol). Thus, nickel plating on the aluminum surface and using high purity gases (isolated from atmosphere or potential contamination sources) seem to have a positive effect on specific activity values obtained when the wet method is used.

[2] Configuration (b) developed a target leak before the plateau was established.

3.2 Methylation reactions starting from cyclotron produced [^{11}C]CH_4

3.2.1 [^{11}C]CH_4 production

The irradiation of nitrogen/hydrogen gas mixtures at sufficient beam (proton) energies yields large amounts of [^{11}C]methane (Christman et al., 1975). During irradiation, ^{14}N is converted into ^{11}C via the ^{14}N(p, α)^{11}C nuclear reaction (Epherre and Seide, 1971). From the reaction of hot recoil carbon atoms with nitrogen molecules, [^{11}C]CN and [^{11}C]CN_2 can be produced (Dubrin et al., 1964), and of these [^{11}C]CN is the most probable final stable species. Upon the addition of small amounts of hydrogen to the target gas, a second (and very fast) reaction gives [^{11}C]HCN (Ache & Wolf, 1968), which is readily reduced via a radiation induced mechanism to yield [^{11}C]CH_4. Unfortunately, increasing the beam current and irradiation lengths results in a significant drop in the amount of [^{11}C]CH_4, probably due to beam-wall interactions and high probability of the radioactive species sticking in the target walls, resulting in a reduction in recoverable yield. Due to these observed interactions with the target walls, large volume targets (flow through design in some cases) where beam wall interactions are less likely, produce results more in line with theory. Thus, the choice of target material in small- to medium-sized targets is therefore proposed to be one of the most important factors for optimizing [^{11}C]methane yields (Koziorowski et al., 2010). Buckley et al. (2004) explored the viability of using a niobium target chamber with a cylindrical shape (15 mm in diameter and 120 mm in length, energy of the proton beam = 12 MeV) for the production of [^{11}C]CH_4 from a gas mixture of N_2/H_2; 95/5 and 90/10. In table 3, the amount of radioactivity (in GBq) and saturation yields (in GBq/μA) for 20 μA irradiations are shown.

Time (min)	Yield (GBq)*	Saturation Yield (GBq/μA)
5	12.47	3.66
10	20.02	3.29
20	32.19	3.18
30	39.22	3.03
40	43.81	2.92
60	48.47	2.78

Table 3. Target yields in GBq and production rate at saturation in GBq/μA for the production of [^{11}C]CH_4 at 20 μA for the Nb chamber (loaded with N_2/H_2; 90/10). Nominal target loading pressure was 2067 kPa.

When beam was performed on 5% hydrogen at 20 μA for 20 min, 26.94 GBq (EOB) were produced (saturation yield of 2.70 GBq/μA). These results are not as good as the 10% values (32.19 GBq, 3.18 GBq/μA) but comparable to 10% results reported for the aluminum target chamber. Although the yields from the niobium target chamber were found to be better than those from the aluminum target chamber, the production rate was found to diminish with time.

In a recent work, the use of quartz as a target material (due to its chemical inertness) was proposed (Koziorowski et al., 2010); the use of such material should also improve the specific activity of produced [^{11}C]CH_4 due to its low carbon content and the fact that it is manufactured without the use of any potential carbon sources, such as lubricants. In this work, the authors designed and constructed a target based on an aluminum body fitted with a quartz liner. A mixture N_2/H_2 (90/10) was used (filling pressure = 26 bar). As previously reported, an increasing deviation from theoretical yields with increased irradiation dose (μAh) was seen (see Figure 5), both when irradiation time and irradiation current were increased. The authors concluded that this drop in yields should be explained by the presence of radioactive species adsorbed to the target, although the underlying mechanism(s) of this phenomenon has yet to be elucidated.

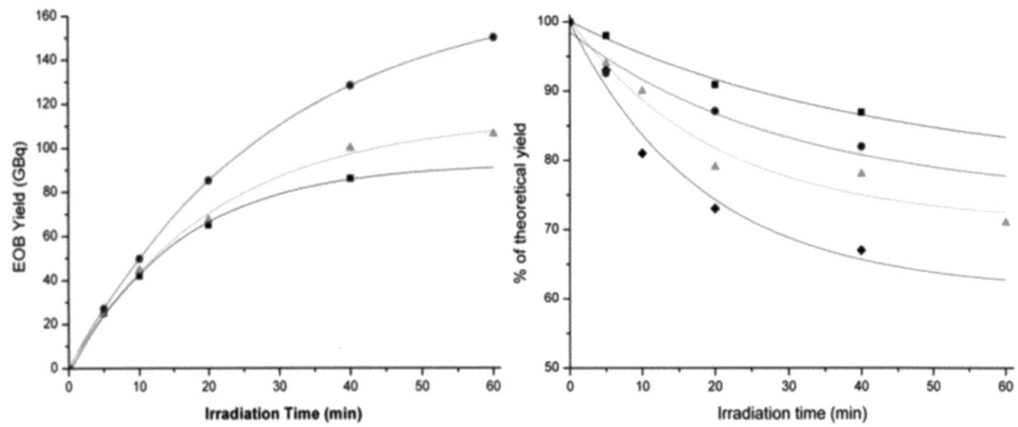

Fig. 5. (A) Theoretical and production yields expressed as GBq at EOB with a beam current of 25 μA. Theoretical yield (●); target with quartz insert (▲); target without quartz insert (■); (B) Production yields expressed as percentage of the theoretical yield for 10 μA with (■) and without quartz insert (●) and for 25 μA with (▲) and without quartz insert (◆).

Buckley et al. (2004) had previously proposed an exponential equation which target production data could be fitted to:

$$Y = A\, e^{-at}\, I\, SF \qquad (3)$$

Where Y is the decay-corrected yield (mCi), A the fitted pre-exponential term (mCi/μA, term representing production rates in the target), a the fitted exponential term (min^{-1}, representing losses due to activity retained in the target), I the beam current, t the irradiation time (min) and SF the saturation correction factor ($1-e^{-\lambda t}$).

The results obtained after fitting the data obtained by Koziorowski and coworkers are shown in Table 4, and compared to those previously obtained with the niobium target (Buckley et al., 2004). As can be seen, the quartz-lined target chamber performs well compared with the niobium target chamber, while the pure aluminum chamber performs slightly less well.

Target chamber	*A*	*a* (x 10000)
Niobium cylinder†	95 ± 2	40 ± 4
Quartz-lined aluminum cylinder‡	170 ± 6	45 ± 11
Aluminum cylinder*	168 ± 10	85 ± 26
Aluminum cone*	78 ± 9	135 ± 44
Nickel cone*	65 ± 9	527 ± 67
Stainless Steel cylinder*	71 ± 11	64 ± 62
Large Aluminum cylinder*	70 ± 9	180 ± 52

Table 4. Fitted parameters *A* and *a* for targets used for production of [^{11}C]CH_4. †Buckley et al., 2004; ‡ Koziorowski et al., 2010; * Buckley et al., 2000.

3.2.2 [^{11}C]CH_3I production and methylation

The general reaction pathway followed for the preparation of ^{11}C-labelled radiopharmaceuticals via methylation using [^{11}C]CH_3I (or [^{11}C]CH_3OTf) produced from [^{11}C]CH_4 can be summarized in 5 steps: (i) [^{11}C]CH_4 is generated in a cyclotron via the ^{14}N(p,α)^{11}C nuclear reaction by bombarding a N_2/H_2 mixture with high energy protons; (ii) the target content is transferred to a hot cell and trapped in Carbosphere 60/80 at low T (approximatelly-140°C); (iii) [^{11}C]CH_4 is desorbed by heating (~80°C) and allowed to react with iodine at 720°C to form [^{11}C]methyl iodide in a gas circulating process. At this step, due to the low efficiency of the iodination reaction, [^{11}C]methyl iodide is selectively retained in a trap (Porapak™ Q, 50-80 mesh) at room temperature, while unreacted [^{11}C]CH_4 is allowed to recirculate until reaction is complete (~80% conversion). (iv) After several recirculations, the Porapak™ Q trap is heated (~190°C) and [^{11}C]methyl iodide is distilled under continuous inert gas flow (20 mL/min); (v) the gas stream is directed to a reactor pre-filled with a solution of the precursor and methylation reaction takes place. A single pass gas phase method (where [^{11}C]CH_4 is not recirculated but reacted with I_2 in a single step) was first reported (Prenant & Crouzel, 1991). Later the method was improved by changing the single-pass to recirculation, starting with either cyclotron produced [^{11}C]CO_2 (converted to [^{11}C]CH_4 by hydrogen reduction in the presence of a nickel catalyst) or[^{11}C]CH_4 (Larsen et al., 1997) reporting yields up to 83%, decay corrected.

3.2.3 Search for the sources of ^{12}C in methylation reactions starting from [^{11}C]CO_2 and [^{11}C]CH_4 via the gas phase method

When the latter procedure (reduction of [^{11}C]CO_2 with a catalyst to produce [^{11}C]CH_4) is used, the same problems associated to the introduction of carrier carbon as in the case of producing [^{11}C]CH_3I from [^{11}C]CO_2 via the wet method can be found: (i) CO, CH_4 and other carbon sources in the target gas can be transformed into CO_2 during irradiations and (ii) CO_2 absorbed on the inner surface of the target chamber or transfer lines can be released to the reaction environment. By using this method, Mock (2006) reported a maximum in specific activity of ~925 GBq/µmol, by using a RDS-111 Eclipse cyclotron and bombarding N_2/O_2; 99/1 mixture. The amount of carrier in the irradiated gas increased with irradiation time and also when the target remained pressurized (even without irradiation). Moreover, specific activity dropped for irradiations > 20µAh due to excessive carrier release from the target.

To overcome the problems associated to the use of [^{11}C]CO_2 at any step of the synthesis, an automated synthesis device using the single pass I_2 method coupled with the in situ [^{11}C]CH_4 production method (irradiation of N_2/H_2; 95/5) was developed, and the experimental conditions for the production of ultra high specific activity [^{11}C]CH_3I were optimized (Noguchi & Suzuki, 2003). The target body (aluminum A5056, metallic seal, length 150 mm, inlet aperture 20 mm, outlet aperture 30 mm) was carefully machined without oil and polished with sandpaper AA-400. All the parts for the target assembly were washed with HCl, Milli-Q water and acetone, and dried at 350°C under vacuum. The target chamber was then assembled quickly in an air-tight glove box filled with pure N_2 gas and connected to the production line. The production route was cleaned carefully by sweeping it under heating with a target gas or helium. Before irradiation for the production of radiotracers, the target chamber was loaded/unloaded a few times without irradiation and three times with irradiation (20 μA, 5 minutes). By following this procedure, specific activities of 4700 ± 2500 GBq/μmol (2900-9700 GBq/μmol) were achieved. However, as reported later (Zhang & Suzuki, 2005), an immediate decrease of such values was occasionally encountered. The authors analyzed the sources of carrier carbon in the previously developed system, assuming that some organic reagents (contaminants in the synthetic line) may react with I_2 vapor to yield CH_3I in the heated quartz tube, resulting in a significant decrease of the specific activity of [^{11}C]CH_3I. The authors found that traces of organic reagents, such as acetone, methanol, silicone oil and paraffin, reacted with I_2 to yield CH_3I in the heated quartz tube, resulting in a significant decrease of the specific activity of [^{11}C]CH_3I. Therefore, prior to production, sufficient washing and drying of the device components and sufficient flushing of the synthetic lines with a pure inert gas were suggested to improve specific activity. In this sense, Koziorowski & Gillings (2010) found that when specific activity of (cyclotron generated) CH_4 was measured by on-line conversion to HCN, values higher than 13000 GBq/μmol were encountered. These results suggest that the A_S of ^{11}C-labelled radiotracers synthesized by the gas phase method is lowered downstream from the target, i.e. during [^{11}C]CH_4 to [^{11}C]CH_3I conversion, which is consistent with the results of Zhang & Suzuki (2005).

Recently, a quartz-lined aluminum target for the production of [^{11}C]methane was developed (Koziorowski et al., 2010). On top of producing [^{11}C]CH_4 in excellent yields and reducing losses of radioactivity significantly (when compared with the aluminum target), the authors were able to produce radiopharmaceuticals with specific radioactivities up to 9000 GBq/μmol at end of bombardment (EOB). In Figure 6, the values of specific activity obtained by Koziorowski's group are depicted. These values were initially (already) a factor of four to five higher compared with the conical, aluminum 750 mL volume target. By installing an inline gas purifier, the specific activities further increased. Additionally, specific activity was seen to increase with repeated irradiations and radiosyntheses on the same day. This fact (which can be attributed to a conditioning effect) has been seen also by the authors of this chapter in a recently performed set of experiments with an Aluminum target (Unpublished results). Seven consecutive 0.25 μAh irradiations were performed in an aluminum target filled with N_2/H_2; 95/5 (P = 16 atm) at 22 μA. As can be seen in Figure 7A, the specific activity (corrected to EOB) increased from ~61 GBq/μmol (beam number 1) up to ~571 GBq/μmol (beam number 7) within one day. When experiments were performed the following day, the same pattern was obtained. A plateau seems to be achieved after 4 runs, which is a clear indication that contamination in the surface of the target walls/window is accumulated while the target is not used (it is maintained unpressurized) and is slowly released as the number of experiments increase. In a second set of experiments, three consecutive irradiations (under the experimental conditions stated above) were performed but the target was kept pressurized (P = 16 bar, N_2/H_2; 95/5) overnight to prevent contamination from the atmosphere. Higher values of A_S were obtained even in the first irradiation of the day (~ 557 GBq/μmol) and were maintained in consecutive runs (Figure 7B). Although the performance of the target was not (apparently) affected in terms of amount of activity obtained at the end of the synthesis, more experiments are still required to assess the potential degradation of the target due to long term exposure of Aluminum to the N_2/H_2 mixture.

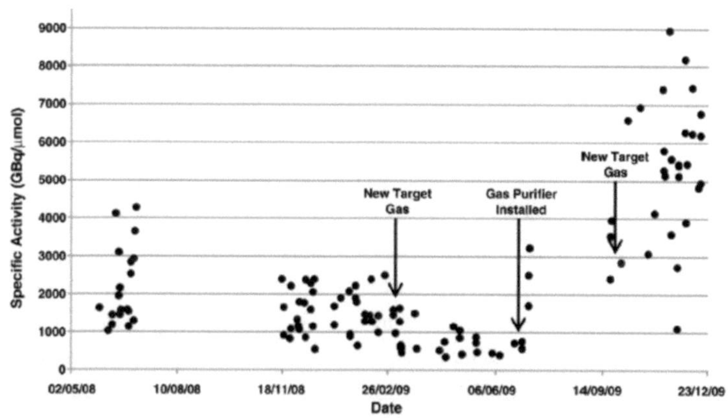

Fig. 6. Specific activities of [^{11}C]radiopharmaceuticals (EOB) produced from [^{11}C]methane.

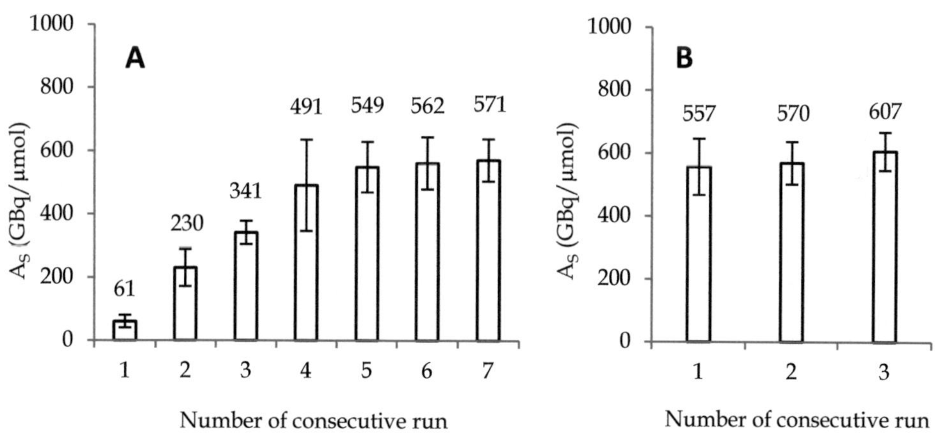

Fig. 7. (A) Specific activities of [^{11}C]anisole (EOB) produced from [^{11}C]methane within 1 day (integrated current = 0.25 μAh, beam intensity = 22 μA, filling pressure = 16 atm, aluminium target). (B) Specific activities of [^{11}C]anisole (EOB) produced from [^{11}C]methane within 1 day (same irradiation conditions, target filled with N_2/H_2 overnight).

4. General discussion and conclusions

As can be concluded from all the previous works, the discussion regarding the origin of non radioactive carbon and the procedures to minimize contamination effects (independently of the production process followed to generate carbon-11 and the reaction pathway followed afterwards) have been lasting for years. Although different sources have been encountered and their individual contribution somehow quantified, it seems clear that the final specific activity of ^{11}C-labelled radiotracers is extremely dependent of site-specific configuration and minimal alteration of experimental conditions can lead to considerable effects on specific activity values, especially when such specific activities are high.

Tables 5 and 6 show specific activity values reported in the literature for syntheses of ^{11}C-labelled radiotracers synthesized either from cyclotron generated $[^{11}C]CO_2$ or $[^{11}C]CH_4$ using either the wet method or the gas phase method. It is absolutely impossible to include every single reported value, and thus a selection has been performed while trying to include representative data. In order to get comparable results, values at EOB are shown, although values at EOS are also included. In the case that one of the values was not reported in the original publications but synthesis time was included, decay corrected values have been calculated and included in the tables.

As can be seen in table 5, specific activity values (EOS) are in the range 5.92-357 GBq/μmol (except for entrance 16, where extremely and unusually high A_S values were obtained, as discussed above). In most cases where high values (relative to average) were reported, specific procedures to prevent external contamination were applied. Thus, Matarrese and co-workers (2003) obtained high A_S values at EOB (217-357 GBq/μmol) by optimizing the amount of $LiAlH_4$ solution, flushing the target with gas several times before beam, checking (and correcting) leaks, carefully cleaning and drying the synthesis system and flushing the lines from the cyclotron to the synthesis boxes continuously during irradiations. However, no special actions were taken with the target itself. When these results are compared to those included in table 6, it can be concluded that higher specific activity values are obtained (in general terms) when the gas phase method is used, independently of the radioactive specie generated in the cyclotron (62-740 GBq/μmol for $[^{11}C]CO_2$, 74-5479 GBq/μmol for $[^{11}C]CH_4$), although higher values are obtained when cyclotron generated $[^{11}C]CH_4$ is used. This is due, partially, to the high concentration of CO_2 in the atmosphere which constitutes an important source of contamination. For instance, by switching from $[^{11}C]CO_2$ target to the $[^{11}C]CH_4$ target and using the gas phase method in both cases, a 6-17 fold increase of specific activity was found in the preparation of some ^{11}C-labelled radiotracers ($[^{11}C]$Raclopride, $[^{11}C]$MADAM, $[^{11}C]$PE2I and $[^{11}C]$FLB457 (Andersson et al., 2009)). In this case, the authors attributed this finding to $[^{11}C]CO_2$ being more sensitive to isotopic dilution from CO_2 in the air, than what the influence of environmental contamination of CH_4 is likely to have on the specific activity. Considering that the concentration of CO_2 and CH_4 in air are 365ppm and 1745ppb, respectively, a 200 times higher specific activity would be expected when using $[^{11}C]CH_4$. As long as the mentioned 200-fold increase is never found in real conditions, one can conclude that specific activity is lowered by carbon introduced not only from the air, but also from the system, all the way from the target gas to the reaction vessel. This is consistent with all previous works that have been referenced all along this chapter.

Entry	Radiotracer	A_S EOB (GBq/μmol)	A_S EOS (GBq/μmol)	Cyclotron	Reference
1	[^{11}C]DMT	13.32‡	3.4	18 MeV	Iwata et al., 1988
2	[^{11}C]MPTP	5.92‡	1.51	18 MeV	Iwata et al., 1988
3	Dilthiazhem	8.51‡	2.17	18 MeV	Iwata et al., 1988
4	[^{11}C]YM-09151-2	37‡	9.44	18 MeV	Iwata et al., 1988
5	[^{11}C]CH_3I	219 ± 88	185 ± 74	CTI-RDS-112	Matarrese et al., 2003
6	[^{11}C]*m*-hydroxy-ephedrine	357 ± 103	152 ± 44	CTI-RDS-112	Matarrese et al., 2003
7	[^{11}C]Flumazenil	304 ± 43	129.5 ± 18.5	CTI-RDS-112	Matarrese et al., 2003
8	[^{11}C]PNU 167760	217 ± 87	92.5 ± 37	CTI-RDS-112	Matarrese et al., 2003
9	[^{11}C]VC-195	258 ± 103	92.5 ± 44	CTI-RDS-112	Matarrese et al., 2003
10	[^{11}C](*R*)MDL-100907	-	392 ± 166	CTI-RDS-112	Matarrese et al., 2003
11	^{11}C-labelled Adrenoceptor antagonists	70	-	Scanditronix RNP 16	Balle et al., 2004
12	^{11}C-labelled *(S)*-thionisoxetine	74-111	22-33	IBA 18 MeV	Filannino et al., 2007
13	[^{11}C]CH_3I	42‡	30	IBA 18 MeV	Gómez-Vallejo et al., 2009
14	[^{11}C]DAC	37-170	-	CYPRIS HM18	Yui et al., 2011
15	[^{11}C]Verapamil	100-170	-	CYPRIS HM18	Yui et al., 2011
16	[^{11}C]TCH346	40-5700		GE PETtrace*	Ermert et al, 2008
17	[^{11}C]SKF 75670	86-305	26-92	Scanditronix MC 17	Da Silva et al., 1996
18	^{11}C-labelled 1-methyl-4-piperidyl-4'-fluorobenzoate	-	26	TCC CS30	Bormans et al., 1996
19	[^{11}C]ketamine	13-17	3.3-4.2	Not specified	Shiue et al., 1997
20	[^{11}C]SKF 82957	115	37	Scanditronix MC 17	Da Silva et al., 1999

Entry	Radiotracer	A_S EOB (GBq/µmol)	A_S EOS (GBq/µmol)	Cyclotron	Reference
21	[^{11}C]MeNER	82-153	35-65	Scanditronix MC 17	Wilson et al., 2003
22	[^{11}C]DAA1106	191-331	90-156	CYPRIS HM18	Zhang et al., 2003
23	^{11}C-labelled MAO-B imaging agents	145	37	Not specified	Vasdev et al., 2011
24	[^{11}C]DACA	163	41.5	Not specified	Brady et al., 1997
25	[^{11}C](L)-deprenyl	37	-	Japan Steel works 41-inch	Ferrieri et al., 1999
26	^{11}C-labelled flutamide derivatives	-	148	Not specified	Jacobson et al., 2006

Table 5. Specific activity values reported in the literature for ^{11}C-labelled radiotracers synthesized from [^{11}C]CO_2 and wet method. ‡corrected to end of transfer of activity, transfer time 3-12 min. *Modified target gas according to Qaim et al., 1993.

Entry	Radiotracer	Precursor†	A_S EOB (GBq/µmol)	A_S EOS (GBq/µmol)	Cyclotron	Reference
1	[^{11}C]MHED	[^{11}C]CO_2	444	360	13 MeV	Link et al., 1997
2	[^{11}C]Ro-15-4513	[^{11}C]CH_4	4700 ± 2500	2000 ± 1060	HM18 cyclotron	Noguchi & Suzuki, 2003
3	[^{11}C]Raclopride	[^{11}C]CH_4	74-370	-	TR13	Buckley et al., 2004
4	[^{11}C]Flumazenil	[^{11}C]CH_4	5730	2440	CYPRIS HM18	Zhang & Suzuki, 2005
5	[^{11}C]HOMADAM	[^{11}C]CO_2	221.1	28.5	Siemens RDS 112	Jarkas et al., 2005
6	[^{11}C]Raclopride	[^{11}C]CH_4	4880 ± 2360	1690 ± 818	CYPRIS HM18	Noguchi et al., 2008
7	[^{11}C]raclopride	[^{11}C]CO_2	124	36,27	GEMs PETtrace	Andersson et al., 2009
8	[^{11}C]raclopride	[^{11}C]CH_4	2335	784,67	GEMs PETtrace	Andersson et al., 2009
9	[^{11}C]MADAM	[^{11}C]CO_2	162	50,74	GEMs PETtrace	Andersson et al., 2009
10	[^{11}C]MADAM	[^{11}C]CH_4	2332	836,53	GEMs PETtrace	Andersson et al., 2009
11	[^{11}C]PE2I	[^{11}C]CO_2	183	59,31	GEMs PETtrace	Andersson et al., 2009

Entry	Radiotracer	Precursor†	A_S EOB (GBq/µmol)	A_S EOS (GBq/µmol)	Cyclotron	Reference
12	[^{11}C]PE2I	[^{11}C]CH_4	1097	683,54	GEMs PETtrace	Andersson et al., 2009
13	[^{11}C]FLB457	[^{11}C]CO_2	176	61,07	GEMs PETtrace	Andersson et al., 2009
14	[^{11}C]FLB457	[^{11}C]CH_4	1313	439,28	GEMs PETtrace	Andersson et al., 2009
15	Not especified	[^{11}C]CH_4	5479 ± 1735	-	Scanditronix MC 32	Koziorowski et al., 2010
16	[^{11}C]DAC	[^{11}C]CH_4	3670-4450	-	CYPRIS HM18	Yui et al., 2011
17	^{11}C-labelled styryl dyes	[^{11}C]CO_2	173.76-260.65	74-111	CTI 11 MeV Siemens	Wang et al., 2009
18	^{11}C-labelled tetrahydroiso-quinoline derivatives	[^{11}C]CO_2	148-222	63-94.54	CTI 11 MeV Siemens	Wang et al., 2007
19	^{11}C-labelled tetrahidroiso-quinolinium derivatives	[^{11}C]CO_2	62-123.50	37-74	CTI 11 MeV Siemens	Gao et al., 2008

Table 6. Specific activity values reported in the literature for ^{11}C-labelled radiotracers synthesized via gas phase method (starting either from [^{11}C]CH_4 or [^{11}C]CO_2).

Although (as previously discussed) the sources of contamination are extremely dependent on the particular configuration of the systems involved in the production process of each particular site, and despite the everlasting discussion among scientists to find out (and control) the main factors contributing to a decrease in the specific activity of ^{11}C-labelled radiotracers, there are general procedures that, independently of the employed radioactive precursor and the synthetic route, might help to improve specific activity. However, it has to be taken into account that contamination can come at any step of the synthesis process, and therefore precautions should be taken at each single step.

1. Generation of the radioactive precursor in the cyclotron; at this step, the purity of the gases, the material of the target chamber, the windows and the o-rings (and the procedure followed for their machining and polishing), the size of the target chamber and the quality of the irradiated gas have been found to have important effects on the introduction of carrier carbon. Beam time and beam current should also be considered. The use of high purity gases (with a purification column between the gas source and the target), careful cleaning of the target chamber components, the use of metallic o-rings

and recovering the target chamber with materials which minimize beam-wall interactions lead usually to improvement in A_S. Increasing beam time and/or current (up to a certain level) offers usually satisfactory results. Preparation protocols have been also historically used, e.g. loading and unloading the target before irradiation, discarding the first 1-3 irradiations of the day and keeping the target under pressure between runs.

2. Transfer of the irradiated gas to the synthesis box; increasing time decreases specific activity, and thus minimizing transfer time leads to higher specific activity values. The material of transfer lines (pipes and connections) and the carrier gas (if used) could also introduce non radioactive carbon into the reaction environment. This should be considered when chosing dimensions (i.e inner diameter; ID) for the transport line: the smaller the ID the less the material, but longer empying/delivery time. Keeping the lines pressurized with high purity gases and avoiding carbon-rich materials should help, thus, to increase A_S.
3. Synthesis process; at this step, the use of high purity reagents is the most important factor. All traps can be activated before synthesis, and reagents should be prepared and stored under adequate inert conditions to prevent contamination from the atmosphere. Reagents and solvents should be used in minimal amounts, especially in those cases where they are supposed to be potential sources of carrier carbon (e.g. $LiAlH_4$ in the wet method). Special attention should be paid to the purity of the non radioactive precursor, which could be contaminated (*ab initio*) with the methylated species. The synthesis box should be also cleaned and dried thoroughly and kept isolated from atmosphere; traces of solvents and direct contact with air contribute to decreased A_S.

5. References

Ache, H. J. & Wolf, A. P. (1968). Effect of Radiation on the Reactions of Recoil Carbon-11 in the Nitrogen-Oxigen System. *The Journal of Physical Chemistry*, Vol. 72, No. 6, (June 1968), pp. 1988-1993, ISSN 0022-2623

Andersson, J., Truong, P., & Halldin, C. (2009). In-Target Produced [^{11}C] Methane: Increased Specific Radioactivity. *Applied Radiation and Isotopes,* Vol. 67, No. 1, (January 2009), pp. 106-110, ISSN 0969-8043

Balle, T., Halldin, C., Andersen, L., Alifrangis, L.H., Badolo, L., Jensen, K.G., Chou, Y., Andersen, K., Perregaard, J., & Farde, L. (2004). New α_1 - Adrenoceptor Antagonists Derived from the Antipsychotic Sertindole-Carbon-11 Labelling and Pet Examination of Brain Uptake in the Cynomolgus Monkey. *Nuclear Medicine and Biology,* Vol. 31, No. 3, (April 2004), pp. 327-336, ISSN 0969-8051

Bernhardt, P., Kölby, L., Johanson, V., Nilsson, O., Ahlman, H., & Forssell-Aronssona, E. (2003). Biodistribution of ^{111}In-DTPA-D-Phe1-octreotide in Tumor-Bearing Nude Mice: Influence of Amount Injected and Route of Administration. *Nuclear Medicine and Biology,* Vol. 30, No. 3, (April 2003), pp. 253–260, ISSN 0969-8051

Bonardi, M.L. (2003). Terminology, Quantities and Units Concerning Production and Applications of Radionuclides in Radiopharmaceutical and Radioanalytical Chemistry, In*: IUPAC,* 03.08.2011, Available from http://www.iupac.org/web/ins/2003-015-2-500

Bormans, G., Sherman, P., Snyder, S.E., & Kilbourn, M.R. (1996). Synthesis of Carbon-11 and Fluorine-18-Labeled 1-Methyl-4-Piperidyl-4'-Fluorobenzoate and their Distribution in Mice. *Nuclear Medicine and biology*, Vol. 23, No. 4, (May 1996), pp. 513-517, ISSN 0969-8051

Brady, F., Luthra, S., Brown, G., Osman, S., Harte, R., Denny, W., Baguley, E., Jonnes, T., & Price, P. (1997). Carbon-11 Labelling of the Antitumour Agent N-[2-(Dimethylamino)ethyl)]acridine-4-carboxamide (DACA) and Determination of Plasma Metabolites in Man, *Applied Radiation and Isotopes*, Vol. 48, No. 4, (April 1997), pp. 487-497, ISSN 0969-8043

Buckley, K.R., Huser, J., Jivan, S., Chun, K.S., & Ruth, T.J. (2000). ^{11}C-Methane Production in Small Volume, High Pressure Gas Targets. *Radiochimica Acta,* Vol. 88, No. 3-4, (Alfred P. Wolf Memorial 2000), pp. 201, ISSN 0033-8230

Buckley, K.R., Jivan, S., & Ruth, T.J. (2004). Improved Yields for the in Situ Production of [^{11}C]CH_4 Using a Niobium Target Chamber. *Nuclear Medicine and biology*, Vol. 31, No. 6, (August 2004), pp. 825–827, ISSN 0969-8051

Catafau, A.M., Suarez, M., Bullich, S., Llop, J., Nucci, G., Gunn, R.N., Britain, C., & Laruelle, M. (2009). Within-subject Comparison of Striatal D2 Receptor Occupancy Measurements Using [^{123}I]IBZM SPECT and [^{11}C]Raclopride PET. *NeuroImage*, Vol. 46, No. 2, (June 2009), pp. 447-458, ISSN 1053-8119

Christman, D.R., Finn, R.D., Karlstrom, K.I., & Wolf, A.P. (1975). The Production of Ultra High ^{11}C-Labeled Hydrogen Cyanide, Carbon Dioxide, Carbon Monoxide and Methane Via the ^{14}N(p,α)^{11}C Reaction (XV). *The International Journal of Applied Radiation and Isotopes,* Vol. 26, No. 8, (August 1975), pp. 435–442, ISSN 0020-708X

Crouzel, C., Langstrom, B., Pike, V.W., & Coenen, H.H. (1987). Recommendations for a Practical Production of [^{11}C]Methyl Iodide. *Applied Radiation and Isotopes,* Vol. 38, No. 8, (January 1987), pp. 601–603, ISSN 0969-8043

DaSilva, J.N., Wilson, A.A., Nobrega, J.N., Jiwa, D., & Houle, S. (1996). Synthesis and Autoradiographic Localization of the Dopamine-1 Agonists [^{11}C]SKF-75670 and [^{11}C]-SKF 82957 as Potential Pet Radioligands. *Applied Radiation and Isotopes,* Vol. 47, No. 3, (March 1996), pp. 279-284, ISSN 0969-8043.

DaSilva, J.N., Swartz, R.A., Greenwald, E.R., Lorenco, C.M., Wilson, A.A., & Houle, S. (1999). Dopamine D1 Agonist R-[^{11}C]SKF-82957: Synthesis and in Vivo Characterization in Rat. *Nuclear Medicine and Biology,* Vol. 26, No. 5, (July 1999), pp. 537-542, ISSN 0969-8051

Dahl, J. R., & Schlyer D. J. (1985). Target Materials. *Proceedings of The First Workshop on Targetry and Target Chemistry,* Institut fur Nuklearmedizin, Heidelberg, West Germany, October 1985.

Dubrin, J., Mackay, C., Pandow, M. L., & Wolfgang, R. (1964). Reactions of Atomic Carbon with π-Bonded Inorganic Molecules. *Journal of Inorganic and Nuclear Chemistry*, Vol. 26, No. 12, (December 1964), pp. 2113-2122, ISSN 0022-1902.

Ehrin, E., Farde, L., De Paulis, T., Eriksson, L., Greitz, T., Johnström, P., Litton, J.E., Lars, J., Nilsson, G., Sedvall, G., Stone-Elander, S., & Ögren, S.O. (1985). Preparation of ^{11}C-Labelled Raclopride, a New Potent Dopamine Receptor Antagonist: Preliminary PET Studies of Cerebral Dopamine Receptors in the Monkey. *The International*

Journal of Applied Radiation and Isotopes, Vol. 36, No. 4, (April 1985), pp. 269-273, ISSN 0020-708X

Ehrlich, P. On immunity, with special reference to cell-life (Croonian Lecture, Royal Society of London, 1990), reprinted in Collected Papers of Ehrlich P, vol 2, ed Himmelweit, New York

Elsinga, P.H., Hatano, K., & Ishiwata, K. (2006). PET Tracers for Imaging of the Dopaminergic System. *Current Medicinal Chemistry,* Vol. 13, No. 18, (2006), pp. 2139–2152, ISSN 0929-8673

Epherre, M., & Seide, C. (1971). Excitation Functions of ^{7}Be and ^{11}C Produced in Nitrogen by Low-Energy Protons. *Physical Review C,* Vol. 3, No. 6, (1971), pp. 2167-2171, ISSN 0556-2813

Eriksson, J., Mooij, R., Buijs, F. L., Lambert, B., Van Rooij, L. F., Kruijer, P. S., & Windhorst, A.D. (2009). In Pursuit of [^{11}C]Carbon Dioxide with Increased Specific Activity. *Journal of Labelled Compounds and Radiopharmaceuticals,* Vol. 52, No. S1,(June 2009), pp. S57–S63, ISSN 1099-1344

Ermert, J., Stüsgen, S., Lang, M., Roden, W., & Coenen, H.H. (2008). High Molar Activity of [11C]TCH346 Via [11C]Methyl Triflate Using the "Wet" [^{11}C]CO_2 Reduction Method. *Applied Radiation and Isotopes,* Vol. 66, No. 5, (May 2008), pp. 619-624, ISSN 0969-8043

Ferrieri, R.A., Alexoff D.L., Schyler D. J., McDonald, K., & Wolf, A. P. (1993). Target Design Considerations for High Specific Activity [^{11}C]CO_2. *Proceedings of the Fifth International Workshop on Targetry and Target Chemistry,* Brookhaven National Laboratory & North Shore University Hospital, Upton, New York, USA, September 1993

Ferrieri, R.A., Garcia, I., Fowler, J.S., & Wolf, A.P. (1999). Investigations of Acetonitrile Solvent Cluster Formation in Supercritical Carbon Dioxide, and its Impact on Microscale Syntheses of Carbon-11 Labeled Radiotracers for PET. *Nuclear Medicine and Biology,* Vol. 26, No. 4, (May 1999), pp. 443-454, ISSN 0969-8051

Filannino, M., Matarresse, M., Turolla, E., Masiello, V., Moresco, R.M., Todde, S., Verza, E., Magni, F., Cattaneo, A., Bachi, A., Kienle, M.G., & Fazio, F. (2007). Synthesis and Carbon-11 Labeling of (R)- and (S)-Thionisoxetine, Norepirephrine Reuptake Inhibitors, Potential Radioligands for Positron Emission Tomography. *Applied Radiation and Isotopes,* Vol. 65, No. 11, (November 2007), pp. 1232-1239, ISSN 0969-8043

Gao, M., Wang, M., & Zheng, Q.H. (2008). Synthesis of Carbon-11-Labeled 1-(3,4-dimethoxybenzyl)-2,2-dimethyl-1,2,3,4-tetrahydroisoquinolimium as New Potential PET Skca Channel Imaging Agents. *Applied Radiation and Isotopes,* Vol. 66, No. 2, (February 2008), pp. 194-202, ISSN 0969-8043

Gómez-Vallejo, V., & Llop, J. (2009). Specific Activity of [^{11}C]CH_3I Synthesized by the Wet Method: Main Sources of Non-Radioactive Carbon. *Applied Radiation and Isotopes,* Vol. 67, No. 1, (January 2009), pp. 111-114, ISSN 0969-8043

Hashimoto, K., Inoue, O., Suzuki, K., Yamasaki, T., & Kojima, M. (1989). Synthesis and Evaluation of ^{11}C-PK 11195 For in Vivo Study of Peripheral-Type Benzodiazepine

Receptors Using Position Emission Tomography. *Annals of Nuclear Medicine,* Vol. 3, No. 2, (August 2009), pp. 63-71, ISSN 1864-6433

Itsenko, O., Kihlberg, T., & Långström, B. (2006). Labeling of Aliphatic Carboxylic Acids using [^{11}C] Carbon Monoxide. *Nature Protocols,* Vol. 1, No. 2, (July 2006), pp. 798-802, ISSN 1754-2189.

Iwata, R,. Ido, T., Ujiie, A., Takahashi, T., Ishiwata, K., Hatano, K., & Sugahara, M. (1988). Comparative Study of Specific Activity of [11C]Methyl Iodide: A Search for the Source of Carrier Carbon. *International Journal of Radiation Applications and Instrumentation. Part A. Applied Radiation and Isotopes,* Vol. 39, No. 1, (1988), pp. 1-7, ISSN 0969-8043

Jacobson, O., Laky, D., Carlson, K., Elgavish, S., Gozin, M., Even-Sapir, E., Leibovitc, E., Gutman, M., Chisin, R., Katzenellenbogen, J.A., & Mishani, E. (2006). Chiral Dimethylamine Flutamide Derivatives-Modeling, Synthesis Androgen Receptor Affinities and Carbon-11 Labeling. *Nuclear Medicine and Biology,* Vol. 33, No. 6, (August 2006), pp. 695-674, ISSN 0969-8051

Jarkas, N., Votaw, J., Voll, J., Williams, L., Camp, V.M., Owens, M.J., Purselle, P.C., Bremmer, J.D., Kilts, C.D., Nemeroff, C.B., & Goodman, M.M. (2005). Carbon-11 HOMADAM: A Novel PET Radiotraces for Imaging Serotonin Transportes. *Nuclear Medicine and biology,* Vol. 32, No. 3, (April 2005), pp. 211-224, ISSN 0969-8051

Jewett, D.M. (1992). A Simple Synthesis of [^{11}C]Methyl Triflate. *International Journal of Radiation Applications and Instrumentation. Part A. Applied Radiation and Isotopes,* Vol. 43, No. 11, (November 1992), pp. 1383-1385, ISSN 0969-8043

de Jong, M., Breeman, W.A.P., Bernard, B.F., Van Gameren, A., De Bruin, E., Bakker, W.H., Van der Pluijm, M. E., Visser, T. J., Mäcke, H. R., & Krenning, E.P.(1999). Tumour Uptake of the Radiolabelled Somatostatin Analogue [DOTA0,TYR3]Octreotide is Dependent on the Peptide Amount. *European Journal of Nuclear Medicine,* Vol 26, No. 7, (June 1999), pp. 693–698, ISSN 1619-7070.

Karimi, F., Kihlberg, T., & Långström, B. (2001). [^{11}C] / (^{13}C) Carbon Monoxide in Palladium-Mediated Synthesis of Imides. *Journal of the Chemical Society, Perkin Transactions1,* Vol. 2001, No. 13, (2001), pp 1528-1531, ISSN 1472-7781

Koziorowski, J., Larsen, P., & Gillings, N. (2010). A Quartz-Lined Carbon-11 Target: Striving for Increased Yield and Specific Activity. *Nuclear Medicine and Biology,* Vol. 37, No. 8, (November 2010), pp. 943–948, ISSN 0969-8051

Koziorowski, J., & Gillings, N. (2010). Streamlined Measurement of the Specific Radioactivity of in Target Produced [^{11}C]Methane by On-line Conversion to [^{11}C]Hydrogen Cyanide, proceedings of the 13th WTTC, Risoe, Denmark, July, 2010

Langstrom, B., & Lundqvist, H. (1976). The Preparation of ^{11}C-Methyl Iodine and its Use in the Synthesis of ^{11}C-Methyl-L-Methionine. *The International Journal of Applied Radiation and Isotopes,* Vol. 27, No. 7, (July 1976), pp. 357-363, ISSN 0020-708X

Larsen, P., Ulin, J., Dahlström, K., & Jensen, M. (1997). Synthesis of [^{11}C]Iodomethane by Iodination of [^{11}C]Methane. *Applied Radiation and Isotopes,* Vol. 48, No. 2, (February 1997), pp. 153-157, ISSN 0969-8043

Link, J. M., Krohn, K. A., & Clark, J. C. (1997). Production of [^{11}C]CH_3I by Single Pass Reaction of [^{11}C]CH_4 with I_2. *Nuclear Medicine and Biology*, Vol. 24, No. 1, (January 1997), pp. 93-97, ISSN 0969-8051

Matarrase, M., Soloviev, D., Todde, S., Neutro, F., Petta, P., Carpinelli, A., Brüssermann, M., Kniele, M.G., & Fazio, F. (2003). Preparation of [^{11}C]Radioligands with High Specific Radioactivity on a Commercial PET Tracer Synthesizer. *Nuclear Medicine and Biology*, Vol. 30, No. 1, (January 2003), pp. 79-83, ISSN 0969-8051

Mathis, C.A., Wang, Y., Holt, D.P., Huang, G.F., Debnath, M.L., & Klunk, W.E. (2003). Synthesis and Evaluation of ^{11}C-Labelled 6-Substituted 2-Arylbenzothiazoles as Amyloid Imaging Agents. *Journal of Medicinal Chemistry*, Vol. 46, No 13, (June 2003), pp 2740–2754, ISSN 0022-2623

Mock, B.H., Vavrek, T., & Mulholland, G.K. (1995). Solid-Phase Reversible Trap for [^{11}C] Carbon Dioxide Using Carbon Molecules Sieves. *Nuclear Medicine and Biology*, Vol. 22, No. 5, (July 1995), pp. 667-670, ISSN 0969-8051

Mock, B.H. (2006). The Search for Carrier [^{12}C]Carbon: A User's Experience with the RDS-111 Eclipse Target. *Eleventh International Workshop on Targetry and Target Chemistry*, Robinson College, Cambridge, August 2006

Noguchi, J., & Suzuki, K. (2003). Automated Synthesis of the Ultra High Specific Activity of [^{11}C]Ro154513 and its Application in an Extremely Low Concentration Region to an ARG Study. *Nuclear Medicine and Biology*, Vol. 30, No. 3, (April 2003), pp. 335-343, ISSN 0969-8051

Noguchi, J., Zhang, M.R., Yanamoto, K., Nakao, R., & Suzuki, K. (2008). In Vitro Binding of [^{11}C]Raclopride with Ultra High Specific Activity in Rat Brain Determined by Homogenate Assay and Autorradiography. *Nuclear Medicine and Biology*, Vol.35, No. 1, (January 2008), pp. 19-27, ISSN 0969-8051

Pandit-Taskar, N., O'Donoghue, J.A., Morris, M.J., Wills, E.A., Schwartz, L.H., Gonen, M., Scher, H.I., Larson, S.M., & Divgi, C.R. (2008). Antibody Mass Escalation Study in Patients with Castration-Resistant Prostate Cancer Using ^{111}In-J591: Lesion Detectability and Dosimetric Projections for 90Y Radioimmunotherapy. *The Journal of Nuclear Medicine*, Vol. 49, No. 7, (July 2008), pp. 1066-1074, ISSN 0161-5505

Prenant, C., & Crouzel, C. (1991). A new simple and attractive method of [^{11}C]halogenomethanes production (Br^{11}CH_3, I^{11}CH_3). *Journal of Labelled Compounds and Radiopharmaceuticals*, Vol. 30, No. 1, (December 1991), pp. 125, ISSN 1099-1344

Qaim, S.M., Clark, J.C., Crouzel, C., Guillaume, M., Helmeke, H.J., Nebeling, B., Pike, V.W., & Stöcklin, G. (1993). PET radionuclide production. In: *Radiopharmaceuticals for PET*, Kluwer Academic Publishers, Dordrecht, pp. 15–26

Rahman, O., Kihlberg, T., & Bengt Långström, B. (2003). Aryl Triflates and [^{11}C]/(^{13}C)Carbon Monoxide in the Synthesis of ^{11}C-/^{13}C-Amides. *The Journal of Organic Chemistry*, Vol. 68, No. 9, pp. 3558–3562, ISSN 0022-3263

Shiue, C., Vallabhahosula, S., Wolf, A.P., Dewey, S.L., Fowler, J.S., Schlyer, D. J., Arnett, C.D., & Zhou, Y.C. (1997). Carbon-11 Labelled Ketamine: Synthesis, Distribution in Mice and PET Studies in Baboons. *Nuclear Medicine and Biology*, Vol. 24, No. 2, (February 1997), pp. 145-150, ISSN 0969-8051

Schlyer, D. J., & Plascjak, P. S. (1991). Small Angle Multiple Scattering of Charged Particles in Cyclotron Target Foils - a Comparison of Experiment with Simple Theory. *Nuclear Instruments and Methods in Physics Research Section B: Beam Interactions with Materials and Atoms,* Vol. 56-57, No. 1, pp. 464-468, ISSN 0168-583X

Schuhmacher, J., Zhang, H., Doll, J., Mäcke, H.R., Matys, R., Hauser, H., Henze, M., Haberkorn, U., & Eisenhut, M. (2005). GRP Receptor-Targeted PET of a Rat Pancreas Carcinoma Xenograft in Nude Mice with a ^{68}Ga-Labeled Bombesin (6-14) Analog. *The Journal of Nuclear Medicine,* Vol. 46, No. 4, (April 2005), pp. 691-699, ISSN 0161-5505

Van Laere, K., Clerinx, K., D'Hondt, E., De Groot, T., & Vandenberghe, W. (2010). Combined Striatal Binding and Cerebral Influx Analysis of Dynamic ^{11}C-Raclopride PET Improves Early Differentiation Between Multiple-System Atrophy and Parkinson Disease. *The Journal of Nuclear Medicine,* Vol. 51, No. 4, (April 2010), pp. 588-595, ISSN 0161-5505

Vasdev, N., Sadovski, O., Moran, M.D., Parkes, J., Meyer, J.H., Houle, S., & Wilson, A.A. (2011). Development of New Radiopharmaceutical for Imaging Monoamine Oxidase B. *Nuclear Medicine and Biology,* Article in Press, Corrected Proof (2011), ISSN 0969-8051

Velikyan, I., Sundin, A., Eriksson, B., Lundqvist, H., Sörensen, J., Bergström, M., & Långström, B. (2010). In Vivo Binding of [^{68}Ga]-DOTATOC to Somatostatin Receptors in Neuroendocrine Tumours-Impact of Peptide Mass. *Nuclear Medicine and Biology,* Vol. 37, No. 3, (April 2010), pp. 265-275, ISSN 0969-8051

Wagner, R., Stöcklin, G., & Schaack, W. (1981). Production of Carbon-11 Labelled Methyl Iodide by Direct Recoil Synthesis. *Journal of Labelled Compounds and Radiopharmaceuticals,* Vol. 18, No. 11, (November 1981), pp. 1557–1566, ISSN 1099-1344

Wang, M., Gao, M., Miller, K.D., Sledge, G.W., & Zheng, Q.H. (2007). Synthesis of Carbon-11 Labeled Biaryl 1,2,3,4-Tetrahydroisoquinoline Derivatives and Conformationally Flexible Analogues as New Potential PET Glioma Tumor Imaging Agents. *Applied Radiation and Isotopes,* Vol. 65, No. 10, (October 2007), pp. 1152-1159, ISSN 0969-8043

Wang, M., Gao, M., Miller, K.D., Sledge, G.W., & Zheng, Q.H. (2009). Simple Synthesis of Carbon-11 Labeled Styryl Dyes as New Potential PET RNA-Specific, Living Cells Imaging Probes. *European Journal of Medicinal Chemistry,* Vol.44, No. 5, (May 2009), pp. 2300-2306, ISSN 0223-5234.

Wilson, A.A., Johnson, D.P., Mozley, D., Hussey, D., Ginovart, N., Nobrega, J., Garcia, A., Meyer, J., & Houle, S. (2003). Synthesis and in Vivo Evaluation of Novel Radiotracers for the in Vivo Imaging of the Norepirephrine Transporter. *Nuclear Imaging and Biology,* Vol. 30, No. 2, (2003), pp. 85-92

Yui, J., Hatori, A., Kawamura, K., Yanamoto, K., Yamasaki, T., Ogawa, M., Yoshida, Y., Kumata, K., Fujinaga, M., Nengaki, N., Fukumura, T., Suzuki, K., & Zhang, M.R. (2011). Visualiton of Early Infarction in Rat Brain After Ischemia Using a Translocator Protein (18 KDa) PET Ligand [^{11}C]DAC with Ultra High Specific Activity. *NeuroImage,* Vol. 54, No. 1, (January 2011), pp. 123-130, ISSN 1053-8119

Zhang, M.R., Kida, T., Noguchi, J., Furutsuka, K., Maeda, J., Suhara, T., & Suzuki, K. (2003). [^{11}C]DAA1106: Radiosynthesis and in Vivo Binding to Peripheral Benzodiazepine Receptors in Mouse Brain. *Nuclear Medicine and Biology*, Vol. 30, No. 5, (May 2003), pp. 513-519, ISSN 0969-8051

Zhang, M.R., & Suzuki, K. (2005). Sources of Carbon which Decrease the Specific Activity of [^{11}C]CH3I Synthesized by the Single Pass I2 Method. *Applied Radiation and Isotopes*, Vol. 62, No. 3, (March 2005), pp. 447-450, ISSN 0969-8043

Part 3

Clinical Application and Diagnosis

8

Potential of Positron Emission Tomography for Neurogenic Tumors and Spinal Disorders

Kenichiro Kakutani, Koichiro Maeno,
Yuki Iwama, Masahiro Kurosaka and Kotaro Nishida
Department of Orthopaedic Surgery, Kobe University Graduate School of Medicine
Japan

1. Introduction

Positron emission tomography (PET) is a three-dimensional nuclear medicine imaging technique that provides metabolic information about the body. This technique was first introduced by Kuhl et al. (Kuhl, Chamberlain et al. 1956). The basic principle of this system is to detect pairs of gamma rays emitted indirectly by a positron-emitting radionuclide (tracer), which is introduced into the body on a biologically active molecule. The metabolic information as three-dimensional imaging is obtained from the positional information of the tracer, obtained by computer analysis of the gamma rays. The metabolic information obtained is considered a functional imaging technique, whereas computed tomography (CT) and magnetic resonance imaging (MRI) are regarded as morphologic imaging techniques. Moreover, the fusion of PET with CT (PET-CT) has further elevated the precision of functional imaging techniques. Clinical applications of PET have increased in the last decade and have proven to be vital in the evaluation and diagnosis of diseases. The broad scope, versatility and sensitivity of PET make it the most powerful molecular imaging technique currently available for clinical use.

2. Clinical use of PET

PET is currently employed for preliminary diagnosis, evaluation of therapy and to determine the aggressiveness of a disease. Its most common and beneficial use is in oncology. The therapeutic strategy used in oncology must be developed according to the stage of the malignancy. The importance of staging derives from the clinical finding that the prognosis of patients with localized malignant disease is generally much better than those with metastases throughout the body. PET is also used for assessment of a viable myocardium that may respond to reperfusion and for medically refractory epilepsy.

The measurement of glucose metabolic rate is one of the prime measures of physiology in the human body. Anaerobic glycolysis is an early indicator of malignant transformation of cells (Schlyer 2004). Whole-body PET imaging with ^{18}F-fluoro-2′-deoxy-D-glucose (^{18}FDG), enables the evaluation of glucose metabolism throughout the entire body in a single examination to improve the detection and staging of a cancer, selection of therapy, and assessment of therapeutic response. Clinical indications for ^{18}FDG-PET imaging are well documented for many solid tumors in adults. Several studies have established that ^{18}FDG-PET techniques have higher specificity than CT (Czernin 2002).

This article focuses on the clinical use of PET in spine surgery. First, we describe the feasibility of using PET for obtaining a preliminary diagnosis, including peripheral benign nerve tumors. Second, the use of PET to assess the functional impairment of the spinal cord in patients with cervical myelopathy is described.

3. Feasibility of the use of PET for preliminary diagnosis

In clinical situations, spine surgeons often encounter patients demonstrating intractable pain or progressive neurologic deficits of unknown origin that cannot be detected by conventional imaging tools. We have had two cases for which PET provided helpful evidence in obtaining a definitive diagnosis.

3.1 Case report (intractable pain)

A 37-year old woman experienced severe sciatica after hitting her left buttock with great force on the edge of a bathtub. A physical examination demonstrated intense radiating pain from the left buttock to the lateral calf. There was weakness in the sciatic nerve innervated musculature. She was diagnosed with Piriformis syndrome by a local hospital. However, her symptoms remained unchanged after surgery to release the Piriformis. Conventional imaging of the sciatica, including plain radiographs, CT and MRI of the spine, showed no abnormal findings. ^{18}FDG-PET detected an abnormal lesion in the sciatic nerve in the posterior compartment of the patient's left thigh, indicating an intraneural tumor in the sciatic nerve. Subtotal resection was achieved and the histological evaluation of the specimen showed typical features of nodular fasciitis (Figure 1). After surgery, the patient was relieved of all symptoms with no evidence of recurrence at a recent two-year follow-up (Kakutani, Doita et al.).

3.2 Case report (Wegener's granulomatosis)

A 61-year old woman presented with progressive back pain, low-grade fever and gait disturbance. She was admitted to our hospital with paralysis of the left lower limb and bladder and rectal disturbances. A neurological examination revealed hyper-reflexia of the left patella and Achilles tendons, a positive Babinski's reflex, muscle weakness in the left lower extremities, foot drop and hypoesthesia below the T3 dermatome. The cranial nerve was not impaired. MRI of the thoracic spine revealed a diffuse space-occupying lesion at the anterior spinal cord in Th2-7. The lesion was hypointense on T1–weighted images and hyperintese on T2–weighted images. The lesion was enhanced after administration of contrast medium. ^{18}FDG-PET detected high uptake in the thoracic spine, bilateral upper lungs, and surrounding tissue of the abdominal aorta (Figure 2). Despite hospital admission and bed rest, the neurological deficit deteriorated, and the authors performed a laminectomy at Th1-T6 and posterior fusion with instrumentation at C7-Th7, including open biopsy. The histological examination of the surgical specimen showed fibrin deposition and granulation tissue formation with inflammatory infiltrate; no definitive diagnosis could be obtained from the surgery and biopsy. However, in addition to the abnormal ^{18}FDG-PET findings, further examinations revealed elevated levels of MPO-ANCA of 66 U/ml (normal<10.0 U/ml) and we concluded that the epidural spinal tumor was a complication associated with Wegener's granulomatosis. The high uptake in the bilateral upper lungs and surrounding tissue of the abdominal aorta detected by ^{18}FDG-PET was the conclusive evidence for the definitive diagnosis of Wegener's granulomatosis (Kasagi, Saegusa et al.).

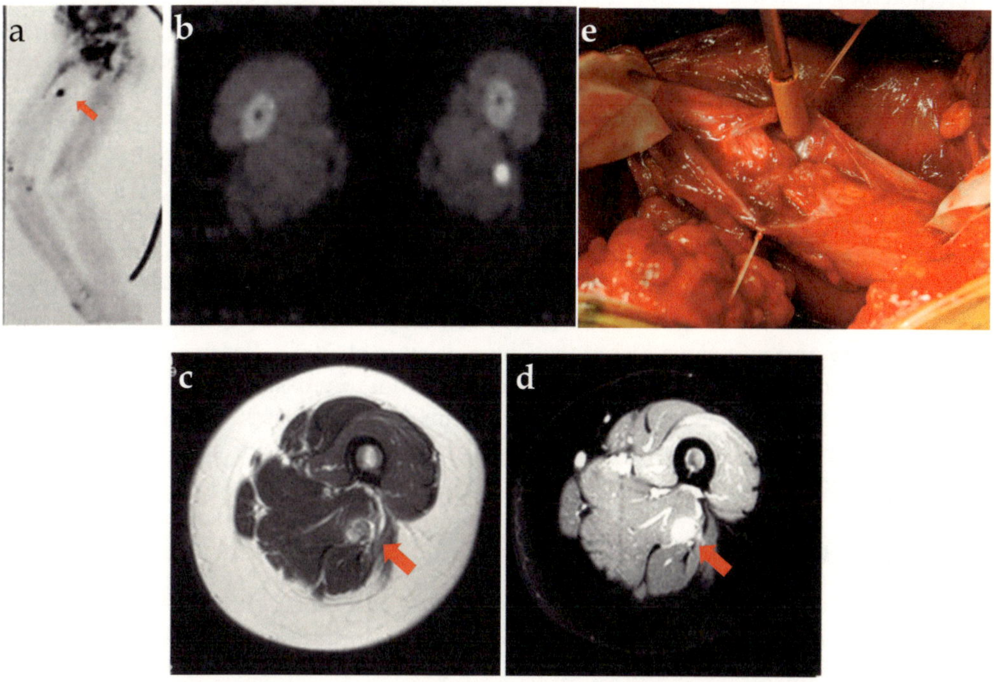

Fig. 1. Nodular fasciitis in the sciatic nerve detected by ^{18}FDG-PET (a,b). T2-weighted MRI (c) and Gd enhanced MRI (d) demonstrated the mass in the right hamstring. After fascicular dissection, the lesion under fascicular of sciatic nerve is disclosed entrapping the perineurium of sciatic nerve(e).

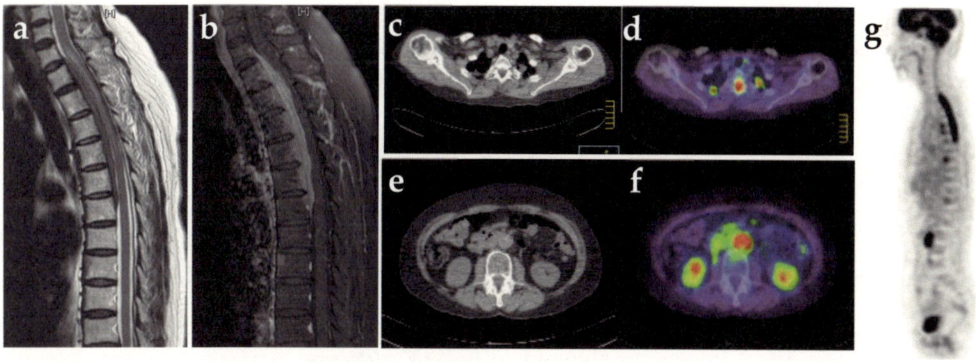

Fig. 2. MRI showing a diffuse space-occupying lesion at the anterior spinal cord: T2-weighted MRI (a); Gd-enhanced (b). Axial CT (c,e); axial PET/CT fusion (d,f) and sagittal PET image (g) demonstrating FDG uptake in the abdominal aorta and bilateral upper lungs.

Although these two case reports represent very rare cases, ^{18}FDG-PET provided helpful diagnostic clues for obtaining the definitive diagnosis. While meticulous physical examinations and the symptoms themselves are usually enough to aid identification of the correct pathomechanism, spine surgeons often encounter patients whose cases are difficult to diagnose using conventional imaging tools, such as MRI and CT. In our cases, the differential diagnosis was intramedullary tumor, extraspinal neurogenic tumor, especially in the pelvis, or inflammatory lesion of the central nervous system (CNS), including the neurosarcoidosis and human T-lymphotropic virus type I-associated myelopathy (HTLV-1 myelopathy). Conventional imaging tools, MRI, CT and scintigraphy, revealed pathological changes consistent with these diagnoses; however MRI without enhancement with gadolinium did not indicate the abnormal findings expected in intramedullary tumor or inflammatory lesion of the CNS. Furthermore, almost all neurogenic tumors are negative with tumor scintigraphy by ^{67}Ga-citrate, ^{201}TICI and Tc-99m. In contrast, PET, providing metabolic information as three-dimensional imaging, can reveal neurogenic tumors in the whole body and CNS inflammatory lesions (Zhuang, Yu et al. 2005). FDG-PET is not only important for detecting malignant tumors, but also has potential for evaluation of a variety of inflammatory and infectious disorders (Zhuang, Yu et al. 2005). Because ^{18}FDG, the most common radiopharmaceutical for PET in oncology, is not tumor-specific, ^{18}FDG-PET cannot differentiate between malignancies and inflammatory processes, a disadvantage for oncological diagnoses. This property is, however, an advantage for screening spinal and neurogenic disorders.

3.3 Tumors and inflammation

Significant tracer accumulation can also occur in viral, bacterial and fungal infections, or in other forms of inflammatory tissue. FDG accumulation in inflammatory tissue may cause false positives during cancer screening. Other PET tracers considered to be proliferation markers may allow improved differential diagnosis of tumor and inflammation. Proliferation activity can be measured by lipid precursors, amino acids, nucleosides and receptor ligands. Only labeled nucleosides incorporated into DNA are true proliferation markers, while amino acid transport, membrane metabolism, enzyme activity and receptor expression can serve as surrogate markers of cellular proliferation based on the tissue kinetics. Established imaging targets for oncology are: (i) glucose transport (^{18}FDG); (ii) choline kinase activity (^{11}choline); (iii) amino acid transport (^{11}C-methionine); and (iv) activity of thymidine kinase 1 (^{18}FLT). Radiolabeled choline, amino acids and nucleosides have been reported to show greater tumor-specificity than ^{18}FDG, both in experimental animals and in humans (van Waarde and Elsinga 2008), although the specificity of any tracer is not absolute. FDG, choline and C-methionine are accumulated in such inflammatory process as bacterial and sterile infections. Although proliferation activity is a key factor of malignancy, cell division can also occur in benign tumors and inflammation processes. Consequently the tumor specificity of PET will never achieve 100%.

Sahlmann et al. reported that the dual time point ^{18}FDG uptake, which was measured at 30 and 90 minutes after injection, showed different pattern between chronic bacterial osteomyelitis and malignant bone tumor. In osteomyelitis, the standard uptake value (SUV) between 30 and 90 minutes post-injection remained stable or decreased, while, in contrast, in malignant bone tumor, the SUV between 30 and 90 minutes post-injection increased

(Sahlmann, Siefker et al. 2004). Moreover, high-grade sarcomas were found to reach peak activity concentration approximately 4 hours after injection of FDG, while benign tumors reached maximum within 30 minutes (Lodge, Lucas et al. 1999). Thus, the dynamic dual time point ^{18}FDG-PET provides is a characteristic pattern in chronic osteomyelitis, similar to inflammatory processes in other locations, differentiating it from malignant tumors. However, clarification of the difference between inflammatory lesions and benign tumors, which have similar uptake patterns, is yet to be accomplished.

3.4 Benign and malignant neurogenic tumors

The cause of nerve pain and neurological deficit is often considered to be extradural tumors, including such neurogenic tumors as schwannoma, neurofibroma, perineurioma, intraneural ganglion and malignant peripheral nerve sheath tumor (MPNST), as well as such intradural tumors as schwannoma, meningioma and ependynoma, etc (Figure 3,4). Generally detection of these benign neurogenic tumors by tumor scintigraphy using ^{67}Ga-citrate, ^{201}TICI or Tc-99m is difficult, as is detection of meningioma except for MPNST.

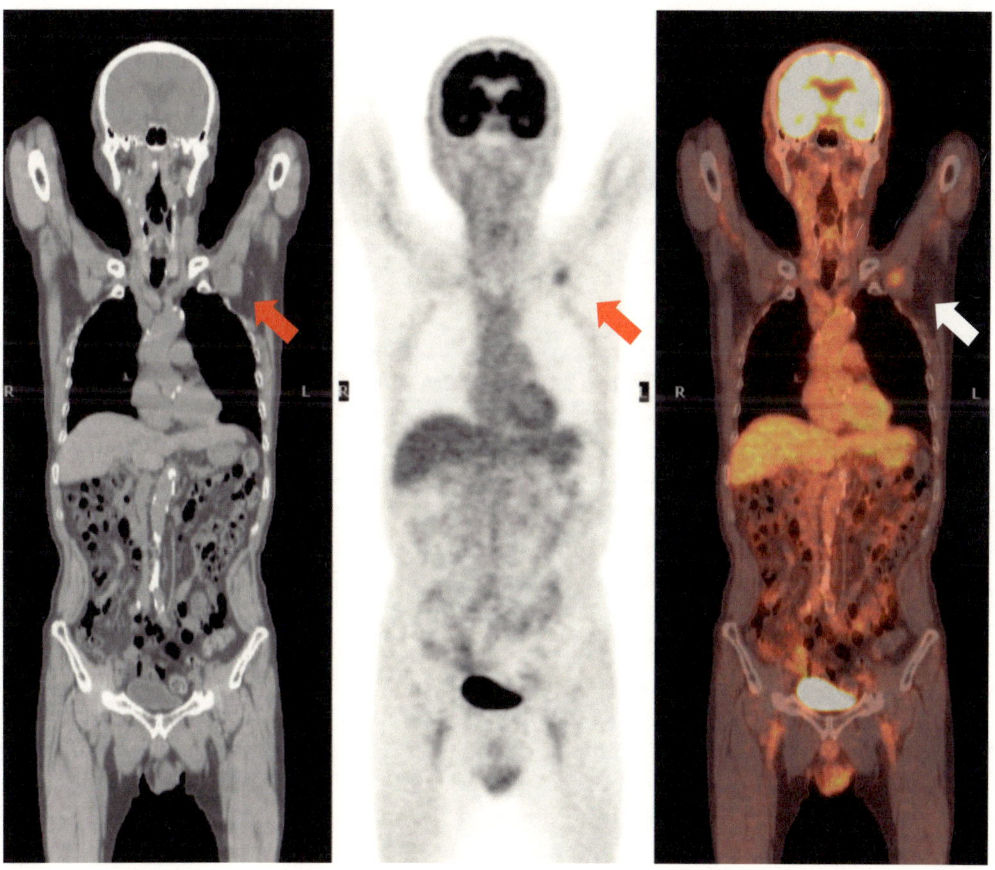

Fig. 3. CT, FDG and PET/CT images showing accidental detection of schwannoma in the left brachial plexus.

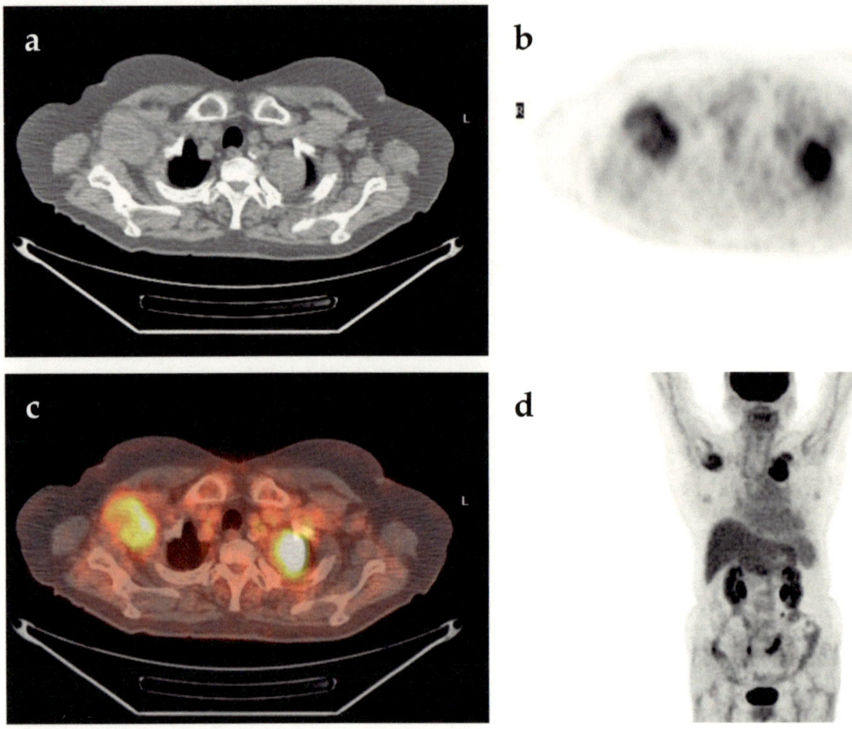

Fig. 4. Malignant peripheral nerve sheath tumor (MPNST) located in the right brachial plexus and the left upper lung demonstrated by axial CT (a), axial PET (b), axial PET/CT fusion (c) and coronal PET (d).

In contrast, ^{18}FDG-PET reveals benign neurogenic tumors and menigiomas in the whole body (Ahmed, Watanabe et al. 2001);(Lippitz, Cremerius et al. 1996; Antoch, Egelhof et al. 2002; Beaulieu, Rubin et al. 2004; Ghodsian, Obrzut et al. 2005; Hamada, Ueda et al. 2005; Halac, Cnaral et al. 2008). Studies have investigated the tumor growth characteristics of schwannoma and meningioma by PET. Ahmed et al. retrospectively reviewed schwannoma of the extremities in 22 patients. They found that ^{18}FDG-PET and ^{18}FMT-PET, in which ^{18}F-fluoro-α-methyl tyrosine (^{18}FMT) is an amino acid tracer to monitor protein metabolism, detected schwannoma in all cases, and reflected proliferation activity of the schwannoma. The authors suggested that ^{18}FMT-PET is more reliable for differentiation between benign schwannoma and malignancy than ^{18}FDG-PET (Ahmed, Watanabe et al. 2001). Kubota et al. studied the feasibility of differentiating benign and malignant schwannomas by dual time point ^{18}FDG-PET, comparing uptake 1 hour post-injection to 2 hours post-injection. Most malignant schwannomas showed greater increase at 2 hours post-injection than at 1 hour post-injection, while most normal tissue showed lower ^{18}FDG uptake at 1 hour than at 2 hours (Kubota, Itoh et al. 2001). In addition, from analysis of the SUV of ^{18}FDG on 55 patients with benign and malignant tumors involving the musculoskeletal system, the cut-off point, 1.9, was calculated and the sensitivity of ^{18}FDG -PET for correctly diagnosing malignancy was 100%, with a specificity of 76.9% and an overall accuracy of 83.0%(Watanabe, Shinozaki et al. 2000). Thus, dual time point PET and the cut-off value of

SUV can furnish useful diagnostic information for differentiating benign and malignant schwannomas.

In contrast, because meningioma cells have high uptake levels for 1,4,7,10-tetraazacyclododecane-N,N',N'',N'''-tetraacetic-acid-D-Phe1-Tyr3-oc treotide (^{68}Ga-DUTATOC), a new PET radiotracer with high specific binding to somatostatin receptors, ^{68}Ga-DUTATOC can be used to image the meningioma (Henze, Schuhmacher et al. 2001). Lipptiz et al. investigated the correlation of ^{18}FDG-uptake with the histopathology, cellularity and proliferation rate of intrancanial meningioma. They found significant differences between ^{18}FDG-uptake in World Health Organization (WHO) grade I vs. grades II and III, low vs. high cellularity and Ki-67 index $< 2\%$ vs. $> 2\%$ intracranial meningomas (Lippitz, Cremerius et al. 1996). These results indicate that a portion of a tumor can be imaged using this specific tracer and dynamic dual time point examination and show that PET is useful not only for screening but also as a noninvasive predictor of tumor growth characteristics of schwannoma and meningioma.

3.5 Inflammatory lesion of spinal cord

When clinical manifestations are more severe than imaging indicates an inflammatory lesion of the spinal cord should be considered in the differential diagnosis. Inflammatory diseases of the spinal cord, such as neurosarcoidosis and HTLV-1 myelopathy, present a wide spectrum of clinical and radiological manifestations, making them difficult to diagnose. Bolat et al. explored the usefulness of PET in the diagnosis of neurosarcoidosis (Bolat, Berding et al. 2009). In addition, Umehara et al. found ^{18}FDG-PET to be helpful for diagnosing HTLV-1 myelopathy (Umehara, Hagiwara et al. 2008). Radu et al. measured experimental autoimmune encephalomyelitis by ^{18}FDG-PET; their results highlighted the potential use of serial ^{18}FDG-PET for monitoring neuroinflammation in encephalomyelitis. They also suggested that similar approaches could be applied to the diagnosis and evaluation of other autoimmune and inflammatory disorders in animal models and humans (Radu, Shu et al. 2007).

4. Prediction of surgical outcomes in cervical sclerotic myelopathy

Conventional morphological imaging with CT and MRI can visualize precisely the location and pathological cause of stenosis and compression; however the severity of morphological stenosis does not necessarily correlate with either the actual functional deficits or the clinical course of the condition. Therefore, alternative diagnostic methods to morphological imaging are needed to better reflect the functional impairment of the cervical cord.

To accurately predict prognosis and neurological improvement after neurosurgical decompression, it is essential to be able to assess spinal cord function in patients with cervical compression myelopathy. Most conventional evaluations focus on morphologic and pathologic changes to the compressed cord, which can be identified on MRI. MRI is a valuable tool because it visualizes not only the magnitude of the spinal cord compression, but also intramedullary signal intensity. Several investigators have reported a correlation between morphologic and pathologic changes on MRI and neurologic status, with most studies suggesting that preoperative MRI findings could be used to predict surgical outcome and prognosis (Okada, Ikata et al. 1993; Wada, Yonenobu et al. 1999; Singh, Crockard et al. 2001; Alafifi, Kern et al. 2007).

The spinal cord is considered to have viscoelastic properties that allow it to return to its original configuration following decompression, leading to recovery of physiologic function of sensorimotor pathways. However, spinal cord atrophy is associated with significantly reduced extensibility and the atrophic spinal cord in patients with profound paresis fails to regain its original configuration after decompression. It has been reported that patients who show early postoperative expansion of the spinal cord tend to have favorable neurologic improvements (Baba, Maezawa et al. 1997). The restoration of the transverse area and sagittal diameter of the spinal cord also correlates with better neurologic improvement (Fukushima, Ikata et al. 1991; Yone, Sakou et al. 1992). An important issue is the significance of changes in MRI intramedullary signal intensity. Increased capillary permeability with subsequent stromal edema and venous congestion can be visualized on T2-weighted MRI. Although it is unclear whether intramedullary signal intensity of the spinal cord on a T2-weighted MRI can be used to predict neurologic recovery following decompression, a number of investigators have suggested that high-signal intensity on T2-weighted MRI is a marker for poor neurologic prognosis (Ramanauskas, Wilner et al. 1989; Mehalic, Pezzuti et al. 1990); (Takahashi, Yamashita et al. 1989).

The central nerve system, brain and spinal cord, is known to mainly utilize glucose for basic metabolism. ^{18}FDG-PET can reflect spinal cord neural cell activity by visualization and measurement of glucose utilization. In myelopathy patients, ^{18}FDG-PET uptake and glucose utilization rate in the cervical spinal cord is variable. Metabolic evaluation of space-occupying and spinal cord-compressing spinal cord abnormalities with ^{18}FDG-PET has been used successfully for more than 25 years, especially for neoplastic disease (Nguyen, Sayed et al. 2008) (Francken, Hong et al. 2005); (Di Chiro, Oldfield et al. 1983; Meltzer, Townsend et al. 1998; Wilmshurst, Barrington et al. 2000; Poggi, Patronas et al. 2001). In all these space-occupying and spinal cord-compressing lesions, ^{18}FDG-PET was used to differentiate between benign and malignant abnormalities or to monitor the biological activity of a condition. Consequently, ^{18}FDG-PET should be considered a contemporary advanced technology for further assessment of chronically damaged spinal cords in patients with cervical myelopathy.

SUV is a potentially suitable parameter for assessment of neurologic status in clinical practice. Kamoto et al. reported that the normal value of metabolic rate of glucose utilization in the cervical spinal cord in healthy Japanese subjects was 1.93 ± 0.23 (Kamoto, Sadato et al. 1998). Although several investigators have reported ^{18}FDG uptake levels in cervical compressive myelopathy, the relationship between metabolic activity and severity of neurologic dysfunction is controversial.

Baba et al. utilized mouse animal models and observed that during the early stages of cord compression, neuropeptide activity in neurons and glial cells was increased by external pressure, thus stimulating glucose utilization by the spinal cord. Chronic compression, however, leads to atrophy and necrosis of anterior grey horn cells, and the loss of glucose-consuming neurons leads to decreased ^{18}FDG uptake of the spinal cord (Baba, Uchida et al. 1999). Uchida et al. reported that patients with mild to moderate myelopathy have a significantly higher SUV, while those with marked and profound tetraparaesis have significantly lower values (Uchida, Kobayashi et al. 2004). Uchida et al. also analyzed the SUV during neurologic improvement of cervical myelopathy, and found that more improved patients had significantly higher preoperative SUV compared to patients with less improvement (Uchida, Nakajima et al. 2009). Interestingly, classification by preoperative SUV did not differ significantly from classification by the intramedullary signal intensity of the spinal cord on MRI. It is possible that the absolute level of the SUV is not decisive for assessment of the metabolic status of the cervical cord. Floeth et al. studied homogenous myelopathy patients with monosegemental chronic degenerative stenosis using ^{18}FDG-PET, and found that patients with chronic compressive myelopathy had normal glucose utilization just above the level of the stenosis but significantly decreased ^{18}FDG uptake below the level of cord compression (Floeth, Stoffels et al.2010). They noted that these results are compatible with those of Baba et al. (Baba, Uchida et al. 1999).

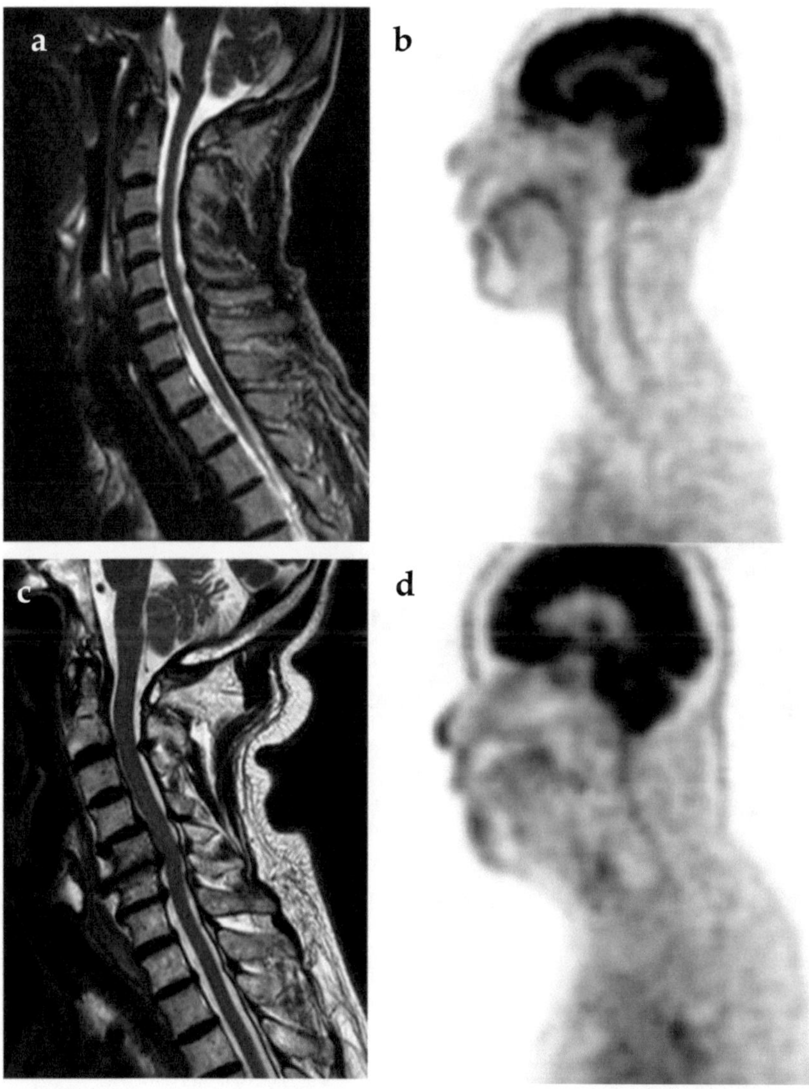

Fig. 5. MRI (a) and PET (b) showing homogenous FDG uptake in a patient with a normal cord, and MRI (c) and PET (d) illustrating reduced FDG uptake at the compression level in a patient with mild myelopathy.

^{18}FDG-PET can reflect the glucose utilization of the spinal cord in spinal disorder patients (Figure 5). It can be an important predictor for prognosis and neurological improvement after neurosurgical decompression. However, ^{18}FDG uptake is affected by the range of stenosis, whether it is bi- or multisegmental stenosis, and duration and severity of symptoms. Further studies in a larger series of patients with chronic and clinically stable myelopathy, and in patients with an acute and rapidly progressing myelopathy are needed.

5. Conclusion

^{18}FDG-PET is important not only for detecting malignant tumors but also for its potential use in the evaluation of a variety of inflammatory and infectious disorders (Zhuang, Yu et al. 2005). For oncology, there is the limitation that ^{18}FDG-PET cannot differentiate between malignant and inflammatory processes. However, this limitation would be considered an advantage when screening for spinal anomalies and benign neurogenic tumors. Therefore, despite the high cost and relative scarcity of PET scanners at institutions, the role of PET in screening for and assessment of benign neurogenic tumors and compressive myelopathies is expected to increase.

6. References

Ahmed, A. R., H. Watanabe, et al. (2001). "Schwannoma of the extremities: the role of PET in preoperative planning." *Eur J Nucl Med* 28(10): 1541-51.

Alafifi, T., R. Kern, et al. (2007). "Clinical and MRI predictors of outcome after surgical intervention for cervical spondylotic myelopathy." *J Neuroimaging* 17(4): 315-22.

Antoch, G., T. Egelhof, et al. (2002). "Recurrent schwannoma: diagnosis with PET/CT." *Neurology* 59(8): 1240.

Baba, H., Y. Maezawa, et al. (1997). "Plasticity of the spinal cord contributes to neurological improvement after treatment by cervical decompression. A magnetic resonance imaging study." *J Neurol* 244(7): 455-60.

Baba, H., K. Uchida, et al. (1999). "Potential usefulness of 18F-2-fluoro-deoxy-D-glucose positron emission tomography in cervical compressive myelopathy." *Spine (Phila Pa 1976)* 24(14): 1449-54.

Beaulieu, S., B. Rubin, et al. (2004). "Positron emission tomography of schwannomas: emphasizing its potential in preoperative planning." *AJR Am J Roentgenol* 182(4): 971-4.

Bolat, S., G. Berding, et al. (2009). "Fluorodeoxyglucose positron emission tomography (FDG-PET) is useful in the diagnosis of neurosarcoidosis." *J Neurol Sci* 287(1-2): 257-9.

Czernin, J. (2002). "Clinical applications of FDG-PET in oncology." *Acta Med Austriaca* 29(5): 162-70.

Di Chiro, G., E. Oldfield, et al. (1983). "Metabolic imaging of the brain stem and spinal cord: studies with positron emission tomography using 18F-2-deoxyglucose in normal and pathological cases." *J Comput Assist Tomogr* 7(6): 937-45.

Floeth, F. W., G. Stoffels, et al. (2010). "Regional impairment of 18F-FDG uptake in the cervical spinal cord in patients with monosegmental chronic cervical myelopathy." *Eur Radiol* 20(12): 2925-32.

Francken, A. B., A. M. Hong, et al. (2005). "Detection of unsuspected spinal cord compression in melanoma patients by 18F-fluorodeoxyglucose-positron emission tomography." *Eur J Surg Oncol* 31(2): 197-204.

Fukushima, T., T. Ikata, et al. (1991). "Magnetic resonance imaging study on spinal cord plasticity in patients with cervical compression myelopathy." *Spine (Phila Pa 1976)* 16(10 Suppl): S534-8.

Ghodsian, M., S. L. Obrzut, et al. (2005). "Evaluation of metastatic meningioma with 2-deoxy-2-[18F]fluoro-D-glucose PET/CT." *Clin Nucl Med* 30(11): 717-20.

Halac, M., F. Cnaral, et al. (2008). "FDG PET/CT findings in recurrent malignant schwannoma." *Clin Nucl Med* 33(3): 172-4.

Hamada, K., T. Ueda, et al. (2005). "Peripheral nerve schwannoma: two cases exhibiting increased FDG uptake in early and delayed PET imaging." *Skeletal Radiol* 34(1): 52-7.

Henze, M., J. Schuhmacher, et al. (2001). "PET imaging of somatostatin receptors using [68GA]DOTA-D-Phe1-Tyr3-octreotide: first results in patients with meningiomas." *J Nucl Med* 42(7): 1053-6.

Kakutani, K., M. Doita, et al. (2010)."Intractable sciatica due to intraneural nodular fasciitis detected by positron emission tomography." *Spine (Phila Pa 1976)* 35(21): E1137-40.

Kamoto, Y., N. Sadato, et al. (1998). "Visualization of the cervical spinal cord with FDG and high-resolution PET." *J Comput Assist Tomogr* 22(3): 487-91.

Kasagi, S., J. Saegusa, et al. (2011). "Epidural spinal tumor and periaortitis as rare complications of Wegener's granulomatosis." *Mod Rheumatol.*

Kubota, K., M. Itoh, et al. (2001). "Advantage of delayed whole-body FDG-PET imaging for tumour detection." *Eur J Nucl Med* 28(6): 696-703.

Kuhl, D. E., R. H. Chamberlain, et al. (1956). "A high-contrast photographic recorder for scintillation counter scanning." *Radiology* 66(5): 730-9.

Lippitz, B., U. Cremerius, et al. (1996). "PET-study of intracranial meningiomas: correlation with histopathology, cellularity and proliferation rate." *Acta Neurochir Suppl* 65: 108-11.

Lodge, M. A., J. D. Lucas, et al. (1999). "A PET study of 18FDG uptake in soft tissue masses." *Eur J Nucl Med* 26(1): 22-30.

Mehalic, T. F., R. T. Pezzuti, et al. (1990). "Magnetic resonance imaging and cervical spondylotic myelopathy." *Neurosurgery* 26(2): 217-26 discussion 226-7.

Meltzer, C. C., D. W. Townsend, et al. (1998). "FDG imaging of spinal cord primitive neuroectodermal tumor." *J Nucl Med* 39(7): 1207-9.

Nguyen, N. C., M. M. Sayed, et al. (2008). "Spinal cord metastases from lung cancer: detection with F-18 FDG PET/CT." *Clin Nucl Med* 33(5): 356-8.

Okada, Y., T. Ikata, et al. (1993). "Magnetic resonance imaging study on the results of surgery for cervical compression myelopathy." *Spine (Phila Pa 1976)* 18(14): 2024-9.

Poggi, M. M., N. Patronas, et al. (2001). "Intramedullary spinal cord metastasis from renal cell carcinoma: detection by positron emission tomography." *Clin Nucl Med* 26(10): 837-9.

Radu, C. G., C. J. Shu, et al. (2007). "Positron emission tomography with computed tomography imaging of neuroinflammation in experimental autoimmune encephalomyelitis." *Proc Natl Acad Sci U S A* 104(6): 1937-42.

Ramanauskas, W. L., H. I. Wilner, et al. (1989). "MR imaging of compressive myelomalacia." *J Comput Assist Tomogr* 13(3): 399-404.

Sahlmann, C. O., U. Siefker, et al. (2004). "Dual time point 2-[18F]fluoro-2'-deoxyglucose positron emission tomography in chronic bacterial osteomyelitis." *Nucl Med Commun* 25(8): 819-23.

Schlyer, D. J. (2004). "PET tracers and radiochemistry." *Ann Acad Med Singapore* 33(2): 146-54.

Singh, A., H. A. Crockard, et al. (2001). "Clinical and radiological correlates of severity and surgery-related outcome in cervical spondylosis." *J Neurosurg* 94(2 Suppl): 189-98.

Takahashi, M., Y. Yamashita, et al. (1989). "Chronic cervical cord compression: clinical significance of increased signal intensity on MR images." *Radiology* 173(1): 219-24.

Uchida, K., S. Kobayashi, et al. (2004). "Metabolic neuroimaging of the cervical spinal cord in patients with compressive myelopathy: a high-resolution positron emission tomography study." *J Neurosurg Spine* 1(1): 72-9.

Uchida, K., H. Nakajima, et al. (2009). "High-resolution magnetic resonance imaging and 18FDG-PET findings of the cervical spinal cord before and after decompressive surgery in patients with compressive myelopathy." *Spine (Phila Pa 1976)* 34(11): 1185-91.

Umehara, F., T. Hagiwara, et al. (2008). "Enlarged, multifocal upper limb neuropathy with HTLV-I associated myelopathy in a patient with chronic adult T-cell leukemia." *J Neurol Sci* 266(1-2): 167-70.

van Waarde, A. and P. H. Elsinga (2008). "Proliferation markers for the differential diagnosis of tumor and inflammation." *Curr Pharm Des* 14(31): 3326-339.

Wada, E., K. Yonenobu, et al. (1999). "Can intramedullary signal change on magnetic resonance imaging predict surgical outcome in cervical spondylotic myelopathy?" *Spine (Phila Pa 1976)* 24(5): 455-61; discussion 462.

Watanabe, H., T. Shinozaki, et al. (2000). "Glucose metabolic analysis of musculoskeletal tumours using 18fluorine-FDG PET as an aid to preoperative planning." *J Bone Joint Surg Br* 82(5): 760-7.

Wilmshurst, J. M., S. F. Barrington, et al. (2000). "Positron emission tomography in imaging spinal cord tumors." *J Child Neurol* 15(7): 465-72.

Yone, K., T. Sakou, et al. (1992). "Preoperative and postoperative magnetic resonance image evaluations of the spinal cord in cervical myelopathy." *Spine (Phila Pa 1976)* 17(10 Suppl): S388-92.

Zhuang, H., J. Q. Yu, et al. (2005). "Applications of fluorodeoxyglucose-PET imaging in the detection of infection and inflammation and other benign disorders." *Radiol Clin North Am* 43(1): 121-34.

9

$[^{18}F]$Fluorodeoxyglucose Positron Emission Tomography in Alzheimer Disease and Related Disorders

Nobuhiko Miyazawa and Toyoaki Shinohara
Department of PET and Nuclear Medicine, Kofu Neurosurgical Hospital
Japan

1. Introduction

The numbers of cases of Alzheimer disease (AD) and related disorders have been increasing with higher life expectancy worldwide. In particular, the incidence has sharply increased in people aged 70 to 80 years, with consequent significant burdens on health care systems and economies. In the 1990s, more than 4% of individuals aged over 65 years were affected by AD (Folstein et al., 1991), and 7–10% of this age group in Japan have been estimated to have AD (Meguro et al., 2002). Worldwide, the estimated number of individuals with AD of 24.3 million in 2001 is expected to increase to 42.3 million by 2020, and to 81.1 million by 2040 (Ferri et al., 2005).

AD is characterized by various definitive histopathological findings including presence of amyloid plaques, neurofibrillary tangles, and microglia in different degrees, and neuronal loss and neurotransmitter changes (Mattson et al., 2004; Thal et al., 2002). A characteristic early sign of pathology is the deposition of amyloid-β (Aβ) peptide in the medial side of the temporal lobe. The diagnosis of AD has been defined by the Diagnostic and Statistical Manual of Mental Disorders, fourth edition, text revision (American Psychiatric Association, 2000) and the National Institute of Neurological and Communicative Disorders and Stroke-Alzheimer's Disease and Related Disorders Association (NINCDS-ADRDA) (McKhann et al., 1984). The definitive diagnosis of AD is based on both the NINCDS-ADRDA criteria and the histopathological findings, but probabilistic clinical diagnosis of AD depends on these criteria without the investigations by magnetic resonance (MR) imaging, positron emission tomography (PET), or other biomarkers (Dubois et al., 2007).

Several potential biomarkers for AD have been proposed, such as biochemical biomarkers based on measurement of the concentration of $A\beta_{42}$ and total tau in the cerebrospinal fluid (CSF), structural neuroimaging biomarker based on MR imaging using specific software, and functional neuroimaging biomarker based on PET using $[^{18}F]$fluorodeoxyglucose (FDG) or $[^{11}C]$Pittsburgh compound B (PIB). Detection of AD based on the concentrations of $A\beta_{42}$ and total tau in patients versus normal individuals achieved sensitivity of 85–94% and specificity of 83–100% (Blennow & Hampel, 2003). Detection of prodromal AD based on the MR imaging measurement of middle temporal lobe volume and lateral temporal lobe or anterior cingulate volume achieved sensitivity of 68–93% and specificity of 48–96% (Convit et al., 2000; Killiany et al., 2000). Discrimination of AD from controls using FDG-PET achieved sensitivity of 94% and specificity of 73–78% (Foster et al., 1983; Herholz et al., 2002b; Ishii et al., 1999; Mielke et al., 1994; Silverman et al., 2001). Therefore, novel criteria have been proposed based on these distinctive and reliable biomarkers of AD as follows. The core diagnostic criterion is the presence of early and significant episodic memory impairment, and the secondary criterion is the detection of at least one or more abnormal findings of the structural neuroimaging biomarker using MR imaging, molecular neuroimaging biomarker using PET, and Aβ or tau protein level using CSF analysis (Dubois et al., 2007).

Several clinical trials have tested drugs aimed at modifying the AD process, such as acetylcholinesterase inhibitor, anti-inflammatory drugs, statins, γ and β secretase inhibitors, immunotherapy, and neuroprotective drugs. However, no large trial has attempted to identify the most powerful diagnostic biomarker, and to monitor disease progression and treatment effects. The Alzheimer's Disease Neuroimaging Initiative (ADNI) is a new multicenter clinical AD research project launched in 2004, and intended to detect neuroimaging parameters and biomarkers associated with the cognitive and functional changes in aged individuals with normal cognition, mild cognitive impairment (MCI), and AD in the United States and Canada (Mueller et al., 2005). ADNI-like trials have also been started in Europe, Australia, Japan, and Korea. Together, these trials could identify the most helpful biomarker and the optimum application for monitoring of the progress of AD and treatment effects.

The present review investigates the potential and feasibility of FDG-PET for the detection and monitoring of AD and related disorders, based on reported cases and our own experience (over 500 cases), and discuss the future applications of FDG-PET to the investigation of AD.

2. FDG-PET imaging of AD

2.1 History

Measurements of cerebral blood flow, and of oxygen and glucose metabolism have been made since the 1970s, and could be performed in dementia patients since the early 1980s (Benson et al., 1981; de Leon et al., 1983; Foster et al., 1984; Frackowiak et al., 1981; Jagust et al., 1985). These studies mainly depended on examination of cross-sectional PET images to detect regional decreases in cerebral blood flow or glucose metabolism in temporal or parietal lobe (Benson et al., 1981; Frackowiak et al., 1981). Development of a novel mapping method based on the three-dimensional stereotactic surface projection (3D-SSP) technique in the mid 1990s revealed preclinical metabolic decrease in the posterior cingulate and cinguloparietal transitional cortices in patients with AD (Minoshima et al., 1994, 1997). The statistical parametric mapping (SPM) technique allowing voxel-by-voxel basis analysis appeared in the early 2000s (Herholz et al., 2002). Such techniques have since been modified, such as the fully automatic diagnostic system using 3D-SSP (Ishii et al., 2006). These modified techniques provide more precise and earlier detection of AD compared with 20 years ago.

2.2 Progress of image analysis

2.2.1 3D-SSP

This technique has been developed to facilitate the diagnosis of AD and AD-related disorders by radiologists who are not specialists in nuclear medicine. The base images are corrected for head rotation and realigned to the standard stereotactic coordinate system. After images from different subjects are standardized in the same coordinate system, parametric analysis can be performed across subjects on a pixel-by-pixel basis. The 3D-SSP is used to exclude false findings caused by residual individual anatomic differences and cortical atrophy that is often present in patients with dementia. After individual PET image sets are standardized in the 3D-SSP format, image data obtained from normal individuals can be averaged to form a normal database. Patient PET image sets processed in the same manner can be compared with the normal database, and deviations of regional metabolic activities from normal values are expressed as Z scores. This method can identify areas of statistically significant reduction of metabolism in AD patients (Burdette et al., 1996; Minoshima et al., 1993, 1994, 2003). This method is routinely used worldwide to obtain consistent diagnostic accuracy using FDG-PET in the diagnosis of AD and AD-related disorders [Fig. 1].

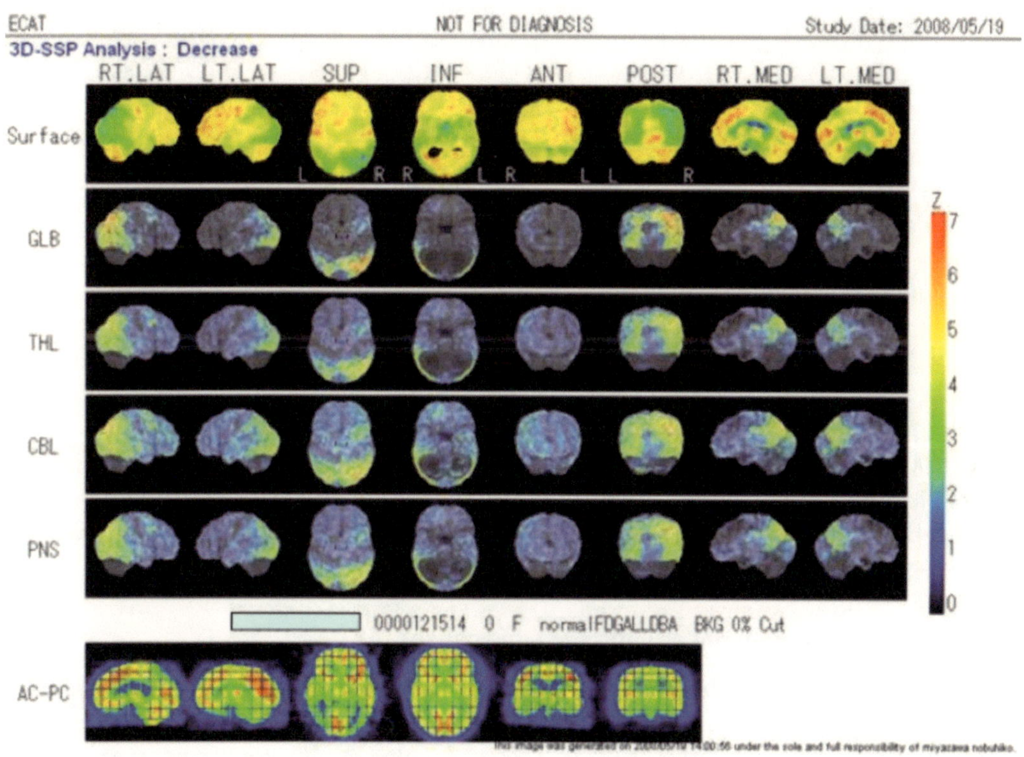

Fig. 1. FDG-PET study of AD patients using 3D-SSP (Minoshima). Z-score mapping compared with normal controls showed decreased glucose metabolism in the bilateral precuneus, posterior cingulate, and temporo-parietal cortices, which is not clearly visible on normal scans by the visual method.

2.2.2 SPM

SPM is also used for analyzing FDG-PET data. MATLAB software (MathWorks, Natick, MA, USA) was utilized for basic image processing with SPM99 software (Wellcome Department of Cognitive Neurology, London, UK) for spatial normalization. Further image analysis was performed with interactive data language programs. MPITool (Advanced Tomo Vision GmbH, Kerpen, Germany) was used for image display and SAS (SAS Institute Inc., Cary, NC, USA) was used for statistical evaluation of results. The t sum, calculated as the sum of t values over all voxels with FDG uptake below the 95% age-adjusted prediction limit, was selected as the global indicator of scan abnormality, and the AD t sum was calculated as the sum over all t values of voxels with FDG uptake below the 95% age-adjusted prediction limit within the AD mask for each individual. Diagnostic accuracy for AD was determined by receiver operating characteristic analysis using the t sum and AD t sum (Herholz et al., 2002a). The usefulness of SPM was recognized by multicenter trials with 395 patients and 110 normal controls (Herholz et al., 2002) [Fig. 2].

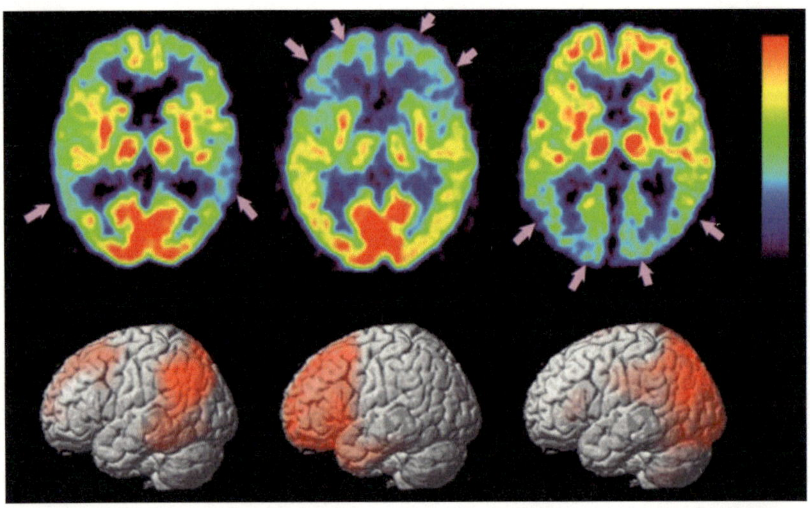

Fig. 2. FDG-PET study of AD (left column), FTD (center column), and DLB (right column) using SPM. Compared to normal scans (upper row), SPM analysis (lower row) disclosed reduced glucose metabolic sites (arrows) clearly and showed the characteristic patterns of 3 major diseases with dementia.

2.3 Distinctive abnormal pattern and possible causes

Reduction of glucose metabolism in AD patients was noted in the temporal and parietal lobes in early studies (Foster et al., 1984) and also in the posterior cingulate cortex (Herholz et al., 2002; Minoshima et al., 1997). Another study confirmed that glucose metabolism is reduced in the parietotemporal, frontal, and posterior cingulate cortices compared with normal individuals, and these reductions accord with the severity of dementia (Mosconi et al., 2005). FDG-PET mainly detects glucose consumption at the synapses (Kadekaro et al., 1985), and these synapses are insulted in the early stage of AD

(Masliah et al., 1991). Early loss of synapses is thought to occur in the hippocampus, especially in the entorhinal cortex. However, reduction of glucose metabolism has not been detected by FDG-PET in such regions. This interesting discordance between histopathological changes and FDG-PET findings may result from overall synaptic loss being milder in the hippocampus and entorhinal cortex than in the frontal or parietal lobe (Masliah et al., 1991).

Reduction of glucose metabolism in these regions remains asymmetric in the earlier stage of AD. As AD progresses, such asymmetrical reduction disappears and frontal involvement become evident (Jagust et al., 1988; Kumar et al., 1991). Other studies disclosed that the cerebellum and large regions of the association cortex are affected in contrast to the relative preservation of the basal ganglia, and motor and sensory cortices in the advanced stage of AD (Herholz et al., 1990; Ishii et al., 1997). Such atypical patterns should be considered as reduction in the bilateral temporal and parietal lobes is less severe in older patients (Grady et al., 1987; Mielke et al., 1992; Small et al., 1989).

The method of FDG-PET provides a highly consistent rate of accuracy compared to normal controls. Using the visual semiquantitative method, sensitivity was 92%, specificity was 83%, and accuracy was 87% (Azari et al., 1993; Burdette et al., 1996; Fazekas et al., 1989; Kippenhan et al., 1992; Scheurich et al., 2005). Quantitative methods showed that overall sensitivity was 94%, specificity was 87%, and accuracy was 91% (Duara et al., 1989; Herholz et al., 1990, 1993; Ishii et al., 2006; Kawachi et al., 2006; Mielke et al., 1994; Minoshima et al., 1995; Mosconi et al., 2005; Ng et al., 2007; Ohyama et al., 2000; Szelies et al., 1994; von Borczyskowski et al., 2006). Overall, the sensitivity was 94%, specificity was 85%, and accuracy was 90% (Ito et al., 2010).

We examined 500 patients with memory impairment by FDG-PET using the 3D-SSP method over approximately 5 years, using 33 subjects with average mini-mental state examination (MMSE) score of 30 as normal controls. The patients were divided into two groups, with MMSE score of 23 or less and 24 or over, to evaluate the age and sex distribution, type of abnormal findings and frequency, and presence of differences in MMSE between AD pattern and normal pattern. To assess the usefulness of FDG-PET for long-term follow up, AD pattern and normal pattern in patients with MMSE score of 24 or over followed up for over 3 years were compared with deterioration of MMSE, and the areas of deterioration were investigated using stereotactic extraction estimation. SPM was used to investigate the differences in the normal database between two institutes. Chi-square test, Fisher's exact test, and Student's t test were utilized to test for significant difference.

The 201 male and 291 female patients were aged from 20 to 90 years (mean 74.9±9.0 years). A total of 359 patients (72%) had MMSE score of 23 or less and 141 patients (28%) had MMSE score of 24 or over, and female predominance was recognized in both groups. The abnormal pattern was recognized in 97.2% of patients with MMSE score of 23 or less, consisting mainly of 77% with the AD pattern, followed by dementia with Lewy bodies (DLB) pattern. The abnormal pattern was recognized in 77% of patients with MMSE score of 24 or over, including 52% with the AD pattern, and 23% with the normal pattern. Significant differences were recognized in MMSE score between the AD pattern and normal pattern, in both patients with MMSE score of 23 or less (p=0.0188) and with MMSE score of 24 or over (p=1.63E-06). Twenty-five patients with MMSE score of 24 or over have been followed up for over 3 years, 8 with the normal pattern and 17 with the AD pattern. No patient with normal pattern had deteriorated MMSE score, but 7 of 17 patients (41%) with AD pattern had deteriorated MMSE score, showing a significant difference (p=0.0324). This study confirmed that FDG-PET using ordinary imaging and statistical imaging can be helpful to identify patients with memory disturbance based on the MMSE score (Miyazawa et al., 2011) [Fig. 3].

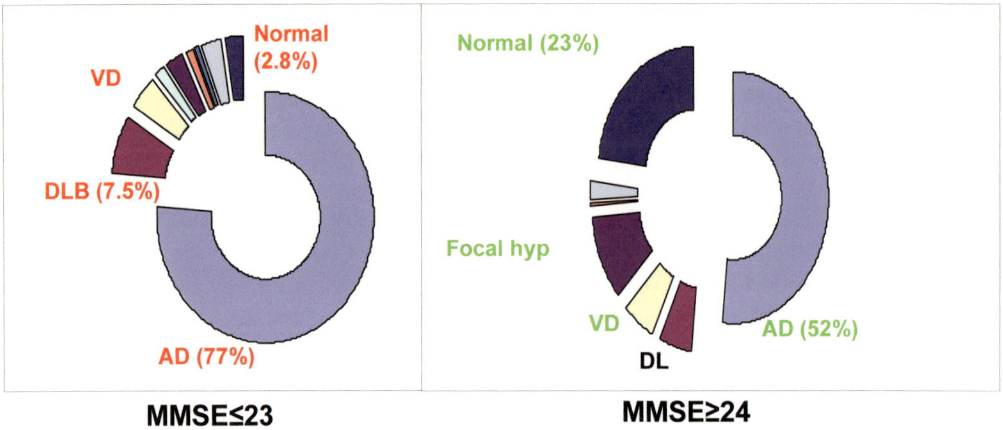

Fig. 3. Incidence of AD and AD-related disorders in 500 cases according to MMSE. In cases with MMSE score of 23 or less, 77% were AD and 2.8% were normal. In cases with MMSE score of 24 or over, 52% were AD and 23% were normal.

2.4 Prediction of deterioration

Prediction of clinical deterioration by FDG-PET may be affected by many bias factors preventing rigorous results, but FDG-PET could predict the occurrence of progressive dementia with sensitivity of 93% and specificity of 76% in 146 cases. Negative FDG-PET finding suggested that the pathological progression of cognitive impairment during a mean 3-year follow-up period was unlikely to occur (Silverman et al., 2001). A prospective longitudinal analysis showed a significant association between initial metabolic impairment and subsequent clinical deterioration. In patients with mild cognitive deficits at entry, the risk of deterioration was up to 4.7 times higher if the metabolism was severely impaired than with mild or absent metabolic impairment (Herholz et al., 1999). Study of a large number of cases (69 probable AD patients, 154 MCI patients, and 79 cognitively normal controls) revealed that the probable AD and MCI groups both had significant declines in 12-month glucose metabolism in the bilateral posterior cingulate, precuneus, medial parietal, lateral parietal, medial temporal, frontal, and occipital cortices (p<0.001). In each of these brain regions, the decline in AD patients was significantly greater than in the normal control group (p<0.001) (Chen et al., 2010). Careful and periodical follow up with PET study may predict the decline of AD patients [Fig. 4].

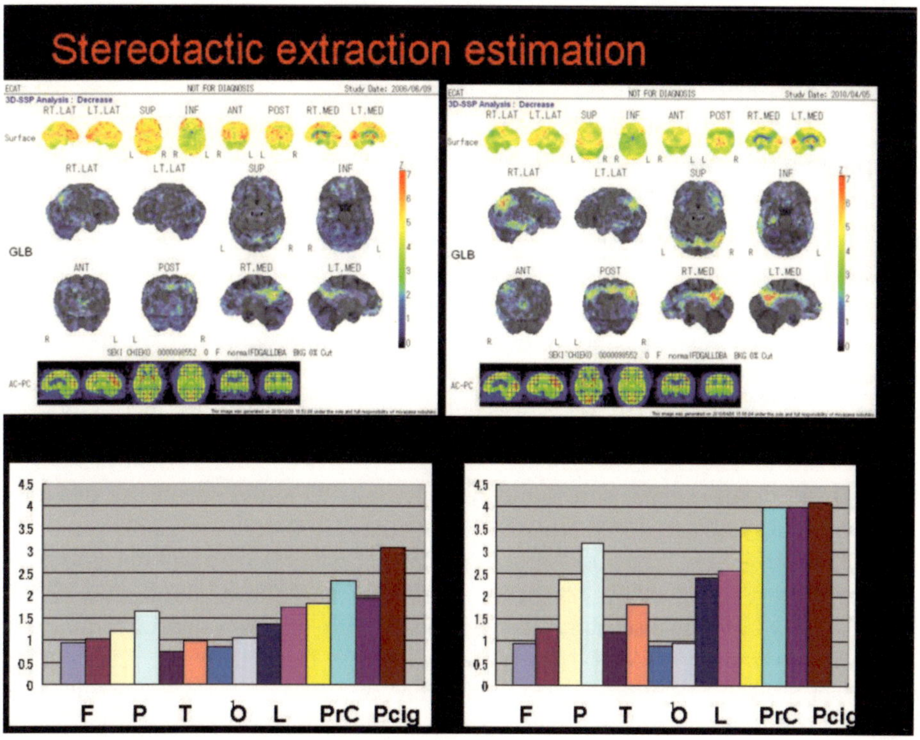

Fig. 4. Longitudinal study of FDG-PET in AD.

2.5 Correlation between FDG-PET and histopathology

Good correlations were found between metabolic reduction in the temporoparietal lobe on FDG-PET and histopathologically verified AD (DeCarli et al., 1992; McGeer et al., 1990; Mielke et al., 1996; Tedeschi et al., 1995). A study of 22 cases investigated whether bilateral temporo-parietal hypometabolism on FDG-PET is the metabolic abnormality associated with AD, and found the sensitivity of 93%, specificity of 63%, and accuracy of 82% could differentiate between AD and other AD-related disorders, confirming that such metabolic reduction is the classic abnormality associated with AD, and patients without AD pattern on FDG-PET should be suspected of AD-related disorders (Hoffman et al., 2000). Another study with 138 patients also reported that FDG-PET could identify AD and AD-related disorders with sensitivity of 94% and specificities of 73% and 78% (Silverman et al, 2001).

2.6 Imaging of treatment response and follow up

FDG-PET is helpful to observe the longitudinal aspect of metabolism in AD and AD-related disorders, as well as the efficacy of drug treatment (Diehl-Schmid et al., 2006; Drzezga et al., 2003; Nordberg et al., 2010). Serial FDG-PET findings elucidated the improvement in specific regions in patients treated with acetylcholinesterase inhibitors (Mega et al., 2001). Treatment effects with rivastigmine, galantamine, and citalopram were also clearly demonstrated by FDG-PET (Kadir et al., 2008; Mega et al., 2005; Smith et al., 2009; Teipel et al., 2006; Tune et al., 2003). Another treatment using implantation of genetically modified neurotrophin-producing autologous fibroblast yielded improvement of glucose metabolism by FDG-PET (Tuszynski et al., 2005).

2.7 Comparison with MR imaging, single photon emission computed tomography (SPECT), and neuropsychiatric testing

Neuropsychiatric testing has sensitivity of 93% and specificity of 99% for the discrimination of patients with mild AD from healthy people (Buschke et al., 1997), but the overall sensitivity and specificity of clinical diagnosis in cases confirmed at autopsy and Class II articles by American Academy of Neurology rating system were 70–81% (Holmes et al., 1999; Jobst et al., 1998; Lim et al., 1999). Many factors involved with PET and clinical testing contribute to the difficulty in judging prevalence, but overall accuracy of PET is no worse than the accuracy of clinical diagnosis (Minoshima, 2003).

Studies with no direct comparison found sensitivity of 93% and specificity of 74% using SPECT (Read et al., 1995), and 96% and 89% (Jobst et al., 1994). Initial regional cerebral blood flow SPECT studies of MCI may be useful in predicting patients who will develop AD in the near future (Hirao et al., 2005). Studies with direct comparison found that PET is the superior modality both for discrimination of patients with AD from normal individuals and predicting deterioration in MCI (Döbert et al., 2005; Herholz et al., 2002). Recently, comparison of SPECT, MR imaging, CSF biomarker, and PET in 207 patients with probable AD found AD findings in 81.6% with SPECT and 93.1% with PET (Morinaga et al., 2010).

Abnormal findings by MR imaging in the entorhinal cortex have a high predictive value for incipient disease in patients with MCI (deToledo-Morrell et al., 2004; Pennanen et al., 2004). Measurements of hippocampal atrophy by MR imaging can distinguish AD patients from cognitively normal elderly people with 80–90% accuracy (Jagust et al., 2006). Studies with direct comparison showed PET provided better diagnostic accuracy than MR imaging for hippocampus atrophy with accuracies of 73% and 73% in normal individuals and MCI patients, respectively, 91% and 83% in normal individuals and AD patients, respectively, and for middle/inferior and superior temporal gyrus atrophy with accuracies of 100% and 78% in normal individuals and AD patients, respectively (De Santi et al., 2001). AD findings were observed in 77.4% with MR imaging, and 93.1% with PET in 207 patients with probable AD (Morinaga et al., 2010). Further investigations and analysis will be needed to confirm the importance of PET.

3. FDG-PET imaging of MCI

3.1 Criteria and clinical importance of MCI

MCI was first proposed to represent subjective memory impairment and memory impairment by memory test, defined as a score of less than 1.5 standard deviations below the age-matched control, with no dementia and preserved activities of daily living (Petersen et al., 1999). MCI was subsequently classified into 3 subtypes, amnestic type, multiple cognitive domains slightly impaired type, and single non-memory domain impaired type in 2001, with Petersen's type equivalent to the amnestic type. New criteria were proposed to include amnestic MCI single domain, amnestic MCI multiple domain, non-amnestic MCI single domain, and non-amnestic MCI multiple domain types (Petersen & Morris, 2005). The prevalence of MCI differs between nations and depends on the definition of MCI, but values of approximately 3% are reported from many countries (Panza et al, 2005).

The annual progression rate of amnestic MCI to AD is around 12%, which is significantly higher than that of age-matched non-MCI subjects over 15 years (Petersen & Morris, 2003). On the other hand, 10% of MCI cases did not progress to AD. Meta-analysis of 19 studies showed the annual conversion rate has an average of 10% (Bruscoli & Loverstone, 2004). Clinical features of high rate conversion are high age, female, low score in MMSE, high score in Clinical Dementia Rating or Geriatric Depression Scale, over 4 in Hachinski Ischemic Score, and presence of allele type of ApoE4 (Morris et al., 2006). Such findings strongly indicate that MCI or amnestic MCI should be followed up to monitor progression to AD.

3.2 Abnormal findings and prediction of MCI progression to AD on FDG-PET

Glucose metabolism in the entorhinal cortex was reported to be the most reliable method for discriminating MCI patients from normal individuals (De Santi et al., 2001). MCI patients also had glucose metabolic reduction in the hippocampus, and this reduction was prominent in amnestic MCI (Clerici et al., 2009; Jauhiainen et al., 2008; Mosconi et al., 2005). After correction for the partial volume effect, glucose metabolism reduction in the temporoparietal cortex has become the core finding in MCI rather than glucose metabolism reduction in the hippocampus (Chételat et al., 2008).

Investigation of the prediction of progression from MCI to AD in a small number of cases examined (17 to 20 cases) found progression occurred in 41% to 50% of cases during 18 months to 3 years, associated with glucose metabolism reduction in the association cortex, bilateral temporoparietal cortices, and left temporal cortex (Arnáiz et al., 2001; Berent et al., 1999; Chételat et al., 2003; Morbelli et al., 2010). Study of a larger number of cases (30 to 85 cases) found progression in 29% to 40% of cases during 16 months to 2 years, associated with glucose metabolism reduction in the bilateral parietal and posterior cingulate cortices, bilateral temporoparietal and posterior cingulate cortices, and posterior cingulate cortex (Anchisi et al., 2005; Drzezga et al., 2005; Landau et al., 2010). In our study, 16 of 30 patients with MCI (53%) progressed to AD during 5 years, associated with glucose metabolism reduction in the posterior cingulate cortex and temporoparietal cortex. Another study showed that glucose metabolism reduction in the frontal lobe might also be predictive of MCI progression to AD, and the ApoE-ε4 genotype may be related to impairment of the frontal cortex (Drzezga et al., 2003; Mosconi et al., 2004).

Longitudinal or comparison trials of brain MR imaging and FDG-PET in 20 amnestic MCI patients and 12 controls with mean follow up of about 2 years identified 9 patients who progressed to AD. The discordant topography between atrophy and hypometabolism reported in AD was already present at the amnestic MCI stage. Posterior cingulate-precuneus hypometabolism seemed to be an early sign of memory deficit, whereas hypometabolism in left temporal cortex marked the progression to AD (Morbelli et al., 2010). A comparison study evaluated ApoE-ε4 allele frequency, CSF proteins, glucose metabolism using FDG-PET, hippocampal volume by MR imaging, and episodic memory performance in patients with amnestic MCI (n=85). Baseline FDG-PET and episodic memory predicted progression to AD. CSF proteins and, marginally, FDG-PET predicted longitudinal cognitive decline (Landau et al., 2010). Estimation of trials using the large number of cases examined suggested 66 AD patients or 217 MCI patients per treatment group were necessary to detect a 25% AD-slowing treatment effect in a 12-month, multi-center randomized clinical trial with 80% power and two-tailed aα=0.05 (Chen et al., 2010). These findings show the advantages of FDG-PET over conventional trials using neuropsychological testing.

4. FDG-PET imaging of normal individuals

Studies of AD and MCI have suggested that early diagnosis is essential to identify and treat individuals at risk before irreversible neuronal damage occurs. Improved brain imaging like FDG-PET and other methods are promising tools for the early detection of dementia and related disorders.

Two studies reported that normal individuals with the ApoE-ε4 allele and family history of AD had reduced glucose metabolism in the temporoparietal association area (Reiman et al., 1996; Small et al., 1995). Another study found individuals with the ApoE-ε4 allele had metabolic reduction in the temporoparietal and posterior cingulate cortices at about 2% per year (Small et al., 2000). MR imaging-guided FDG-PET disclosed that 12 individuals (25%) demonstrated cognitive decline in a 3-year longitudinal study of 48 healthy normal elderly subjects, associated with hypometabolism in the temporal lobe neocortex and hippocampus, and that ApoE E4 carrier showed marked longitudinal temporal neocortex metabolic reduction in subjects who declined (de Leon et al., 2001). A maternal history of AD was a strong association factor in reduced glucose metabolism (Mosconi et al., 2007, 2009). FDG-PET and additional CSF study showed that the combination of CSF and glucose metabolism significantly improved the accuracy of either measure in discriminating ApoE groups (86% accuracy, odds ratio=4.1, p<0.001) and normal ApoE E4 carrier with subjective memory complaint from all other subgroups (86% accuracy, odds ratio= 3.7, p=0.005). Parahippocampal gyrus glucose metabolism was the most accurate discriminator of subjective memory complaint groups (75% accuracy, odds ratio=2.4, p<0.001) (Mosconi et al., 2008). However, a longitudinal assessment of CSF and FDG-PET biomarkers is necessary to determine the usefulness of any combination (Petrie et al., 2009). Another association study with FDG-PET and MR imaging for prediction of cognitive decline in normal individuals disclosed that among 60 cognitively intact older individuals with mean follow up of 3.8 years, 6 subjects (10%) developed incident dementia or cognitive impairment, suggesting that reductions in temporal and parietal glucose metabolism predict decline in global cognitive function, and reductions in medial temporal brain volumes predict memory decline in normal older individuals (Jagust et al., 2006). Investigation of a larger number of cases is necessary to evaluate the efficacy of FDG-PET or other methods.

5. ADNI

Recently, several methods (biomarkers) have been investigated other than FDG-PET, including MR imaging, CSF/blood biochemical marker, amyloid detecting PET (PIB-PET), and genetic biomarker, to improve the accuracy of diagnosis of AD, MCI, and prodromal AD, and to monitor the progression of these diseases and treatment effects. The most reliable and valid biomarker for the treatment of AD should be identified within current limitations, but the number of such biomarkers is unclear.

The ADNI has been launched as described elsewhere (Chen et al., 2010; Mueller et al., 2005; Weiner et al., 2010). Briefly, the ADNI started in October 2004 in USA and Canada as a large, multi-center, longitudinal study of 822 older adults, consisting of 188 with probable AD, 405 with amnestic MCI, and 299 cognitively normal controls, followed up at 58 clinical institutes for 5 years. All patients underwent clinical ratings, neuropsychological testing, 1.5 T volumetric MR imaging, and blood and urine sampling at every visit, half of the subjects also underwent FDG-PET or 3 T MR imaging at every visit, a smaller number underwent PIB-PET, and more than half underwent CSF evaluation. Funding for the ADNI ended on October 1, 2010. Over 60 papers had been published by May 2010 (Weiner et al., 2010).

Baseline regional cerebral metabolic rate for glucose (CMRgl) measurement by FDG-PET was compared in 74 AD patients, 142 amnestic MCI patients, and 82 cognitively normal controls, and a correlation between CMRgl and clinical disease severity was observed, in comparison with normal controls. The AD and amnestic MCI patients had significantly lower CMRgl in the bilateral posterior cingulate, precuneus, parietotemporal, and frontal cortices. Clinical disease severity or lower MMSE scores were also correlated with lower CMRgl (Langbaum et al., 2009). Twelve-month follow-up study estimated the need for 66 AD patients or 217 MCI patients per treatment group to detect a 25% AD-slowing treatment effect in a 12-month, multi-center randomized clinical trial with 80% power and two-tailed α=0.05, roughly one-tenth of the number of patients needed to study MCI patients using clinical endpoints. These findings support the use of FDG-PET, brain-mapping algorithms, and empirically pre-defined statistical regions of interests in the randomized clinical trials of AD-slowing treatments (Chen et al., 2010).

In the near future, the results of ADNI-like studies are expected from Australia, Europe, Korea, and Japan, started since 2007 aiming at total of 600 cases including 300 MCI, 150 AD, and 150 normal controls, and over 460 cases have been enrolled and over 300 cases examined by FDG-PET in January 2011 in Japan. Analysis of the data and also further trials like ADNI-2 will be needed to confirm the findings.

6. FDG-PET imaging of AD-related disorders

6.1 Fronto-temporal dementia (FTD)

Discrimination of AD and FTD currently depend on the clinical history and examination, but FDG-PET shows different patterns of hypometabolism in these disorders that might aid differential diagnosis. A series of 45 patients with pathologically confirmed AD (n=31) or FTD (n=14) were investigated using five separate methods including FDG-PET SSP metabolic and statistical maps. Visual interpretation of SSP images was superior to clinical assessment and had the best inter-rater reliability (mean κ=0.78) and diagnostic accuracy (89.6%), as well as the highest specificity (97.6%) and sensitivity (86%), and positive likelihood ratio for FTD (36.5). The addition of FDG-PET to clinical summaries increased diagnostic accuracy and confidence for both AD and FTD. Visual interpretation of FDG-PET after brief training is more reliable and accurate in distinguishing FTD from AD than only clinical methods. FDG-PET adds important information that appropriately increases diagnostic confidence, even among experienced dementia specialists (Foster et al., 2007).

Twenty-one patients with clinical diagnosis of FTD, 21 patients matched for age, sex, and dementia severity- with probable AD and 21 normal control subjects matched for age and sex were studied by measuring the CMRgl with FDG-PET. In the FTD group, CMRgl was preserved only in the left cerebellum, right sensorimotor area, and occipital lobes. The CMRgl was significantly lower in the FTD group as opposed to the AD group in the hippocampi, orbital gyri, anterior temporal lobes, anterior cingulate gyri, basal ganglia, thalami, middle and superior frontal gyri, and left inferior frontal gyrus. Metabolic abnormality associated with FTD is predominant in the frontal and anterior temporal lobes, and the subcortical structures, but is more widespread than previously believed (Ishii et al., 1998). On the other hand, patients with progressive supranuclear palsy and progressive subcortical gliosis have similar findings (D'Antona et al., 1985; Foster et al., 1986, 1992). The cost of FDG-PET to discriminate AD from FTD has only been covered by insurance in the USA since 2003.

6.2 DLB

The clinical criteria of DLB are rather complicated and the differential diagnosis of Parkinson disease, Parkinson disease dementia, and DLB is difficult. Glucose hypometabolism in the occipital lobe was recognized as a distinctive abnormality in DLB with relative preservation of hippocampal glucose metabolism compared to AD (Higuchi et al., 2000; Imamura et al., 1997; Ishii et al., 1998). The study of morphologic and functional changes in patients with mild DLB compared with patients with AD were investigated in 20 patients with very mild DLB, 20 patients with very mild AD, and 20 healthy volunteers matched for age and sex (normal controls) by both FDG-PET and 3D spoiled gradient echo MR imaging. In DLB patients, volumetric data indicated a significant volume decrease in the striatum, whereas FDG-PET showed significant glucose metabolic reductions in the temporal, parietal, and frontal areas, including the occipital lobe, compared with the normal controls. In contrast, both the hippocampal volume and glucose metabolism were significantly decreased in AD patients, whereas the occipital volume and metabolism were preserved. Comparison of very mild DLB and AD revealed different morphologic and metabolic changes in the medial temporal lobes and the occipital lobe, demonstrating characteristic pathophysiologic differences between these diseases (Ishii et al., 2007).

Parkinson disease dementia and DLB share many similar aspects, and the differential clinical diagnosis relies heavily on an arbitrary criterion, the so-called 1-year rule. One study of 16 patients with Parkinson disease, 13 patients with Parkinson disease dementia, and 7 patients with DLB performed FDG-PET and reconstructed images by iterative reconstruction using computed tomography scans, normalized to a standard template. Compared with patients with Parkinson disease, both Parkinson disease dementia and DLB patients had similar patterns of decreased metabolism in bilateral inferior and medial frontal lobes, and right parietal lobe. In a direct comparison, DLB patients had significant metabolic decrease in the anterior cingulate cortex compared with those with Parkinson disease dementia. These findings support the concept that Parkinson disease dementia and DLB have similar underlying neurobiological characteristics, and can be regarded as a spectrum of Lewy body disorders (Yong et al., 2007). The diagnostic accuracy of FDG-PET -for AD versus DLB confirmed at autopsy was sensitivity of 90% and specificity of 80% (Minoshima, 2003).

An interesting study of occurrence of visual hallucination in DLB revealed that reduction of glucose metabolism in the visual association cortex may be involved in the occurrence of visual hallucination (Perneczky et al., 2008). Furthermore, we reported that the presence of hypermetabolic areas in the cerebellum, basal ganglia, or motor cortex may be related to the occurrence of visual hallucination in 22 DLB patients (Miyazawa et al., 2010) [Fig. 5].

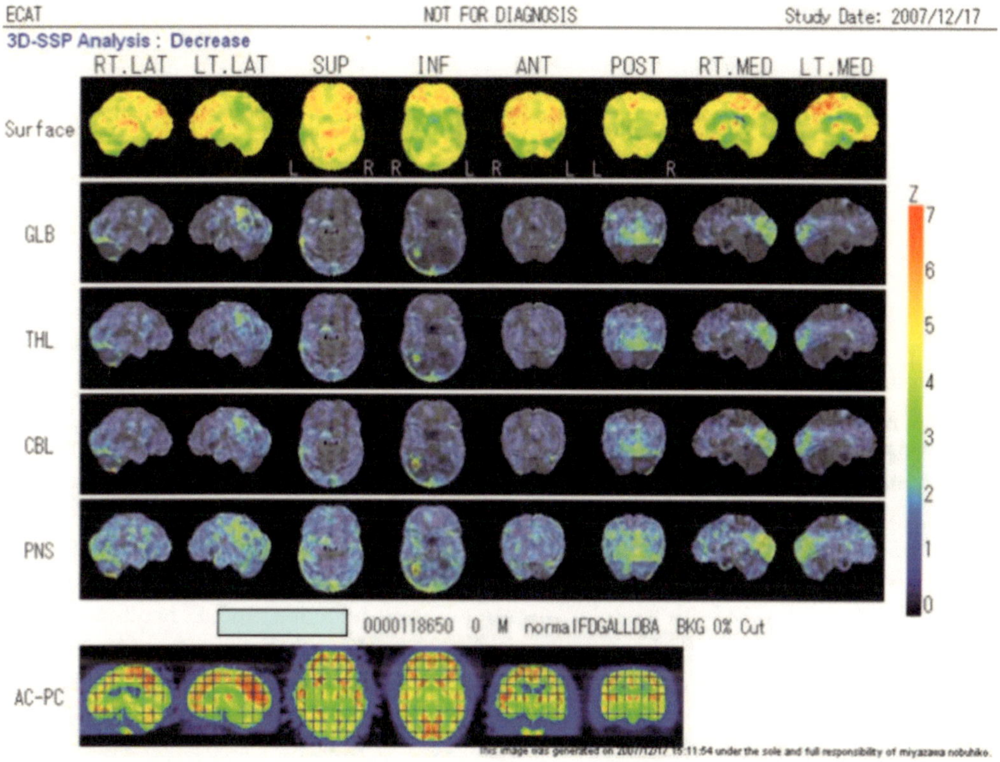

Fig. 5. FDG-PET study of DLB. Hypometabolism in the bilateral occipital lobes and posterior cingulate cortices is clearly detected by Z-score mapping with 3D-SSP.

6.3 Vascular dementia

The diagnosis of vascular dementia by MR imaging or FDG-PET is difficult because pathological changes characteristic of both AD and vascular dementia often co-exist. White matter hyperintensity on MR imaging and lacunar infarction may contribute to reduction in cerebral blood flow and glucose metabolism (DeCarli et al., 1996; Miyazawa et al., 1997). Several studies tried to identify distinctive patterns for vascular dementia on FDG-PET, but due to the limitations of the visual method on FDG-PET, no definitive finding could be obtained (De Reuck et al., 1998; Mielke et al., 1994; Sultzer et al., 1995). However, analysis using SPM and 3-D SSP could detect more precise and subtle differences between AD and vascular dementia. Comparison of the regional metabolic patterns on FDG-PET from 18 patients with subcortical vascular MCI and 25 patients with amnestic MCI matched for age, sex, education, and MMSE score, and 35 healthy subjects, using voxel-wise analysis with SPM 2 for statistical analysis revealed that relative to normal controls, hypometabolic regions in the amnestic MCI patients were located in the bilateral parahippocampal and posterior cingulate cortices, left superior temporal gyri, left inferior parietal lobule, and right inferior frontal gyrus, whereas hypometabolic regions in the subcortical vascular MCI patients were located in the thalamus, insula, superior temporal gyrus, anterior cingulate gyrus, cingulum, right basal ganglia, cerebellum, and brainstem. Further direct comparison of glucose metabolism between subcortical vascular MCI and amnestic MCI showed that glucose hypometabolism in patients with subcortical vascular MCI was more severe in the thalamus, brainstem, and cerebellum, suggesting that subcortical vascular MCI is distinct from amnestic MCI in terms of neuropsychological and PET findings, which may explain their clinical manifestations (Seo et al., 2009). Application of a novel voxel-based multivariate technique to a large FDG-PET data set from 153 subjects, with probable subcortical vascular dementia, probable AD, and normal controls in one third each, showed that lower metabolism differentiating vascular dementia from AD mainly occurred in the deep gray nuclei, cerebellum, primary cortices, middle temporal gyrus, and anterior cingulate gyrus, whereas lower metabolism in AD versus vascular dementia occurred mainly in the hippocampal region and orbitofrontal, posterior cingulate, and posterior parietal cortices. The hypometabolic pattern common to vascular dementia and AD mainly occurred in the posterior parietal, precuneus, posterior cingulate, prefrontal, and anterior hippocampal regions, and linearly correlated with the MMSE. This study shows the potential of voxel-based multivariate methods to highlight independent functional networks in dementia diseases. By maximizing the separation between groups, this method extracted a metabolic pattern that efficiently differentiated vascular dementia and AD with 100% accuracy (Kerrouche et al., 2006). A recent study of 48 subjects (12 with AD, 12 with vascular disease and dementia, 12 with vascular disease without dementia, and 12 healthy controls) with FDG-PET using SPM 2 showed the independent pattern of vascular dementia was glucose metabolic reduction in the thalamus, caudate, and frontal lobe (Pascual et al., 2010). Validation study with postmortem will be needed to confirm these newly-emerged patterns.

6.4 Neurodegenerative disorders showing dementia

6.4.1 Creutzfeldt-Jakob disease

Creutzfeldt-Jakob disease is a rare prion-associated disorder within the dementia spectrum. Only a few cases have been reported in terms of the FDG-PET findings of Creutzfeldt-Jakob disease (Engler et al., 2003; Henkel et al., 2002; Nagasaka et al., 2011). Study with FDG-PET only found that all 8 patients had reduction of CMRgl in at least one temporal or parietal region. The occipital lobe, the cerebellum, or the basal ganglia were involved in another 7 cases. These findings differ from typical patterns of hypometabolism in AD and other neurodegenerative disorders. The distribution was markedly asymmetric in two thirds of the cases. In three of four patients with visual symptoms, FDG uptake was reduced in the bilateral visual cortices. Typical hyperintensity on MR imaging was only found in two of the eight cases at the time of PET studies, which demonstrates that FDG-PET appears to be a sensitive investigation for

Creutzfeldt-Jakob disease and could be useful to differentiate Creutzfeldt-Jakob disease from other neurodegenerative disorders (Henkel et al., 2002). Another study with a relatively large number of cases showed that FDG-PET revealed, in comparison with normal controls, a typical pattern characterized by a pronounced regional decrease in CMRgl in 8 cases, indicative of neuronal dysfunction. These changes were most pronounced in the cerebellum, and the frontal, occipital, and parietal cortices, whereas the pons, the thalamus, and the putamen were less affected, and the temporal cortex appeared unaffected. FDG-PET gave a different pattern in 3 of 15 cases, so hypermetabolism was present in parts of the brain, particularly in the temporal lobes and basal ganglia, which could suggest encephalitis (Engler et al., 2003). We also reported a case with hypermetabolism in the cortical region (Nagasaka et al., 2011). FDG-PET can be used to detect the stage of encephalitis in Creutzfeldt-Jakob disease [Fig. 6].

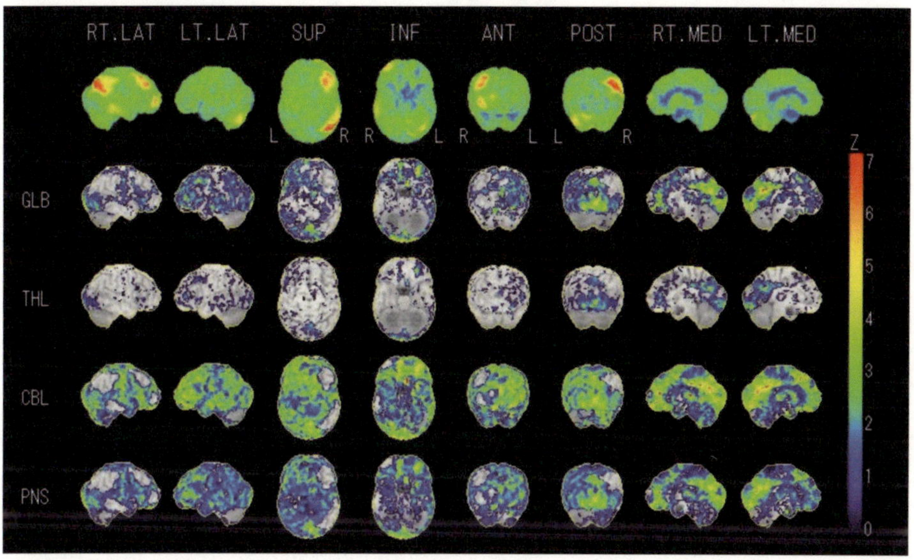

Fig. 6. FDG-PET study of Creutzfeldt-Jakob disease. Hypometabolism and hypermetabolism are both present.

6.4.2 Huntington disease

Huntington disease is another rare hereditary neurodegenerative disorder with characteristic symptoms of cognitive impairment and involuntary movement. FDG-PET of symptomatic Huntington disease found typical metabolic reduction in the striatum (Kuwert et al., 1990; Young et al., 1987) [Fig. 7]. In contrast, the consensus for FDG-PET in presymptomatic individuals at risk or in the early stage has not yet been reached (Hayden et al., 1987; Mazziotta et al., 1987). Cross-sectional study with FDG-PET in 18 presymptomatic individuals and 13 early-stage Huntington disease patients demonstrated significant metabolic covariance patterns characterized by caudate and putaminal glucose hypometabolism and metabolic reduction in the mediotemporal region, as well as relative hypermetabolism in the occipital cortex (Feigin et al., 2001). A longitudinal study of 71 cases in the symptomatic and presymptomatic stages using FDG-PET and MR imaging revealed that individuals at risk and symptomatic Huntington disease patients had significant glucose metabolic reduction in the cortex and striatum, and more importantly that Huntington disease patients had progressive white matter reduction in the preclinical stage, and decreased glucose uptake in the cortex and striatum in affected and preclinical individuals, suggesting that white matter volume reduction may precede gray matter reduction (Ciarmiello et al., 2006). FDG-PET can detect early signs of changes and is especially helpful in longitudinal studies [Table 1].

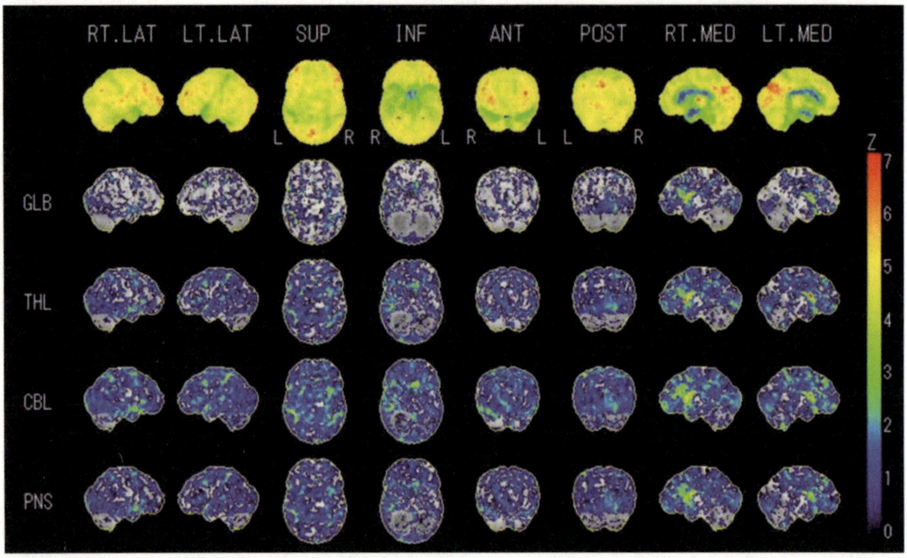

Fig. 7. FDG-PET study of Huntington disease. Hypometabolism is clearly recognized in the caudate and putamen by 3D-SSP.

Name of diseases and disorders	Regions with hypometabolism on FDG-PET
Alzheimer's disease (AD)	precuneus and posterior cingulate cortex temporoparietal association cortex (frontolateral association cortex)
Fronto-temporal dementia (FTD)	frontotemporal cortex
Dementia with Lewy bodies (DLB)	primary visual cortex (same as in AD)
Vascular dementia	dependent on vascular territories affected, usually with laterality
Creutzfeldt-Jakob disease	dependent on cortex affected, similar findings to AD
Huntington disease	putamen and caudate nucleus (thalamus and other basal ganglia)

Table 1. Characteristic findings on FDG-PET in AD and related disorders

7. Conclusion

For 30 years, FDG-PET has been applied to investigate the functional metabolic aspects of AD and related disorders. Approximately 15–10 years ago, the helpfulness of FDG-PET was established using rigorous and valid analyzing software like 3-D SSP or SPM compared to postmortem data, and the sensitivity, specificity, and accuracy of FDG-PET are over 90%. FDG-PET is very useful for the elucidation of the cross-sectional and longitudinal aspects of probable AD, and the monitoring of progression of MCI to AD and normal individuals at risk. Furthermore, differential diagnosis of AD from FTD by FDG-PET is helpful and valid in clinical settings. In parallel with the progress in FDG-PET, other methods like MR imaging using voxel-based volumetry and measuring specific proteins in the blood or CSF have emerged as promising tools for the diagnosis of AD and progression of MCI to AD. The ADNI trial was launched in the USA, and was followed by Europe, Australia, Korea, and Japan. The main concerns are identifying the most powerful probe in future clinical trials and the optimum combinations to minimize the cost burden. Given the several limitations of FDG-PET, this review illustrates that FDG-PET remains a helpful and pivotal tool in clinical studies and trials.

8. References

American Psychiatric Association. (2000). *Diagnostic and Statistical Manual of Mental Disorders, Fourth Edition, Text Revision (DSM-IV-TR)*, American Psychiatric Publishing, ISBN 0-89042-024-6, Arlington, VA

Anchisi, D.; Borroni, B., Franceschi, M., Kerrouche, N., Kalbe, E., Beuthien-Beumann, B., Cappa, S., Lenz, O., Ludecke, S., Marcone, A., Mielke, R., Ortelli, P., Padovani, A., Pelati, O., Pupi, A., Scarpini, E., Weisenbach, S., Herholz, K., Salmon, E., Holthoff, V., Sorbi, S., Fazio, F. & Perani, D. (2005). Heterogeneity of Brain Glucose Metabolism in Mild Cognitive Impairment and Clinical Progression to Alzheimer Disease. *Archives of Neurology*, Vol.62, No.11, (November 2005), pp. 1728-1733, ISSN 0003-9942

Arnáiz, E.; Jelic, V., Almkvist, O., Wahlund, L.O., Winblad, B., Valind, S. & Nordberg, A. (2001). Impaired Cerebral Glucose Metabolism and Cognitive Functioning Predict Deterioration in Mild Cognitive Impairment. *Neuroreport*, Vol.12, No.4, (March 2001), pp. 851-855, ISSN 0959-4965

Azari, N.P.; Pettigrew, K.D., Schapiro, M.B., Haxby, J.V., Grady, C.L., Pietrini, P., Salerno, J.A., Heston, L.L., Rapoport, S.I. & Horwitz, B. (1993). Early Detection of Alzheimer's Disease: a Statistical Approach Using Positron Emission Tomographic Data. *Journal of Cerebral Blood Flow and Metabolism*, Vol.13, No.3, (May 1993), pp. 438-447, ISSN 0271-678X

Benson, D.F.; Kuhl, D.E., Phelps, M.E., Cummings, J.L. & Tsai, S.Y. (1981). Positron Emission Computed Tomography in the Diagnosis of Dementia. *Transactions of the American Neurological Association*, Vol.106, pp. 68-71, ISSN 0065-9479

Berent, S.; Giordani, B., Foster, N., Minoshima, S., Lajiness-O'Neill, R., Koeppe, R. & Kuhl, D.E. (1999). Neuropsychological Function and Cerebral Glucose Utilization in Isolated Memory Impairment and Alzheimer's Disease. *Journal of Psychiatric Research*, Vol.33, No.1, (January-February 1999), pp. 7-16, ISSN 0022-3956

Blennow, K. & Hampel, H. (2003). CSF Markers for Incipient Alzheimer's Disease. *Lancet Neurology*, Vol.2, No.10, (October 2003), pp. 605-613, ISSN 1474-4422

Bruscoli, M. & Lovestone, S. (2004). Is MCI Really Just Early Dementia? A Systematic Review of Conversion Studies. *International Psychogeriatrics / IPA*, Vol.16, No.2, (June 2004), pp. 129-140, ISSN 1041-6102

Burdette, J.H.; Minoshima, S., Vander Borght, T., Tran, D.D. & Kuhl, D.E. (1996). Alzheimer Disease: Improved Visual Interpretation of PET Images by Using Three-Dimensional Stereotaxic Surface Projections. *Radiology*, Vol.198, No.3, (March 1996), pp. 837-843, ISSN 0033-8419

Buschke, H.; Sliwinski, M.J., Kuslansky, G. & Lipton, R.B. (1997). Diagnosis of Early Dementia by the Double Memory Test: Encoding Specificity Improves Diagnostic Sensitivity and Specificity. *Neurology*, Vol.48, No.4, (April 1997), pp. 989-997, ISSN 0028-3878

Chen, K.; Langbaum, J.B., Fleisher, A.S., Ayutyanont, N., Reschke, C., Lee, W., Liu, X., Bandy, D., Alexander, G.E., Thompson, P.M., Foster, N.L., Harvey, D.J., de Leon, M.J., Koeppe, R.A., Jagust, W.J., Weiner, M.W. & Reiman, E.M; Alzheimer's Disease Neuroimaging Initiative. (2010). Twelve-Month Metabolic Declines in Probable Alzheimer's Disease and Amnestic Mild Cognitive Impairment Assessed Using an Empirically Pre-defined Statistical Region-of-Interest: Findings from the Alzheimer's Disease Neuroimaging Initiative. *NeuroImage*, Vol.51, No.2, (June 2010), pp. 654-664, ISSN 1053-8119

Chételat, G.; Desgranges, B., de la Sayette, V., Viader, F., Eustache, F. & Baron, J.C. (2003). Mild Cognitive Impairment: Can FDG-PET Predict Who is to Rapidly Convert to Alzheimer's Disease? *Neurology*, Vol.60, No.8, (April 2003), pp. 1374-1377, ISSN 0028-3878

Chételat, G.; Fouquet, M., Kalpouzos, G., Denghien, I., De la Sayette, V., Viader, F., Mézenge, F., Landeau, B., Baron, J.C., Eustache, F. & Desgranges, B. (2008). Three-Dimensional Surface Mapping of Hippocampal Atrophy Progression from MCI to AD and Over Normal Aging as Assessed Using Voxel-Based Morphometry. *Neuropsychologia*, Vol.46, No.6, pp. 1721-1731, ISSN 0028-3932

Ciarmiello, A.; Cannella, M., Lastoria, S., Simonelli, M., Frati, L., Rubinsztein, D.C. & Squitieri F. (2006). Brain White-Matter Volume Loss and Glucose Hypometabolism Precede the Clinical Symptoms of Huntington's Disease. *Journal of Nuclear Medicine*, Vol.47, No.2, (February 2006), pp. 215-222, ISSN 0161-5505

Clerici, F.; Del Sole, A., Chiti, A., Maggiore, L., Lecchi, M., Pomati, S., Mosconi, L., Lucignani, G. & Mariani, C. (2009). Differences in Hippocampal Metabolism between Amnestic and Non-amnestic MCI Subjects: Automated FDG-PET Image Analysis. *The Quarterly Journal of Nuclear Medicine and Molecular Imaging*, Vol.53, No.6, (December 2009), pp. 646-657, ISSN 1824-4785

Convit, A.; de Asis, J., de Leon, M.J., Tarshish, C.Y., De Santi, S. & Rusinek, H. (2000). Atrophy of the Medial Occipitotemporal, Inferior, and Middle Temporal Gyri in Non-demented Elderly Predict Decline to Alzheimer's Disease. *Neurobiology of Aging*, Vol.21, No.1, (January-February 2000), pp. 19-26, ISSN 0197-4580

D'Antona, R.; Baron, J.C., Samson, Y., Serdaru, M., Viader, F., Agid, Y. & Cambier, J. (1985). Subcortical Dementia. Frontal Cortex Hypometabolism Detected by Positron

Tomography in Patients with Progressive Supranuclear Palsy. *Brain*, Vol.108, Part 3, (September 1985), pp. 785-799, ISSN 0006-8950

de Leon, M.J.; Ferris, S.H., George, A.E., Reisberg, B., Christman, D.R., Kricheff I.I. & Wolf, A.P. (1983). Computed Tomography and Positron Emission Transaxial Tomography Evaluations of Normal Aging and Alzheimer's Disease. *Journal of Cerebral Blood Flow and Metabolism*, Vol.3, No.3, (September 1983), pp. 391-394, ISSN 0271-678X

de Leon, M.J.; Convit, A., Wolf, O.T., Tarshish, C.Y., DeSanti, S., Rusinek, H., Tsui, W., Kandil, E., Scherer, A.J., Roche, A., Imossi, A., Thorn, E., Bobinski, M., Caraos, C., Lesbre, P., Schlyer, D., Poirier, J., Reisberg, B. & Fowler, J. (2001). Prediction of Cognitive Decline in Normal Elderly Subjects with 2-[(18)F]Fluoro-2-Deoxy-D-Glucose/Positron-Emission Tomography (FDG/PET). *Proceedings of the National Academy of Sciences of the United States of America*, Vol.98, No.19, (September 2001), pp. 10966-10971, ISSN 0027-8424

De Reuck, J.; Decoo, D., Marchau, M., Santens, P., Lemahieu, I. & Strijckmans, K. (1998). Positron Emission Tomography in Vascular Dementia. *Journal of the Neurological Sciences*, Vol.154, No.1, (January 1998), pp. 55-61, ISSN 0022-510X

De Santi, S.; de Leon, M.J., Rusinek, H., Convit, A., Tarshish, C.Y., Roche, A., Tsui, W.H., Kandil, E., Boppana, M., Daisley, K., Wang, G.J., Schlyer, D. & Fowler, J. (2001). Hippocampal Formation Glucose Metabolism and Volume Losses in MCI and AD. *Neurobiology of Aging*, Vol.22, No.4, (July-August 2001), pp. 529-539, ISSN 0197-4580

DeCarli, C.; Haxby, J.V., Gillette, J.A., Teichberg, D., Rapoport, S.I. & Schapiro, M.B. (1992). Longitudinal Changes in Lateral Ventricular Volume in Patients with Dementia of the Alzheimer Type. *Neurology*, Vol.42, No.10, (October 1992), pp. 2029-2036, ISSN 0028-3878

DeCarli, C.; Grady, C.L., Clark, C.M., Katz, D.A., Brady, D.R., Murphy, D.G., Haxby, J.V., Salerno, J.A., Gillette, J.A., Gonzalez-Aviles, A. & Rapoport, S.I. (1996). Comparison of Positron Emission Tomography, Cognition, and Brain Volume in Alzheimer's Disease with and without Severe Abnormalities of White Matter. *Journal of Neurology, Neurosurgery, and Psychiatry*, Vol.60, No.2, (February 1996), pp. 158-167, ISSN 0022-3050

deToledo-Morrell, L.; Stoub, T.R., Bulgakova, M., Wilson, R.S., Bennett, D.A., Leurgans, S., Wuu, J. & Turner, D.A. (2004). MRI-Derived Entorhinal Volume is a Good Predictor of Conversion from MCI to AD. *Neurobiology of Aging*, Vol.25, No.9, (October 2004), pp. 1197-1203, ISSN 0197-4580

Diehl-Schmid, J.; Grimmer, T., Drzezga, A., Bornschein, S., Perneczky, R., Forstl, H., Schwaiger, M. & Kurz, A. (2006). Longitudinal Changes of Cerebral Glucose Metabolism in Semantic Dementia. *Dementia and Geriatric Cognitive Disorders*, Vol.22, No.4, pp. 346-351, ISSN 1420-8008

Döbert, N.; Pantel, J., Frölich, L., Hamscho, N., Menzel, C. & Grünwald, F. (2005). Diagnostic Value of FDG-PET and HMPAO-SPET in Patients with Mild Dementia and Mild Cognitive Impairment: Metabolic Index and Perfusion Index. *Dementia and Geriatric Cognitive Disorders*, Vol.20, No.2-3, pp. 63-70, ISSN 1420-8008

Drzezga, A.; Lautenschlager, N., Siebner, H., Riemenschneider, M., Willoch, F., Minoshima, S., Schwaiger, M. & Kurz, A. (2003). Cerebral Metabolic Changes Accompanying

Conversion of Mild Cognitive Impairment into Alzheimer's Disease: a PET Follow-up Study. *European Journal of Nuclear Medicine and Molecular Imaging*, Vol.30, No.8, (August 2003), pp. 1104-1113, ISSN 1619-7070

Drzezga, A.; Grimmer, T., Riemenschneider, M., Lautenschlager, N., Siebner, H., Alexopoulus, P., Minoshima, S., Schwaiger, M. & Kurz, A. (2005). Prediction of Individual Clinical Outcome in MCI by Means of Genetic Assessment and (18)F-FDG PET. *Journal of Nuclear Medicine*, Vol.46, No.10, (October 2005), pp. 1625-1632, ISSN 0161-5505

Duara, R.; Barker, W., Loewenstein, D., Pascal, S. & Bowen, B. (1989). Sensitivity and Specificity of Positron Emission Tomography and Magnetic Resonance Imaging Studies in Alzheimer's Disease and Multi-infarct Dementia. *European Neurology*, Vol.29, Supplement 3, pp. 9-15, ISSN 0014-3022

Dubois, B.; Feldman, H.H., Jacova, C., Dekosky, S.T., Barberger-Gateau, P., Cummings, J., Delacourte, A., Galasko, D., Gauthier, S., Jicha, G., Meguro, K., O'brien, J., Pasquier, F., Robert, P., Rossor, M., Salloway, S., Stern, Y., Visser, P.J. & Scheltens, P. (2007). Research Criteria for the Diagnosis of Alzheimer's Disease: Revising the NINCDS-ADRDA Criteria. *Lancet Neurology*, Vol.6, No.8, (August 2007), pp. 734-46, ISSN 1474-4422

Engler, H.; Lundberg, P.O., Ekbom, K., Nennesmo, I., Nilsson, A., Bergström, M., Tsukada, H., Hartvig, P. & Långström, B. (2003). Multitracer Study with Positron Emission Tomography in Creutzfeldt-Jakob Disease. *European Journal of Nuclear Medicine and Molecular Imaging*, Vol.30, No.1, (January 2003), pp. 85-95, ISSN 1619-7070

Fazekas, F.; Alavi, A., Chawluk, J.B., Zimmerman, R.A., Hackney, D., Bilaniuk, L., Rosen, M., Alves, W.M., Hurtig, H.I., Jamieson, D.G., Kushner, M.J. & Reivich, M. (1989). Comparison of CT, MR, and PET in Alzheimer's Dementia and Normal Aging. *Journal of Nuclear Medicine*, Vol.30, No.10, (October 1989), pp. 1607-1615, ISSN 0161-5505

Feigin, A.; Leenders, K.L., Moeller, J.R., Missimer, J., Kuenig, G., Spetsieris, P., Antonini, A. & Eidelberg, D. (2001). Metabolic Network Abnormalities in Early Huntington's Disease: an [(18)F]FDG PET Study. *Journal of Nuclear Medicine*, Vol.42, No.11, (November 2001), pp. 1591-1595, ISSN 0161-5505

Ferri, C.P.; Prince, M., Brayne, C., Brodaty, H., Fratiglioni, L., Ganguli, M., Hall, K., Hasegawa, K., Hendrie, H., Huang, Y., Jorm, A., Mathers, C., Menezes, P.R., Rimmer, E. & Scazufca, M.; Alzheimer's Disease International. (2005). Global Prevalence of Dementia: a Delphi Consensus Study. *Lancet*, Vol.366, No.9503, (December 2005), pp. 2112-2117, ISSN 0140-6736

Folstein, M.F.; Bassett, S.S., Anthony, J.C., Romanoski, A.J. & Nestadt, G.R. (1991). Dementia: Case Ascertainment in a Community Survey. *Journal of Gerontology*, Vol.46, No.4, (July 1991), pp. M132-M138, ISSN 0022-1422

Foster, N.L.; Chase, T.N., Fedio, P., Patronas, N.J., Brooks, R.A. & Di Chiro, G. (1983). Alzheimer's Disease: Focal Cortical Changes Shown by Positron Emission Tomography. *Neurology*, Vol.33, No.8, (August 1983), pp. 961-965, ISSN 0028-3878

Foster, N.L.; Chase, T.N., Mansi, L., Brooks, R., Fedio, P., Patronas, N.J. & Di Chiro, G. (1984). Cortical Abnormalities in Alzheimer's Disease. *Annals of Neurology*, Vol.16, No.6, (December 1984), pp. 649-654, ISSN 0364-5134

Foster, N.L.; Chase, T.N., Patronas, N.J., Gillespie, M.M. & Fedio, P. (1986). Cerebral Mapping of Apraxia in Alzheimer's Disease by Positron Emission Tomography. *Annals of Neurology*, Vol.19, No.2, (February 1986), pp. 139-143, ISSN 0364-5134

Foster, N.L.; Gilman, S., Berent, S., Sima, A.A., D'Amato, C., Koeppe, R.A. & Hicks, S.P. (1992). Progressive Subcortical Gliosis and Progressive Supranuclear Palsy Can Have Similar Clinical and PET Abnormalities. *Journal of Neurology, Neurosurgery, and Psychiatry*, Vol.55, No.8, (August 1992), pp. 707-713, ISSN 0022-3050

Foster, N.L.; Heidebrink, J.L., Clark, C.M., Jagust, W.J., Arnold, S.E., Barbas, N.R., DeCarli, C.S., Turner, R.S., Koeppe, R.A., Higdon, R. & Minoshima, S. (2007). FDG-PET Improves Accuracy in Distinguishing Frontotemporal Dementia and Alzheimer's Disease. *Brain*, Vol.130, Part 10, (October 2007), pp. 2616-2635, ISSN 0006-8950

Frackowiak, R.S.; Pozzilli, C., Legg, N.J., Du Boulay, G.H., Marshall, J., Lenzi, G.L. & Jones, T. (1981). Regional Cerebral Oxygen Supply and Utilization in Dementia. A Clinical and Physiological Study with Oxygen-15 and Positron Tomography. *Brain*, Vol.104, Part 4, (December 1981), pp. 753-778, ISSN 0006-8950

Grady, C.L.; Haxby, J.V., Horwitz, B., Berg, G. & Rapoport, S.I. (1987). Neuropsychological and Cerebral Metabolic Function in Early vs Late Onset Dementia of the Alzheimer Type. *Neuropsychologia*, Vol.25, No.5, pp. 807-816, ISSN 0028-3932

Hayden, M.R.; Hewitt, J., Stoessl, A.J., Clark, C., Ammann, W. & Martin, W.R. (1987). The Combined Use of Positron Emission Tomography and DNA Polymorphisms for Preclinical Detection of Huntington's Disease. *Neurology*, Vol.37, No.9, (September 1987), pp. 1441-1447, ISSN 0028-3878

Henkel, K.; Zerr, I., Hertel, A., Gratz, K.F., Schröter, A., Tschampa, H.J., Bihl, H., Büll, U., Grünwald, F., Drzezga, A., Spitz, J. & Poser, S. (2002). Positron Emission Tomography with [(18)F]FDG in the Diagnosis of Creutzfeldt-Jakob Disease (CJD). *Journal of Neurology*, Vol.249, No.6, (June 2002), pp. 699-705, ISSN 0340-5354

Herholz, K.; Adams, R., Kessler, J., Szelies, B., Grond, M. & Heiss, W.D. (1990). Criteria for the Diagnosis of Alzheimer's Disease with Positron Emission Tomography. *Dementia and Geriatric Cognitive Disorders*, Vol.1, No.3, pp. 156-164, ISSN 1420-8008

Herholz, K.; Perani, D., Salmon, E., Franck, G., Fazio, F., Heiss, W.D. & Comar, D. (1993). Comparability of FDG PET Studies in Probable Alzheimer's Disease. *Journal of Nuclear Medicine*, Vol.34, No.9, (September 1993), pp. 1460-1466, ISSN 0161-5505

Herholz, K.; Nordberg, A., Salmon, E., Perani, D., Kessler, J., Mielke, R., Halber, M., Jelic, V., Almkvist, O., Collette, F., Alberoni, M., Kennedy, A., Hasselbalch, S., Fazio, F. & Heiss, W.D. (1999) Impairment of Neocortical Metabolism Predicts Progression in Alzheimer's Disease. *Dementia and Geriatric Cognitive Disorders*, Vol.10, No.6, (November-December 1999), pp. 494-504, ISSN 1420-8008

Herholz, K.; Salmon, E., Perani, D., Baron, J.C., Holthoff, V., Frölich, L., Schönknecht, P., Ito, K., Mielke, R., Kalbe, E., Zündorf, G., Delbeuck, X., Pelati, O., Anchisi, D., Fazio, F., Kerrouche, N., Desgranges, B., Eustache, F., Beuthien-Baumann, B., Menzel, C., Schröder, J., Kato, T., Arahata, Y., Henze, M. & Heiss, W.D. (2002a). Discrimination between Alzheimer Dementia and Controls by Automated Analysis of Multicenter FDG PET. *NeuroImage*, Vol.17, No.1, (September 2002), pp. 302-316, ISSN 1053-8119

Herholz, K.; Schopphoff, H., Schmidt, M., Mielke, R., Eschner, W., Scheidhauer, K., Schicha, H., Heiss, W.D. & Ebmeier, K. (2002b). Direct Comparison of Spatially Normalized

PET and SPECT Scans in Alzheimer's Disease. *Journal of Nuclear Medicine*, Vol.43, No.1, (January 2002), pp. 21-26, ISSN 0161-5505

Higuchi, M.; Tashiro, M., Arai, H., Okamura, N., Hara, S., Higuchi, S., Itoh, M., Shin, R.W., Trojanowski, J.Q. & Sasaki, H. (2000). Glucose Hypometabolism and Neuropathological Correlates in Brains of Dementia with Lewy Bodies. *Experimental Neurology*, Vol.162, No.2, (April 2000), pp. 247-256, ISSN 0014-4886

Hirao, K.; Ohnishi, T., Hirata, Y., Yamashita, F., Mori, T., Moriguchi, Y., Matsuda, H., Nemoto, K., Imabayashi, E., Yamada, M., Iwamoto, T., Arima, K. & Asada, T. (2005). The Prediction of Rapid Conversion to Alzheimer's Disease in Mild Cognitive Impairment Using Regional Cerebral Blood Flow SPECT. *NeuroImage*, Vol.28, No.4, (December 2005), pp. 1014-1021, ISSN 1053-8119

Hoffman, J.M.; Welsh-Bohmer, K.A., Hanson, M., Crain, B., Hulette, C., Earl, N. & Coleman, R.E. (2000). FDG PET Imaging in Patients with Pathologically Verified Dementia. *Journal of Nuclear Medicine*, Vol.41, No.11, (November 2000), pp. 1920-1928, ISSN 0161-5505

Holmes, C.; Cairns, N., Lantos, P. & Mann, A. (1999). Validity of Current Clinical Criteria for Alzheimer's Disease, Vascular Dementia and Dementia with Lewy Bodies. *The British Journal of Psychiatry*, Vol.174, (January 1999), pp. 45-50, ISSN 0007-1250

Imamura, T.; Ishii, K., Sasaki, M., Kitagaki, H., Yamaji, S., Hirono, N., Shimomura, T., Hashimoto, M., Tanimukai, S., Kazui, H. & Mori, E. (1997). Regional Cerebral Glucose Metabolism in Dementia with Lewy Bodies and Alzheimer's Disease: a Comparative Study Using Positron Emission Tomography. *Neuroscience Letters*, Vol.235, No.1-2, (October 1997), pp. 49-52, ISSN 0304-3940

Ishii, K.; Sasaki, M., Kitagaki, H., Yamaji, S., Sakamoto, S., Matsuda, K. & Mori, E. (1997). Reduction of Cerebellar Glucose Metabolism in Advanced Alzheimer's Disease. *Journal of Nuclear Medicine*, Vol.38, No.6, (June 1997), pp. 925-928, ISSN 0161-5505

Ishii, K.; Sakamoto, S., Sasaki, M., Kitagaki, H., Yamaji, S., Hashimoto, M., Imamura, T., Shimomura, T., Hirono, N. & Mori, E. (1998). Cerebral Glucose Metabolism in Patients With Frontotemporal Dementia. *Journal of Nuclear Medicine*, Vol.39, No.11, (November 1998), pp. 1875-1878, ISSN 0161-5505

Ishii, K.; Sasaki, M., Sakamoto, S., Yamaji, S., Kitagaki, H. & Mori, E. (1999). Tc-99m Ethyl Cysteinate Dimer SPECT and 2-[F-18]Fluoro-2-Deoxy-D-Glucose PET in Alzheimer's Disease. Comparison of Perfusion and Metabolic Patterns. *Clinical Nuclear Medicine*, Vol.24, No.8, (August 1999), pp. 572-575, ISSN 0363-9762

Ishii, K.; Kono, A.K., Sasaki, H., Miyamoto, N., Fukuda, T., Sakamoto, S. & Mori, E. (2006). Fully Automatic Diagnostic System for Early- and Late-Onset Mild Alzheimer's Disease Using FDG PET and 3D-SSP. *European Journal of Nuclear Medicine and Molecular Imaging*, Vol.33, No.5, (May 2006), pp. 575-583, ISSN 1619-7070

Ishii, K.; Soma, T., Kono, A.K., Sofue, K., Miyamoto, N., Yoshikawa, T., Mori, E. & Murase, K. (2007). Comparison of Regional Brain Volume and Glucose Metabolism between Patients with Mild Dementia with Lewy Bodies and Those with Mild Alzheimer's Disease. *Journal of Nuclear Medicine*, Vol.48, No.5, (May 2007), pp. 704-711, ISSN 0161-5505

Ito, K.; Kato, T. & Torizuka, K. (2010). [Clinical Value of 18F-FDG PET in Assessment of Alzheimer's Disease: Meta-analysis] (Japanese). *Kaku Igaku*, Vol.47, No.1, (March 2010), pp. 1-8, ISSN 0022-7854

Jagust, W.J.; Friedland, R.P. & Budinger, T.F. (1985). Positron Emission Tomography with [18F]Fluorodeoxyglucose Differentiates Normal Pressure Hydrocephalus from Alzheimer-Type Dementia. *Journal of Neurology, Neurosurgery, and Psychiatry*, Vol.48, No.11, (November 1985), pp. 1091-1096, ISSN 0022-3050

Jagust, W.J.; Friedland, R.P., Budinger, T.F., Koss, E. & Ober, B. (1988). Longitudinal Studies of Regional Cerebral Metabolism in Alzheimer's Disease. *Neurology*, Vol.38, No.6):, (June 1988), pp. 909-912, ISSN 0028-3878

Jagust, W.; Gitcho, A., Sun, F., Kuczynski, B., Mungas, D. & Haan, M. (2006). Brain Imaging Evidence of Preclinical Alzheimer's Disease in Normal Aging. *Annals of Neurology*, Vol.59, No.4, (April 2006), pp. 673-681, ISSN 0364-5134

Jauhiainen, A.M.; Kangasmaa, T., Rusanen, M., Niskanen, E., Tervo, S., Kivipelto, M., Vanninen, R.L., Kuikka, J.T. & Soininen, H. (2008). Differential Hypometabolism Patterns According to Mild Cognitive Impairment Subtypes. *Dementia and Geriatric Cognitive Disorders*, Vol.26, No.6, pp. 490-498, ISSN 1420-8008

Jobst, K.A.; Hindley, N.J., King, E. & Smith, A.D. (1994). The Diagnosis of Alzheimer's Disease: a Question of Image? *The Journal of Clinical Psychiatry*, Vol.55, Supplement, (November 1994), pp. 22-31, ISSN 0160-6689

Jobst, K.A.; Barnetson, L.P. & Shepstone, B.J. (1998). Accurate Prediction of Histologically Confirmed Alzheimer's Disease and the Differential Diagnosis of Dementia: the Use of NINCDS-ADRDA and DSM-III-R Criteria, SPECT, X-ray CT, and Apo E4 in Medial Temporal Lobe Dementias. Oxford Project to Investigate Memory and Aging. *International Psychogeriatrics / IPA*, Vol.10, No.3, (September 1998), pp. 271-302, ISSN 1041-6102

Kadekaro, M.; Crane, A.M. & Sokoloff, L. (1985). Differential Effects of Electrical Stimulation of Sciatic Nerve on Metabolic Activity in Spinal Cord and Dorsal Root Ganglion in the Rat. *Proceedings of the National Academy of Sciences of the United States of America*, Vol.82, No.17, (September 1985), pp. 6010-6013, ISSN 0027-8424

Kadir, A.; Darreh-Shori, T., Almkvist, O., Wall, A., Grut, M., Strandberg, B., Ringheim, A., Eriksson, B., Blomquist, G., Långström, B. & Nordberg, A. (2008). PET Imaging of the In Vivo Brain Acetylcholinesterase Activity and Nicotine Binding in Galantamine-Treated Patients with AD. *Neurobiology of Aging*, Vol.29, No.8, (August 2008), pp. 1204-1217, ISSN 0197-4580

Kawachi, T.; Ishii, K., Sakamoto, S., Sasaki, M., Mori, T., Yamashita, F., Matsuda, H. & Mori, E. (2006). Comparison of the Diagnostic Performance of FDG-PET and VBM-MRI in Very Mild Alzheimer's Disease. *European Journal of Nuclear Medicine and Molecular Imaging*, Vol.33, No.7, (July 2006), pp. 801-809, ISSN 1619-7070

Kerrouche, N.; Herholz, K., Mielke, R., Holthoff, V. & Baron, J.C. (2006). 18FDG PET in Vascular Dementia: Differentiation from Alzheimer's Disease Using Voxel-Based Multivariate Analysis. *Journal of Cerebral Blood Flow and Metabolism*, Vol.26, No.9, (September 2006), pp. 1213-1221, ISSN 0271-678X

Killiany, R.J.; Gomez-Isla, T., Moss, M., Kikinis, R., Sandor, T., Jolesz, F., Tanzi, R., Jones, K., Hyman, B.T. & Albert, M.S. (2000). Use of Structural Magnetic Resonance Imaging to Predict Who Will Get Alzheimer's Disease. *Annals of Neurology*, Vol.47, No.4, (April 2000), pp. 430-439, ISSN 0364-5134

Kippenhan, J.S.; Barker, W.W., Pascal, S., Nagel, J. & Duara, R. (1992). Evaluation of a Neural-Network Classifier for PET Scans of Normal and Alzheimer's Disease Subjects. *Journal of Nuclear Medicine*, Vol.33, No.8, (August 1992), pp. 1459-1467, ISSN 0161-5505

Kumar, A.; Schapiro, M.B., Grady, C.L., Matocha, M.F., Haxby, J.V., Moore, A.M., Luxenberg, J.S., St George-Hyslop, P.H., Robinette, C.D., Ball, M.J. & Rapoport, S.I. (1991). Anatomic, Metabolic, Neuropsychological, and Molecular Genetic Studies of Three Pairs of Identical Twins Discordant for Dementia of the Alzheimer's Type. *Archives of Neurology*, Vol.48, No.2, (February 1991), pp. 160-168, ISSN 0003-9942

Kuwert, T.; Lange, H.W,, Langen, K.J., Herzog, H., Aulich, A. & Feinendegen, L.E. (1990). Cortical and Subcortical Glucose Consumption Measured by PET in Patients with Huntington's Disease. *Brain*, Vol.113, Part 5:, (October 1990), pp. 1405-1423, ISSN 0006-8950

Landau, S.M.; Harvey, D., Madison, C.M., Reiman, E.M., Foster, N.L., Aisen, P.S., Petersen, R.C., Shaw, L.M., Trojanowski, J.Q., Jack, C.R Jr., Weiner, M.W. & Jagust, W.J.; Alzheimer's Disease Neuroimaging Initiative. (2010). Comparing Predictors of Conversion and Decline in Mild Cognitive Impairment. *Neurology*, Vol.75, No.3, (July 2010), pp. 230-238, ISSN 0028-3878

Langbaum, J.B.; Chen, K., Lee, W., Reschke, C., Bandy, D., Fleisher, A.S., Alexander, G.E., Foster, N.L., Weiner, M.W., Koeppe, R.A., Jagust, W.J. & Reiman, E.M.; Alzheimer's Disease Neuroimaging Initiative. (2009). Categorical and Correlational Analyses of Baseline Fluorodeoxyglucose Positron Emission Tomography Images from the Alzheimer's Disease Neuroimaging Initiative (ADNI). *NeuroImage*, Vol.45, No.4, (May 2009), pp. 1107-1116, ISSN 1053-8119

Lim, A.; Tsuang, D., Kukull, W., Nochlin, D., Leverenz, J., McCormick, W., Bowen, J., Teri, L., Thompson, J., Peskind, E.R., Raskind, M. & Larson, E.B. (1999). Clinico-neuropathological Correlation of Alzheimer's Disease in a Community-Based Case Series. *Journal of the American Geriatric Society*, Vol.47, No.5, (May 1999), pp. 564-569, ISSN 0002-8614

Masliah, E.; Mallory, M., Hansen, L., Alford, M., Albright, T., DeTeresa, R., Terry, R., Baudier, J., & Saitoh, T. (1991). Patterns of Aberrant Sprouting in Alzheimer's Disease. *Neuron*, Vol.6, No.5, (May 1991), pp. 729-739, ISSN 0896-6273

Mattson, M.P.; Duan, W., Wan, R. & Guo, Z. (2004). Prophylactic Activation of Neuroprotective Stress Response Pathways by Dietary and Behavioral Manipulations. *NeuroRx*, Vol.1, No.1, (January 2004), pp. 111-116, ISSN 1545-5343

Mazziotta, J.C.; Phelps, M.E., Pahl, J.J., Huang, S.C., Baxter, L.R., Riege, W.H., Hoffman, J.M., Kuhl, D.E., Lanto, A.B. Wapenski, J.A. & Markham, C.H. (1987). Reduced Cerebral Glucose Metabolism in Asymptomatic Subjects at Risk for Huntington's Disease. *The New England Journal of Medicine*, Vol.316, No.7, (February 1987), pp. 357-362, ISSN 0028-4793

McGeer, E.G.; Peppard, R.P., McGeer, P.L., Tuokko, H., Crockett, D., Parks, R., Akiyama, H., Calne, D.B., Beattie, B.L. & Harrop, R. (1990). 18Fluorodeoxyglucose Positron Emission Tomography Studies in Presumed Alzheimer Cases, Including 13 Serial

Scans. *The Canadian Journal of Neurological Sciences*, Vol.17, No.1, (February 1990), pp. 1-11, ISSN 0317-1671

McKhann, G.; Drachman, D., Folstein, M., Katzman, R., Price, D. & Stadlan, E.M. (1984). Clinical Diagnosis of Alzheimer's Disease: Report of the NINCDS-ADRDA Work Group under the Auspices of Department of Health and Human Services Task Force on Alzheimer's Disease. *Neurology*, Vol.34, No.7, (July 1984), pp. 939-944, ISSN 0028-3878

Mega, M.S.; Cummings, J.L., O'Connor, S.M., Dinov, I.D., Reback, E., Felix, J., Masterman, D.L., Phelps, M.E., Small, G.W. & Toga, A.W. (2001). Cognitive and Metabolic Responses to Metrifonate Therapy in Alzheimer Disease. *Neuropsychiatry, Neuropsychology, and Behavioral Neurology*, Vol.14, No.1, (January 2001), pp. 63-68, ISSN 0894-878X

Mega, M.S.; Dinov, I.D., Porter, V., Chow, G., Reback, E., Davoodi, P., O'Connor, S.M., Carter, M.F., Amezcua, H. & Cummings, J.L. (2005). Metabolic Patterns Associated with the Clinical Response to Galantamine Therapy: a Fludeoxyglucose F 18 Positron Emission Tomographic Study. *Archives of Neurology*, Vol.62, No.5, (May 2005), pp. 721-728, ISSN 0003-9942

Meguro, K.; Ishii, H., Yamaguchi, S., Ishizaki, J., Shimada, M., Sato, M., Hashimoto, R., Shimada, Y., Meguro, M., Yamadori, A. & Sekita, Y. (2002). Prevalence of Dementia and Dementing Diseases in Japan: the Tajiri Project. *Archives of Neurology*, Vol.59, No.7, (July 2002), pp. 1109-1114, ISSN 0003-9942

Mielke, R.; Herholz, K, Grond, M., Kessler, J. & Heiss, W.D. (1992). Differences of Regional Cerebral Glucose Metabolism between Presenile and Senile Dementia of Alzheimer Type. *Neurobiology of Aging*, Vol.13, No.1, (January-February 1992), pp. 93-98, ISSN 0197-4580

Mielke, R.; Pietrzyk, U., Jacobs, A., Fink, G.R., Ichimiya, A., Kessler, J., Herholz, K. & Heiss, W.D. (1994). HMPAO SPET and FDG PET in Alzheimer's Disease and Vascular Dementia: Comparison of Perfusion and Metabolic Pattern. *European Journal of Nuclear Medicine*, Vol.21, No.10, (October 1994), pp. 1052-1060, ISSN 0340-6997

Mielke, R.; Schröder, R., Fink, G.R., Kessler, J., Herholz, K. & Heiss, W.D. (1996). Regional Cerebral Glucose Metabolism and Postmortem Pathology in Alzheimer's Disease. *Acta Neuropathologica*, Vol.91, No.2, pp. 174-179, ISSN 0001-6322

Minoshima, S.; Koeppe, R.A., Mintun, M.A., Berger, K.L., Taylor, S.F., Frey, K.A. & Kuhl, D.E. (1993). Automated Detection of the Intercommissural Line for Stereotactic Localization of Functional Brain Images. *Journal of Nuclear Medicine*, Vol.34, No.2, (February 1993), pp. 322-329, ISSN 0161-5505

Minoshima, S.; Foster, N.L. & Kuhl, D.E. (1994). Posterior Cingulate Cortex in Alzheimer's Disease. *Lancet*, Vol.344, No.8926, (September 1994), p. 895, ISSN 0140-6736

Minoshima, S.; Frey, K.A., Koeppe, R.A., Foster, N.L. & Kuhl, D.E. (1995). A Diagnostic Approach in Alzheimer's Disease Using Three-Dimensional Stereotactic Surface Projections of Fluorine-18-FDG PET. *Journal of Nuclear Medicine*, Vol.36, No.7, (July 1995), pp. 1238-1248, ISSN 0161-5505

Minoshima, S.; Giordani, B., Berent, S., Frey, K.A., Foster, N.L. & Kuhl, D.E. (1997). Metabolic Reduction in the Posterior Cingulate Cortex in Very Early Alzheimer's Disease. *Annals of Neurology*, Vol.42, No.1, (July 1997), pp. 85-94, ISSN 0364-5134

Minoshima, S. (2003). Imaging Alzheimer's Disease: Clinical Applications. *Neuroimaging Clinics of North America*, Vol.13, No.4, (November 2003), pp. 769-780, ISSN 1052-5149

Miyazawa, N.; Satoh, T., Hashizume, K. & Fukamachi, A. (1997). Xenon Contrast CT-CBF Measurements in High-Intensity Foci on T2-Weighted MR Images in Centrum Semiovale of Asymptomatic Individuals. *Stroke*, Vol.28, No.5, (May 1997), pp. 984-987, ISSN 0039-2499

Miyazawa, N.; Shinohara, T., Nagasaka, T. & Hayashi, M. (2010). Hypermetabolism in Patients with Dementia with Lewy Bodies. *Clinical Nuclear Medicine*, Vol.35, No.7, (July 2010), pp. 490-493, ISSN 0363-9762

Miyazawa, N.; Shinohara, T., Kobayasi, R. & Nagasaka, T. (2011). Application of F-18 FDG-PET by Ordinary and Statistical Images and Methods to Patients with Memory Disturbance: Analysis of its Usefulness with 500 Consecutive Cases. *Nuclear Medicine in Clinic* (in press)

Morbelli, S.; Piccardo, A., Villavecchia, G., Dessi, B., Brugnolo, A., Piccini, A., Caroli, A., Frisoni, G., Rodriguez, G. & Nobili, F. (2010). Mapping Brain Morphological and Functional Conversion Patterns in Amnestic MCI: a Voxel-Based MRI and FDG-PET Study. *European Journal of Nuclear Medicine and Molecular Imaging*, Vol.37, No.1, (January 2010), pp. 36-45, ISSN 1619-7070

Morinaga, A.; Ono, K., Ikeda, T., Ikeda, Y., Shima, K., Noguchi-Shinohara, M., Samuraki, M., Yanase, D., Yoshita, M., Iwasa, K., Mastunari, I. & Yamada, M. (2010). A Comparison of the Diagnostic Sensitivity of MRI, CBF-SPECT, FDG-PET and Cerebrospinal Fluid Biomarkers for Detecting Alzheimer's Disease in a Memory Clinic. *Dementia and Geriatric Cognitive Disorders*, Vol.30, No.4, pp. 285-292, ISSN 1420-8008

Morris, J.C.; Weintraub, S., Chui, H.C., Cummings, J., Decarli, C., Ferris, S., Foster, N.L., Galasko, D., Graff-Radford, N., Peskind, E.R., Beekly, D., Ramos, E.M. & Kukull, W.A. (2006). The Uniform Data Set (UDS): Clinical and Cognitive Variables and Descriptive Data from Alzheimer Disease Centers. *Alzheimer Disease and Associated Disorders*, Vol.20, No.4, (October-December 2006), pp. 210-216, ISSN 0893-0341

Mosconi, L.; Perani, D., Sorbi, S., Herholz, K., Nacmias, B., Holthoff, V., Salmon, E., Baron, J.C., De Cristofaro, M.T., Padovani, A., Borroni, B., Franceschi, M., Bracco, L. & Pupi, A. (2004). MCI Conversion to Dementia and the APOE Genotype: a Prediction Study with FDG-PET. *Neurology*, Vol.63, No.12, (December 2004), pp. 2332-2340, ISSN 0028-3878

Mosconi, L.; Tsui, W.H., De Santi, S., Li, J., Rusinek, H., Convit, A., Li, Y., Boppana, M. & de Leon, M.J. (2005). Reduced Hippocampal Metabolism in MCI and AD: Automated FDG-PET Image Analysis. *Neurology*, Vol.64, No.11, (June 2005), pp. 1860-1867, ISSN 0028-3878

Mosconi, L.; Brys, M., Switalski, R., Mistur, R., Glodzik, L., Pirraglia, E., Tsui, W., De Santi, S. & de Leon, M.J. (2007). Maternal Family History of Alzheimer's Disease Predisposes to Reduced Brain Glucose Metabolism. *Proceedings of the National Academy of Sciences of the United States of America*, Vol.104, No.48, (November 2007), pp. 19067-19072, ISSN 0027-8424

Mosconi, L.; De Santi, S., Brys, M., Tsui, W.H., Pirraglia, E., Glodzik-Sobanska, L., Rich, K.E., Switalski, R., Mehta, P.D., Pratico, D., Zinkowski, R., Blennow, K. & de Leon, M.J. (2008). Hypometabolism and Altered Cerebrospinal Fluid Markers in Normal Apolipoprotein E E4 Carriers with Subjective Memory Complaints. *Biological Psychiatry*, Vol.63, No.6, (March 2008), pp. 609-618, ISSN 0006-3223

Mosconi, L.; Mistur, R., Switalski, R., Brys, M., Glodzik, L., Rich, K., Pirraglia, E., Tsui, W., De Santi, S. & de Leon, M.J. (2009). Declining Brain Glucose Metabolism in Normal Individuals with a Maternal History of Alzheimer Disease. *Neurology*, Vol.72, No.6, (February 2009), pp. 513-520, ISSN 0028-3878

Mueller, S.G.; Weiner, M.W., Thal, L.J., Petersen, R.C., Jack, C.R., Jagust, W., Trojanowski, J.Q., Toga, A.W. & Beckett, L. (2005). Ways Toward an Early Diagnosis in Alzheimer's Disease: the Alzheimer's Disease Neuroimaging Initiative (ADNI). *Alzheimer's & Dementia*, Vol.1, No.1, (July 2005), pp. 55-66, ISSN 1552-5260

Nagasaka, T.; Nagasaka, K., Ohta, E., Shindo, K., Takiyama, Y., Shiozawa, Z., Miyazawa, N., Yamasaki, N., Mori, N., Onda, H. & Shinohara, T. (2011). Cerebral Hypermetabolism Demonstrated by FDG PET in Familial Creutzfeldt-Jakob Disease. *Clinical Nuclear Medicine*, Vol.36, No.8, (August 2011), pp. 725-727, ISSN 0363-9762

Ng, S.; Villemagne, V.L., Berlangieri, S., Lee, S.T., Cherk, M., Gong, S.J., Ackermann, U., Saunder, T., Tochon-Danguy, H., Jones, G., Smith, C., O'Keefe, G., Masters, C.L. & Rowe, C.C. (2007). Visual Assessment Versus Quantitative Assessment of 11C-PIB PET and 18F-FDG PET for Detection of Alzheimer's Disease. *Journal of Nuclear Medicine*, Vol.48, No.4, (April 2007), pp. 547-552, ISSN 0161-5505

Nordberg, A.; Rinne, J.O., Kadir, A. & Långström, B. (2010). The Use of PET in Alzheimer Disease. *Nature Reviews. Neurology*, Vol.6, No.2, (February 2010), pp. 78-87, ISSN 1759-4758

Ohyama, M.; Senda, M., Mishina, M., Kitamura, S., Tanizaki, N., Ishii, K. & Katayama, Y. (2000). Semi-automatic ROI Placement System for Analysis of Brain PET Images Based on Elastic Model: Application to Diagnosis of Alzheimer's Disease. *The Keio Journal of Medicine*, Vol.49, Supplement 1, (February 2000), pp. A105-A106, ISSN 0022-9717

Panza, F.; D'Introno, A., Colacicco, A.M., Capurso, C., Del Parigi, A., Caselli, R.J., Pilotto, A., Argentieri, G., Scapicchio, P.L., Scafato, E., Capurso, A. & Solfrizzi, V. (2005). Current Epidemiology of Mild Cognitive Impairment and Other Predementia Syndromes. *The American Journal of Geriatric Psychiatry*, Vol.13, No.8, (August 2005), pp. 633-644, ISSN 1064-7481

Pascual, B.; Prieto, E., Arbizu, J., Marti-Climent, J., Olier, J. & Masdeu, J.C. (2010). Brain Glucose Metabolism in Vascular White Matter Disease with Dementia: Differentiation from Alzheimer Disease. *Stroke*, Vol.41, No.12, (December 2010), pp. 2889-2893, ISSN 0039-2499

Pennanen, C.; Kivipelto, M., Tuomainen, S., Hartikainen, P., Hänninen, T., Laakso, M.P., Hallikainen, M., Vanhanen, M., Nissinen, A., Helkala, E.L., Vainio, P., Vanninen, R., Partanen, K. & Soininen, H. (2004). Hippocampus and Entorhinal Cortex in Mild Cognitive Impairment and Early AD. *Neurobiology of Aging*, Vol.25, No.3, (March 2004), pp. 303-310, ISSN 0197-4580

Perneczky, R.; Drzezga, A., Boecker, H., Förstl, H., Kurz, A. & Häussermann, P. (2008). Cerebral Metabolic Dysfunction in Patients with Dementia with Lewy Bodies and Visual Hallucinations. *Dementia and Geriatric Cognitive Disorders*, Vol.25, No.6, pp. 531-538, ISSN 1420-8008

Petersen, R.C.; Smith, G.E., Waring, S.C., Ivnik, R.J., Tangalos, E.G. & Kokmen, E. (1999). Mild Cognitive Impairment: Clinical Characterization and Outcome. *Archives of Neurology*, Vol.56, No.3, (March 1999), pp. 303-308, ISSN 0003-9942

Petersen, R.C. & Morris, J.C. (2003). Clinical Features, In: *Mild Cognitive Impairment*, R.C. Petersen, (Ed.), 15-39, Oxford University Press, ISBN 0-19-512342-5, New York, NY, USA

Petersen, R.C. & Morris, J.C. (2005). Mild Cognitive Impairment as a Clinical Entity and Treatment Target. *Archives of Neurology*, Vol.62, No.7, (July 2005), pp. 1160-1167, ISSN 0003-9942

Petrie, E.C.; Cross, D.J., Galasko, D., Schellenberg, G.D., Raskind, M.A., Peskind, E.R. & Minoshima, S. (2009). Preclinical Evidence of Alzheimer Changes: Convergent Cerebrospinal Fluid Biomarker and Fluorodeoxyglucose Positron Emission Tomography Findings. *Archives of Neurology*, Vol.66, No.5, (May 2009), pp. 632-637, ISSN 0003-9942

Read, S.L.; Miller, B.L., Mena, I., Kim, R., Itabashi, H. & Darby, A. (1995). SPECT in Dementia: Clinical and Pathological Correlation. *Journal of the American Geriatrics Society*, Vol.43, No.11, (November 1995), pp. 1243-1247, ISSN 0002-8614

Reiman, E.M.; Caselli, R.J., Yun, L.S., Chen, K., Bandy, D., Minoshima, S., Thibodeau, S.N. & Osborne, D. (1996). Preclinical Evidence of Alzheimer's Disease in Persons Homozygous for the Epsilon 4 Allele for Apolipoprotein E. *The New England Journal of Medicine*, Vol.334, No.12, (March 1996), pp. 752-758, ISSN 0028-4793

Scheurich, A.; Muller, M.J., Siessmeier, T., Bartenstein, P., Schmidt, L.G. & Fellgiebel, A. (2005). Validating the DemTect with 18-Fluoro-2-Deoxy-Glucose Positron Emission Tomography as a Sensitive Neuropsychological Screening Test for Early Alzheimer Disease in Patients of a Memory Clinic. *Dementia and Geriatric Cognitive Disorders*, Vol.20, No.5, pp. 271-277., ISSN 1420-8008

Seo, S.W.; Cho, S.S., Park, A., Chin, J. & Na, D.L. (2009). Subcortical Vascular Versus Amnestic Mild Cognitive Impairment: Comparison of Cerebral Glucose Metabolism. *Journal of Neuroimaging*, Vol.19, No.3, (July 2009), pp. 213-219, ISSN 1051-2284

Silverman, D.H.; Small, G.W., Chang, C.Y., Lu, C.S., Kung De Aburto, M.A., Chen, W., Czernin, J., Rapoport, S.I., Pietrini, P., Alexander, G.E., Schapiro, M.B., Jagust, W.J., Hoffman, J.M., Welsh-Bohmer, K.A., Alavi, A., Clark, C.M., Salmon, E., de Leon, M.J., Mielke, R., Cummings, J.L., Kowell, A.P., Gambhir, S.S., Hoh, C.K. & Phelps, M.E. (2001). Positron Emission Tomography in Evaluation of Dementia: Regional Brain Metabolism and Long-Term Outcome. *JAMA*, Vol.286, No.17, (November 2001), pp. 2120-2027, ISSN 0098-7484

Small, G.W.; Kuhl, D.E., Riege, W.H., Fujikawa, D.G., Ashford, J.W., Metter, E.J. & Mazziotta, J.C. (1989). Cerebral Glucose Metabolic Patterns in Alzheimer's Disease. Effect of Gender and Age at Dementia Onset. *Archives of General Psychiatry*, Vol.46, No.6, (June 1989), pp. 527-532, ISSN 0003-990X

Small, G.W.; La Rue, A., Komo, S., Kaplan, A. & Mandelkern, M.A. (1995). Predictors of Cognitive Change in Middle-Aged and Older Adults with Memory Loss. *The American Journal of Psychiatry*, Vol.152, No.12, (December 1995), pp. 1757-1764, ISSN 0002-953X

Small, G.W.; Ercoli, L.M., Silverman, D.H., Huang, S.C., Komo, S., Bookheimer, S.Y., Lavretsky, H., Miller, K., Siddarth, P., Rasgon, N.L., Mazziotta, J.C., Saxena, S., Wu, H.M., Mega, M.S., Cummings, J.L., Saunders, A.M., Pericak-Vance, M.A., Roses, A.D., Barrio, J.R. & Phelps, M.E. (2000). Cerebral Metabolic and Cognitive Decline in Persons at Genetic Risk for Alzheimer's Disease. *Proceedings of the National Academy of Sciences of the United States of America*, Vol.97, No.11, (May 2000), pp. 6037-6042, ISSN 0027-8424

Smith, G.S.; Kramer, E., Ma, Y., Hermann, C.R., Dhawan, V., Chaly, T. & Eidelberg, D. (2009). Cholinergic Modulation of the Cerebral Metabolic Response to Citalopram in Alzheimer's Disease. *Brain*, Vol.132, Part 2, (February 2009), pp. 392-401, ISSN 0006-8950

Sultzer, D.L.; Mahler, M.E., Cummings, J.L., Van Gorp, W.G., Hinkin, C.H. & Brown, C. (1995). Cortical Abnormalities Associated with Subcortical Lesions in Vascular Dementia. Clinical and Position Emission Tomographic Findings. *Archives of Neurology*, Vol.52, No.8, (August 1995), pp. 773-780, ISSN 0003-9942

Szelies, B.; Mielke, R., Herholz, K. & Heiss, W.D. (1994). Quantitative Topographical EEG Compared to FDG PET for Classification of Vascular and Degenerative Dementia. *Electroencephalography and Clinical Neurophysiology*, Vol.91, No.2, (August 1994), pp. 131-139, ISSN 0013-4694

Tedeschi, E.; Hasselbalch, S.G., Waldemar, G., Juhler, M., Høgh, P., Holm, S., Garde, L., Knudsen, L.L., Klinken, L. & Gjerris, F. (1995). Heterogeneous Cerebral Glucose Metabolism in Normal Pressure Hydrocephalus. *Journal of Neurology, Neurosurgery, and Psychiatry*, Vol.59, No.6, (December 1995), pp. 608-615, ISSN 0022-3050

Teipel, S.J.; Drzezga, A., Bartenstein, P., Möller, H.J., Schwaiger, M. & Hampel, H. (2006). Effects of Donepezil on Cortical Metabolic Response to Activation during (18)FDG-PET in Alzheimer's Disease: a Double-Blind Cross-Over Trial. *Psychopharmacology*, Vol.187, No.1, (July 2006), pp. 86-94, ISSN 0033-3158

Thal, DR.; Rüb, U., Orantes, M., & Braak, H. (2002). Phases of A Beta-Deposition in the Human Brain and its Relevance for the Development of AD. *Neurology*, Vol.58, No.12, (June 2002), pp. 1791-1800, ISSN 0028-3878

Tune, L.; Tiseo, P.J., Ieni, J., Perdomo, C., Pratt, R.D., Votaw, J.R., Jewart, R.D. & Hoffman, J.M. (2003). Donepezil HCl (E2020) Maintains Functional Brain Activity in Patients with Alzheimer Disease: Results of a 24-Week, Double-Blind, Placebo-Controlled Study. *The American Journal of Geriatric Psychiatry*, Vol.11, No.2, (March-April 2003), pp. 169-177, ISSN 1064-7481

Tuszynski, M.H.; Thal, L., Pay, M., Salmon, D.P., U, H.S., Bakay, R., Patel, P., Blesch, A., Vahlsing, H.L., Ho, G., Tong, G., Potkin, S.G., Fallon, J., Hansen, L., Mufson, E.J., Kordower, J.H., Gall, C. & Conner, J. (2005). A Phase 1 Clinical Trial of Nerve Growth Factor Gene Therapy for Alzheimer Disease. *Nature Medicine*, Vol.11, No.5, (May 2005), pp. 551-555, ISSN 1078-8956 von Borczyskowski, D.; Wilke, F., Martin, B., Brenner, W., Clausen, M., Mester, J. & Buchert, R. (2006). Evaluation of a New Expert System for Fully Automated Detection of the Alzheimer's Dementia Pattern in FDG PET. *Nuclear Medicine Communications*, Vol.27, No.9, (September 2006), pp. 739-743, ISSN 0143-3636

Weiner, M.W.; Aisen, P.S., Jack, C.R. Jr., Jagust, W.J., Trojanowski, J.Q., Shaw, L., Saykin, A.J., Morris, J.C., Cairns, N., Beckett, L.A., Toga, A., Green, R., Walter, S., Soares, H., Snyder, P., Siemers, E., Potter, W., Cole, P.E. & Schmidt, M.; Alzheimer's Disease Neuroimaging Initiative. (2010). The Alzheimer's Disease Neuroimaging Initiative: Progress Report and Future Plans. *Alzheimer's & Dementia*, Vol.6, No.3, (May 2010), pp. 202-211.e7, ISSN 1552-5260

Yong, S.W.; Yoon, J.K., An, Y.S. & Lee, P.H. (2007). A Comparison of Cerebral Glucose Metabolism in Parkinson's Disease, Parkinson's Disease Dementia and Dementia with Lewy Bodies. *European Journal of Neurology*, Vol.14, No.12, (December 2007), pp. 1357-1362, ISSN 1351-5101

Young, A.B.; Penney, J.B., Starosta-Rubinstein, S., Markel, D., Berent, S., Rothley, J., Betley, A. & Hichwa, R. (1987). Normal Caudate Glucose Metabolism in Persons at Risk for Huntington's Disease. *Archives of Neurology*, Vol.44, No.3, (March 1987), pp. 254-257, ISSN 0003-9942

10

Amyloid Imaging PET Ligands as Biomarkers for Alzheimer's Disease, Preclinical Evaluation

Marie Svedberg[1,2], Ewa Hellström-Lindahl[2], Obaidur Rahman[3] and Håkan Hall[1,2]
[1,2]Uppsala University, Uppsala
[1]Department of Public Health and Caring Sciences, Molecular Geriatrics
[2]Department of Medicinal Chemistry, Preclinical PET Platform
[3]Norwegian Medical Cyclotron Center, Oslo University Hospital, Oslo
[1,2]Sweden
[3]Norway

1. Introduction

Alzheimer's disease (AD) is the most common form of dementia in the aging population. It is a complex disease that affects many brain functions and is characterized by a progressive impairment of cognitive abilities, such as memory, learning and social skills. AD was first described over hundred years ago by the German psychiatrist Dr. Alois Alzheimer, reporting of the in due course characteristic pathological changes postmortem discovered in his 56 years old patient Auguste D (Alzheimer, 1907). The disease is obviously devastating for the patients and affects everyday life for both patients and their families, but it also generates economical challenges for the heath-care system and the society as the elderly population is growing (Wimo & Winblad, 2008). Although research regarding AD is intensive worldwide and new results do get a greater understanding of the causes of the disease, the exact mechanisms and underlying cause behind AD are still unsolved. The disease progresses over decades leading to premature death. There are no disease-modifying therapies for AD available, and the current treatment might provide symptomatic relief and slower disease progression.

The new imaging technologies based on structural and functional processes in the brain enable early diagnosis and may also differentiate between types and severity of neurodegeneration. Mild cognitive impairment (MCI) is closely related to AD and can be considered as a transitional stage between normal cognition and dementia. MCI is characterized by either isolated memory impairment or impairment in several cognitive domains, but not of sufficient severity to meet diagnostic criteria for AD (Petersen et al., 2001). Although MCI is associated with an increased risk of developing AD, about half of MCI patients progress to AD at a rate of approximately 10%-15% per year, but approximately half do not develop AD even after follow-up periods as long as 10 years (Ewers et al., 2010; Ganguli & Petersen, 2008; Ganguli et al., 2011).

A clinical diagnosis of AD is assessed by several investigations including medical history and neuropsychological criteria such as the NINCDS-ADRDA (National Institute of Neurological and Communicative Disorders and Stroke and the Alzheimer's disease and Related Disorders Association) (McKhann et al., 1984), but a definite diagnosis of AD can only be done postmortem. Therefore, development of efficient prevention therapies for AD would greatly benefit from a diagnosis at a prodromal stage of the disease. Positron emission tomography (PET) is considered a unique diagnostic tool that enables early detection of pathology that facilitates prediction of AD and following the progression *in vivo* (Långström et al., 2007). Highly specific and sensitive biomarkers are of great value to assess therapeutic efficacy clinically and in terms of clearance of histopathological lesions and decelerated neurodegeneration.

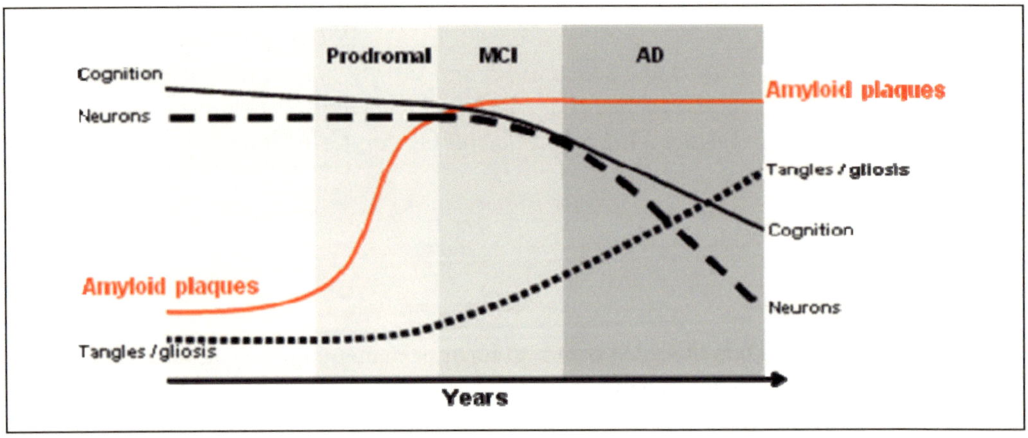

Fig. 1. Model of the temporal pattern of neuropathologic changes in AD neocortex. The figure shows that there is increase in amyloid plaques (Aβ) in the prodromal phase, followed by a progressive loss of neurons and a formation of neurofibrillary tangles in parallel with deteriorating cognitive capacities in the intermediate cognition state, MCI and later in AD. Figure adapted from Långström et al. (2007).

2. Pathology

AD is characterized neuropathologically by cerebral neuronal loss and the main histopathological hallmarks are intracellular neurofibrillary tangles consisting of hyperphosphorylated tau and extracellular β-amyloid (Aβ) deposits found as senile plaques in the brain parenchyma. These plaques are formed from insoluble Aβ peptides, fibrils and oligomers, that originate through processing of the larger Amyloid Precursor Protein (APP) (Selkoe & Schenk, 2003).

2.1 Pathological protein, Aβ

The Aβ containing plaques induce cell death and are formed during early disease progression long before the patient feels any symptoms in the prodromal phase of the disease (Braak et al., 1998; Ingelsson et al., 2004) (figure 1). Whether the formation of plaques is the major underlying event of the neurogenerative process in AD is a matter of debate. The amyloid cascade hypothesis is today one of the leading theories and suggests that Aβ depositions in the brain are the central lesion in the pathogenesis of AD (Korczyn, 2008). However, although the Aβ plaques appear in the brain prior to the neurofibrillary tangles, it has been demonstrated that the neurofibrillary tangles are better correlated with neuronal loss and cognitive decline than to Aβ plaques (Schönheit et al., 2004). Furthermore, plaques are present in cognitively normal elderly subjects without any signs of neurodegeneration (Hellström-Lindahl et al., 2004; Villemagne et al., 2008). Nonetheless, there is evidence that amyloid are associated with severity of dementia (Näslund et al., 2000).

Since it became possible to measure Aβ *in vivo* in the brain by PET (Klunk et al., 2004), Aβ plaques has became a disease-defining pathologic marker of AD. However, the plaques might play an important role in the pathophysiological mechanisms of the disease. Various strategies to prevent aggregation, increase Aβ clearance or alter APP metabolism sought for the development of new treatment strategies of AD

2.1.1 Amyloid imaging

Amyloid imaging using PET has developed rapidly in recent years. With the development of the amyloid-imaging PET tracer [^{11}C]PIB (N-methyl-[^{11}C]-2-(4-methylaminophenyl)-6-hydroxy-benzothiazole), a derivate of the widely used dye for plaques thioflavin-T, the possibility to study the presence of amyloid in the brains of AD patients in early stages of the disease with PET became an important tool (Archer et al., 2006; Klunk et al., 2004; Mintun et al., 2006; Nordberg, 2004). [^{11}C]PIB has a high affinity for aggregated Aβ, crosses the blood brain barrier (BBB) easily, has low toxicity and makes it possible to visualize plaque and vascular amyloid deposits in the brain. [^{11}C]PIB is today the most commonly used radioligand in the assessment of amyloid plaques in the living human brain using PET, although several new compounds are under development (see table 1) (Henriksen et al., 2008; Ono, 2009). However, the exact nature of the mechanism for the binding of [^{11}C]PIB and other amyloid ligands to Aβ in the form of β-pleated sheets is still unknown.

One of the central issues regarding the PIB-amyloid binding in the AD brain is thus to understand the mechanisms and binding properties of the ligand. It has been demonstrated that [^{11}C]PIB has high affinity for fibrillar Aβ and binds to the β-sheet structure of the Aβ fibrils (Klunk et al., 2003). It has also been shown that [^{11}C]PIB in nanomolar concentrations does not bind to neurofibrillary tangles (Bacskai et al., 2007; Ikonomovic et al., 2008; Kadir et al., 2011; Rosen et al., 2011).

2.1.2 Neuroinflammation (gliosis)

The widespread cellular degeneration and neuronal loss in AD is accompanied by reactive gliosis (Kadir et al., 2011). Close to the amyloid plaques both astrocytes and microglia are clustered, probably as a result of a starting neuroinflammatory process (Akiyama et al., 2000). Activated microglia accumulate in order to remove the plaques by phagocytosis (Streit, 2004). However, the cluster of microglia produce a number of various neurotoxic substances thereby inducing inflammatory processes, possibly contributing to the neurodegeneration process (Akiyama et al., 2000; Streit, 2004). Astrocytes proliferate as a reaction to neuronal insults, and astrogliosis is thus also a phenomenon in the AD brain (Porchet et al., 2003). Moreover, astrocytes may impair the efficacy of microglia to remove the plaques (Akiyama et al., 2000).

Molecular imaging of the entities involved in neuroinflammation process that follows plaque formation is today possible, as a result of the development of a number of new different radiotracers labeling microglia or astrocytes (Akiyama et al., 2000). For the study of activated microglia, ligands labeling the peripheral benzodiazepine receptor (translocator protein 18 kDa) are used, such as PK11195 and analogues (Banati, 2002; Cagnin et al., 2002). Astrocytes, which also are involved in the neuroinflammatory process, may be studied using a tracer labeling the monoamine oxidase B (MAO-B) enzyme, such as deprenyl. However, deprenyl is rapidly metabolized *in vivo*, which can be diminished by using a di-deuteriated deprenyl (Bergström et al., 1998; Fowler et al., 1988; Logan et al., 2000).

3. Chemistry

The highly conjugated fluorescent staining agents Congo red and chrysamine G (figure 2) were the first selected target molecules for the development of Aβ imaging ligands. However, those compounds were not suitable *in vivo* due to their low brain penetration ability (Klunk et al., 1994; Klunk et al., 1995). A number of other compounds with various chemical structures and promising Aβ binding abilities have been developed during last couple of years (Henriksen et al., 2008; Ono, 2009). Among those the most successful one so far is [^{11}C]PIB or [^{11}C]6-OH-BTA-1. All these compounds are small molecules with a central lipophilic group, a secondary or tertiary amine at one end and a polar or non-polar group at the other end. The terminal amine group and the middle lipophilic group which are the common features of all so far published molecules might have some impact on their amyloid binding properties. A list of available Aβ imaging PET ligands together with their chemical names and structures is presented in table 1.

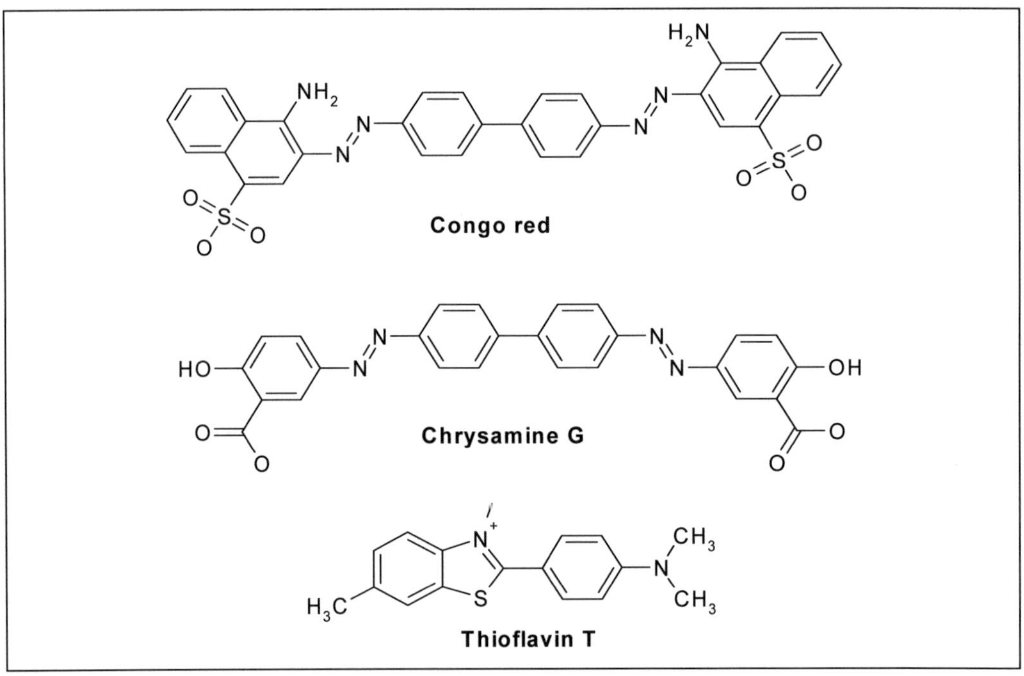

Fig. 2. Chemical structures of Congo red, chrysamine G and thioflavin T.

Short names	Chemical names	Structures
[^{11}C]AZD2184	*N*-[^{11}C]methyl)-2-(6-methylamino-pyridin-3-yl)-benzo[d]thiazol-6-ol	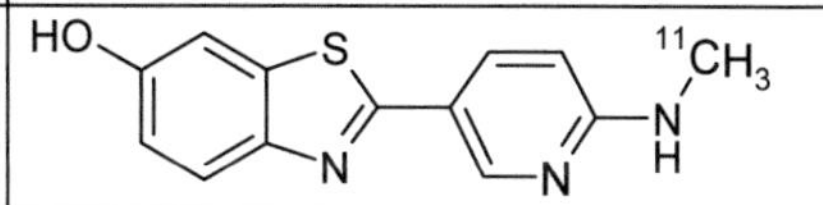
[^{11}C]BF-145	2-(4-[*N*-Methyl-^{11}C]methylaminostyryl)-5-fluorobenzoxazole	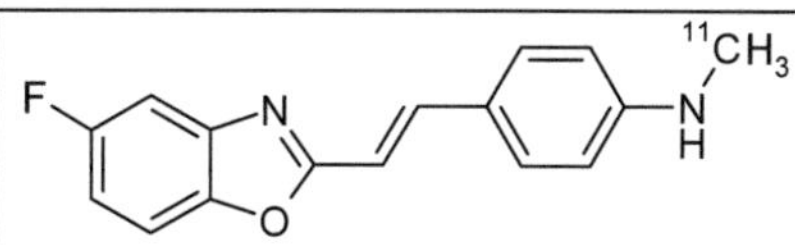
[^{18}F]BF-168	2-(4-methylaminostyryl)-6-(2-[^{18}F]fluoroethoxy)benzoxazole	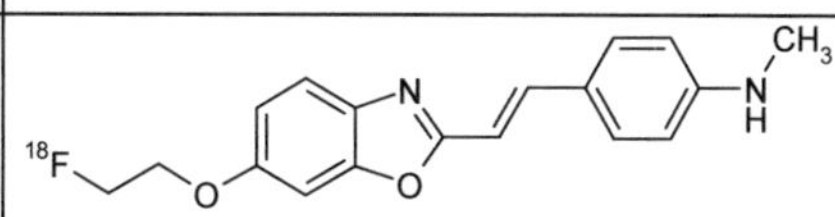
[^{18}F]BF-227	2-(2-[2-dimethylaminothiazol-5-yl]ethenyl)-6-(2-[^{18}F]fluoroethoxy)benzoxazole	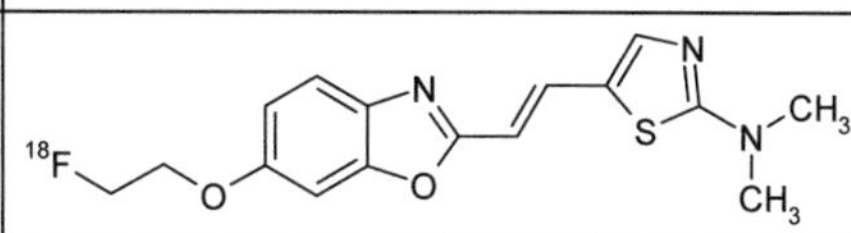
[^{11}C]BF-227	[^{11}C]2-(2-[2-dimethylaminothiazol-5-yl]ethenyl)-6-(2-fluoroethoxy)benzoxazole	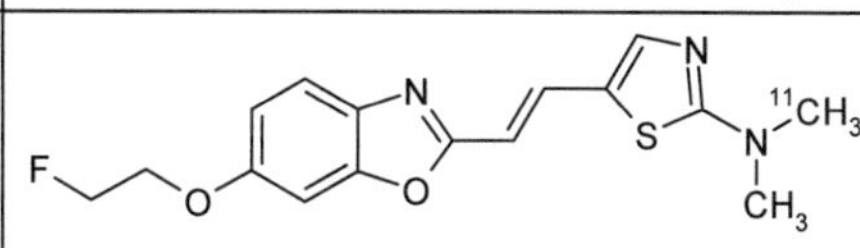
[^{18}F]FDDNP	2-(1-(2-(*N*-(2-[^{18}F]fluoroethyl)-*N*-methylamino)naphthalene-6-yl)ethylidene)malononitrile	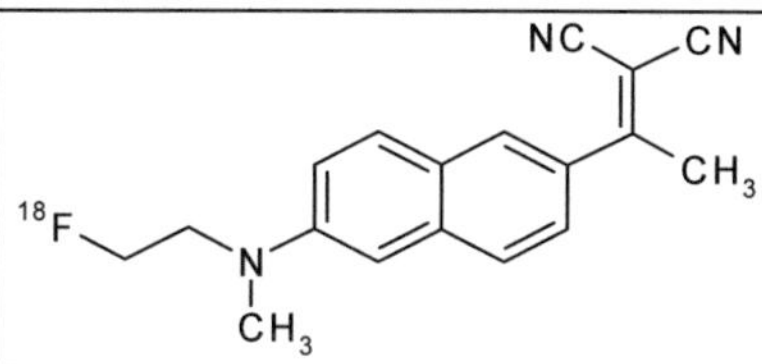
[^{18}F]FEM-IMPY	6-iodo-2-[4´-*N*-(2-[^{18}F]fluoroethyl)methylamino] phenyl-imidazo[1,2-a]pyridine	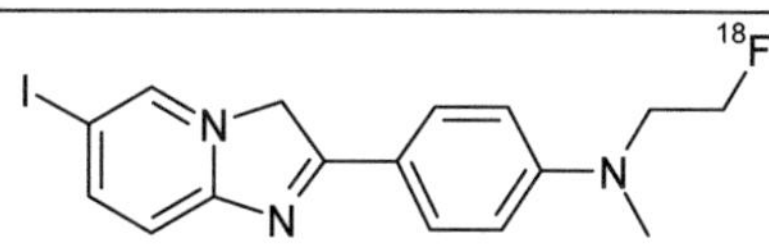
[^{18}F]FPM-IMPY	6-iodo-2-[4´-*N*-(2-[^{18}F]fluoropropyl)methylamino] phenyl-imidazo[1,2-a]pyridine	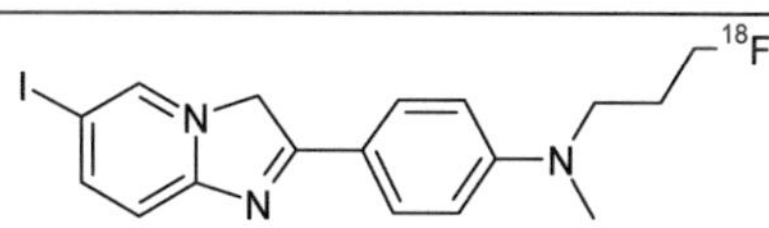
[^{18}F]florbetaben ([^{18}F]BAY94-9172)	4-(*N*-methylamino)-4´-(2-(2-(2-[^{18}F]fluoroethoxy)-ethoxy)-ethoxy)-stilbene	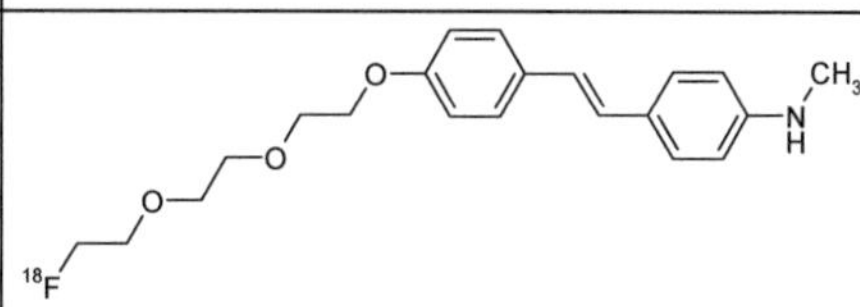
[^{18}F]florbetapir ([^{18}F]AV-45)	*N*-{4-[2-(4-{2-[2-(2-[^{18}F]fluoroethoxy)ethoxy] ethoxy}-phenyl)vinyl]phenyl}-*N*-methylamine	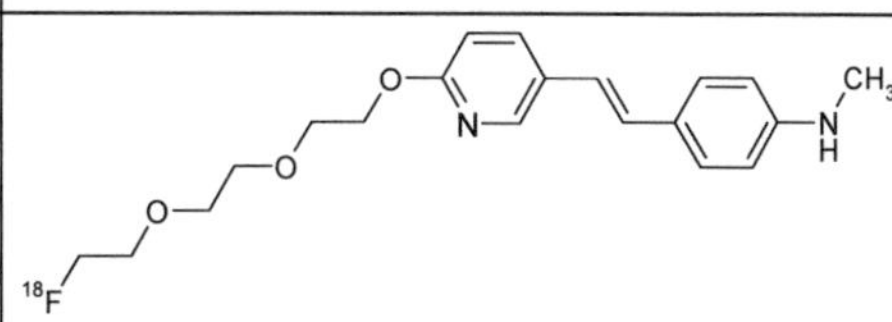
[^{18}F]flutemeta-mol	2-[3-[^{18}F]fluoro-4-(methylamino)phenyl]1,3-benzothiazol-6-ol	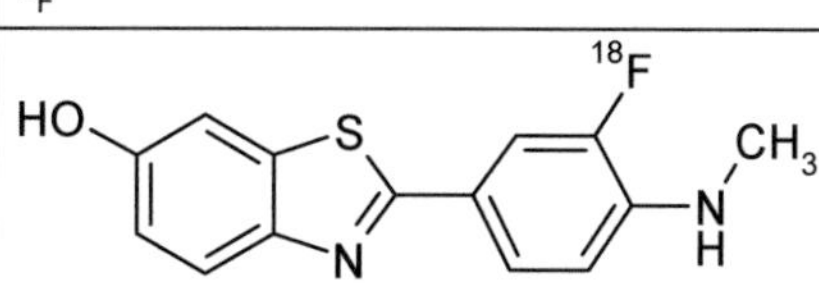

Short names	Chemical names	Structures
[^{11}C]MeS-IMPY	[*S*-methyl-^{11}C]*N*,*N*-dimethyl-4-(6-(methylthio)imidazo[1,2-a]pyridine-2-yl)aniline	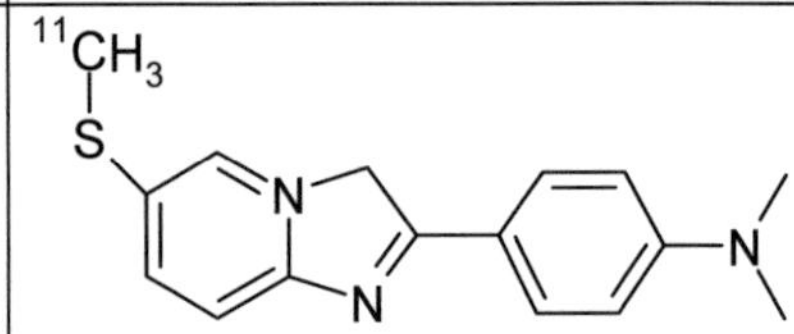
[^{11}C]PIB	[^{11}C]-2-4-(methylaminophenyl)-6-hydroxybenzothiazole	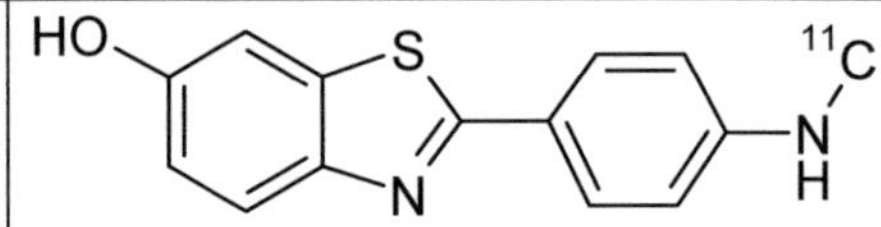
[^{11}C]SB-13	[^{11}C]4-*N*-methylamino-4´-hydroxystilbene	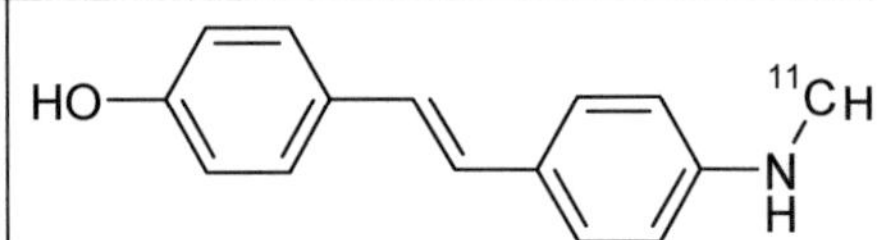

Table 1. Aβ imaging PET ligands

3.1 Synthesis of ^{11}C-and ^{18}F-labeled Aβ binding PET ligands

The Aβ binding PET ligands have been labeled with the ideal positron emitting radionuclides ^{11}C or ^{18}F, and the terminal amino or hydroxyl group of the molecule is mainly selected as the suitable ^{11}C or ^{18}F-labeling position. In case of [^{18}F]flutemetamol, the labeling strategy was different and one of the aromatic ring of the lipophilic part of the molecule was selected for that purpose.

3.1.1 Synthesis of ^{11}C-labeled ligands

The commonly used method for the synthesis of ^{11}C-labeled Aβ binding PET ligands is the methylation using [^{11}C]methyl iodide or [^{11}C]methyl triflate. The cyclotron produced [^{11}C]carbon dioxide is first converted to [^{11}C]methyl iodide or [^{11}C]methyl triflate which react with the desmethyl precursor of the corresponding target molecule to give the final ^{11}C-labeled product. A typical example of methylation using [^{11}C]methyl iodide is the synthesis of [^{11}C]PIB or [^{11}C]6-OH-BTA-1. *N*-Methylation of methoxymethyl (MOM) protected BTA using [^{11}C]methyl iodide in presence of potassium hydroxide followed by deprotection of MOM by treating with 50:50 mixture of methanol and concentrated hydrochloric acid gave the target compound [^{11}C]PIB (Scheme 1) (Mathis et al., 2003). Other Aβ binding PET ligands prepared by methylation using [^{11}C]methyl iodide are [^{11}C]AZD2184 (Andersson et al., 2010), [^{11}C]BF-145 (Shimadzu et al., 2004) and [^{11}C]MeS-IMPY (Seneca et al., 2007).

The synthesis of the ^{11}C-labeled stilbene derivative [^{11}C]SB-13 is an example of methylation using [^{11}C]methyl triflate. The synthesis was performed in a HPLC sample loop (Scheme 1) (Ono et al., 2003). Some other known Aβ binding PET ligands prepared by methylation using [^{11}C]methyl triflate are [^{11}C]BF-227 (Kudo et al., 2007), [^{11}C]IMPY (Cai et al., 2008), benzofuran derivatives (Ono et al., 2006) and analogues of aminophenylbenzothiazoles with a fluorine substituted phenyl ring (Henriksen et al., 2007).

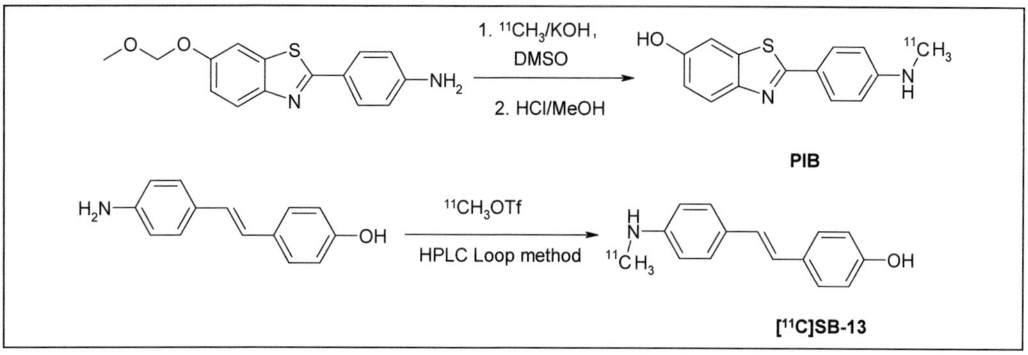

Scheme 1. Synthesis of [^{11}C]PIB and [^{11}C]SB-13

3.1.2 Synthesis of ^{18}F-labeled ligands

The commonly used ^{18}F-labeling strategy for Aβ binding PET ligands is the aliphatic nucleophilic fluorination of the corresponding tosylate or mesylate precursors of the target molecules using non carrier added [^{18}F]fluoride. A number of ligands have been prepared using this method and the followings are examples of such Aβ ligands. Two benzoxazole derivatives [^{18}F]BF-168 (Shimadzu et al., 2004) and [^{18}F]BF-227 (Okamura et al., 2007) were prepared by aliphatic nucleophilic fluorination of the corresponding 6-(2-tosyloxyethoxy)-benzoxazole derivatives using [^{18}F]fluoride ion in presence of potassium carbonate and kryptofix (Scheme 2). Other ^{18}F-labeled Aβ ligands prepared by aliphatic nucleophilic fluorination are [^{18}F]fluoropegylated stilbene derivatives [^{18}F]florbetapir ([^{18}F]AV-45) (Yao et al., 2010) and [^{18}F]florbetaben ([^{18}F]BAY 94-9172) (Wang et al., 2011; Zhang et al., 2005), amino naphthalene derivative [^{18}F]FDDNP (Klok et al., 2008; Liu et al., 2007), and phenylimidazole derivatives [^{18}F]FEM-IMPY and [^{18}F]FPM-IMPY (Cai et al., 2004). Only one of all amyloid binding ligands published so far has been prepared by aromatic nucleophilic fluorination. This ligand is a ^{18}F-labeled analogue of BTA known as [^{18}F]flutemetamol (or [^{18}F]FPIB, [^{18}F]GE-067). The precursor contains a nitro group situated ortho to a carboxamide group on one of the aromatic ring which is substituted by no-carrier added [^{18}F]fluoride to give the target compound (Scheme 3) (Koole et al., 2009; Storey et al., 2007).

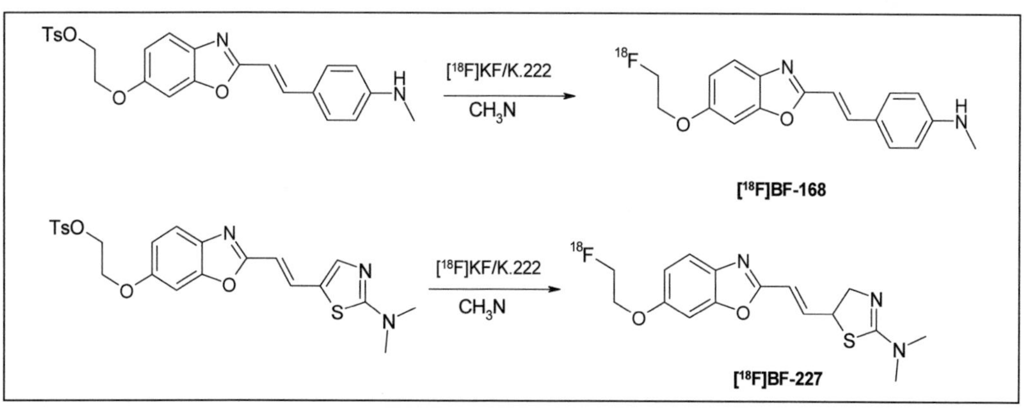

Scheme 2. Synthesis of [^{18}F]BF-168 and [^{18}F]BF-227

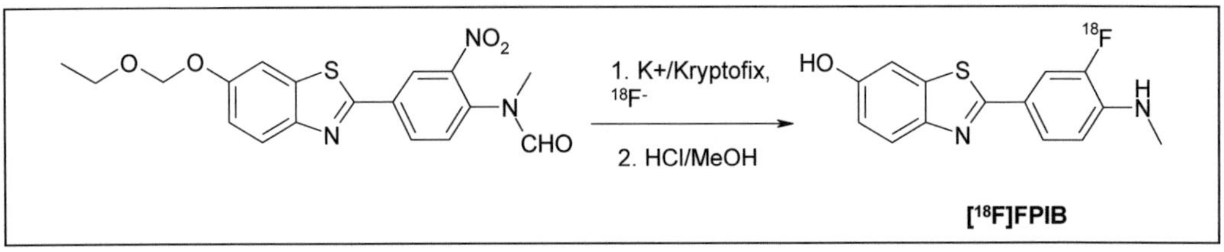

Scheme 3. Synthesis of [^{18}F]flutemetamol ([^{18}F]FPIB)

4. Evaluation of amyloid binding PET ligands

An important part of the development of new potential tracers for visualizing amyloid with PET is the preclinical evaluation of these compounds. Several complementary *in vitro* and *in vivo* animal techniques are used for the evaluation which has to be performed before the new tracer can be given to humans. These techniques aim at finding compounds with optimal affinity for the target (Aβ), while having as low binding as possible to other targets. Moreover, the kinetics needs to be suitable for PET, i.e. the binding equilibrium should be reached in the time frame of a PET experiment. These and other important criteria for a suitable PET ligand need to be studied in the preclinical evaluation phase.

Homogenate binding assay is a standard technique for the determination of affinity and selectivity of any compound. However, many of the parameters obtained in homogenate binding studies can also be obtained using *in vitro* cryosection autoradiography. After the process of evaluating the binding properties of a compound to be developed into a tracer to be used in PET or SPECT, homogenate binding studies may be used for determining of the absolute density of amyloid plaques in a tissue homogenate.

Autoradiography is a commonly used method in the study of radioligands for use in PET or SPECT, as direct comparisons of *in vitro* autoradiography images can be made with *in vivo* PET images labeled with ^{11}C and ^{18}F. Autoradiography gives information on distribution, selectivity and nonspecific binding, as well as a number of kinetic parameters which all are parameters indicative of usefulness for *in vivo* molecular imaging. With regard to visualization of amyloid plaques *in vivo*, cryosection autoradiography is often used in comparison of different potential ligands, for example in structure activity relationship studies. Furthermore, the much higher resolution with *in vitro* autoradiography as compared with *in vivo* PET makes the former technique a complementary technique.

It is obvious that certain parameters can be determined solely by an *in vivo* administration. For example, of great importance with regard to visualization of amyloid plaques *in vivo* is the extent of BBB penetration. In this case, "*ex vivo*" autoradiography could be preferred. Here "*ex vivo*" is defined as administration of the radioligand *in vivo* followed by autoradiography *in vitro*, and at least some of the above mentioned parameters can be determined. On the other hand, some parameters might be very difficult, if not impossible, to determine *in vivo*, such as to determine if an interaction really is saturable or not. Many of the compounds developed as tracers cannot be given in high enough concentrations to determine this, due to known toxicity or lack of toxicity information. For example, in spite of the numerous clinical studies performed with [^{11}C]PIB, saturating amounts of [^{11}C]PIB cannot be given to living subjects, and from *in vivo* PET it is not known if all [^{11}C]PIB binding can be blocked by excess unlabeled PIB *in vivo*. Using *in vitro* autoradiography the binding was blocked totally by adding 1000-fold higher concentration with unlabeled PIB (figure 3) (Långström et al., 2007; Svedberg et al., 2009).

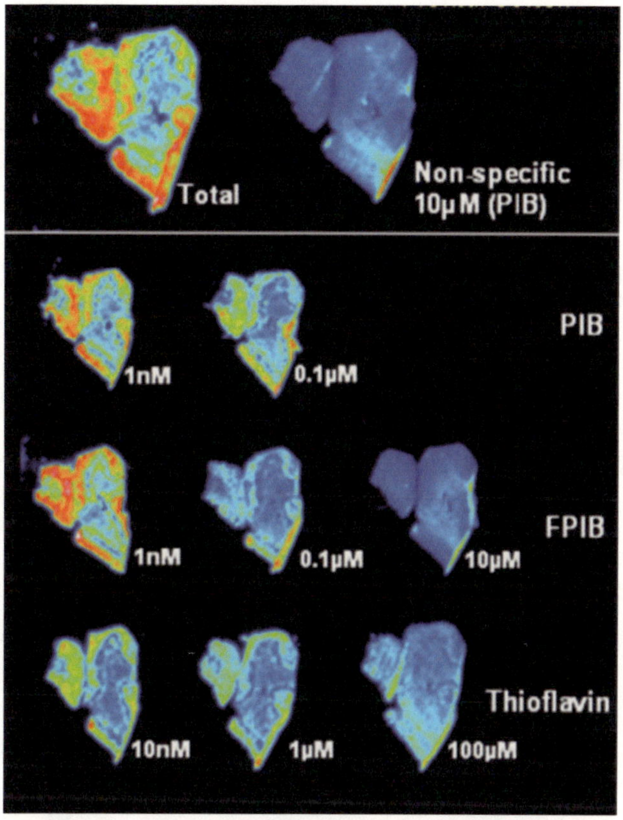

Fig. 3. Autoradiograms showing effects of PIB, flutemetamol (FPIB) and thioflavin on [18F]flutemetamol binding to sections of the temporal cortex of an AD patient.

5. Results

5.1 *In vitro* binding of PIB to postmortem AD brain

Binding of [3H]PIB binding to insoluble Aβ deposits in postmortem brain obtained from AD patients has been reported by several investigators. *In vitro* studies have shown that the Kd for [3H]PIB binding to AD brain (3-4 nM) is similar to the Kd for binding synthetic Aβ1-40 and Aβ1-42 fibrils (1 nM) (Fodero-Tavoletti et al., 2007; Ikonomovic et al., 2008; Kadir et al., 2011; Klunk et al., 2005). In some AD and control brain homogenates as well as with Aβ synthetic fibrils a lower-affinity [3H]PIB binding site with Kd values of 75-250 nM have been observed (Ikonomovic et al., 2008; Klunk et al., 2005). However, these low-affinity sites would not contribute significantly to *in vivo* binding at [11C]PIB concentrations around 1 nM. No significant correlation of [3H]PIB binding with soluble Aβ peptides has been observed (Ikonomovic et al., 2008; Klunk et al., 2005). The requirement that Aβ be in fibrillar form for PIB binding was verified by showing that the highly fluorescent PIB derivative 6-CN-PIB labeled both Aβ42 -and Aβ40-immunoreactive plaques whereas no labeling was detected in tissue sections pre-treated with formic acid which disrupts β-pleated sheets (Ikonomovic et al., 2008).

Several studies have reported correlations between *in vivo* [^{11}C]PIB retention and with region-matched postmortem quantification of [^{3}H]PIB binding, Aβ plaque loads and Aβ peptide levels but not with neurofibrillar tangles (Bacskai et al., 2007; Ikonomovic et al., 2008; Kadir et al., 2011; Rosen et al., 2011). In addition, a direct correlation between [^{11}C]PIB binding and insoluble Aβ levels determined by ELISA in homogenates of AD brain has been observed (Ikonomovic et al., 2008; Kadir et al., 2011; Klunk et al., 2005; Rosen et al., 2011; Svedberg et al., 2009).

Although several clinical PET studies with [^{11}C]PIB have been performed (Engler et al., 2003; Engler et al., 2006; Klunk et al., 2003; Klunk et al., 2004), *in vitro* evaluation studies have provided us with important new information. In agreement with others (Fodero-Tavoletti et al., 2007; Klunk et al., 2005; Rosen et al., 2011) our recent *in vitro* study (Svedberg et al., 2009) revealed significantly higher binding of PIB in AD brain compared to control brain when using [^{11}C]PIB autoradiography and [^{11}C]PIB radioligand assay. Moreover, we observed no specific [^{11}C]PIB binding in the cerebellum which is often used as a reference region for quantification of [^{11}C]PIB retention in PET studies. For example, the distribution of [^{11}C]PIB was investigated using autoradiography on tissue from patients that suffered from AD (Svedberg et al., 2009), which demonstrated that the binding is confined to external layers of the cerebral cortex, which due to a lower resolution is not seen in PET (figure 4).

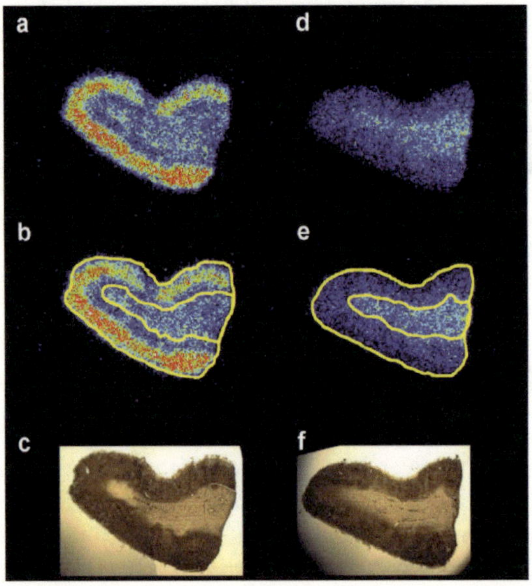

Fig. 4. [^{11}C]PIB binding in the temporal cortex of an AD patient and microscopic images of the sections used. Autoradiograms depicting total (a and b) and nonspecific binding (d and e) of [^{11}C]PIB in the temporal cortex of a patient with AD and microscopic images of the sections used (c and f). The yellow lines in B and E were drawn as regions of interest; the gray and the white matter area, respectively, on the microscopic images and were transferred to the autoradiograms. From Svedberg et al. (2009).

By using a combination of autoradiography and histochemical techniques Lockhart et al. (2007) showed that PIB, in addition to binding senile plaques (dense core plaques) also bound to cerebral amyloid angiopathy (CAA) and some diffuse plaques. In contrast to senile plaques where Aβ42 are much more abundant (Hellström-Lindahl et al., 2004; Näslund et al., 2000), the major amyloid peptide species in CAA is Aβ40 with less amounts of Aβ42 (Mann et al., 1996). CAA is present in 80% or more of AD patients (Jellinger, 2002) and may therefore contribute significantly to the *in vivo* [^{11}C]PIB signal and *in vitro* binding of PIB (Bacskai et al., 2007; Johnson et al., 2007; Svedberg et al., 2009).

PIB binds only weakly to Aβ deposits in nonhuman species (Klunk et al., 2005; Rosen et al., 2011). Recently, Rosen et al (2011) showed that despite levels of Aβ in cortical extracts that sometimes exceeded those in AD brain, high-affinity [^{3}H]PIB *in vitro* binding in nonhuman primates (aged chimpanzees, rhesus macaques, and squirrel monkeys) was strikingly less than that in humans with AD. Similarly, less [^{3}H]PIB binding was detected in homogenates of transgenic PS1/APP mouse brain compared to AD brain, despite higher Aβ levels (Klunk et al., 2005). A substantial difference in the intensity of [^{11}C]PIB labeling between AD brain and APP transgenic mice has also been shown by ex vivo autoradiography (Maeda et al., 2007).

5.2 *In vivo* animal studies

Two major *in vivo* modalities are of importance in the evaluation of new PET ligands. One is organ distribution studies in normal mice or rats, which gives information on to where the compound and its metabolites distribute. Organ distribution studies are also used in calculation of dosimetry, i.e. how much of a radiolabeled compound can be given without reaching radioactive doses that may risk damages due to radiation.

A more obvious modality is the use of animal PET. In order to study binding to Aβ plaques transgenic animals are required, as plaques are not found naturally in old rats or mice (Philipson et al., 2010). Transgenic mouse models have become an important and valuable research tool in neurodegenerative disorders like AD. Attempts to model and study in detail longitudinal pathological processes in living brains and molecular mechanisms involved in the pathogenesis of the disease can provide insight into disease progression in AD patients.

Transgenic mice of different types have been developed, all with amyloid plaques in the brain (Elder et al., 2010; Lannfelt et al., 1993; Morrissette et al., 2009). In the early animal PET studies using transgenic animals no binding of [^{11}C]PIB was seen, in spite of a high amyloid load in the animal brains (Klunk et al., 2005; Toyama et al., 2005; Ye et al., 2006), The inconsistency between AD patients and transgenic mice models was for long unclear and explained by fewer binding sites or lower binding affinity of [^{11}C]PIB for Aβ plaques in transgenic mice (Klunk et al., 2005; Toyama et al., 2005) and/or that the Aβ containing plaques in the mice resembles synthetic Aβ, where low [^{11}C]PIB binding was demonstrated (Ye et al., 2006). It was demonstrated that intrinsic mouse Aβ is formed and deposited in significant amounts in the brain of an AD mouse model and is deposited together with human Aβ, and this might also explain the low efficacy of PIB binding in transgenic mice brain tissue (van Groen et al., 2006). Few years later it was demonstrated that the specific radioactivity of the tracer significantly contributed to the detection of the amyloid deposits in the mouse brain. High-level retention of [^{11}C]PIB in APP transgenic mice brain regions known to contain amyloid was obtained when high-specific activity [^{11}C]PIB was administrated (Maeda et al., 2007). It might also depend on the type of transgenic animal used, as ex vivo studies using [^{3}H]PIB and a new transgenic animal model, ARTE10, clearly showed intense labeling of the amyloid in these animals (Willuweit et al., 2009).

Senile plaques are generally enriched in Aβ 1-42 species and are additionally subjected to a wide range of post-translational and post-deposition modifications, such as N-and C-terminal truncation, oxidation, and isomerization (Lockhart, 2006). The N-terminally truncated and modified Aβ, AβN3-pyroglutamate, has been identified in AD brain (Wirths et al., 2010) and suggested to be a major contributor to PIB binding (Maeda et al., 2007). Compared to AD brain, this Aβ subtype is not so abundant in transgenic mice (Güntert et al., 2006; Kawarabayashi et al., 2001), and the levels of AβN3-pyroglutamate may therefore provide another plausible explanation for the difference in [^{11}C]PIB binding between humans and mice.

5.3 Clinical PET

[^{11}C]PIB, developed in collaboration between Uppsala University in Sweden and University of Pittsburgh School of Medicine, PA, USA, was the first tracer to detect Aβ in the brain of living patients (figure 5) (Klunk et al., 2004). The results demonstrated an increased [^{11}C]PIB retention in several brain regions known to contain Aβ in AD and none in controls (Klunk et al., 2004). The [^{11}C]PIB signal in the cortex was approximately 1.5-2 fold higher in the AD patients compared to the control subjects (Klunk et al., 2004). Interestingly enough, postmortem studies of the same patients that showed elevated [^{11}C]PIB retention *in vivo* during their life correlates significantly with regional *in vitro* measures of Aβ pathology found at autopsy (Ikonomovic et al., 2008; Kadir et al., 2011).

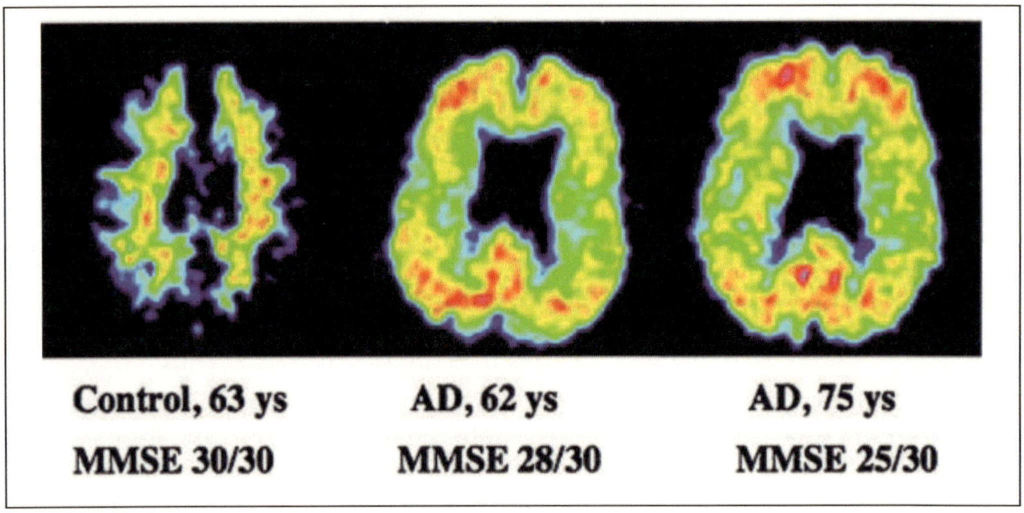

Fig. 5. [^{11}C]PIB amyloid binding to the brains of two AD patients and one healthy control (sagittal sections). Red indicates high, yellow medium, blue low [^{11}C]PIB retention. MMSE Mini-Mental- State-Examination, vs. years. Figure adapted from Nordberg (2008).

Since the study reported by Klunk et al. (2004) several selective amyloid ligands are under study or have been studied *in vivo* in living patients (see table 1). Regardless of compelling results with [^{11}C]PIB the short half-life limits the use of PIB and other ^{11}C-ligands. This emphasizes the need for ^{18}F-ligands, with longer half-life, to implement a broader Aβ PET imaging. Recently, [^{18}F]AV-45 PET imaging was performed in AD patients and control subjects (Wong et al., 2010). The results revealed an increase in [^{18}F]AV-45 retention in the cortical gray matter in the AD patients, areas that expected to have high Aβ accumulation and none in the control subjects (Wong et al., 2010) similar to previously reported for [^{11}C]PIB.

6. Conclusion

The development of plaques are very early events in the course of events leading to AD (Ingelsson et al., 2004; Långström et al., 2007), and imaging plaques in early stages of the disease would be of great value for the treatment. However, the "ceiling effect", i.e. that the amount of amyloid plaques reaches maximum already early in the disease (Engler et al., 2006; Nordberg, 2007), makes it difficult to follow the slow progression of the disease using *in vivo* imaging of amyloid plaques. The large number of compounds that are under development or are today used in *in vivo* PET or SPECT investigations of amyloid plaques all aim at visualizing the same entities, and will hardly overcome this problem. New ligands that visualize the formation of plaques earlier in the course of disease are therefore needed. The presently available compounds bind to plaques, but some are also binding to earlier stages in the formation of plaques, such as to fibrils and oligomers, and might therefore be of great value for finding new treatment of AD and thus also for the individual patients.

There is also great interest in finding a specific radioligand for the visualization of neurofibrillary tangles, which is another hallmark seen in AD. Some of the ligands binding to the amyloid plaques also bind to some extent to tangles, and further development of these compounds may lead to ligands also labeling tangles (see e.g Barrio et al., 2008; Okamura et al., 2005; Shoghi-Jadid et al., 2002; Åslund et al., 2009). The development of tracers labeling tangles should be complementing the tracers labeling amyloid discussed above.

It can be concluded that the use of PET in the evaluation of AD has alleviated the diagnosis of the disease considerably. The development of new tracers with even better properties and tracers labeling amyloid fibrils and neurofibrillary tangles is therefore still a highly prioritized research area.

7. Acknowledgment

We are grateful for valuable discussions with Prof. Bengt Långström and our colleagues at Uppsala University. This study was performed when authors OR and HH were employed at Uppsala Applied Science Lab, GE Healthcare. We are grateful to a SAMBIO funding from Vinnova, Sweden.

8. References

Akiyama, H., Barger, S., Barnum, S., Bradt, B., Bauer, J., Cole, G.M., Cooper, N.R., Eikelenboom, P., Emmerling, M., Fiebich, B.L., Finch, C.E., Frautschy, S., Griffin, W.S., Hampel, H., Hull, M., Landreth, G., Lue, L., Mrak, R., Mackenzie, I.R.,

McGeer, P.L., O'Banion, M.K., Pachter, J., Pasinetti, G., Plata-Salaman, C., Rogers, J., Rydel, R., Shen, Y., Streit, W., Strohmeyer, R., Tooyoma, I., Van Muiswinkel, F.L., Veerhuis, R., Walker, D., Webster, S., Wegrzyniak, B., Wenk, G. & Wyss-Coray, T. (2000) Inflammation and Alzheimer's disease. *Neurobiology of Aging,* Vol. 21, No. 3, pp. 383-421, 0197-4580 (Print), 0197-4580 (Linking).

Alzheimer, A. (1907) Über eine eigenartige Erkrankung der Hirnrinde. *Allegemeine Zeitschrift für Psychiatrie und Psychisch-Gerchtliche Medizin,* Vol. 64, No. pp. 146-148.

Andersson, J.D., Varnäs, K., Cselenyi, Z., Gulyas, B., Wensbo, D., Finnema, S.J., Swahn, B.-M., Svensson, S., Nyberg, S., Farde, L. & Halldin, C. (2010) Radiosynthesis of the candidate beta-amyloid radioligand [^{11}C]AZD2184: Positron emission tomography examination and metabolite analysis in cynomolgus monkeys. *Synapse,* Vol. 64, No. 10, pp. 733-741.

Archer, H.A., Edison, P., Brooks, D.J., Barnes, J., Frost, C., Yeatman, T., Fox, N.C. & Rossor, M.N. (2006) Amyloid load and cerebral atrophy in Alzheimer's disease: an ^{11}C-PIB positron emission tomography study. *Annals of Neurology,* Vol. 60, No. 1, pp. 145-147, 0364-5134 (Print), 0364-5134 (Linking).

Bacskai, B.J., Frosch, M.P., Freeman, S.H., Raymond, S.B., Augustinack, J.C., Johnson, K.A., Irizarry, M.C., Klunk, W.E., Mathis, C.A., Dekosky, S.T., Greenberg, S.M., Hyman, B.T. & Growdon, J.H. (2007) Molecular imaging with Pittsburgh Compound B confirmed at autopsy: a case report. *Archives of Neurology,* Vol. 64, No. 3, pp. 431-434.

Banati, R.B. (2002) Visualising microglial activation in vivo. *Glia,* Vol. 40, No. 2, pp. 206-217, 0894-1491 (Print), 0894-1491 (Linking).

Barrio, J.R., Kepe, V., Satyamurthy, N., Huang, S.C. & Small, G. (2008) Amyloid and tau imaging, neuronal losses and function in mild cognitive impairment. *The Journal of Nutrition, Health & Aging,* Vol. 12, No. 1, pp. 61S-65S, 1279-7707 (Print), 1279-7707 (Linking).

Bergström, M., Kumlien, E., Lilja, A., Tyrefors, N., Westerberg, G. & Långström, B. (1998) Temporal lobe epilepsy visualized with PET with ^{11}C-L-deuterium-deprenyl--analysis of kinetic data. *Acta Neurologica Scandinavica,* Vol. 98, No. 4, pp. 224-231, 0001-6314 (Print), 0001-6314 (Linking).

Braak, H., de Vos, R.A., Jansen, E.N., Bratzke, H. & Braak, E. (1998) Neuropathological hallmarks of Alzheimer's and Parkinson's diseases. *Progress in Brain Research,* Vol. 117, No. pp. 267-285.

Cagnin, A., Gerhard, A. & Banati, R.B. (2002) In vivo imaging of neuroinflammation. *European Neuropsychopharmacology,* Vol. 12, No. 6, pp. 581-586, 0924-977X (Print), 0924-977X (Linking).

Cai, L., Chin, F.T., Pike, V.W., Toyama, H., Liow, J.S., Zoghbi, S.S., Modell, K., Briard, E., Shetty, H.U., Sinclair, K., Donohue, S., Tipre, D., Kung, M.P., Dagostin, C., Widdowson, D.A., Green, M., Gao, W., Herman, M.M., Ichise, M. & Innis, R.B. (2004) Synthesis and evaluation of two ^{18}F-labeled 6-iodo-2-(4'-N,N-dimethyl-amino)phenylimidazo[1,2-a]pyridine derivatives as prospective radioligands for β-amyloid in Alzheimer's disease. *Journal of Medicinal Chemistry,* Vol. 47, No. 9, pp. 2208-2218.

Cai, L., Liow, J.-S., Zoghbi, S.S., Cuevas, J., Baetas, C., Hong, J., Shetty, H.U., Seneca, N.M., Brown, A.K., Gladding, R., Temme, S.S., Herman, M.M., Innis, R.B. & Pike, V.W. (2008) Synthesis and evaluation of N-methyl and S-methyl ^{11}C-labeled 6-

methylthio-2-(4'-N,N-dimethylamino)phenylimidazo[1,2-a]pyridines as radioligands for Imaging β-amyloid plaques in Alzheimer's disease. *Journal of Medicinal Chemistry,* Vol. 51, No. 1, pp. 148-158.

Elder, G.A., Gama Sosa, M.A. & De Gasperi, R. (2010) Transgenic mouse models of Alzheimer's disease. *Mount Sinai Journal of Medicine,* Vol. 77, No. 1, pp. 69-81, 1931-7581 (Electronic), 0027-2507 (Linking).

Engler, H., Lundberg, P.O., Ekbom, K., Nennesmo, I., Nilsson, A., Bergström, M., Tsukada, H., Hartvig, P. & Långström, B. (2003) Multitracer study with positron emission tomography in Creutzfeldt-Jakob disease. *European Journal of Nuclear Medicine and Molecular Imaging,* Vol. 30, No. 1, pp. 85-95, 1619-7070 (Print), 1619-7070 (Linking).

Engler, H., Forsberg, A., Almkvist, O., Blomquist, G., Larsson, E., Savitcheva, I., Wall, A., Ringheim, A., Långström, B. & Nordberg, A. (2006) Two-year follow-up of amyloid deposition in patients with Alzheimer's disease. *Brain,* Vol. 129, No. Pt 11, pp. 2856-2866.

Ewers, M., Walsh, C., Trojanowski, J.Q., Shaw, L.M., Petersen, R.C., Jack, C.R., Jr., Feldman, H.H., Bokde, A.L., Alexander, G.E., Scheltens, P., Vellas, B., Dubois, B., Weiner, M. & Hampel, H. (2010) Prediction of conversion from mild cognitive impairment to Alzheimer's disease dementia based upon biomarkers and neuropsychological test performance. *Neurobiology of Aging,* Vol. No. pp. 1558-1497 (Electronic), 0197-4580 (Linking).

Fodero-Tavoletti, M.T., Smith, D.P., McLean, C.A., Adlard, P.A., Barnham, K.J., Foster, L.E., Leone, L., Perez, K., Cortes, M., Culvenor, J.G., Li, Q.X., Laughton, K.M., Rowe, C.C., Masters, C.L., Cappai, R. & Villemagne, V.L. (2007) In vitro characterization of Pittsburgh compound-B binding to Lewy bodies. *Journal of Neurochemistry,* Vol. 27, No. 39, pp. 10365-10371, 1529-2401 (Electronic), 0270-6474 (Linking).

Fowler, J.S., Wolf, A.P., MacGregor, R.R., Dewey, S.L., Logan, J., Schlyer, D.J. & Långström, B. (1988) Mechanistic positron emission tomography studies: demonstration of a deuterium isotope effect in the monoamine oxidase-catalyzed binding of [^{11}C]L-deprenyl in living baboon brain. *Journal of Neurochemistry,* Vol. 51, No. 5, pp. 1524-1534, 0022-3042 (Print), 0022-3042 (Linking).

Ganguli, M. & Petersen, R.C. (2008) Mild cognitive impairment: challenging issues. *American Journal of Geriatric Psychiatry,* Vol. 16, No. 5, pp. 339-342, 1545-7214 (Electronic), 1064-7481 (Linking).

Ganguli, M., Blacker, D., Blazer, D.G., Grant, I., Jeste, D.V., Paulsen, J.S., Petersen, R.C. & Sachdev, P.S. (2011) Classification of neurocognitive disorders in DSM-5: a work in progress. *American Journal of Geriatric Psychiatry,* Vol. 19, No. 3, pp. 205-210, 1545-7214 (Electronic), 1064-7481 (Linking).

Güntert, A., Döbeli, H. & Bohrmann, B. (2006) High sensitivity analysis of amyloid-beta peptide composition in amyloid deposits from human and PS2APP mouse brain. *Neuroscience,* Vol. 143, No. 2, pp. 461-475, 0306-4522 (Print), 0306-4522 (Linking).

Hellström-Lindahl, E., Mousavi, M., Ravid, R. & Nordberg, A. (2004) Reduced levels of Abeta 40 and Abeta 42 in brains of smoking controls and Alzheimer's patients. *Neurobiology of Disease,* Vol. 15, No. 2, pp. 351-360.

Henriksen, G., Hauser, A.I., Westwell, A.D., Yousefi, B.H., Schwaiger, M., Drzezga, A. & Wester, H.-J. (2007) Metabolically stabilized benzothiazoles for imaging of amyloid plaques. *Journal of Medicinal Chemistry,* Vol. 50, No. 6, pp. 1087-1089.

Henriksen, G., Yousefi, B.H., Drzezga, A. & Wester, H.-J. (2008) Development and evaluation of compounds for imaging of beta-amyloid plaque by means of positron emission tomography. *European Journal of Nuclear Medicine and Molecular Imaging,* Vol. 35, No. Suppl 1, pp. S75-S81.

Ikonomovic, M.D., Klunk, W.E., Abrahamson, E.E., Mathis, C.A., Price, J.C., Tsopelas, N.D., Lopresti, B.J., Ziolko, S., Bi, W., Paljug, W.R., Debnath, M.L., Hope, C.E., Isanski, B.A., Hamilton, R.L. & DeKosky, S.T. (2008) Post-mortem correlates of in vivo PiB-PET amyloid imaging in a typical case of Alzheimer's disease. *Brain,* Vol. 131, No. Pt 6, pp. 1630-1645, 1460-2156 (Electronic).

Ingelsson, M., Fukumoto, H., Newell, K.L., Growdon, J.H., Hedley-Whyte, E.T., Frosch, M.P., Albert, M.S., Hyman, B.T. & Irizarry, M.C. (2004) Early Abeta accumulation and progressive synaptic loss, gliosis, and tangle formation in AD brain. *Neurology,* Vol. 62, No. 6, pp. 925-931.

Jellinger, K.A. (2002) Alzheimer disease and cerebrovascular pathology: an update. *Journal of Neural Transmission,* Vol. 109, No. 5-6, pp. 813-836, 0300-9564 (Print), 0300-9564 (Linking).

Johnson, K.A., Gregas, M., Becker, J.A., Kinnecom, C., Salat, D.H., Moran, E.K., Smith, E.E., Rosand, J., Rentz, D.M., Klunk, W.E., Mathis, C.A., Price, J.C., Dekosky, S.T., Fischman, A.J. & Greenberg, S.M. (2007) Imaging of amyloid burden and distribution in cerebral amyloid angiopathy. *Annals of Neurology,* Vol. 62, No. 3, pp. 229-234, 0364-5134 (Print), 0364-5134 (Linking).

Kadir, A., Marutle, A., Gonzalez, D., Scholl, M., Almkvist, O., Mousavi, M., Mustafiz, T., Darreh-Shori, T., Nennesmo, I. & Nordberg, A. (2011) Positron emission tomography imaging and clinical progression in relation to molecular pathology in the first Pittsburgh Compound B positron emission tomography patient with Alzheimer's disease. *Brain,* Vol. 134, No. Pt 1, pp. 301-317, 1460-2156 (Electronic), 0006-8950 (Linking).

Kawarabayashi, T., Younkin, L.H., Saido, T.C., Shoji, M., Ashe, K.H. & Younkin, S.G. (2001) Age-dependent changes in brain, CSF, and plasma amyloid (beta) protein in the Tg2576 transgenic mouse model of Alzheimer's disease. *Journal of Neuroscience,* Vol. 21, No. 2, pp. 372-381.

Klok, R.P., Klein, P.J., van Berckel, B.N.M., Tolboom, N., Lammertsma, A.A. & Windhorst, A.D. (2008) Synthesis of 2-(1,1-dicyanopropen-2-yl)-6-(2-[^{18}F]-fluoroethyl)-methylamino-naphthalene ([^{18}F]FDDNP). *Applied Radiation and Isotopes,* Vol. 66, No. pp. 203-207.

Klunk, W.E., Debnath, M.L. & Pettegrew, J.W. (1994) Development of small molecule probes for the beta-amyloid protein of Alzheimer's disease. *Neurobiology of Aging,* Vol. 15, No. pp. 691-698.

Klunk, W.E., Debnath, M.L. & Pettegrew, J.W. (1995) Chrysamine-G binding to Alzheimer and control brain: Autopsy study of new amyloid probe. *Neurobiology of Aging,* Vol. 16, No. 4, pp. 541-548.

Klunk, W.E., Engler, H., Nordberg, A., Bacskai, B.J., Wang, Y., Price, J.C., Bergström, M., Hyman, B.T., Långström, B. & Mathis, C.A. (2003) Imaging the pathology of Alzheimer's disease: amyloid-imaging with positron emission tomography. *Neuroimaging Clinics of North America,* Vol. 13, No. 4, pp. 781-789, ix.

Klunk, W.E., Engler, H., Nordberg, A., Wang, Y., Blomqvist, G., Holt, D.P., Bergström, M., Savitcheva, I., Huang, G.F., Estrada, S., Ausen, B., Debnath, M.L., Barletta, J., Price,

J.C., Sandell, J., Lopresti, B.J., Wall, A., Koivisto, P., Antoni, G., Mathis, C.A. & Långström, B. (2004) Imaging brain amyloid in Alzheimer's disease with Pittsburgh Compound-B. *Annals of Neurology,* Vol. 55, No. 3, pp. 306-319.

Klunk, W.E., Lopresti, B.J., Ikonomovic, M.D., Lefterov, I.M., Koldamova, R.P., Abrahamson, E.E., Debnath, M.L., Holt, D.P., Huang, G.F., Shao, L., DeKosky, S.T., Price, J.C. & Mathis, C.A. (2005) Binding of the positron emission tomography tracer Pittsburgh compound-B reflects the amount of amyloid-beta in Alzheimer's disease brain but not in transgenic mouse brain. *Journal of Neuroscience,* Vol. 25, No. 46, pp. 10598-10606.

Koole, M., Lewis, D.M., Buckley, C., Nelissen, N., Vandenbulcke, M., Brooks, D.J., Vandenberghe, R. & Van Laere, K. (2009) Whole-body biodistribution and radiation dosimetry of ^{18}F-GE067: a radioligand for in vivo brain amyloid imaging. *Journal of Nuclear Medicine,* Vol. 50, No. 5, pp. 818-822, 0161-5505 (Print).

Korczyn, A.D. (2008) The amyloid cascade hypothesis. *Alzheimers & Dementia,* Vol. 4, No. 3, pp. 176-178, 1552-5279 (Electronic), 1552-5260 (Linking).

Kudo, Y., Okamura, N., Furumoto, S., Tashiro, M., Furukawa, K., Maruyama, M., Itoh, M., Iwata, R., Yanai, K. & Arai, H. (2007) 2-(2-[2-Dimethylaminothiazol-5-yl]ethenyl)-6-(2-[fluoro]ethoxy)benzoxazole: a novel PET agent for in vivo detection of dense amyloid plaques in Alzheimer's disease patients. *Journal of Nuclear Medicine,* Vol. 48, No. 4, pp. 553-561, 0161-5505 (Print), 0161-5505 (Linking).

Lannfelt, L., Folkesson, R., Mohammed, A.H., Winblad, B., Hellgren, D., Duff, K. & Hardy, J. (1993) Alzheimer's disease: molecular genetics and transgenic animal models. *Behavioural Brain Research,* Vol. 57, No. 2, pp. 207-213, 0166-4328 (Print), 0166-4328 (Linking).

Liu, J., Kepe, V., Zabjek, A., Petric, A., Padgett, H.C., Satyamurthy, N. & Barrio, J.R. (2007) High-yield, automated radiosynthesis of 2-(1-{6-[(2-[^{18}F]fluoroethyl)(methyl) amino]-2-naphthyl}ethylidene)malononi trile ([^{18}F]FDDNP) ready for animal or human administration. *Molecular Imaging and Biology,* Vol. 9, No. pp. 6-16.

Lockhart, A. (2006) Imaging Alzheimer's disease pathology: one target, many ligands. *Drug Discovery Today,* Vol. 11, No. 23-24, pp. 1093-1099.

Logan, J., Fowler, J.S., Volkow, N.D., Wang, G.J., MacGregor, R.R. & Shea, C. (2000) Reproducibility of repeated measures of deuterium substituted [^{11}C]L-deprenyl ([^{11}C]L-deprenyl-D2) binding in the human brain. *Nuclear Medicine and Biology,* Vol. 27, No. 1, pp. 43-49, 0969-8051 (Print), 0969-8051 (Linking).

Långström, B., Andrén, P.E., Lindhe, Ö., Svedberg, M.M. & Hall, H. (2007) In vitro imaging techniques in neurodegenerative diseases. *Molecular Imaging and Biology,* Vol. 9, No. 4, pp. 161-175, 1536-1632 (Print), 1536-1632 (Linking).

Maeda, J., Ji, B., Irie, T., Tomiyama, T., Maruyama, M., Okauchi, T., Staufenbiel, M., Iwata, N., Ono, M., Saido, T.C., Suzuki, K., Mori, H., Higuchi, M. & Suhara, T. (2007) Longitudinal, quantitative assessment of amyloid, neuroinflammation, and anti-amyloid treatment in a living mouse model of Alzheimer's disease enabled by positron emission tomography. *Journal of Neuroscience,* Vol. 27, No. 41, pp. 10957-10968, 1529-2401 (Electronic), 0270-6474 (Linking).

Mann, D.M., Iwatsubo, T., Ihara, Y., Cairns, N.J., Lantos, P.L., Bogdanovic, N., Lannfelt, L., Winblad, B., Maat-Schieman, M.L. & Rossor, M.N. (1996) Predominant deposition of amyloid-beta 42(43) in plaques in cases of Alzheimer's disease and hereditary cerebral hemorrhage associated with mutations in the amyloid precursor protein gene. *American Journal of Pathology,* Vol. 148, No. 4, pp. 1257-1266.

Mathis, C.A., Wang, Y., Holt, D.P., Huang, G.F., Debnath, M.L. & Klunk, W.E. (2003) Synthesis and evaluation of ^{11}C-labeled 6-substituted 2-arylbenzothiazoles as amyloid imaging agents. *Journal of Medicinal Chemistry,* Vol. 46, No. 13, pp. 2740-2754.

McKhann, G., Drachman, D., Folstein, M., Katzman, R., Price, D. & Stadlan, E.M. (1984) Clinical diagnosis of Alzheimer's disease: report of the NINCDS-ADRDA Work Group under the auspices of Department of Health and Human Services Task Force on Alzheimer's Disease. *Neurology,* Vol. 34, No. 7, pp. 939-944.

Mintun, M.A., Larossa, G.N., Sheline, Y.I., Dence, C.S., Lee, S.Y., Mach, R.H., Klunk, W.E., Mathis, C.A., DeKosky, S.T. & Morris, J.C. (2006) [^{11}C]PIB in a nondemented population: potential antecedent marker of Alzheimer disease. *Neurology,* Vol. 67, No. 3, pp. 446-452.

Morrissette, D.A., Parachikova, A., Green, K.N. & LaFerla, F.M. (2009) Relevance of transgenic mouse models to human Alzheimer disease. *Journal of Biological Chemistry,* Vol. 284, No. 10, pp. 6033-6037, 0021-9258 (Print), 0021-9258 (Linking).

Nordberg, A. (2004) PET imaging of amyloid in Alzheimer's disease. *Lancet Neurology,* Vol. 3, No. 9, pp. 519-527.

Nordberg, A. (2007) Amyloid imaging in Alzheimer's disease. *Current Opinion in Neurology,* Vol. 20, No. 4, pp. 398-402.

Nordberg, A. (2008) Amyloid plaque imaging in vivo: current achievement and future prospects. *European Journal of Nuclear Medicine and Molecular Imaging,* Vol. 35 Suppl 1, No. pp. S46-50, 1619-7070 (Print), 1619-7070 (Linking).

Näslund, J., Haroutunian, V., Mohs, R., Davis, K.L., Davies, P., Greengard, P. & Buxbaum, J.D. (2000) Correlation between elevated levels of amyloid beta-peptide in the brain and cognitive decline. *JAMA, The Journal of American Medical Association,* Vol. 283, No. 12, pp. 1571-1577.

Okamura, N., Suemoto, T., Furumoto, S., Suzuki, M., Shimadzu, H., Akatsu, H., Yamamoto, T., Fujiwara, H., Nemoto, M., Maruyama, M., Arai, H., Yanai, K., Sawada, T. & Kudo, Y. (2005) Quinoline and benzimidazole derivatives: candidate probes for in vivo imaging of tau pathology in Alzheimer's disease. *The Journal of Neuroscience,* Vol. 25, No. 47, pp. 10857-10862, 1529-2401 (Electronic).

Okamura, N., Furmoto, S., Funaki, Y., Suemoto, T., Kato, M., Ishikawa, Y., Ito, S., Akatsu, H., Yamamoto, T., Swada, T., Arai, H., Kudo, Y. & Yanai, K. (2007) binding and safety profile of novel derivative for in vivo imaging of amyloid deposite in Alzheimer's disease. *Geriatrics & Gerontology International,* Vol. 7, No. pp. 393-400.

Ono, M., Wilson, A., Nobrega, J., Westaway, D., Verhoeff, P., Zhuang, Z.-P., Kung, M.-P. & Kung, H.F. (2003) ^{11}C-Labeled stilbene derivatives as A-beta aggregate specific PET imaging agents for Alzheimer's disease. *Nuclear Medicine and Biology,* Vol. 30, No. pp. 565-571.

Ono, M., Kawashima, H., Nonaka, A., Kawai, T., Haratake, M., Mori, H., Kung, M.-P., Kung, H.F., Saji, H. & Nakayama, M. (2006) Novel benzofuran derivatives for PET imaging of .beta.-amyloid plaques in Alzheimer's disease brains. *Journal of Medicinal Chemistry,* Vol. 49, No. 9, pp. 2725-2730.

Ono, M. (2009) Development of positron-emission tomography/single-photon emission computed tomography imaging probes for in vivo detection of β-amyloid plaques in Alzheimer's brains. *Chemical & Pharmaceutical Bulletin,* Vol. 57, No. 10, pp. 1029-1039.

Petersen, R.C., Doody, R., Kurz, A., Mohs, R.C., Morris, J.C., Rabins, P.V., Ritchie, K., Rossor, M., Thal, L. & Winblad, B. (2001) Current concepts in mild cognitive impairment. *Archives of Neurology,* Vol. 58, No. 12, pp. 1985-1992.

Philipson, O., Lord, A., Gumucio, A., O'Callaghan, P., Lannfelt, L. & Nilsson, L.N. (2010) Animal models of amyloid-beta-related pathologies in Alzheimer's disease. *FEBS Journal,* Vol. 277, No. 6, pp. 1389-1409, 1742-4658 (Electronic), 1742-464X (Linking).

Porchet, R., Probst, A., Bouras, C., Draberova, E., Draber, P. & Riederer, B.M. (2003) Analysis of glial acidic fibrillary protein in the human entorhinal cortex during aging and in Alzheimer's disease. *Proteomics,* Vol. 3, No. 8, pp. 1476-1485, 1615-9853 (Print), 1615-9853 (Linking).

Rosen, R.F., Walker, L.C. & Levine, H., 3rd. (2011) PIB binding in aged primate brain: enrichment of high-affinity sites in humans with Alzheimer's disease. *Neurobiology of Aging,* Vol. 32, No. 2, pp. 223-234, 1558-1497 (Electronic), 0197-4580 (Linking).

Schönheit, B., Zarski, R. & Ohm, T.G. (2004) Spatial and temporal relationships between plaques and tangles in Alzheimer-pathology. *Neurobiology of Aging,* Vol. 25, No. 6, pp. 697-711.

Selkoe, D.J. & Schenk, D. (2003) Alzheimer's disease: molecular understanding predicts amyloid-based therapeutics. *Annual Review of Pharmacology and Toxicology,* Vol. 43, No. pp. 545-584, 0362-1642 (Print), 0362-1642 (Linking).

Seneca, N., Cai, L., Liow, J.-S., Zoghbi, S.S., Gladding, R.L., Hong, J., Pike, V.W. & Innis, R.B. (2007) Brain and whole-body imaging in nonhuman primates with [^{11}C]MeS-IMPY, a candidate radioligand for .beta.-amyloid plaques. *Nuclear Medicine and Biology,* Vol. 34, No. 6, pp. 681-689.

Shimadzu, H., Suemoto, T., Suzuki, M., Shiomitsu, T., Okamura, N., Kudo, Y. & Sawada, T. (2004) Novel probes for imaging amyloid-b: F-18 and C-11 labeling of 2-(4-aminostyryl)benzoxazole derivatives. *Journal of Labelled Compounds and Radiopharmaceuticals.,* Vol. 47, No. pp. 181-190.

Shoghi-Jadid, K., Small, G.W., Agdeppa, E.D., Kepe, V., Ercoli, L.M., Siddarth, P., Read, S., Satyamurthy, N., Petric, A., Huang, S.C. & Barrio, J.R. (2002) Localization of neurofibrillary tangles and β-amyloid plaques in the brains of living patients with Alzheimer disease. *The American Journal of Geriatric Psychiatry,* Vol. 10, No. 1, pp. 24-35, 1064-7481 (Print).

Storey, A.E., Jones, C.L., Bouvet, D.R.C., Lasbistes, N., Fairway, S.M., Williams, L., Gibson, A.M., Nairne, R.J., Karimi, F. & Långström, B. (2007) Process for fluorination of anilides. *PCT international applications WO 2006-GB3009 20060811,* Vol. No. pp. 45.

Streit, W.J. (2004) Microglia and Alzheimer's disease pathogenesis. *Journal of Neuroscience Research,* Vol. 77, No. 1, pp. 1-8, 0360-4012 (Print), 0360-4012 (Linking).

Svedberg, M.M., Hall, H., Hellström-Lindahl, E., Estrada, S., Guan, Z., Nordberg, A. & Långström, B. (2009) [^{11}C]PIB-amyloid binding and levels of Abeta40 and Abeta42 in postmortem brain tissue from Alzheimer patients. *Neurochemistry International,* Vol. 54, No. 5-6, pp. 347-357, 1872-9754 (Electronic).

Toyama, H., Ye, D., Ichise, M., Liow, J.S., Cai, L., Jacobowitz, D., Musachio, J.L., Hong, J., Crescenzo, M., Tipre, D., Lu, J.Q., Zoghbi, S., Vines, D.C., Seidel, J., Katada, K., Green, M.V., Pike, V.W., Cohen, R.M. & Innis, R.B. (2005) PET imaging of brain with the beta-amyloid probe, [^{11}C]6-OH-BTA-1, in a transgenic mouse model of

Alzheimer's disease. *European Journal of Nuclear Medicine and Molecular Imaging,* Vol. 32, No. 5, pp. 593-600, 1619-7070 (Print), 1619-7070 (Linking).

van Groen, T., Kiliaan, A.J. & Kadish, I. (2006) Deposition of mouse amyloid β in human APP/PS1 double and single AD model transgenic mice. *Neurobiology of Disease,* Vol. 23, No. 3, pp. 653-662.

Wang, H., Shi, H., Yu, H., Jiang, S. & Tang, G. (2011) Facile and rapid one-step radiosynthesis of [^{18}F]BAY94-9172 with a new precursor. *Nuclear Medicine and Biology,* Vol. 38, No. pp. 121-127.

Villemagne, V.L., Pike, K.E., Darby, D., Maruff, P., Savage, G., Ng, S., Ackermann, U., Cowie, T.F., Currie, J., Chan, S.G., Jones, G., Tochon-Danguy, H., O'Keefe, G., Masters, C.L. & Rowe, C.C. (2008) Abeta deposits in older non-demented individuals with cognitive decline are indicative of preclinical Alzheimer's disease. *Neuropsychologia,* Vol. 46, No. 6, pp. 1688-1697, 0028-3932 (Print), 0028-3932 (Linking).

Willuweit, A., Velden, J., Godemann, R., Manook, A., Jetzek, F., Tintrup, H., Kauselmann, G., Zevnik, B., Henriksen, G., Drzezga, A., Pohlner, J., Schoor, M., Kemp, J.A. & von der Kammer, H. (2009) Early-onset and robust amyloid pathology in a new homozygous mouse model of Alzheimer's disease. *PLoS One,* Vol. 4, No. 11, pp. e7931, 1932-6203 (Electronic), 1932-6203 (Linking).

Wimo, A. & Winblad, B. (2008) Economical aspects of dementia. *Handbook of Clinical Neurology,* Vol. 89, No. pp. 137-146, 0072-9752 (Print), 0072-9752 (Linking).

Wirths, O., Bethge, T., Marcello, A., Harmeier, A., Jawhar, S., Lucassen, P.J., Multhaup, G., Brody, D.L., Esparza, T., Ingelsson, M., Kalimo, H., Lannfelt, L. & Bayer, T.A. (2010) Pyroglutamate Abeta pathology in APP/PS1KI mice, sporadic and familial Alzheimer's disease cases. *Journal of Neural Transmission,* Vol. 117, No. 1, pp. 85-96, 1435-1463 (Electronic), 0300-9564 (Linking).

Wong, D.F., Rosenberg, P.B., Zhou, Y., Kumar, A., Raymont, V., Ravert, H.T., Dannals, R.F., Nandi, A., Brasic, J.R., Ye, W., Hilton, J., Lyketsos, C., Kung, H.F., Joshi, A.D., Skovronsky, D.M. & Pontecorvo, M.J. (2010) In vivo imaging of amyloid deposition in Alzheimer disease using the radioligand ^{18}F-AV-45 (florbetapir [corrected] F 18). *Journal of Nuclear Medicine,* Vol. 51, No. 6, pp. 913-920, 1535-5667 (Electronic), 0161-5505 (Linking).

Yao, C.-H., Lin, K.-J., Weng, C.-C., Hsiao, I.-T., Ting, Y.-S., Yen, T.-C., Jan, T.-R., Skovronsky, D., Kung, M.-P. & Wey, S.-P. (2010) GMP-compliant automated synthesis of [^{18}F]AV-45 (Florbetapir F-18) for imaging beta-amyloid plaques in human brain. *Applied Radiation and Isotopes,* Vol. 68, No. pp. 2293-2297.

Ye, L., Morgenstern, J.L., Lamb, J.R. & Lockhart, A. (2006) Characterisation of the binding of amyloid imaging tracers to rodent Aβ fibrils and rodent-human Aβ co-polymers. *Biochemical and Biophysical Research Communications,* Vol. 347, No. 3, pp. 669-677.

Zhang, W., Oya, S., Kung, M.P., Hou, C., Maier, D.L. & Kung, H.F. (2005) F-18 stilbenes as PET imaging agents for detecting beta-amyloid plaques in the brain. *Journal of Medicinal Chemistry,* Vol. 48, No. 19, pp. 5980-5988, 0022-2623 (Print), 0022-2623 (Linking).

Åslund, A., Sigurdson, C.J., Klingstedt, T., Grathwohl, S., Bolmont, T., Dickstein, D.L., Glimsdal, E., Prokop, S., Lindgren, M., Konradsson, P., Holtzman, D.M., Hof, P.R., Heppner, F.L., Gandy, S., Jucker, M., Aguzzi, A., Hammarström, P. & Nilsson, K.P. (2009) Novel pentameric thiophene derivatives for in vitro and in vivo optical imaging of a plethora of protein aggregates in cerebral amyloidoses. *Acs Chemical Biology,* Vol. 4, No. 8, pp. 673-684, 1554-8937 (Electronic), 1554-8929 (Linking).

11

Monitoring of Chemotherapy Response in Malignant Pleural Mesothelioma

Tatsuo Kimura, Shinzoh Kudoh and Kazuto Hirata
Department of Respiratory Medicine, Graduate School of Medicine
Osaka City University
Japan

1. Introduction

Malignant pleural mesothelioma (MPM), typically associated with asbestos exposure, is an insidious neoplasm with findings of malignant unilateral pleural effusion or increase in pleural thickness (Jaurand and Fleury-Feith, 2005; Sterman and Albelda, 2005). Currently, imaging techniques such as computed tomography (CT) and magnetic resonance imaging (MRI) are widely used to evaluate the effects of chemotherapy on thoracic tumors. However, evaluation of the clinical response of MPM is difficult because it exhibits a non-spherical growth pattern and irregular edges.

MPM shows some technical problems to measure sizes of tumors in determining the response to chemotherapy. Cross-sectional CT or MRI appears inadequate for measuring the size of non-spherical tumors such as MPM. Response evaluation criteria in solid tumor (RECIST) criteria determine the method for measuring the longest diameter of the tumor (Therasse et al., 2000), but the appropriateness of these methods to MPM has not been determined. Recently, modified RECIST criteria were reported (Byrne and Nowak, 2004). Modified RECIST criteria determine the method of measuring tumor thickness perpendicularly to the chest wall or mediastinum in nonspherical tumors.

In positron emission tomography (PET), altered glucose metabolism is visualized using the radiolabeled glucose analogue ^{18}F-fluoro-2-deoxy-D-glucose (FDG). Evaluation of glucose metabolism using FDG-PET plays a critical role in early tumor diagnosis, staging, therapeutic strategy, and prognosis prediction (Kalff et al., 2001; Pieterman et al., 2000; Swisher et al., 2004; Vansteenkiste et al., 1998). FDG-PET imaging to evaluate responses to chemotherapy or irradiation is useful for patients with a variety of carcinomas (Kostakoglu and Goldsmith, 2003; Mac Manus et al., 2003). However, few studies involving MPM patients have been performed to assess the usefulness of FDG-PET for monitoring treatment responses (Ceresoli et al., 2006; Francis et al., 2007; Steinert et al., 2005; Veit-Haibach et al., 2010). Here, we present a case involving the use of FDG-PET for monitoring responses to chemotherapy in a patient with MPM. FDG-PET and CT were performed before chemotherapy and after the first and second courses of chemotherapy. The tumor lesion exhibited shrinkage according to CT and a decrease in the SUVmax after the first course of chemotherapy, but exhibited size enlargement with an increase in SUVmax after the second course of chemotherapy. These findings suggest that quantification of metabolic responses using FDG-PET may be related to the objective response as determined by modified RECIST in patients with MPM. We also discuss current data regarding FDG-PET in the clinical management of MPM.

2. Case

A 56-year-old non-smoking man was referred to our medical center for further examination of massive pleural effusion in the right lobe according to chest radiography. He had a 6-month history of dyspnea and had been diagnosed with tuberculous pleuritis. He was treated with tuberculous drugs without improvement. His height was 162 cm, and his body weight was 63.5 kg, with no body weight loss in the preceding 6 months. He worked as a bus driver for 30 years without known asbestos exposure. Results of physical examination were nearly normal, and he exhibited no weakness of breath sounds in the right lung. Results of full hematological and biochemistry testing were all within normal limits, except for γGTP of 67 IU/L due to fatty liver. CRP was not elevated, and tumor markers CEA, NSE, and pro-GRP were all within normal ranges; CYFRA 21-1 was elevated to 6.7 ng/mL. A chest wall biopsy specimen obtained upon admission revealed biphasic-type MPM. Thoracic drainage of pleural effusion and OK-432 was performed. Pleural thickening was noted in the upper right hemithorax on chest computed tomography (Fig. 1a). FDG-PET scanning was performed as a part of a study of the usefulness of functional imaging of MPM at the Osaka City University Hospital (Osaka, Japan) (Kimura et al., 2008). FDG-PET imaging and CT scanning were performed before chemotherapy, as well as after the first and second courses of chemotherapy, with written informed consent.

Upon completion of each scan, the patient was injected with intravenous FDG 185-370 MBq. The degree of FDG accumulation was evaluated using scanned images acquired 40 to 55 minutes after injection. FDG was produced using an NKK-Oxford superconducting cyclotron and an NKK synthesis system (AMFG01, NKK, Muroran, Japan). PET images were obtained using a PET scanner (HEADTOME IV; Shimadzu, Kyoto, Japan) with 4 detector rings providing 7 contiguous slices at 13-mm intervals and an intrinsic resolution of 4.5-mm full width at half maximum (FWHM). Attenuation correction of reconstructed images was accomplished through a patient-specific transmission study using a 68 Ge ring source. FDG-PET images were compared with the corresponding CT images, allowing accurate identification of tumors by using anatomical landmarks. For quantitative evaluation, a region of interest (ROI) (circle 6 mm in diameter) was placed on the area of maximum FDG uptake within the lesion. A background ROI was then placed on a non-tumorous region of the lung. The standardized uptake value (SUV), a quantitative measure of activity in the region of interest (ROI), was determined using the following formula:

$$SUV = \frac{\text{Radioactivity Concentration in ROI (Bq / mL)}}{\text{Injected dose (Bq) / body weight (g)}}$$

He received chemotherapy with cisplatin and irinotecan. Severe diarrhea due to irinotecan, a different chemotherapy regimen, including cisplatin and docetaxel, was administered as a second course. The tumor lesion exhibited shrinkage according to CT images (Fig. 1), and SUVmax (Table 1) decreased after the first course of chemotherapy; however, size enlargement and an increase in SUVmax after the second course of chemotherapy occurred. Progression-free survival and overall survival were 90 days and 320 days, respectively.

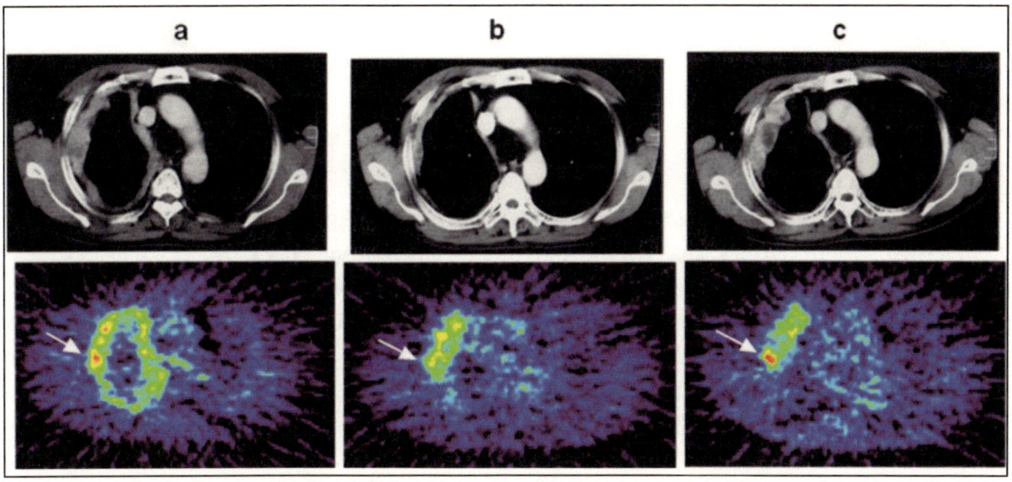

Fig. 1. Monitoring chemotherapy response of malignant pleural mesothelioma using CT-based modified RECIST criteria and FDG-PET-based SUVmax. CT and PET monitoring before chemotherapy (a), after the first course of chemotherapy (b), and after the second course of chemotherapy (c). Arrows show the target lesions.

	a	b	c
SUVmax	3.78	2.47	3.67
Modified RECIST	10.38	6.45	10.08

Table 1. Comparison of SUVmax and Modified RECIST in Fig 1.

3. Brief reviews

3.1 Differentiating malignant from benign disease

Pleural disease has 3 fundamental pathologic features: effusion, thickening, and calcification of pleural surfaces, with overlapping radiological findings. Differentiation of malignant from benign lesions on the basis of clinical findings alone is often difficult. Furthermore, the results of thoracentesis, percutaneous biopsy, and even thoracotomy may be ambiguous, and nonfatal complications can occur in up to 10% of patients undergoing such procedures. FDG-PET imaging is highly accurate and reliable in differentiating malignant from benign pleural effusion and/or involvement (Gupta et al., 2002; Mavi et al., 2009). When an SUV cut-off of 2.0 was used to differentiate malignant from benign disease, a sensitivity of 91% and specificity of 100% were achieved, although the activity in some epithelial mesotheliomas was close to the threshold value (Benard et al., 1998). Another study found that PET scanning sensitivity was 96.8% and specificity was 88.5% in distinguishing benign from malignant pleural disease (Duysinx et al., 2004). Additionally, another study showed that a cut-off value of 2.2 for SUV provided the best accuracy, with 94.1% and 100% for sensitivity and specificity (Yildirim et al., 2009). Furthermore, the usefulness of dual time point FDG-PET imaging in distinguishing malignant from benign localizing pleural disease has been reported (Mavi et al., 2009). The SUVmax and its change over time in MPM patients were significantly higher than those in the benign pleural disease group ($P < 0.0001$). Yamamoto also described the usefulness of dual time point FDG-PET (Yamamoto et al., 2009). Sensitivity, specificity, and accuracy in detecting MPM by using both early and delayed PET were 88%. Mean values of SUVearly and SUVdelayed in MPM were significantly higher than the corresponding values in benign pleural disease ($P < 0.01$, respectively).

We also treated a 66-year-old man with the benign pleural thickness with no tumor involvement. Pleural thickness was found during an annual check-up. He was an office worker and had smoked 20 cigarettes per day for 40 years; he had not been exposed to asbestos and did not complain of symptoms. However, his father had been exposed to asbestos for a long period of time. CT-guided needle biopsy of left side pleura revealed an increase in the collagen structure and infiltration of lymphocytes with no tumor involvement. CT, PET, and PET-CT images are shown in Fig. 2. Bilateral pleural thickness was shown in CT image(Fig 2a,c). Almost normal FDG uptake in the bilateral pleural thickness was shown in PET images (Fig 2b,d). A Biograph 16 (Siemens Medical, Germany), which has 39 detector ring providing 81 contiguous slices at 2-mm intervals, was employed for PET-CT examination.

Thus, a combination of metabolic and anatomical information is useful for differentiating malignant from benign tissue. CT scans are most commonly used, although the use of PET scans has increased. Although multi procedures are valuable, false negative findings occur with both. These methods can be used in combination for a more accurate diagnosis.

3.2 International TNM staging system for MPM

For the past 30 years, several staging systems have been used for MPM. The TNM system is used to evaluate tumor size, lymph nodes, and distant metastasis. The clear need for an internationally accepted staging system prompted a group of International Mesothelioma Interest Group (IMIG) members to hold a consensus meeting in June 1994, and the new International TNM Staging System for MPM was developed as a result of this meeting. These guidelines reconcile the multiple previous staging systems, provide a staging system similar to those used for other solid tumors, and take into consideration recent data regarding the influence of T and N status on overall survival in MPM (Rusch, 1995). The TNM system of MPM consists of 4 stages. In Stage I, the MPM is in the membrane lining the chest (right or left pleura), and the MPM has not spread to the lymph nodes. In Stage II, the MPM involves the right or left pleura lining the chest. The MPM has also spread from the lining of the chest into the outer lining of the lung, into the diaphragm, or into the lung. In addition to involvement of the chest pleura, Stage III MPM has spread into the first layer of the chest wall, part of the mediastinum (the chest cavity behind the breastbone that lies between the lungs), or a single location in the chest wall. It may have also spread to the outer covering layer of the heart or to the lymph nodes on one side of the chest. In Stage IV MPM, the disease has advanced to other organs in the body such as the liver, brain, or bone or to lymph nodes on both sides of the chest. Tables 2 and 3 show TNM staging definitions and descriptions.

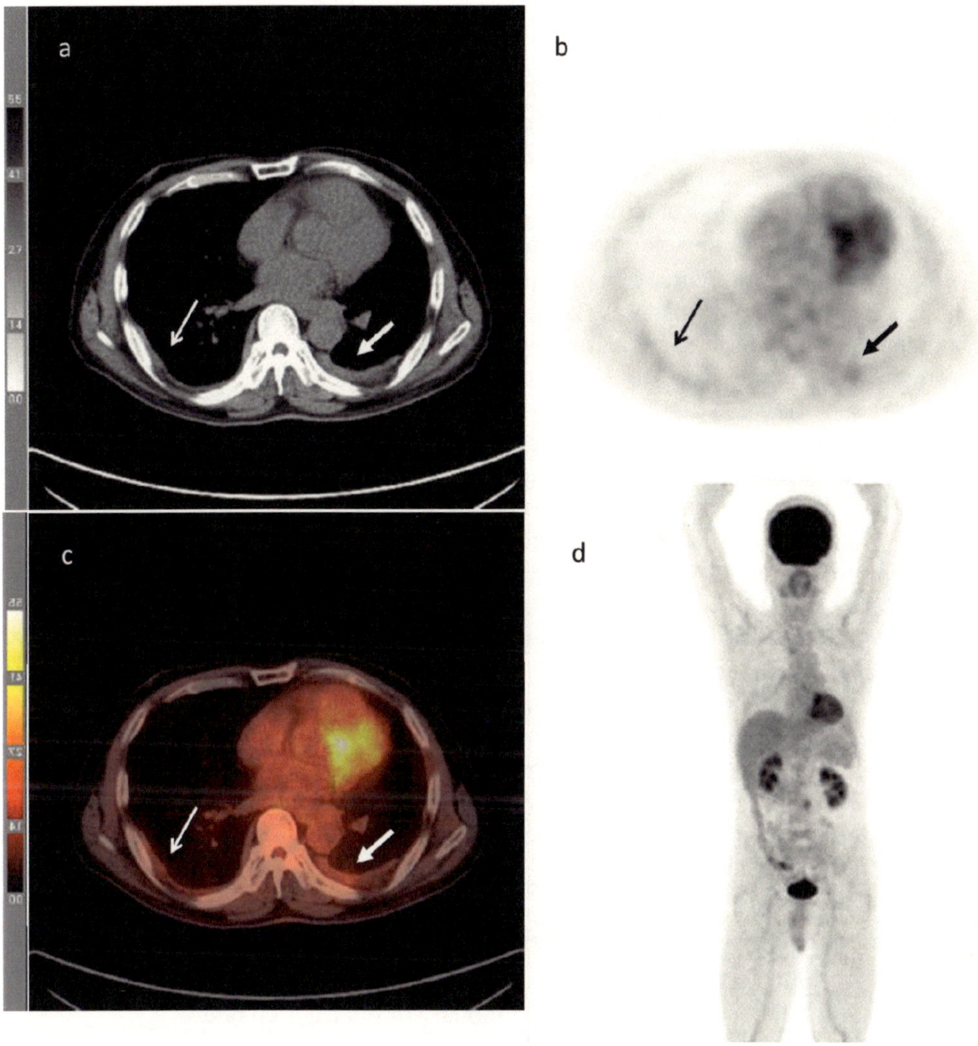

Fig. 2. Benign pleural thickness with no tumor involvement. PET-CT images of bilateral pleural thickness (narrow and large arrows). The trans-axial views of CT image (a), PET image (b) and PET-CT image (c), and coronal view of whole-body PET image (d). The SUVmax of the left side pleura (large arrow) and the right side pleura (narrow arrow) were 2.019 and 1.452, respectively.

T	
T1a	Tumor limited to the ipsilateral parietal pleura, including mediastinal and diaphragmatic pleura No involvement of the visceral pleura
T1b	Tumor involving the ipsilateral parietal pleura, including mediastinal and diaphragmatic pleura Scattered foci of tumor also involving the visceral pleura
T2	Tumor involving each of the ipsilateral pleural surfaces (parietal, mediastinal, diaphragmatic, and visceral pleura) with at least one of the following features: involvement of diaphragmatic muscle confluent visceral pleural tumor (including fissures) or extension of tumor from visceral pleura into the underlying pulmonary parenchyma
T3	Describes locally advanced but potentially resectable tumor Tumor involving all ipsilateral pleural surfaces (parietal, mediastinal, diaphragmatic, and visceral pleura) with at least one of the following features: involvement of the endothoracic fascia extension into the mediastinal fat solitary, completely resectable focus of tumor extending into the soft tissues of the chest wall nontransmural involvement of the pericardium
T4	Describes locally advanced technically unresectable tumor Tumor involving all ipsilateral pleural surfaces (parietal, mediastinal, diaphragmatic, and visceral) with at least one of the following features: diffuse extension or multifocal masses of tumor in the chest wall, with or without associated rib destruction direct extension of tumor to the contralateral pleura direct extension of tumor to one or more mediastinal organs direct extension of tumor into the spine tumor extending through to the internal surface of the pericardium with or without a pericardialeffusion; or tumor involving the myocardium
N	
NX	Regional lymph nodes cannot be assessed
N0	No regional lymph node metastases
N1	Metastases in the ipsilateral bronchopulmonary or hilar lymph nodes
N2	Metastases in the subcarinal or the ipsilateral mediastinal lymph nodes, including the ipsilateral internal mammary nodes
N3	Metastases in the contralateral mediastinal, contralateral internal mammary, ipsilateral, or contralateral supraclavicular lymph nodes
M	
MX	Presence of distant metastases cannot be assessed
M0	No distant metastasis
M1	Distant metastasis present

Table 2. New International Staging System for diffuse MPM

Stage	T	N	M
I	T1	N0	M0
Ia	T1a	N0	M0
Ib	T1b	N0	M0
II	T2	N0	M0
III	T1, T2	N1	M0
	T1,T2	N2	M0
	T3	N0,N1,N2	M0
IV	T4	Any N	M0
	Any T	N3	M0
	Any T	AnyN	M1

Table 3. Stage by tumor (T), lymph node (N), metastasis (M), and Description of International TNM staging system for diffuse MPM

3.3 PET for staging and preoperative evaluation for MPM

The combination of metabolic and anatomical information provided by PET is useful in determining the stage and conducting a preoperative evaluation of MPM. Recent studies indicate the potential in the use of PET in diagnosing MPM and determining MPM staging or the extent to which tumors have spread. In a comparative study by Plathow et al., the diagnostic values of CT, PET, PET/CT, and MRI for staging were evaluated in 54 patients with limited MPM (Plathow et al., 2008). The accuracies of CT, PET, MRI, and PET/CT were 0.77, 0.86, 0.8, and 1.0, respectively, for limited MPM patients, and 0.75, 0.83, 0.9, and 1.0, respectively, for patients in Stages II and III. FDG-PET/CT is significantly more accurate in Stages II and III compared with all other techniques.

In addition, FDG-PET is particularly useful for identifying occult distant metastases. Twenty-eight consecutive patients referred for the evaluation of suspected MPM underwent FDG-PET imaging at the University of Pennsylvania Medical Center (Benard et al., 1998). PET imaging was compared with thoracoscopy and surgical biopsies and was found to successfully indicate the presence of disease in 24 patients and of benign conditions in the remaining 4 patients. FDG uptake was significantly higher in diseased cells, and PET analysis showed tumors in the lymph nodes of 9 patients. Lymph nodes appeared normal based on CT scans. Another study at Brigham and Women's Hospital and Harvard Medical School in Boston evaluated 15 patients, 11 of whom had MPM and 4 who were disease-free (Gerbaudo et al., 2002). PET results were compared with laboratory analysis of biopsied fluids and tissues. PET was used to detect all 11 primary tumors and confirm the absence of disease in the other 4 patients. For biopsied lesions, overall sensitivity, specificity, and accuracies for FDG-PET were 97%, 80%, and 94%, respectively, compared with 83%, 80%, and 82%, respectively, for CT. FDG-PET was used to identify extrathoracic metastases in 5 patients, excluding these patients from surgical therapy. Sorensen et al. compared the accuracy of preoperative staging with different imaging modalities and found that non-curative surgery could be avoided in 29% of 42 MPM patients using preoperative PET/CT and in another 14% by employing mediastinoscopy (Sorensen et al., 2008). Wilcox et al. reported the utility of PET/CT in the initial staging and assessed 35 patients with MPM included in the Mayo clinic database. PET/CT excluded 14 of 35 patients from surgical intervention (Wilcox et al., 2009). Upstaging from PET/CT was noted in 70% of patients when surgical pathology was available.

These studies indicate that although CT scans are a standard test for evaluating MPM patients, PET can also be used for MPM diagnosis. PET/CT increases staging accuracy in patients with MPM and improves patient selection for curative surgical procedures. Distant metastases have historically been considered to be an uncommon late manifestation of MPM (Truong et al., 2006). But, accurate determination of the presence or absence of distant metastases is crucial for potentially curative surgical resection of MPM.

3.4 PET for restaging and survival

Accurate restaging of disease after treatment has also implications for survival. Two retrospective studies have concluded that FDG-PET/CT is useful for detecting metastases. The first was reported by Tan et al. and involved the evaluation of 44 patients using PET/CT after multimodality therapy for MPM (Tan, 2010). The other study was reported by Lee and was a retrospective study involving 46 patients who were evaluated using PET/CT for staging or re-staging after therapy for MPM (Lee et al., 2009). Both studies concluded that detecting extrathoracic metastases using FDG-PET/CT indicates poor prognosis in patients with MPM.

A correlation between PET parameters and prognosis has been shown in some reports. Nowak et al. reported that 93 patients underwent PET/CT assessments at baseline; these patients were then treated clinically and survival was followed (Nowak et al., 2010). In univariate analysis, significant prognostic factors included total glycolytic volume (TGV), sarcomatous history, weight loss, CT stage, and European Organization for Research and Treatment of Cancer (EORTC) good prognosis category. In multivariate analysis, TGV and weight loss remained as significant prognostic factors in patients with non-sarcomatoid histology and no pleurodesis. Gerbaudo et al. reported 50 patients subjected to PET/CT assessments after therapy, and survival after relapse was independently predicted based on the pattern of FDG uptake and PET nodal status; overall survival was predicted based on the maximum standard uptake value (Gerbaudo et al., 2011).

3.5 PET for response assessment

3.5.1 Modified RECIST criteria

Modified RECIST criteria have been published with particular reference to MPM (Byrne and Nowak, 2004). Response to treatment is evaluated by measuring uni-dimensional tumor thickness perpendicular to the chest wall in 2 positions at 3 different levels on CT. The sum of these 6 measurements is defined as the pleural uni-dimensional measure. Transverse cuts at least 1 cm apart and related to anatomical landmarks in the thorax were chosen to allow reproducible assessment at later time points. If a measurable tumor was present, transverse cuts in the upper thorax, above the level of the main bronchi division were preferred. At reassessment, pleural thickness was measured at the same position and at the same level by the same observer. This measurement did not necessarily represent the greatest tumor thickness at the level. Nodal, subcutaneous, and other bi-dimensionally measurable lesions were measured uni-dimensionally based on the RECIST criteria. Uni-dimensional measurements were included to obtain the total tumor measurement. The RECIST definition is listed in Table 4. A confirmed response required repeat observation on 2 occasions 4 weeks apart.

Complete response (CR)	Disappearance of all target lesions with no evidence of tumors elsewhere
Partial response (PR)	At least a 30%reduction in the total tumor measurement
Progressive disease (PD)	Increase of at least 20% in the total tumor measurement over the nadir measurement or the appearance of one or more new lesions
Stable disease (SD)	Those who fulfilled the criteria for neither PR and PD

Table 4. Response criteria of Modified RECIST

3.5.2 PET in RECIST version 1.1

Currently, most clinical trials evaluating cancer treatments for objective responses in solid tumors are using RECIST. The RECIST Working Group, consisting of clinicians with expertise in early drug development from academic research organizations, government, and industry, together with imaging specialists and statisticians, has met regularly to set an agenda to update RECIST, determine the evidence needed to justify various changes made, and to review emerging evidence (Eisenhauer et al., 2009). RECIST 1.1, published in January 2009, is an update to the original criteria. A critical aspect of the revision process was to create a database of prospectively documented solid tumor measurement data obtained from industry and academic group trials. However, the Working Group and particularly those involved in imaging research, did not believe that there was sufficient standardization and widespread availability to recommend adoption of either volumetric anatomical assessment or to functional assessment (e.g. dynamic contrast enhanced MRI, CT, or FDG-PET techniques assessing tumor metabolism). The only exception to this is the use of FDG-PET imaging as an adjunct to determine progression. The RECIST Working Group looks forward to such data emerging in the next few years to allow appropriate changes to be made to the next iteration of the RECIST criteria.

3.5.3 PERCIST— Positron Emission tomography Response Criteria In Solid Tumors

Therapy monitoring with FDG-PET is generally based on consensus criteria from the European Organization for Research and Treatment of Cancer (EORTC) (Young et al., 1999). Based on the extensive literature now supporting the use of ^{18}F-FDG PET as well as the known limitations of anatomic imaging to assess early treatment response, updated draft PET criteria have been proposed that may be useful for consideration in clinical trials and potentially in clinical practice. We refer to these draft criteria as "PERCIST"—Positron Emission tomography Response Criteria In Solid Tumors (Wahl et al., 2009). The premise of the PERCIST 1.0 criteria is that cancer response as assessed by PET is a continuous and time-dependent variable. A tumor may be evaluated at a number of times during treatment and glucose use may rise or fall from baseline values. SUV will likely vary for the same tumor and the same treatment at different times. For example, tracer uptake by a tumor is expected to decline over time with effective treatment. Thus, capturing and reporting the fractional change in SUV from the starting value and when the scan was obtained are important.

Complete metabolic response (CMR)	Complete resolution of ^{18}F-FDG uptake within a measurable target lesion such that it is less than the mean liver activity and indistinguishable from surrounding background blood-pool levels. Disappearance of all other lesions to background blood-pool levels.
Partial metabolic response (PMR)	Reduction by a minimum of 30% in target measurable tumor ^{18}F-FDG SUL peak. Absolute drop in SUL must be at least 0.8 S UL units as well. Measurement is commonly in same lesion as baseline but can be another lesion if that lesion was previously present and is the most active lesion after treatment. Reduction in the extent of tumor 18F-FDG uptake is not a requirement for PMR.
Progressive metabolic disease (PMD)	>30% increase in ^{18}F-FDG SUL peak, with >0.8 SUL unit increase in tumor SUV peak from baseline scan in pattern typical of a tumor and not of infection/treatment effect OR: visible increase in extent of ^{18}F-FDG tumor uptake (75% in TLG volume with no decline in SUL OR: new ^{18}F-FDG–avid lesions.
Stable metabolic disease (SMD)	Not CMR, PMR, or PMD.

Table 5. Response criteria of PERCIST

Patients should fast for at least 4 to 6 h before undergoing scanning, and the measured serum glucose level (no correction) must be less than 200 mg/dL. Patients may be on an oral hypoglycaemic but not on insulin. A baseline PET scan should be obtained 50 to 70 min after tracer injection. A follow-up scan should be obtained within 15 min (but always 50 min or later) of the baseline scan. All scans should be performed using the same PET scanner with the same injected dose ±20% of radioactivity. Appropriate attenuation correction along with evaluation for proper PET and CT registration of the quantitated areas should be performed. Lean body mass (SUL) is determined for up to 5 tumors (up to 2 per organ) with the most intense ^{18}F-FDG uptake. These will typically be lesions identified using RECIST 1.1. The SUV peak (this is a sphere with a diameter of approximately 1.2 cm to produce a 1-cm^3-volume spherical ROI) centered near the hottest point in the tumor foci should be determined and the image planes and coordinates should be noted (SUL peak). This SUL peak ROI will typically include the maximal SUL pixel (which should also be recorded) but is not necessarily centered on the maximal SUL pixel. Tumor sizes should be noted and should be 2 cm or larger in diameter for accurate measurement, although smaller lesions of sufficient ^{18}F-FDG uptake, including those not well observed anatomically, can be assessed. Each baseline (pretreatment) tumor SUL peak must be 1.5 × mean liver SUL + 2 SDs of mean SUL. If the liver is diseased, 2.0 × blood-pool ^{18}F-FDG activity + 2 SDs in the mediastinum is suggested as the minimal metabolically measurable tumor activity. In PERCIST, the response to therapy is assessed as a continuous variable and expressed as the percentage change in SUL peak (or sum of lesion SULs) between pre- and post-treatment scans. After chemotherapy, waiting a minimum of 10 d before performing FDG-PET is advised. This time permits bypassing of the chemotherapeutic effect and of transient fluctuations in ^{18}F-FDG uptake that may occur early after treatment, including stunning or flaring of tumor uptake. The response criteria are listed in Table 5.

3.6 PET for therapeutic response assessment in MPM

PET and CT examinations can play important roles in the management of patients with MPM. Particularly, an emerging role for FDG-PET/CT is that of therapeutic response assessment. Steinert et al. performed assessments on 17 patients after 3 cycles of chemotherapy and reported that total lesion glycolysis (TLG), defined as (SUVmax) × (Vol), more accurately identifies patients responding to chemotherapy (Steinert et al., 2005). Ceresoli et al. measured CT and PET responses in 22 patients after 2 cycles of chemotherapy and found that an early metabolic response as a 25% decrease in SUVmax was significantly correlated to median time-to-tumor progression and was tended to be associated with longer overall survival (Ceresoli et al., 2006). Francic et al. reported a prospective study, including patients who had undergone both FDG-PET and conventional radiological response assessment before and after 1 cycle of chemotherapy (Francis et al., 2007). Twenty-three patients were evaluated and a statistically significant relationship between a fall in TGV and improved patient survival was shown. Veit-Haibach et al. reported a study involving 41 patients evaluated by FDG-PET/CT at baseline and after 3 cycles of pemetrexed plus platinum-based chemotherapy (Veit-Haibach et al., 2010). Neither SUVmax-response nor SUVmean-response was related to survival; however, a decrease in TLG and PETvol was found to be significantly predictive of survival. Flores et al. reported a statistically significant association between a decrease in SUV after chemotherapy and overall survival in 24 MPM patients treated with cisplatin-based induction chemotherapy and surgery (Flores et al., 2005).

Our group conducted a small study involving 11 patients with MPM (Kimura et al., 2005). FDG-PET scanning was performed at the Osaka City University Hospital (Osaka, Japan) as part of a prospective study to examine the usefulness of functional imaging of MPM. This study was conducted between March 1999 and December 2004 and all patients had a proven histological diagnosis of MPM treated using chemotherapy. Each patient underwent both FDG-PET imaging and CT scanning before treatment and after the first courses of chemotherapy. Written informed consent was obtained from all patients. A total of 33 lesions in 11 patients with MPM were studied. The Spearman rank correlation test was used to compare ratios of pre-therapy to post-therapy SUVs. In an examination of CT evaluation, the mean SUV of the 8 lesions exhibiting a clinical response after the first course of the chemotherapy significantly decreased from 4.03 + 1.28 SD to 2.83 + 0.69 SD ($P = 0.050$) (Fig. 3a). The mean SUV of the 5 lesions exhibiting clinical progression after the first course of chemotherapy tended to increase from 2.42 + 0.90 SD to 2.74 + 0.88 SD ($P = 0.072$) (Fig. 3b). The mean SUV of the 20 lesions exhibiting no clinical change after the first course of chemotherapy significantly decreased from 3.71 + 1.85 SD to 3.03 + 1.63 SD ($P = 0.0002$) (Fig. 3c).

Thus, some PET parameters used to evaluate metabolic response may be associated with overall survival as well as predict anatomical response. The differences between these studies are the timing of assessments for early evaluation of metabolic response. The best timing and best parameters in patients with MPM remain to be clearly determined. Further clinical studies are necessary to determine the usefulness of FDG-PET as a monitoring method for response to chemotherapy.

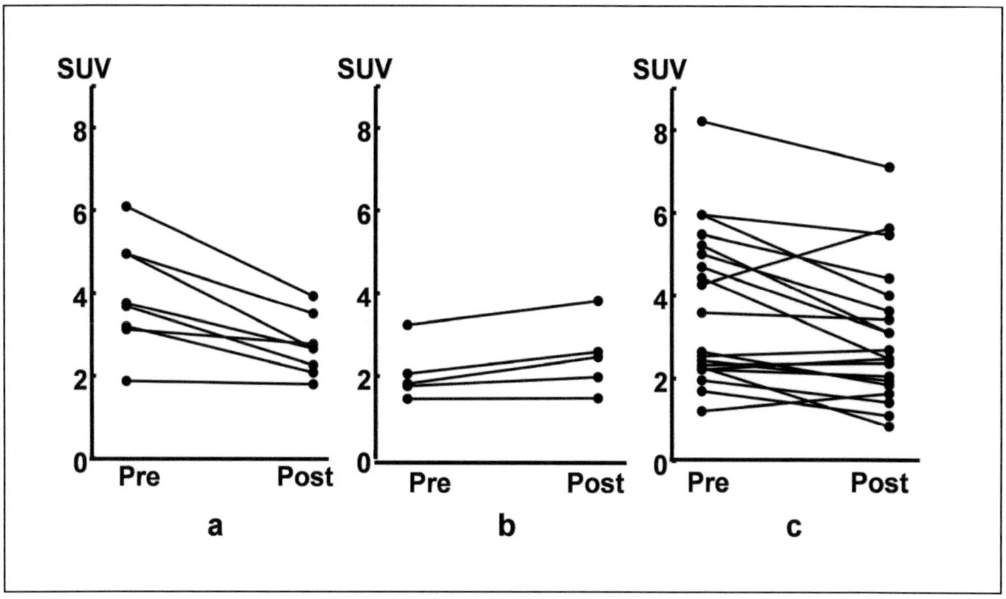

Fig. 3. FDG uptake (SUV) changes assorted to CT responses. Lesions exhibiting clinical response (a), clinical progression (b), and without change (c) before and after the first course of chemotherapy.

4. Limitations and pitfalls

FDG-PET has been reported to yield false-negative results for lesions smaller than 1 cm and false-positive results for lesions with inflammatory change (Kostakoglu and Goldsmith, 2003). In the current state of technology, it is impossible to detect small clusters of tumor cells that will cause a clinically detectable recurrence of disease in the future (Hueltenschmidt et al., 2001). Tumors exhibit heterogeneous biological activity in single tumors; however, it is difficult to obtain cytological and histological materials from patients with MPM from multiple lesions at multiple time points and histological confirmation of metabolic response. Unfortunately, in this chapter, it has been impossible to cite all references referring to the use of FDG-PET in MPM.

5. Conclusion

The present case suggests that the results of quantification of metabolic response by FDG-PET may be related to objective response as determined by modified RECIST in patients with MPM. It also is important to acknowledge that SUVs are not strictly quantitative, and repeated biopsies are sometimes required. Information derived from FDG-PET during treatment may require assessment based on standard follow-up procedures. Final interpretations of images reported are based on total analysis and not SUV alone.

6. Acknowledgment

We thank the invaluable assistance of Dr. Shigeki Mitsuoka, Dr. Hiroshi Kamoi, and all of the colleagues in the Department of Respiratory Medicine, Osaka City University. We also thank radiological technologist Mr. Hideki Kawahata, radiologists Dr. Koichi Koyama in the Deparmtnet of Radiology and Dr. Shigeaki Higashiyama, Dr. Joji Kawabe, and Prof. Susumu Shiomi in the Deparmtnet of Nuclear Medicine, Osaka City University for providing clinical resources, image annotation, and inspection of the results.

7. References

Benard, F.; Sterman, D.; Smith, R. J.; Kaiser, L. R.; Albelda, S. M. & Alavi, A. (1998). Metabolic imaging of malignant pleural mesothelioma with fluorodeoxyglucose positron emission tomography. *Chest.*, Vol.114, pp.713-722. ISSN: 0012-3692.

Byrne, M. J. & Nowak, A. K. (2004). Modified RECIST criteria for assessment of response in malignant pleural mesothelioma. *Ann Oncol.*, Vol.15, pp.257-260. ISSN: 0923-7534.

Ceresoli, G. L.; Chiti, A.; Zucali, P. A.; Rodari, M.; Lutman, R. F.; Salamina, S.; Incarbone, M.; Alloisio, M. & Santoro, A. (2006). Early response evaluation in malignant pleural mesothelioma by positron emission tomography with [18F]fluorodeoxyglucose. *J Clin Oncol.*, Vol.24, pp.4587-4593. ISSN: 1527-7755.

Duysinx, B., Nguyen, D.; Louis, R.; Cataldo, D.; Belhocine, T.; Bartsch, P. & Bury, T. (2004). Evaluation of pleural disease with 18-fluorodeoxyglucose positron emission tomography imaging. *Chest.*, Vol.125, pp.489-493. ISSN: 0012-3692.

Eisenhauer, E. A.; Therasse, P.; Bogaerts, J.; Schwartz, L. H.; Sargent, D.; Ford, R.; Dancey, J.; Arbuck, S.; Gwyther, S.; Mooney, M.; Rubinstein, L.; Shankar, L.; Dodd, L.; Kaplan, R.; Lacombe, D. & Verweij, J.. (2009). New response evaluation criteria in solid tumours: revised RECIST guideline (version 1.1). *Eur J Cancer.*, Vol.45, pp.228-247. ISSN: 1879-0852.

Flores, R. M.; Akhurst, T.; Krug, L.; Gonen, M.; Dycoco, J.; Rosenzweig, K.; Larson, S. M.; Downey, R. J. & Rusch, V. W. (2005)*Proceedings of American Society of Clinical Oncology Annual Meeting.* Vol 23, No. 16S, Part I of II (June 1 Supplement), (abstract 7066). Orlando, Florida. May, 2005.

Francis, R. J.; Byrne, M. J.; van der Schaaf, A. A.; Boucek, J. A.; Nowak, A. K.; Phillips, M.; Price, R.; Patrikeos, A. P.; Musk, A. W. & Millward, M. J. (2007). Early prediction of response to chemotherapy and survival in malignant pleural mesothelioma using a novel semiautomated 3-dimensional volume-based analysis of serial 18F-FDG PET scans. *J Nucl Med.*, Vol.48, pp.1449-1458. ISSN: 0161-5505.

Gerbaudo, V. H.; Mamede, M.; Trotman-Dickenson, B.; Hatabu, H. & Sugarbaker, D. J. (2011). FDG PET/CT patterns of treatment failure of malignant pleural mesothelioma: relationship to histologic type, treatment algorithm, and survival. *Eur J Nucl Med Mol Imaging.*, Vol.38, pp.810-821. ISSN: 1619-7089.

Gerbaudo, V. H.; Sugarbaker, D. J.; Britz-Cunningham, S.; Di Carli, M. F.; Mauceri, C. & Treves, S. T. (2002). Assessment of malignant pleural mesothelioma with (18)F-FDG dual-head gamma-camera coincidence imaging: comparison with histopathology. *J Nucl Med.*, Vol.43, pp.1144-1149. ISSN: 0161-5505.

Gupta, N. C.; Rogers, J. S.; Graeber, G. M.; Gregory, J. L.; Waheed, U.; Mullet, D. & Atkins, M. (2002). Clinical role of F-18 fluorodeoxyglucose positron emission tomography imaging in patients with lung cancer and suspected malignant pleural effusion. *Chest.*, Vol.122, pp.1918-1924. ISSN: 0012-3692.

Hueltenschmidt, B.; Sautter-Bihl, M. L.; Lang, O.; Maul, F. D.; Fischer, J.; Mergenthaler, H. G. and Bihl, H. (2001). Whole body positron emission tomography in the treatment of Hodgkin disease. *Cancer.*, Vol.91, pp.302-310. ISSN: 0008-543X.

Jaurand, M. C. & Fleury-Feith, J. (2005). Pathogenesis of malignant pleural mesothelioma. *Respirology.*, Vol.10, pp.2-8. ISSN: 1323-7799.

Kalff, V.; Hicks, R. J.; MacManus, M. P.; Binns, D. S.; McKenzie, A. F.; Ware, R. E.; Hogg, A. & Ball, D. L. (2001). Clinical impact of (18)F fluorodeoxyglucose positron emission tomography in patients with non-small-cell lung cancer: a prospective study. *J Clin Oncol.*, Vol.19, pp.111-118. ISSN: 0732-183X.

Kimura, T.; Koyama, K.; Kudoh, S.; Kawabe, J.; Yoshimura, N.; Mitsuoka, S.; Shiomi, S. & Hirata, K. (2008). Monitoring of chemotherapy response in malignant pleural mesothelioma using fluorodeoxyglucose positron emission tomography. *Intern Med.*, Vol.47, pp.2053-2056. ISSN: 1349-7235.

Kimura, T.; Kudoh, S.; Yoshimura, N.; Mitsuoka, S.; Matuura, K.; Koyama, K.; kawabe, J.; Okamura, M.; Hirata, K.; Shiomi, S. &Yoshikawa, J. (2005) Monitoring of chemotherapy response in multiple disseminated malignant pleural mesothelioma using fluorodeoxyglucose positron emission tomography. *Proceedings of American Society of Clinical Oncology Annual Meeting.* Vol 23, No. 16S, Part I of II (June 1 Supplement), (abstract 7177). Orlando, Florida. May, 2005.

Kostakoglu, L. & Goldsmith, S. J. (2003). 18F-FDG PET evaluation of the response to therapy for lymphoma and for breast, lung, and colorectal carcinoma. *J Nucl Med.*, Vol.44, pp.224-239. ISSN: 0161-5505.

Lee, S. T.; Ghanem, M.; Herbertson, R. A.; Berlangieri, S. U.; Byrne, A. J.; Tabone, K.; Mitchell, P.; Knight, S. R.; Feigen, M, & Scott, A. M. (2009). Prognostic value of 18F-FDG PET/CT in patients with malignant pleural mesothelioma. *Mol Imaging Biol.*, Vol.11, pp.473-479. ISSN: 1860-2002.

Mac Manus, M. P.; Hicks, R. J.; Matthews, J. P.; McKenzie, A.; Rischin, D.; Salminen, E. K. & Ball, D. L. (2003). Positron emission tomography is superior to computed tomography scanning for response-assessment after radical radiotherapy or chemoradiotherapy in patients with non-small-cell lung cancer. *J Clin Oncol.*, Vol.21, pp.1285-1292. ISSN: 0732-183X.

Mavi, A.; Basu, S.; Cermik, T. F.; Urhan, M.; Bathaii, M.; Thiruvenkatasamy, D.; Houseni, M.; Dadparvar, S. & Alavi, A. (2009). Potential of dual time point FDG-PET imaging in differentiating malignant from benign pleural disease. *Mol Imaging Biol.*, Vol.11, pp.369-378. ISSN: 1860-2002.

Nowak, A. K.; Francis, R. J.; Phillips, M. J.; Millward, M. J.; van der Schaaf, A. A.; Boucek, J.; Musk, A. W.; McCoy, M. J.; Segal, A.; Robins, P. & Byrne, M. J. (2010). A novel prognostic model for malignant mesothelioma incorporating quantitative FDG-PET imaging with clinical parameters. *Clin Cancer Res.*, Vol.16, pp.2409-2417. ISSN: 1078-0432.

Pieterman, R; M., van Putten, J. W.; Meuzelaar, J. J.; Mooyaart, E. L.; Vaalburg, W.; Koeter, G. H.; Fidler, V.; Pruim, J. & Groen, H. J. (2000). Preoperative staging of non-small-cell lung cancer with positron-emission tomography. *N Engl J Med.*, Vol.343,pp. 254-261. ISSN: 0028-4793.

Plathow, C.; Staab, A.; Schmaehl, A.; Aschoff, P.; Zuna, I.; Pfannenberg, C.; Peter, S. H.; Eschmann, S. & Klopp, M. (2008). Computed tomography, positron emission tomography, positron emission tomography/computed tomography, and magnetic resonance imaging for staging of limited pleural mesothelioma: initial results. *Invest Radiol.*, Vol.43, pp.737-744. ISSN: 1536-0210.

Rusch, V. W. (1995). A proposed new international TNM staging system for malignant pleural mesothelioma. From the International Mesothelioma Interest Group. *Chest.*, Vol.108, pp.1122-1128. ISSN: 0012-3692.

Sorensen, J. B.; Ravn, J.; Loft, A.; Brenoe, J. & Berthelsen, A. K. (2008). Preoperative staging of mesothelioma by 18F-fluoro-2-deoxy-D-glucose positron emission tomography/computed tomography fused imaging and mediastinoscopy compared to pathological findings after extrapleural pneumonectomy. *Eur J Cardiothorac Surg.*, Vol.34, pp.1090-1096. ISSN: 1873-734X.

Steinert, H. C.; Santos Dellea, M. M.; Burger, C. & Stahel, R. (2005). Therapy response evaluation in malignant pleural mesothelioma with integrated PET-CT imaging. *Lung Cancer.*, Vol.49 Suppl 1, pp.S33-35. ISSN: 0169-5002.

Sterman, D. H. & Albelda, S. M. (2005). Advances in the diagnosis, evaluation, and management of malignant pleural mesothelioma. *Respirology.*, Vol.10, pp.266-283. ISSN: 1323-7799.

Swisher, S. G.; Erasmus, J.; Maish, M.; Correa, A. M.; Macapinlac, H.; Ajani, J. A.; Cox, J. D.; Komaki, R. R.; Hong, D.; Lee, H. K.; Putnam, J. B., Jr.; Rice, D. C.; Smythe, W. R.; Thai, L.; Vaporciyan, A. A.; Walsh, G. L.; Wu, T. T. & Roth, J. A. (2004). 2-Fluoro-2-deoxy-D-glucose positron emission tomography imaging is predictive of pathologic response and survival after preoperative chemoradiation in patients with esophageal carcinoma. *Cancer.*, Vol.101, pp.1776-1785. ISSN: 0008-543X.

Therasse, P.; Arbuck, S. G.; Eisenhauer, E. A.; Wanders, J.; Kaplan, R. S.; Rubinstein, L.; Verweij, J.; Van Glabbeke, M.; van Oosterom, A. T.; Christian, M. C. & Gwyther, S. G. (2000). New guidelines to evaluate the response to treatment in solid tumors. European Organization for Research and Treatment of Cancer, National Cancer Institute of the United States, National Cancer Institute of Canada. *J Natl Cancer Inst.*, Vol.92, pp.205-216. ISSN: 0027-8874.

Truong, M. T.; Marom, E. M. & Erasmus, J. J. (2006). Preoperative evaluation of patients with malignant pleural mesothelioma: role of integrated CT-PET imaging. *J Thorac Imaging.*,Vol. 21, pp.146-153. ISSN: 0883-5993.

Vansteenkiste, J. F.; Stroobants, S. G.; De Leyn, P. R.; Dupont, P. J.; Bogaert, J.; Maes, A.; Deneffe, G. J.; Nackaerts, K. L.; Verschakelen, J. A.; Lerut, T. E.; Mortelmans, L. A. & Demedts, M. G. (1998). Lymph node staging in non-small-cell lung cancer with FDG-PET scan: a prospective study on 690 lymph node stations from 68 patients. *J Clin Oncol.*, Vol.16, pp.2142-2149. ISSN: 0732-183X.

Veit-Haibach, P.; Schaefer, N. G.; Steinert, H. C.; Soyka, J. D.; Seifert, B. & Stahel, R. A. (2010). Combined FDG-PET/CT in response evaluation of malignant pleural mesothelioma. *Lung Cancer.*, Vol.67, pp.311-317. ISSN: 1872-8332.

Wahl, R. L.; Jacene, H.; Kasamon, Y. & Lodge, M. A. (2009). From RECIST to PERCIST: Evolving Considerations for PET response criteria in solid tumors. J Nucl Med., Vol.50 Suppl 1, pp.122S-150S. ISSN: 0161-5505.

Wilcox, B. E.; Subramaniam, R. M.; Peller, P. J.; Aughenbaugh, G. L.; Nichols Iii, F. C.; Aubry, M. C. & Jett, J. R. (2009). Utility of integrated computed tomography-positron emission tomography for selection of operable malignant pleural mesothelioma. *Clin Lung Cancer.*, Vol.10, pp.244-248. ISSN: 1938-0690

Yamamoto, Y.; Kameyama, R.; Togami, T.; Kimura, N.; Ishikawa, S. & Nishiyama, Y. (2009). Dual time point FDG PET for evaluation of malignant pleural mesothelioma. *Nucl Med Commun.*, Vol.30, pp.25-29. ISSN: 0143-3636.

Yildirim, H.; Metintas, M.; Entok, E.; Ak, G.; Ak, I.; Dundar, E. & Erginel, S. (2009). Clinical value of fluorodeoxyglucose-positron emission tomography/computed tomography in differentiation of malignant mesothelioma from asbestos-related benign pleural disease: an observational pilot study. *J Thorac Oncol.*, Vol.4, pp.1480-1484. ISSN: 1556-1380.

Young, H.; Baum, R.; Cremerius, U.; Herholz, K.; Hoekstra, O.; Lammertsma, A. A.; Pruim, J. & Price, P. (1999). Measurement of clinical and subclinical tumour response using [18F]-fluorodeoxyglucose and positron emission tomography: review and 1999 EORTC recommendations. European Organization for Research and Treatment of Cancer (EORTC) PET Study Group. *Eur J Cancer.*, Vol.35, pp.1773-1782. ISSN: 0959-8049.

12

Tumour Markers and Molecular Imaging with FDG PET/CT in Breast Cancer: Their Combination for Improving the Prediction of Disease Relapse

Laura Evangelista[1], Zora Baretta[1], Lorenzo Vinante[1],
Guido Sotti[1] and Pier Carlo Muzzio[1,2]
[1]*Istituto Oncologico Veneto, IOV – IRCCS, Padua*
[2]*University of Padua, Padua,*
Italy

1. Introduction

The aims of this chapter are to describe:

1. the actual role of tumour markers in the follow-up for breast cancer;
2. the use of tumour markers as an indicator of positron emission tomography (PET) execution and as a predictor of PET positivity;
3. the diagnostic accuracy of tumour markers, PET or PET/computed tomography (CT), and their combination;
4. the clinical and therapeutic impacts of tumour markers and nuclear medicine imaging;
5. the future prospective for breast cancer follow-up.

In this chapter we will bring together various reports on these subjects, and propose the use of tumour markers as a guide for the use of PET/CT, in particular to define the risk categories for breast cancer patients and the correct algorithm for follow-up.

2. Background

The definition of tumour markers is extremely broad, as tumour cells may express certain molecules at different rates from normal cells. These substances are released into the blood stream or other biological fluids. It would be justified to assert that biochemical measurement of the serum marker level in patients with a cancer diagnosis can give dynamic information about the clinical evolution of neoplastic processes and reflect the biological rather than the structural behaviour of the tumour. Even though their use in the follow-up of cancer patients has the advantages of being simple, objective, reproducible and cost-effective, the main problem is the lack of both sensitivity and specificity. In fact, the optimal tumour markers should only increase in the presence of a tumour and in the early phases of tumour growth, but none of the tumour markers currently available completely meet these requirements.

2.1 The role of serum markers in the management of patients with breast cancer

In breast cancer, the role of serum markers has remained unclear. Their potential uses in breast cancer include early diagnosis, determination of the prognosis, prediction of response or resistance to specific therapies, monitoring of the treatment in patients with metastatic disease and follow-up after primary treatment. Cancer antigen 15.3 (CA 15.3) and CA 27.29 are well-characterized assays that allow the detection of circulating MUC-1 antigen in peripheral blood. Carcinoembryogenic antigen (CEA) levels are less commonly elevated than the levels of MUC-1 assays, CA 27.29 or CA 15.3. Only 50% - 60% of patients with metastatic disease will have elevated CEA levels (sensitivity varies from 30 - 70% for visceral and skeletal metastases, with a positive predictive value ranging from 18% - 26%, respectively) compared to 75% - 90% who have elevated levels of the MUC-1 antigens. For this reason CA 15.3 is considered to be more specific than CEA in monitoring breast cancer evolution, and this latter marker is usually considered a poor predictor of breast cancer recurrence.

Unfortunately, aspecific elevation of both CEA and CA 15.3 can also be found in patients with inflammatory disease (e.g. diverticulitis, bronchitis), autoimmune disease (e.g. sarcoidosis) and other benign diseases (e.g. hepatitis, cirrhosis, hypothyroidism) in the presence of lung, gastrointestinal or neuroendocrine tumours, as well as in smokers and the elderly (Lumachi et al., 2004; Duffy et al., 2006).

Many attempts have been made in the past to provide evidence of the ability of CA 15.3 elevation at diagnosis to predict shorter survival rates, both disease-free and overall, but results are conflicting, and statistical significance was often lost at multivariate analysis. CA 15.3 is not therefore an independent prognostic factor in predicting the risk of recurrence, and it has no clinical value in the early detection of local recurrence or second cancer, due to low sensitivity in the presence of localized disease. The importance of detecting locally-recurrent breast cancer at an early stage arises from the fact that an increasing rate of distant metastases and a poor outcome are usually associated with local failure in breast cancer therapy (Fortin et al., 2006).

2.2 Monitoring response to treatment in breast cancer

Traditionally, the response to systemic treatment in patients with metastatic breast cancer is evaluated using criteria from the International Union Against Cancer (UICC). The UICC criteria includes physical examination, measurement of lesions, radiology and isotope scanning (Hayward et al., 1977). Two multi-centre trials, however, have shown that changes in serial concentrations of tumour markers correlate with therapy response based on the UICC criteria (Robertson et al., 1999; Van Dalen et al., 2004). Tampellini et al. (Tampellini et al., 2006) performed a large single institution study with the aim of measuring serum CA 15.3 at baseline, and at three and six months during anthracycline-based first-line chemotherapy in 526 patients with advanced breast cancer who had been prospectively enrolled in five phase II-III trials. A significant relationship between changes in CA 15.3 level and clinical response was found; and at multivariate analysis, CA 15.3 variation at six months was found to be an independent prognostic indicator for time to progression and overall survival. The early detection of disease progression and of resistance to ongoing treatment is considered an important issue in metastatic patients, because the target of therapy in this patient subset is the palliation. Therefore, tolerability and quality of life are fundamental in therapeutic decisions, and should be balanced against potential gains in disease regression and global survival. A lead time of 1-10 months has been reported when the assessment of treatment response, according to the UICC criteria, was made using blood markers. This finding can be explained by the fact that the international criteria reflect structural change: a metastasis needs to reach a significant size to be detectable by radiological exams; otherwise, blood tumour markers reflect the total tumour burden which is be measurable from the summation of numerous sub-clinical metastases (Cheug et al., 2000). Tumour markers can give important information concerning the response of cancer to ongoing treatment, even if they cannot be used alone for monitoring therapy in patients with advanced breast cancer. An increase of tumour markers can be detected even when the tumour has been responding to treatment; this phenomenon is known as a "tumour marker spike" (Yasasever et al., 1997; Hayes et al., 1988) and represents a transient increase in serum CA 15.3 levels following the initiation of effective therapy for metastatic disease. The peak usually occurs 15-30 days after the initiation of treatment, although spikes may last as long as 90 days. The return to a normal value, or to below baseline level, is consistent with response to therapy.

Although the studies available show encouraging data, the American Society of Clinical Oncology (ASCO) panel stated that CA 15.3 and CEA alone cannot be employed to define response to treatment (Harris L et al., 2007). Conversely, both the European Group on Tumour Markers (EGTM) and the National Academy of Clinical Biochemistry (NACB) panels recommend the use of CA 15.3 for monitoring therapy in patients with metastatic breast cancer (Molina et al., 2005; Fleisher et al., 2002).

2.3 Tumour markers and surveillance after primary treatment

In breast cancer, not only the use of serum markers, but also the follow-up in general, is not generally established. Two multi-centre randomized prospective trials (The GIVIO Investigators, 1994 and Rosselli et al. 1994), and a systematic review (Collins et al., 2004), compared the outcome in patients followed with clinical visits and mammography, with those followed up with an intensive regime including radiology and traditional laboratory testing. All reports concluded that the use of an intensive follow-up programme failed to improve either the outcome or quality of life. However, in these studies, some limitations with respect to management of patients with breast cancer are reported: 1) the use of old and insensitive biochemical tests and/or radiological exams, and 2) the unavailability of new treatments such as taxanes, aromatase inhibitors and trastuzumab for recurrence treatment (Duffy et al., 2006). The current ASCO guidelines recommend only careful history taking, physical examination and a regular mammography for appropriate detection of breast cancer recurrence (Khatcheressian et al., 2006). The purpose of an intensive follow-up with radiological exams and serial tumour markers determination is the early detection of recurrent or metastatic disease, which can enhance the chances of appropriate treatment and survival. Although serial CA 15.3 concentrations can anticipate the diagnosis of recurrent/metastatic disease with a lead time of between 2 - 9 months (Safi et al., 1989; Colomer et al., 1989; Nicolini et al., 1991; Repetto et al., 1993; al-Jarallah et al., 1993; Sölétormos et al., 1993), it is unclear whether the introduction of early treatment based on this lead time actually improves disease-free survival, overall survival, or quality of life for patients. In an attempt to address these issues, several small-scale studies have been carried out. In one of the first of these, Jager et al. (Jager et al.,

1995) randomized patients who had no evidence of metastatic disease, with increasing concentrations of tumour markers (CA 15-3 or CEA) to receive (n = 21) or not receive (n = 26) medroxyprogesterone acetate, reporting that for the untreated patients, the median time interval between increase in marker concentration and detectable metastasis was four months, while for the treated patients it was >36 months. Kovner et al. (Kovner et al., 1994) randomized asymptomatic patients with increasing mammary cancer antigen concentrations to receive (n = 23) or not receive tamoxifen (n = 26). After an average follow-up of 11 months, 7 out of 29 patients (24%) in the control group had relapsed, whereas none of the 23 patients who had received treatment developed a recurrence (p= 0.012). Nicolini et al. (Nicolini et al., 1997; 2004) compared the outcomes in 36 asymptomatic patients who received salvage treatment based on tumour marker increases (CA 15-3, CEA, or TPA) with 32 patients who were given treatment only after radiologic confirmation of metastasis. Survival from both the time of mastectomy and salvage treatment was significantly improved in the group with tumour marker–guided treatment than in those treated conservatively. These studies suggested that an early treatment of recurrent or metastatic disease based exclusively on an increase of tumour markers can improve the outcome, but the numbers of patients in the studies are too small to recommend this approach. In fact, the ASCO (Harris et al. 2007), the European Society of Clinical Oncology (Kataja et al., 2009) and the National Comprehensive Cancer Network (NCCN 2010) do not recommend their use. Furthermore, in some studies the value of tumour markers resulted positive in two thirds of patients with a recurrence of disease, while for the remaining third it either did not become positive or became positive late, thus showing both low sensitivity and positive predictive value (PPV) (Duffy et al., 2006; Anonymous et al., 1996). Therefore, in patients suspected of having a breast cancer relapse, low levels of markers do not exclude the presence of malignancy; whereas, high levels of markers almost certainly indicate the presence of metastatic disease (Soletormos et al., 2004; Given et al., 2000).

Sutterlin et al. (Sutterlin et al., 1999) evaluated 1228 serum samples from 664 women with a history of breast cancer, with accuracy and predictive values of CEA and CA 15.3. Seventy-six of the 664 women had had a relapse; the diagnostic accuracies of CEA and CA 15.3 were 83% and 88%, with a PPV of 27% and 47% and a negative predictive value (NPV) of 91% and 93%, respectively. The low PPV and sensitivity of CEA and CA 15.3 clearly limit their clinical utility. The effectiveness of routine determinations during the follow-up seems questionable, and the choice of the best marker is also unclear. Given et al. compared the diagnostic accuracy of CA 15.3, CEA and tissue polypeptide antigen (TPS) in the detection of breast cancer recurrences in 1448 patients (Given M et al., 2000). The results are summarized in **Table 1**:

	Sensitivity			**Specificity**			**PPV**			**NPV**		
	Vis	**Bone**	**Loc**	**Vis**	**Bone**	**Loc**	**Vis**	**Bone**	**Loc**	**Vis**	**Bone**	**Loc**
CA 15.3	68%	69%	23%	92%	92%	86%	47%	54%	22%	94%	96%	86%
TPS	64%	51%	17%	88%	88%	79%	25%	21%	16%	91%	93%	78%
CEA	27%	46%	11%	92%	92%	76%	18%	26%	13%	90%	92%	84%

Vis: visceral recurrence; Bone: bone recurrence; Loc: loco-regional recurrence; PPV: positive predictive value; NPV: negative predictive value

Table 1. A summary of results based on lesion sites

As shown in **Table 1**, the role of CA 15.3 as the tumour marker remains the better choice as it is useful as a predictor of recurrence in breast cancer, although it has low sensitivity and PPV for loco-regional recurrence, and neither TPS nor CEA complemented its sensitivity or PPV. In conclusion, even if expert panels have different positions on the matter, the actual main utility of CEA and CA 15.3 is in monitoring patients with advanced breast cancer, especially in women with non-valuable disease. Insufficient data has been published to suggest that the use of tumour markers during follow-up can change the course of breast cancer patients. Prospective randomized trials are needed to answer this question definitively.

3. Why is PET associated with tumour markers?

Multiple metastatic disease and a large tumour burden correlate with high marker values (Bast et al., 2001; Berruti et al., 1994).Metastatic disease, especially in the liver, bones and lungs, and metastatic pleural effusions, can give rise to pathological CA 15.3 values (Tampellini et al., 1997). Imaging modalities are important not only for seeing tumour lesions in the case of cancer , but also in evaluating the size of the tumour for staging and restaging assessment, in monitoring the therapy responses, and during follow-up (Ugrinska et al., 2002). The link between imaging and CA 15.3 can be found in the report by Tampellini et al. (Tampellini et al., 1997). The authors demonstrate that the supranormal value of CA 15.3 was positive more frequently in patients with liver metastases (74.6%), pleural effusion (75.7%), and oestrogen receptor (ER)-positive tumours, and in patients with a larger extent of the disease than in patient subgroups with recurrence in the bones (65%), lungs (61.8%) or soft tissue (47.1%). At multivariable logistic regression, the pleural effusion, ER status and disease extent were confirmed as independent variables in determining CA 15.3 positivity. Considering overall survival as the end-point, the multivariable survival analysis calculated with the COX regression model showed that ER status, disease extent and liver metastases were independent variables, and when the disease extent variable was removed, the CA 15.3 values became an independent variable associated with poor prognosis (Tampellini et al., 1997). Thus the extent of the disease represents a marker of poor prognosis, and the use of an imaging tool allows it to be assessed; however if this is not possible, tumour marker values can be used. An asymptomatic patient with elevated tumour markers is quite common in daily practice. Elevated tumour marker levels (both CEA and CA 15.3) are associated with an increased risk of recurrence (Nakamura et al., 2005), but localization of metastases or recurrent disease remains a challenge, which often requires an extensive diagnostic workup. The management of cancer patients has improved in the last few decades with the introduction of 18F-FDG PET (Zangheri et al., 2004). Tumour cells have an increased metabolism of glucose (Warburg et al. 1931), which has been shown to be true for breast cancer cells (Adler et al., 1993; Wahl et al., 1991; Nieweg et al., 1993; Avril et al., 2001). Glucose metabolism can be imaged by metabolic diagnostic modality, such as FDG PET. The imaging tool permits a complete tumour staging with a single whole-body investigation, even allowing the diagnosis of a significant number of metastases, which would be missed or incorrectly diagnosed by computed tomography (CT), magnetic resonance imaging (MRI) and bone scintigraphy. This indicates that a whole-body PET can be fundamental in the search for metastasis, especially when recurrences are suspected due to a progressive increase in circulating tumour markers (Hoh et al., 1999). Circulating tumour markers are biochemical products of the same alterations imaged by nuclear medicine (such as the overexpression and production of tumour-associated antigens on the membrane surface and in the bloodstream), or, alternatively, resulting from completely different pathways.

Recent data suggests that FDG PET is a useful technique for detecting recurrent breast cancer suspected on the basis of an asymptomatically elevated tumour marker level and negative conventional imaging results (Siggenkolw et al., 2004; Liu et al., 2002). In the last few years, PET/CT, as an integrated instrument for the evaluation of suspected disease relapse for various tumours (e.g. lymphomas), has become routinely used, showing to be superior to PET alone in re-staging the disease in patients who have been previously treated, particularly when the only indicator of recurrence is a rise in serum tumour markers (such as CA 15.3) (Suarez et al., 2002; Flamen et al., 2001). At present, as described by Siggelkow et al. (Siggelkow et al., 2004), PET should only be performed in cases where tumour marker is increasing and conventional imaging is unclear. In **Figure 1** are shown two examples of PET and PET/CT scan in breast cancer patients.

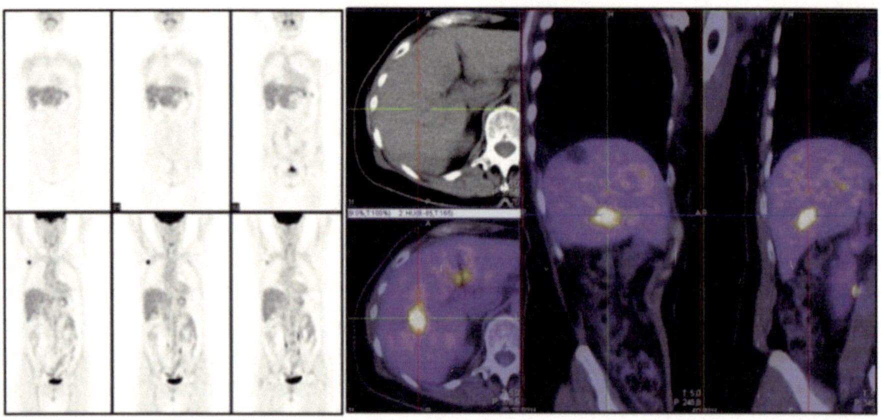

Fig. 1. Left: coronal images of PET scan. Right: PET/CT images on the three planes (transverse, sagittal and coronal)

4. A summary of articles concerning PET and PET/CT in patients with rising tumour markers

Elevated levels of tumour markers are frequently registered in the follow-up of breast cancer patients. This presents a diagnostic challenge, often requiring some conventional diagnostic tests to localize the metastases or recurrent disease. Cases of asymptomatic patients with elevated tumour marker levels have demonstrated a high rate of false-negatives with conventional morphological imaging modalities (Haug et al., 2007). In a review by Lamy et al. (Lamy et al., 2005), the authors summarized the results of a set of some studies in colorectal, breast and ovarian cancer. They stressed that one of the major indications of tumour marker is the detection of occult disease; less than 20% of tumour marker elevations are associated with clinical and radiological findings. Such elevations have led the medical community to doubt the value of tumour marker-based follow-up, such as CA 15.3 in breast cancer. PET with FDG using metabolic parameters of malignant cells allows tumour recurrences to be seen at the early stages of development, before any morphologic changes can be seen by radiological examinations. The authors underlined that, given the early positives they find, and that they are non-invasive and cost-effective, tumour markers have become an invaluable guide to the prescription of 18F-FDG PET in oncology, giving a 'map' of widespread disease. Suarez et al (Suarez et al., 2002) reported that values of CA 15.3 above 60 UI/ml were always associated with positive PET results and values below 50 UI/ml were accompanied by negative PET results. In the interval from 50 to 60 UI/ml the PET could be either positive or negative. Symptomatic patients, or those with suspected disease relapse, despite negative markers or both negative markers and CT, can nevertheless present with disease recurrence. Some authors have proposed that whole-body PET may become the method of choice for the assessment of asymptomatic patients with elevated tumour marker levels (Ugrinska et al., 2002; Siggelkow et al., 2004; Trampal et al., 2000). Shen et al. (Shen et al., 2003) screened 1283 patients who underwent whole-body FDG PET studies with the additional help of the serum levels of tumour markers. The final diagnoses were obtained by other imaging modalities of pathological findings. The authors concluded that the whole-body FDG PET, with the additional help of tumour markers, could reduce false negative and false positive results of FDG PET in all types of cancer.

In detail, we will consider an accurate description of various reports published concerning the employment of PET or PET/CT in the detection of breast cancer recurrence based on tumour marker levels, making some observations.

4.1 Tumour markers and PET alone

Lonneaux et al. (Lonneaux et al., 2000) were the first authors to evaluate the place of whole-body FDG PET in women presenting symptoms of recurrence, with a special focus on patients with an isolated increase in tumour markers. They studied 39 patients, 34 of whom were selected due to their increase in tumour markers. They found an overall sensitivity of 94%, specificity of 50%, NPV of 60%, PPV of 91% and accuracy of 87%. The high accuracy was related to the discovery of recurrence in 37 out of 39 patients (two false negative diseases were due to lymphedema of the arm and carcinomatosis that developed after some months). They demonstrated that FDG PET is useful in the evaluation of women suspected of a distant recurrence of breast cancer. PET allows for an earlier diagnosis of recurrence, which can lead to earlier therapy. As far as patient management is concerned, their results suggest that, as it is a non-invasive and highly sensitive imaging procedure, whole-body PET FDG should be performed as first line imaging when a recurrence of breast cancer is suspected on the basis of clinical symptoms or biological signs. In the second place, and only when patient management could be affected, dedicated and oriented CT or MRI could confirm precisely the anatomical localization of the sites with increased FDG uptake. Indeed there is no need for additional imaging procedures if PET shows disseminated bone disease or multiple lymph node metastases. On the contrary, the cases of equivocal PET findings should be checked by appropriate procedures.

Trampal et al. (Trampal et al., 2000) studied 72 patients with different types of cancer, 23 of whom had breast cancer. FDG PET detected lesions in 85% of the patients, and at the end of the study this was confirmed for 33 of the patients. PET sensitivity and specificity were 96.4% and 75.6%, respectively. They concluded that PET was an accurate tool in the diagnosis of recurrent tumoural disease in patients with rising tumour marker levels and negative conventional imaging, which could change the form of therapeutic management.

Pecking et al. (Pecking et al., 2000) reported that 1) blood tumour marker are widely used in the follow-up of patients treated for a malignant tumour and 2) in many cases where the tumour associated marker increases, the clinical and radiological evaluations remain normal. FDG PET and CT-scan have proven to be powerful tools in oncology, and their use in such situations may give a new appraisal on the development of the disease. They tested 70 patients with isolated increasing in tumour markers (CEA, CA 19.9, CA 15.3, CA 125). Focusing on breast cancer and CA 15.3, as well as ovarian cancers and CA 125, the sensitivity and predictive value reached 100%. Patients exhibiting a tumour target associated with an increase in blood tumour markers can be treated earlier with dedicated protocols. They concluded that where occult metastasis is detected by blood marker measurements, the tumour volume is smaller than when the patient presents overt symptoms; the treatment should therefore be more effective, and the use of imaging is advised. The same authors, after one year, (Peching et al., 2001) evaluated the efficacy of PET in clinically disease-free breast cancer patients in whom occult disease was suspected on the basis of increased blood tumour markers. They studied 132 patients who had received a totally negative follow-up evaluation, but who had a persistent increase in blood CA 15.3 confirmed by serial measurements. The confirmation of disease relapse was given by fine needle biopsy or surgical biopsy no later than two months later, or by imaging follow-up performed 6-12 months later. Ninety-two out of 119 eligible patients had a recurrence of disease after two months, while 102 out of 119 had a recurrence after 12 months, thus the sensitivity of PET/CT was 92.9% and 93.6%, respectively. The increase between the early and delayed recurrence of disease was more evident for specificity and PPV (30 vs. 60% and 86.8 vs. 96.2%) than accuracy (83.2 vs. 90.7%) and NPV (46.1 vs. 46.1%). Moreover, PPVs of PET increased with the serum CA 15.3 levels (diagnostic accuracy after 12 mo. was CA 15.3 <30 and ≤ 50 U/ml = 84.0% vs. serum CA 15.3 $>$ 75 U/ml = 90.3%). They concluded that when rising serum CA 15.3 is confirmed, positive FDG imaging can be significantly associated with recurrence, becoming significantly associated to recurrence or metastatic disease within one year ($p=0.036$ for 12 mo. vs. 0.046 for 2 mo.). Moreover, they suggested designing new therapeutic protocols based on positive FDG imaging in disease-free patients with an elevated serum CA 15.3 marker.

Spanish authors (Suarez et al., 2002) retrospectively studied 45 women with a histological diagnosis of breast cancer who had undergone a tumour marker-guided whole-body FDG PET. All patients were in remission, and without any other clinical symptoms or instrumental signs of relapse, except for the progressive elevation of CA 15.3 and/or CEA, tested during follow-up. FDG PET was obtained in 38 out of 45 patients, with 24 true-positives and 3 false positives. In total, 54 sites of FDG accumulation were revealed and 48 out of 54 patients were confirmed as metastases. The performances of tumour marker-guided FDG PET per patient were as follows: sensitivity = 92%, specificity = 78%, PPV = 89%, NPV = 82%, accuracy = 89%. They concluded that tumour marker-guided PET in the follow-up of breast cancer patients is of clinical utility. PET/CT was also able to identify three new neoplasms (ovary, contralateral breast and endometrium cancers). The inclusion of PET in the diagnostic algorithm allowed the clinical management to be modified (the change was shown in 24 out of 38 patients, or 63%) in those patients in whom a tumour relapse or unexpected primary neoplasm was discovered. It should be noted that tumour marker-guided PET led oncologists to adequate therapeutic decisions - performing different treatments - when three unknown primary cancers were detected.

Liu et al. (Liu et al., 2002) studied 30 patients with recurrent breast cancer after primary treatment. They evaluated both CA 15.3 and CEA, dosing the same day as FDG PET. They used the threshold of 32 UI/mL and 5 UI/mL respectively for CA 15.3 and CEA, useful to address PET. Employing this cut-off value, they found that PET had a high sensitivity and specificity (96 and 90%, respectively), identifying the presence of disease in 25 out of 28 recurrent patients, with only one false-negative result and two false positives. Their conclusion was that FDG PET is a useful technique for detecting recurrent breast cancer suspected from asymptomatically elevated tumour marker levels and negative or equivocal other imaging modality results.

Galloswitch et al. (Gallonswitch et al., 2003) studied 62 patients with breast cancer who were evaluated with both conventional imaging and FDG PET for disease relapse. A patient-based and lesion-based analysis was performed. The concordance of the conventional imaging and FDG PET were computed. Furthermore, patients were divided in two groups (with negative and positive tumour markers; CA 15.3 and CEA). PET in both subsets of patients showed a higher diagnostic accuracy than conventional imaging (87 vs. 90.3% and 61.5 vs. 90.3% respectively in patients with pathologic and normal tumour markers). They concluded that 18F-FDG PET demonstrates apparent advantages in the diagnosis of metastases in patients with breast cancer compared with conventional imaging on a patient base. On a lesion base, significantly more lymph nodes and fewer bone metastases can be detected using 18F-FDG PET compared with conventional imaging, including bone scan. Concerning bone metastases, sclerotic lesions are predominantly detected by bone scan. On the other hand, there are several patients with more FDG positive bone lesions and also mixed FDG positive/Tc-99m MDP negative and FDG negative/Tc-99m MDP positive metastases. In patients with clinically-suspicious, but negative, tumour marker profiles, FDG PET seems to be a reliable imaging tool for the detection of tumour recurrence or metastases.

Kamel et al. (Kamel et al., 2003) studied 43 breast cancer patients with suspected disease relapse. Twenty-five of those patients had available value of tumour markers that had been collected within two weeks of their PET scan. Among the 25 patients, 19 were proven to have disease relapse, while six patients were categorized as being free from any tumour-related manifestation. Eight patients with local recurrence (n=3), distant metastases (n=1), or both (n=4) did not show elevated values (an average of 12.4 U/ml) despite the true positive PET findings. However, in 11 patients both PET findings and tumour marker status (median 42 U/ml) indicated disease recurrence. Three of these 11 patients had characteristically increased value of CA 15.3 (1394 U/ml, 666 U/ml, 185 U/ml), and PET revealed extensive disease relapse, while four had normal tumour markers (an average of 16.6) and two had slightly elevated values (an average of 21.5 U/ml). FDG PET was more sensitive than serum marker CA 15.3 in detecting relapsed breast cancer, CA 15.3 levels were normal in eight out 19 (42%) patients with true positive PET findings.

Siggelkow et al., (Siggelkow et al., 2003) studied 35 patients suspected of having recurrent disease or elevated tumour markers. Depending on the region of suspicion, conventional imaging included chest X-ray, MRI, CT and US. All patients had had at least 12 months of follow-up treatment. In the patients who were examined due to elevated CA 15.3, PET was able to detect recurrence or metastatic disease in six of the eight patients (sensitivity = 75%). PET missed three tumour sites in three patients: two supraclavicular lymph node metastases and one lung metastasis. The overall sensitivity and specificity for PET for the whole series of patients was 80.6% and 97.6%, respectively. The same authors (Siggelkow et al. 2004) declared in a review that few studies have gathered sufficient data on the value of FDG PET in a patient with asymptomatically elevated tumour marker levels during follow-up for breast cancer.

Eubank et al. (Eubank et al., 2004) retrospectively analysed 125 consecutive patients with breast cancer with the aim of 1) evaluating the impact of FDG PET on defining the extent of disease and 2) evaluating the impact of FDG PET on patient management. The patients were referred for FDG PET for the following reasons: evaluation of disease response or viability after therapy (n=43; 35%), local recurrence with intent of aggressive local treatment (n=39; 31%), equivocal findings on conventional imaging (n=25; 20%), evaluation of the extent of the disease in patients with known metastases (n=13; 10%) and elevated tumour markers with unknown disease site (n=5; 4%). In this latter subset of patients, the authors found that PET enabled the therapeutic management to be changed in three out of five patients (60%); in particular, one patient received systemic therapy other than surgery (intermodality change) and two patients were treated with systemic chemotherapy (intramodality change). For the whole group, the overall sensitivity, specificity, and accuracy of FDG PET was 94%, 91% and 92%, respectively. The final conclusions of the study were: 1) FDG PET helped to define the extent of disease and determine the treatment plan in a significant number of patients with advanced breast cancer; 2) the treatment plan was altered by FDG PET findings most frequently in patients who had loco-regional recurrence and an increase in tumour markers.

The findings of the articles mentioned above are summarized in **Table 2:**

Study	**No. of patients/ proven recurrence**	**Sensitivity (%)**	**Specificity (%)**
Lonneux et al., 2000	33/31	-	-
Pecking et al., 2000	132/92	93.6	-
Liu et al., 2002	30/28	96	90
Suarez et al., 2002	38/27	92	75
Kamel et al., 2003	25/19	-	-

Table 2. A summary of current studies on the impact of FDGPET in patients with elevated tumour marker levels

Current reports univocally indicate that the use of FDG PET is rational in patients with asymptomatically elevated tumour marker levels and equivocal findings on conventional imaging. Both FDG PET and tumour marker status are biological tools that characterize the functional state of existing tumour tissue, but the tumour marker status was previously reported to be too insensitive to identify the existence of tumour tissue with a relatively smaller burden (Kokko et al., 2002). However, FDG PET is not sensitive enough for the detection of micrometastases, yet it remains the most accurate imaging device for early breast cancer recurrence detection. In fact, although FDG PET cannot rule out microscopic disease, it nevertheless has particular value in providing a reliable assessment of the true extent of the disease in a single examination (Vranjesevic et al., 2002; Haug et al., 2007).

4.2 PET *vs.* PET/CT and tumour markers

A PET scan alone has certain limitations, for example the exact localization of pathologically-increased focal glucose metabolism can be crucial, and physiological accumulation of FDG without precise anatomical localization can be misinterpreted as pathological. Conversely, CT permits exact anatomical localization of small physiological and pathological foci, but does not provide any information with regard to tissue metabolism. Combining both morphological and functional imaging technologies in a single scanner can be expected to overcome the respective limitations of CT, MRI, and PET, and provide the additional advantage of simultaneous data acquisition, obviating the need for patient repositioning, and so on. Haug et al. (Haug et al., 2007) studied patients with an isolated increase of tumour markers, who were asymptomatic but with suspected disease recurrence. Thirty-four patients were studied, five of whom were symptomatic and 29 asymptomatic. The authors compared PET, CT and PET/CT in a subset of patients with high levels of tumour markers (both CEA and CA 15.3), showing that the combined modality is associated with a higher diagnostic accuracy than when considered alone. PET/CT was able to identify 149 malignant foci in 24 patients (71%); CT identified 96 foci and PET 124 foci, in 18 and 17 patients respectively. The PET results were no different to the CT results, but both were significantly different from the PET/CT results (all $p<0.01$) (see **Table 3**).

	Sensitivity (%)	Specificity (%)
PET	88	78
CT	96	78
PET/CT	96	89

Table 3. Diagnostic accuracy of PET alone, CT alone and PET/CT

The authors concluded that PET/CT is a valuable modality for the follow-up of patients with suspected breast cancer relapse and elevated levels of tumour markers.

4.3 PET/CT and tumour markers

Fueger et al. (Fueger et al., 2005) made a comparison between PET and PET/CT for diagnostic accuracy and the advantages for patients with a recurrence of breast cancer. They studied 58 patients with suspected disease recurrence, including the elevation of tumour marker levels (21/58 patients). They suggested that integrated PET/CT restages breast cancer patients with a higher accuracy than PET alone, but only marginally ($p=0.059$). This observation emphasizes the need for a careful evaluation of the entire CT data set for an appropriate interpretation of PET/CT studies.

Saad et al. (Saad et al., 2005) in their retrospective study evaluated 35 patients with metastatic breast cancer. The results of PET/CT were compared with CA 27.29 and circulating tumour cells (CTC). A correlation between the results of PET/CT scans, CA 27.29 and CTC was found. CA 27.29 and CTC had poor sensitivity (59 and 55%, respectively) and NPV (24 and 33%, respectively) to detect metastatic disease observed on PET/CT scan, therefore PET remains the most sensitive test in detecting metastatic disease.

Radan et al. (Radan et al., 2006) retrospectively evaluated 47 patients with elevated tumour markers, 1 - 21 years from diagnosis. Thirty patients had had a recurrence of disease and 16 had not. Sensitivity, specificity and accuracy were 90%, 71% and 83%, respectively. PET/CT was compared to contrast enhancement CT demonstrating a higher sensitivity (85 vs. 70%), specificity (76 vs. 47%) and accuracy (81 vs. 59%). The impact of PET/CT on management was found in 51% of the patients. In conclusion, PET/CT had high performance indices and was superior to CT for the diagnosis of tumour recurrence in patients with breast cancer and rising tumour markers.

An Italian group (Grassetto et al., 2010) retrospectively studied 89 breast cancer patients with high values of CA 15.3 and inconclusive or negative PET/CT findings. Forty out of 89 patients (45%) had evidence of disease at FDG PET/CT, 23 had a solitary FDG-positive small lesion multiple cancer deposits were found in 14 of the 23 patients, and three patients were negative. The authors found that PET/CT may be able to detect occult metastatic and recurrent disease in post-therapy breast cancer patients with rising CA 15.3 levels and negative conventional imaging. They suggested that it could be reasonable to use tumour markers for guiding the performance of PET with the purpose of identifying the site of relapse in order to choose the most appropriate treatment.

Filippi et al. (Filippi et al., 2011) evaluated the role of FDG PET/CT in recurrent breast cancer detection in the presence of high levels of tumour markers and equivocal or negative conventional imaging. They studied 46 patients without any other clinical or laboratorial sign of disease; conventional imaging was negative in 29 patients and inconclusive in 17. FDG PET/CT resulted positive in 34 out of 46 patients. True-positive findings were found in 33 out of 46 patients (sensitivity = 86.8%, PPV = 97.1%) while false-positive and false-negative results were shown in six patients (specificity = 87.5%, NPV = 58.3%). The global diagnostic accuracy of PET/CT for disease detection was 86.9%. Change in clinical management was obtained in 50% of cases (23 out of 46), performing selective therapy in a number of patients. They concluded that the FDG PET/CT scan plays an important role in restaging breast cancer patients with rising tumour markers and negative or equivocal findings in conventional imaging techniques, with a consequent significant clinical impact on further management in these patients.

Champion et al. (Champion et al., 2011) studied 368 patients, 228 of whom had increased CA 15.3 and/or CEA. The cut-off value of CA 15.3 serum level was 60 UI/mL, as previously defined by various studies (Suarez et al., 2002; and Aide et al., 2007; Molina et al., 2005). The average CA 15.3 serum level was significantly higher in the true positive group than in the false negative one (166±115 vs. 77±52 UI/mL; $p<0.001$) and the true-negative one (166±115 vs. 65±56 UI/mL; $p<0.001$) **(Figure 2).** In asymptomatic patients with rising tumour markers, FDG PET/CT imaging is an accurate modality to screen for breast cancer recurrence. It is more sensitive than a conventional imaging workup; showing the extent of disease, it enables further treatment to be adjusted, proving a general picture in a high performance "one stop-shop" procedure.

In a study performed at our Nuclear Medicine Unit (Evangelista et al., 2011), we assessed the role of tumour markers, CT and 18F-FDG PET/CT in identifying disease relapse in patients with breast cancer which had already been treated, and the impact of PET/CT findings on patient management. We studied 111 patients with breast cancer with clinical-biochemical signs of loco-regional and distant recurrence of disease. Within three months, all patients performed CA 15.3, CT and PET/CT imaging for the evaluation of the extent of the disease. Recurrence was found in 32 out of the 111 patients, and PET/CT recognized the majority of patients with disease relapse, irrespective of the value of CA 15.3 and CT findings, identifying 81% of cancer recurrence and missing only 19%, with a gain of 30% toward tumour markers and 10% toward CT (see **Table 3**). The change in management was significantly important after PET/CT evaluation (change in 56% vs. 34%, respectively for PET/CT and CA 15.3). Furthermore, no advantage was obtained by reducing the value of the abnormal cut-off point of CA 15.3 from 31.0 to 19.1 U/mL, increasing the detection of recurrence by only 6%.

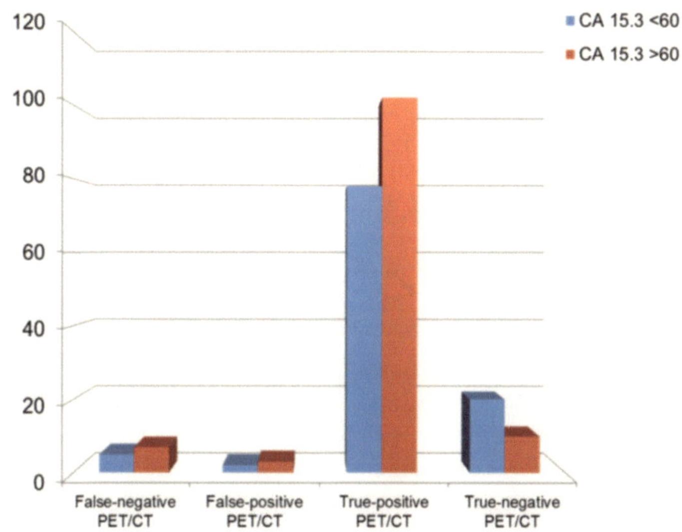

Fig. 2. A histogram showing the different groups of PET/CT results expressed as the number of patients against the CA 15-3 blood level (cut-off, 60 UI/mL) (from Champion et al., 2011).

	Sensitivity (%)	Specificity (%)	PPV (%)	NPV (%)	Accuracy (%)
Tumour markers	50	69	40	77	64
CT	72	37	32	76	47
PET/CT	81	62	41	87	60
Elevated tumour markers					
CT	69	93	50	72	60
PET/CT	88	33	47	80	55
Normal tumour markers					
CT	75	29	24	80	39
PET/CT	75	60	35	89	63

PPV, positive predictive value; NPV, negative predictive value

Table 3. Diagnostic accuracy of tumour marker (CA 15.3), CT and PET/CT in detecting relapse of disease

There is a general consensus in literature that steadily rising levels of CEA and CA 15.3 value must be regarded as a significant sign of change in tumour cell growth; this means that tumour marker determination during follow-up in breast cancer patients who have been radically operated on could anticipate the clinical diagnosis of cancer relapse. In our opinion, the use of PET/CT in patients with breast cancer could improve accuracy in the determination of the extent of the disease in case of an increase of tumour markers, but it is important to evaluate the trend of the increase in tumour marker rather than its single value. In fact, several non-cancerous conditions (benign breast or ovarian disease, endometriosis, pelvic inflammatory disease and hepatitis) can raise levels of CA 15.3, thus reducing the specificity of biochemical relapse; on the contrary, PET/CT can identify the disease before it becomes clinically manifested, even when the value of tumour markers is in a normal range.

5. Doubling timing and serial determinations

A discrepancy exists between the high positivity rate of serological markers in metastatic disease *vs.* the low positivity rate of serological markers in metastatic disease and the low positivity rate related to early relapse, when the results of tumour marker assays are interpreted by means of a dichotomous positive/negative cut-off point. This latter criteria, although easy to use and well accepted in clinical practice, is not powerful enough for the detection of early biological relapse: *a relevant quantity of tumour tissue is necessary to produce a sufficient quantity of tumour markers to exceed the cut-off point.* Dynamic interpretation based on serial samples might provide earlier diagnostic information, so a significant increase could be detected before exceeding the cut-off level, i.e. the difference between the values in three consecutive determinations should be at least two fold the inter-assay coefficient of variation (20%). The interval between the serial tests should be at least one month.

Mariani et al. (Mariani et al., 2009) recommended that the tumour markers should be considered as an indicator of disease presence, not only a tumour marker value above the normal limit (dichotomic criteria) but also a difference between two consecutive measurements greater than a critical value (dynamic criteria). Serial CA 15.3 measurements may be an efficient and cost-effective method of monitoring disease progression, and this is a potentially powerful means of obtaining information about breast cancer whilst causing minimal morbidity, inconvenience and cost (Buffaz et al., 1999). Both CA 15.3 and PET are based on metabolic changes due to tumour activity; they provide information on disease progression in a different way to conventional imaging. The advantage of adding PET or PET/CT in combination with constant elevation of CA 15.3 (15) could be translated into a more valuable method of identifying earlier metabolic changes (which is the basis of the PET principle) even before the morphological changes (noticeable with ultrasound and CT) occur.

Aide et al. (Aide et al., 2007) retrospectively evaluated 35 FDG PET examinations in 32 patients with CA 15.3 blood level above the normal range, and negative conventional imaging within three months before a PET exam. CA 15.3 assays were performed prior to the PET examinations and, all using the same techniques, were collected and used for doubling time calculation if 1) no therapeutic modification occurred in the meantime, and 2) the delay between assays was less than six months. Median CA 15.3 blood levels were higher in the positive PET group (100 U/ml) than in the negative group (65 U/ml) (p=0.04).

The likelihood of depicting recurrence was higher in patients with a short doubling time (<180 days) (p=0.05), a CA 15.3 blood level >60 U/ml (p=0.05), and when a short doubling time was associated with a CA 15.3 blood level >60 U/ml (p=0.03). The authors concluded that the likelihood of recurrence was influenced by CA 15.3 blood level and doubling time.

In our recent report (Evangelista et al., 2011) we assessed the relationship between serial measures of CA 15.3 and FDG PET/CT findings in the follow-up of patients who had already been treated for breast cancer. In sixty patients, three serial measures of CA 15.3 were collected within one year of the PET/CT examination. Coefficient of variation of the CA 15.3 serial determinations was significantly higher in patients with positive than negative PET/CT (39 vs. 24%, $p < 0.05$). ROC analyses showed that an increase of CA 15.3 between the second and third measures have better individuated positive PET/CT and disease relapse (AUC 0.65 and 0.64, respectively; $p < 0.05$). We concluded that an increase of CA 15.3 could be considered optimal in addressing FDG PET/CT examination during breast cancer patients' follow-up. PET/CT performed just on time might allow disease relapse in breast cancer patients to be detected earlier and with higher diagnostic accuracy.

6. The current recommendations according to the American and European societies

Approximately 30-50% of breast cancer patients have a recurrence of disease within ten years after diagnosis. Several international guidelines help physicians using tumour markers to give practical recommendations for the appropriate interpretation of circulating tumour markers. Due to low levels of evidence; the ASCO recommendations for the use of tumour markers do not support the determination of CA 15.3 during the follow-up of patients who have been treated for breast cancer, for monitoring the recurrence of disease (Harris et al., 2007). In clinical practice, disease relapse is suspected if there is positive clinical findings, the appearance of new lesions on imaging examinations, and/or unclear and persistent elevation of tumour markers. The "biochemical evidence" of a possible cancer relapse suggested by increased tumour markers leads oncologists to discover or exclude the sites of the cancer lesions through conventional radiological imaging techniques or nuclear medicine modalities (Strauss et al., 1991; Brown et al., 1996). The early individuation of disease relapse could improve the prognosis and allow for better management, through starting a new treatment or changing the ongoing therapy. Currently, according to ASCO guidelines (Khatcheressian et al., 2006), the follow-up of breast cancer patients should involve only physical examination and conventional mammography; whereas in the presence of new symptoms oncologists recommend performing conventional imaging, such as a chest-X ray, CT or MRI and PET scan. The European Group on Tumour Marker (EGTM) (Molina et al., 2005) panel suggests the following approach during the follow-up of asymptomatic women: tumour markers should be determined every two - four months (according to the risk of recurrence) during the initial five years after diagnosis, and at yearly intervals thereafter. This practice could be considered to be the most useful for monitoring disease development and reducing the lead time.

PET is a rapidly evolving field at both national and international level, with sometimes striking differences between its use in individual countries (Boellaard et al., 2009). The indications for PET and PET/CT are constantly changing, and require updating over time. Based on the current recommendations by the European Association of Nuclear Medicine (EANM guidelines), other than staging and restaging by PET/CT, establishing and localizing disease sites as a cause for elevated serum markers in some tumours (e.g. colorectal, thyroid, ovarian, cervix, melanoma, breast and germ-cell tumour) are also considered important aims.

7. Discussion

There are several patients in whom tumour marker levels are either high or progressively increasing, and neither physical examination nor diagnostic imaging are able to detect the tumour. In these cases the level of tumour markers (biochemical occult disease) serves as a guide to studying the patient with more powerful instruments (tumour marker-guided imaging) (**Figure 3**).

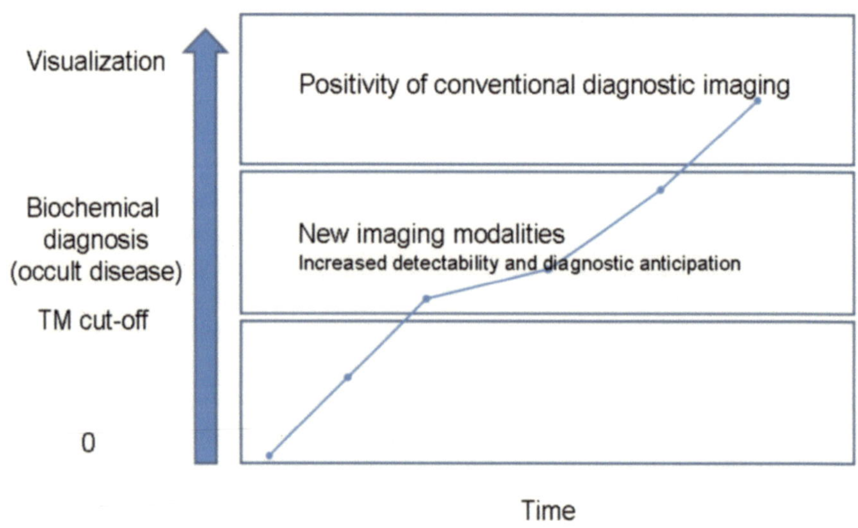

Fig. 3. The impact of technical implementation of diagnostic imaging (from Prof. Bombardieri Emilio, 1stImmunometry Congress ; 27 March 2009, Bari, Italy)

As previously mentioned, PET and PET/CT have proven to be useful imaging devices for earlier detection of disease recurrence, especially when tumour markers are increasing.

The main question is: when is the association of tumour markers and PET or PET/CT (tumour marker-guided imaging) useful? It is undoubtedly useful at early presentation for patients at high risk of metastases, in the diagnosis of tumour relapse/restaging, and for monitoring tumour response (Prof. Bombardieri Emilio, 1st Immunometry Congress ; 27 March 2009, Bari, Italy). In **Table 4** the advantages and limitations of tumour markers as a guide for PET/CT imaging are summarized:

	Added value	Limitations
Diagnosis of metastases at tumour presentation	PET seems more accurate than conventional imaging in the diagnosis of metastases at cancer presentation (in particular for internal chain lymph nodes).	PET usefulness is related to the stage of disease, being more accurate for stage II-III. The sensitivity of tumour markers is very low at early stages. tumour markers tests are not recommended at tumour presentation in low-risk patients.
Detection of recurrent Disease	Limited sensitivity of PET and tumour markers in depiction of loco-regional recurrences High accuracy (~90%) for the detection of metastatic disease.	Inadequate detection by PET of anatomical details. PET/CT overcomes this problem and increases the diagnostic accuracy (with a gain of ~ 10% in diagnostic accuracy, Haug et al., 2007).
Unclear elevation of tumour markers in asymptomatic patients during follow-up	High sensitivity (> 90%) for the detection of occult recurrence in asymptomatic patients with a progressive increase of tumour markers levels.	Some false negative results in breast cancer with low metabolism (lobular carcinoma). Additional conventional imaging is sometimes necessary.

Table 4. A summary of the advantages and limitations of tumour markers as a guide for PET/CT imaging (from Prof. Bombardieri Emilio, 1stImmunometry Congress ; 27 March 2009, Bari, Italy)

Tumour marker tests are a metabolic measure of tumour growth and tumour activity, and well integrate the metabolic imaging information. The association of tumour marker with PET/CT appears to be perfect giving qualitative and quantitative metabolic information, in particular tumour marker concentrations express the blood measure of the tumour products, and the pixel content of morphologic images is related to tumour uptake.

7.1 Considerations

1. In the majority of reports analysed, tumour marker-guided PET and PET/CT have shown a high diagnostic accuracy in the early detection of breast cancer recurrence;
2. PET and PET/CT can be considered to be accurate and powerful tools in detecting disease recurrence even when tumour markers are low or in a normal range;

3. The association of tumour markers and PET/CT also has an impact on patient management; many reports have described a change in planned therapy of about 50%. In a review, Yu et al. (Yu et al. 2007) discussed cancer biomarker development, opportunities for PET to elucidate tumour biology, and the potential role of PET in clinical research and practice. They underlined that the practice of oncology has been changing, with novel biologic agents broadening the therapeutic armamentarium. The concept of individualized cancer care, where therapies are selected based on the unique characteristics of the patient's tumour, is gaining favour as an approach to address the heterogeneity of cancer; for this reason they were incited to discover biomarkers with prognostic and predictive value to improve drug selection, alteration and cancer development. For this purpose, the combination of metabolic data and molecular imaging with PET or PET/CT is at the forefront of this critical field.

8. Conclusions

Tumour marker-guided PET during the follow-up of patients who have already been treated for cancer has not yet been investigated sufficiently. The questions to be solved are: 1) Can the combination of tumour markers and PET scans substitute all other conventional modalities currently used in follow-up? 2) Can this approach affect the survival of patients? Considering the need for stricter integration between laboratory tests and metabolic imaging, in particular FDG PET, we will hopefully be able to answer these questions in the near future.

However, the use of CA 15.3 tests in breast cancer follow-up could involve a considerable risk of over-diagnosis and lead time. When the test result is positive but there is no other confirmation of metastatic disease, decision-making is difficult as to whether to treat or not (Kokko et al., 2002).

As documented in the "Recommended Breast Cancer Surveillance Guidelines" adopted by ASCO, the achievement of survival benefit with clinical follow-up is one of the most important documents that did not confirm the necessary of more aggressive follow-up strategies (Levels of evidence). However, the majority of the studies were carried out 10-20 years ago when many of the current drug regimens were not available. The Association of Breast Surgery to The British Association of Surgical Oncology has noted the above report and made a number of recommendations. One of the most important recommendations states that "follow-up should be stratified according to disease risk". The follow-up management of breast cancer patients based on different risk category of recurrence should therefore be appropriately defined. We suggest considering three categories of patients:

1. Low risk of recurrence (ductal carcinoma in situ, DCIS; lobular carcinoma in situ, LCIS)
2. Intermediate risk (hormone receptor positive cancer; invasive ductal cancer, IDC; invasive lobular cancer; HER-2 negative cancer)
3. High risk (triple negative, advanced stage at diagnosis, cancer associated with familiar genetic mutations, and any remaining categories)

Figure 4 shows a possible clinical and diagnostic algorithm during follow-up:

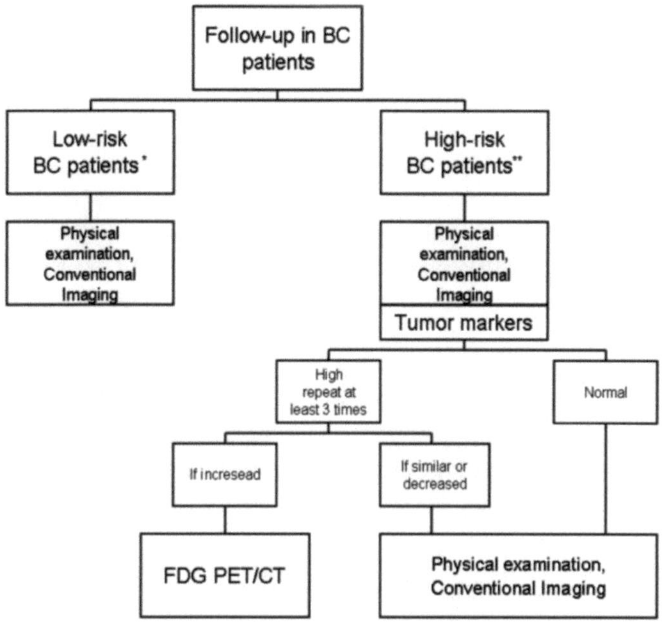

BC = breast cancer

Fig. 4. A follow-up algorithm in breast cancer patients based on risk category (*low-risk and **high risk breast cancer patients are referred to the above definitions)

The clinical experience in breast cancer management and different studies support the following concepts: a) a tumour marker test is not useful in the diagnosis of primary breast cancer, due to their very low sensitivity at cancer presentation; b) there is a correlation between CA 15.3 levels and the presence of bone and visceral metastases; c) the combination of tumour markers with diagnostic imaging can improve the diagnostic sensitivity and the PPV; d) tumour markers may be helpful in the interpretation of equivocal bone scans or any other equivocal imaging modality; e) bone scintigraphy cannot be precluded on the basis of normal tumour marker tests in the presence of suspicious skeletal metastases alone; f) some bone metabolic markers might be helpful in the evaluation of "flare phenomenon" and monitoring therapy response; g) even if tumour marker-guided PET still has to be extensively evaluated, the current experience demonstrates the potential of FDG-PET in discovering occult soft and bone metastases in the presence of a progressive increase of serum tumour markers (Ugrinska et al., 2002).

Some limitations of this article should be remembered: 1) many of the revised articles were retrospective; 2) we reported studies which considered both patients who underwent FDG PET alone and PET/CT imaging for increase in tumour markers, 3) the imaged field of view for whole-body PET/CT protocols is not already standardized and varies by institution (Huston et al. 2010), thus the heterogeneity of the analysis could be skewed the conclusions. Some considerations can be enhanced, firstly in literature there are not prospectively randomized studies which compared the standard follow-up procedures with new imaging technologies (e.g. FDG PET) and secondly the worldwide diffusion of hybrid PET/CT is approximately recent, thus reducing the available results.

9. The future prospective in the follow-up for breast cancer

In an editorial, Hortobangyi et al. (Hortobangyi et al., 2002) hypothesized that a multimodality therapy administered to a group of patients (1-3%) with limited metastatic breast cancer could produce long-term disease-free survival or cure. He concluded that, in this patient subset, the approach should be curative and not palliative. Consequently, intensive postoperative monitoring should be revisited, and large prospective trials are needed to identify the optimal candidates. Nevertheless, the subsequent ASCO guidelines (Khatcheressian et al., 2006) did not take in these indications. As previously mentioned, it is currently recommended that the follow-up of breast cancer patients involves only physical examination and conventional mammography; other examinations are recommended only in the presence of new symptoms. In the last few years we have seen great developments in the biological characterization of breast cancer and in diagnostic technology. These last improvements have profoundly changed breast cancer treatment but whether they can modify the follow-up for breast cancer treatment in the near future is still unclear. Breast cancer is a heterogeneous disease, showing many biological subtypes with different clinical features. For example, the positivity to hormone receptors requires different therapeutic management to the expression of human epidermal growth factor receptor 2 (HER2)-positive or a triple negative breast cancer; furthermore, the prognosis is differs widely from one case to another. Could the future strategy for breast cancer follow-up be adapted to biological characterization? Esserman et al. (Esserman et al., 2011)retrospectively evaluated the hormone receptor, the HER2-receptor and the grade from archival blocks of 23 years minimum follow-up breast cancer to establish if these features were related to risk and timing to recurrence. They observed that in 683 patients with negative-node involvement, the outcome risk for hormone receptor-positive and HER2-negative cancer was partitioned by tumour grade: lower grade cases had very low early recurrence risk but a 20% fall in ten or more years after diagnosis, and higher grade cases had a risk over 20 years. On the contrary, triple-negative and HER2-positive cancer showed a primary recurrence within the first five years, independently from the grade. Thus the recurrence of disease can be stratified based on cancer characteristics.

The site of relapse can also be different in these subtypes; e.g. Musolino et al. (Musolino et al., 2011) conducted a large epidemiological study, concluding that patients with HER2-positive breast cancer have a significantly higher incidence of central nervous system metastasis, especially after treatment with trastuzumab (Herceptin®). Concerning the loco-regional relapse, breast cancer subtypes have a different risk. Gabos et al. (Gabos et al., 2010)identified the hormone receptor negative/HER-2 positive status and the triple negative status as risks for local relapse, and suggested the possibility of a different follow-up and loco-regional treatment for these subtypes. Montagna et al. (Montagna et al., 2011) concluded that loco-regional relapse correlates with a high risk of subsequent events, and death in particular, in patients with the triple-negative subtype. Based on these observations, we can assume that a biological features based approach should be considered for follow-up too.

The technological development in diagnostic techniques could also have a role in follow-up changeling. Regarding conventional radiological imaging, MRI could have a role in surveillance especially for BRCA1 or BRCA2 positive breast cancer, but currently the best way to integrate mammography and breast MRI and their frequencies are unresolved areas of controversy. The major innovations come from nuclear medicine, e.g. the last introduction of hybrid devices (e.g. PET/CT and PET/MRI) useful for the evaluation of disease represents a great technology development. Furthermore, new devices such as positron emission mammography (PEM) represent a technological challenge both in primary diagnosis and in loco-regional recurrence, especially in women treated with conservative surgery. Moreover, the innovations from the radiopharmaceutical field with the introduction, in clinical practice, of new tracers such as 18F-fluoroestradiol (known as FES), which is mainly employed for evaluating the hormone receptor expression, a specific target for hormonal therapy.

10. References

Adler, L.P., Crowe, J.P., al-Kaisi, N.K. & Sunshine, J.L. (1993). Evaluation of breast masses and axillary lymph nodes with [F-18] 2-deoxy-2-fluoro-D-glucose PET. /Radiology, /Vol. 187, No. 3, (June 1993) pp. (743-750), ISSN

Al-Jarallah, M.A., Behbehani, A.E., el-Nass, S.A., Temim, L., Ebraheem, A.K., Ali, M.A. & Szymendera, J.J. (1993). Serum CA-15.3 and CEA patterns in postsurgical follow-up, and in monitoring clinical course of metastatic cancer in patients with breast carcinoma. /Eur J Surg Oncol. /Vol. 19, No. 1, (February 1993), pp. (74-9), ISSN

Aide, N., Huchet, V., Switsers, O., Heutte N., Delozier T., Hardouin A. &Badet S. (2007). Influence of CA 15.3 blood level and doubling time on diagnostic performances of 18F-FDG PET in breast cancer patients with occult recurrence. /Nucl Med Communication /Vol. 28, No. 4, (April 2007), pp. (267-272), ISSN

Anonymous. (1996). Clinical practice guidelines for the use of tumour markers in breast and colorectal cancer. Adopted on May 17, 1996 by the American Society of Clinical Oncology. /J Clin Oncol., /Vol. 14, No. 10, (October 1996), pp. (2843-2877), ISSN.

Avril, N., Menzel, M., Dose, J., Schelling, M., Weber, W., Jänicke, F., Nathrath, W. & Schwaiger, M. (2001). Glucose metabolism of breast cancer assessed by 18F-FDG PET: histologic and immunohistochemical tissue analysis. /J Nucl Med, /Vol. 42, No. 1, (January 2001), pp. (9-16), ISSN

Baum, R.P. & Przetak, C. (2001). Evaluation of therapy response in breast and ovarian cancer patients by positron emission tomography (PET). /Q J Nucl Med, /Vol. 45, No. 3, (September 2001), pp. (257-68), ISSN

Bast, R.C. Jr., Ravdin, P., Hayes, D.F., Bates, S., Fritsche, H. Jr.,m Jessup, J.M.; Kemeny, N.; Locker, G.Y.; Mennel, R.G. & Somerfield, M.R. American Society of Clinical Oncology Tumor Markers Expert Panel. (2001). Update of recommendations for the use of tumor markers in breast and colorectal cancer: clinical practice guidelines of the American Society of Clinical Oncology. /J Clin Oncol., /Vol. 15, No. 6, (March 2001), pp. 1865-78; PMID 11251019.

Berruti, A., Tampellini, M., Torta, M., Buniva, T., Gorzegno, G. & Dogliotti, L. (1994). Prognostic value in predicting overall survival of two mucinous markers: CA 15-3 and CA 125 in breast cancer patients at first relapse of disease. /Eur J Cancer, /Vol. 30A, No. 14, (1994), pp. (2082-2084). ISSN

Boellaard, R., O'Doherty, M.J., Wolfgang, A.W., Mottaghy, F.M., Lonsdale, M.N., Stroobants, S.G., Oyen, W.J.G., Kotzerke, J., Hoekstra, O.S., Pruim, J., Marsden, P.K., Tatsch, K.,

Hoekstra, C.J., Visser, E.P., Arends, B., Verzijlbergen, F.J., Zijlstra, J.M., Comans, E.F.I., Lammertsma, A.A., Paans, A.M., Willemsen, A.T., Beyer, T., Bockisch, A., Schaefer-Prokop, C., Delbeke, D., Baum, R.P., Chiti, A. & Krause, B.J. (2009). FDG PET and PET/CT: EANM procedure guidelines for tumour PET imaging: version 1.0. In Eur J Nucl Med Mol Imaging 2009. Available from https://www.eanm.org/scientific_info/guidelines/gl_onco_fdgpet.pdf

Brown, R.S., Leug, J.Y., Fisher, S.J., Frey, K.A., Ethier, S.P. & Wahl, R.L. (1996). Intratumoral distribution of treated-FDG in breast carcinoma: correlation between Glut-I expression and FDG uptake. / J Nucl Med, /Vol. 37, No. 6, (June 1996), pp. (1042-47), ISSN

Buffaz, P.D., Gauchez, A.S., Caravel, J.P., Vuillez, J.P., Cura, C., Agnius-Delord, C. & Fagret D. (1999). Can tumour marker assays be a guide in the prescription of bone scan for breast and lung cancers? /Eur J Nucl Med, /Vol. 26, No. 1, (January 1999), pp. (8-11), ISSN

Champion, L., Brain, E., Giraudet, A.L., Le Stanc, E., Wartski, M., Edeline, V., Madar, O., Bellet, D., Pecking, A. & Alberini, J.L. (2011). Breast cancer recurrence diagnosis suspected on tumor marker rising: value of whole-body 18FDG-PET/CT imaging and impact on patient management. /Cancer, /Vol. 15, No. 8, (April 2011), pp. (1621-1629), ISSN

Cheung, K.L., Graves, C.R. & Robertson, J.F. (2000). Tumour marker measurements in the diagnosis and monitoring of breast cancer. /Cancer Treat Rev, /Vol. 26, No. 2, (2000), pp. (91-102), ISSN

Colomer, R., Ruibal, A., Genollá, J., Rubio, D., Del Campo, J.M., Bodi, R. & Salvador, L. (1989). Circulating CA 15-3 levels in the postsurgical follow-up of breast cancer patients and in non-malignant diseases. /Breast Cancer Res Treat, /Vol. 12, No. 2, (March 1989), pp. (123-33), ISSN

Collins, R.F., Bekker, H.L. & Dodwell, D.J. (2004). Follow-up care of patients treated for breast cancer: a structured review. /Cancer Treat Rev, /Vol. 30, No. 1, (February 2004), pp. (19-35), ISSN

Duffy, M.J. (2006). Serum tumor markers in breast cancer: are they of clinical value? /Clin Chem, /Vol. 52, No. 3, (March 2006), pp. (345-51), ISSN

Esserman, L.J., Moore, D.H., Tsing, P.J., Chu, P.W., Yau, C., Ozanne, E., Chung, R.E., Tandon, V.J., Park, J.W., Baehner, F.L., Kreps, S., Tutt, A.N., Gillett, C.E. & Benz, C.C. (2011). Biologic markers determine both the risk and the timing of recurrence in breast cancer. /Breast Cancer Res Treat, /(May 2011), ISSN

Eubank, W.B., Mankoff, D., Bhattacharya, M., Gralow, J., Linden, H., Ellis, G., Lindsley, S., Austin-seymour, M. & Livingston, R. (2004). Impact of FDG PET on Defining the Extent of Disease and on the Treatment of Patients with Recurrent or Metastatic Breast Cancer. /AJR, /Vol. 183, No. 2, (August 2004), pp. (479-486), ISSN

Evangelista, L., Baretta, Z., Vinante, L., Cervino, A.R., Gregianin, M., Ghiotto, C., Saladini, G. & Sotti, G. (2011). Tumour markers and FDG PET/CT for prediction of disease relapse in patients with breast cancer. /Eur J Nucl Med Mol Imaging, /Vol. 38, No. 2, (January 2011), pp. (293-301), ISSN.

Evangelista, L., Baretta, Z., Vinante, L., Cervino, A.R., Gregianin, M., Ghiotto, C., Bozza, F. & Saladini, G. (2011). Could the serial determination of Ca15.3 serum improve the diagnostic accuracy of PET/CT? Results from small population with previous breast cancer. /Ann Nucl Med, /(April 2011), 2011, ISSN

Filippi, V., Malamitsi, J., Vlachou, F., Laspas, F., Georgiou, E., Prassopoulos, V. & Andreeou, J. (2011). The impact of FDG PET/CT on the management of breast cancer patients with elevated tumor markers and negative or equivocal conventional imaging modalities. /Nucl Med Commun, /Vol. 32, No. 2, (February 2011), pp. (85-90), ISSN

Flamen, P., Hoekstra, O.S., Homans, F., Van Custem, E., Maes, A., Stroobants, S., Peeters, M., Penninckx, F., Filez, L., Bleichrodt, R.P. & Montelmans, L. (2001) Unexpleined rising carcinoembryonic antigen (CEA) in the postoperative surveillance of colorectal cancer: The utility of positron emission tomography (PET). /Eur J Cancer, /Vol. 37, No. 7, (May 2011), pp. (862-869), ISSN

Fleisher, M., Dnistrian, A.M., Sturgeon, C.M., Lamerz, R. & Wittliff, J. (2002). Practice guidelines and recommendations for use of tumor markers in clinical applications. /AACC Press Chicago, /(2002), pp. (33-63), ISNN

Fortin, A., Larochelle, M., Laverdière, J., Lavertu, S. & Tremblay D. (1999). Local failure is responsible for the decrease in survival for patients with breast cancer treated with conservative surgery and postoperative radiotherapy. /J ClinOncol, /Vol. 17, No. 1, (January 1999), pp. (101-9), ISSN

Fueger, B.J., Wolfgang, A.W., Quon, A., Crawford, T.L., Allen-Auerbach, M.S., Halpern, B.S., Ratib, O., Phelps, M.E. & Czernin, J. (2005). Performance of 2-Deoxy-2-(F-18) fluoro-D-glucose Positron Emission Tomography and Integrated PET/CT in restaged Breast cancer patients. /Mol Imaging Biol, /Vol. 7, No. 5, (September-October 2005), pp. (369-76), ISSN

Gabos, Z., Thoms, J., Ghosh, S., Hanson, J., Deschênes, J., Sabri, S. & Abdulkarim, B. (2010). The association between biological subtype and loco-regional recurrence in newly diagnosed breast cancer. /Breast Cancer Res Treat, /Vol. 124, No. 1, (November 2010), pp. (187-94), ISSN

Gallowitsch, H.J., Kresnik, E., Gasser, J., Kumnig, G., Igerc, I., Mikosch, P. & Lind, P. (2003). F-18 fluorodeoxyglucose positron-emission tomography in the diagnosis of tumor recurrence and metastases in the follow-up of patients with breast carcinoma: a comparison to conventional imaging. /Invest Radiol, /Vol. 38, No. 5, (May 2003), pp. (250-6), ISSN

Given, M., Scott, M., McGrath, J.P. & Given, H.F. (2000). The predictive value of tumour markers Ca 15.3, TPS and CEA in breast cancer recurrence. /The Breast, /Vol. 9, No. 5, (October 2000), pp. (277-80), ISSN

Grassetto, G., Fornasiero, A., Otello, D., Bonciarelli, G., Rossi, E., Nashimben, O., Minicozzi, A.M., Crepaldi, G., Pasini, F., Facci, E., Mandoliti, G., Marzola, M.C., Al-Nahhas, A. & Rubello, D. (2011). (18)F-FDG-PET/CT in patients with breast cancer and rising Ca 15-3 with negative conventional imaging: A multicentre study. /Eur J Radiol,/ (May 2010), ISSN

Harris, L., Fritsche, H., Mennel, R., Norton, L., Ravdin, P., Taube, S., Somerfield, M.R., Hayes, D.F. & Bast, R.C. Jr. (2007). American Society of Clinical Oncology. American Society of Clinical Oncology 2007 update of recommendations for the use of tumor markers in breast cancer. /J Clin Oncol, /Vol. 25, No. 33, (November 2007), pp. (287-312), ISSN

Haug, A.R., Schmidt, G.P., Klingenstein, A., Heinemann, V., Stieber, P., Priebe, M., la Fougère, C., Becker, C. & Hahn, K. (2007). Tiling R.F-18-fluoro-2-deoxyglucose positron emission tomography/computed tomography in the follow-up of breast cancer with elevated levels of tumor markers. /J Comput Assist Tomogr, /Vol. 31, No. 4, (July-August 2007), pp. (629-34), ISSN

Hayes, D.F., Kiang, D.T., Korzum, A., Tondini, C., Wood, W. & Kufe, D. (1988). CA 15.3 and CEA spikes during chemotherapy for metastatic breast cancer. /Proc Am Soc Clin Oncol, /Vol. 7, (1988), pp. (38), ISSN

Hayward, J.L., Carbone, P.P., Heusen, J.C., Kumaoka, S., Segaloff, A. & Rubens, R.D. (1977). Assessment of response to therapy in advanced breast cancer. /Br J Cancer, /Vol. 35, No. 3, (March 1977), pp. (292-98), ISSN

Hoh, C.K. & Schiepers, C. (1999). 18FDG imaging in breast cancer. /Semin Nucl Med, /Vol. 29, No. 1, (January 1999), pp. (49-56), ISSN

Hortobagyi, G.N. (2001). Overview of treatment results with trastuzumab (Herceptin) in metastatic breast cancer. /Semin Oncol, /Vol. 28, No. 6, (December 2001), pp. (43–7), ISSN

Hortobagyi, G.N. (2002). Can we cure limited metastatic breast cancer? /J Clin Oncol, /Vol. 20, No. 3, (February 2002), pp. (620-3), ISSN

Huston, S.F., Adelmalik, A.G., Nguyen, N.C., Farghaly, H.R. & Osman, M.M. Whole-body 18F-FDG PET/CT: The Need for a Standardized Field of View-A Referring-Physician Aid. /J Nucl Med Technol,/Vol. 38, No.3, (September 2010), pp. 123-127, ISSN

Jager, W. (1995). Disseminated breast cancer: does early treatment prolong survival without symptoms? [abstract]. / Breast, /Vol. 4, (1995), pp.(65), ISSN

Kamel, E.M., Wyss, M.T., Fehr, M.K., von Schulthess, G.K. & Goerres, G.W. (2003). [18F]-Fluorodeoxyglucose positron emission tomography in patients with suspected recurrence of breast cancer. /J Cancer Res Clin Oncol, /Vol. 129, No. 3, (March 2003), pp. (147-53), ISSN

Kataja, V. & Castiglione, M. (2009). ESMO Guideline Working Group. Primary breast cancer: ESMO clinical recommendations for diagnosis, treatment and follow-up. /Ann Oncol, /Vol. 20, (May 2009), pp. (10-4), ISSN

Khatcheressian, J.L., Wolff, A.C., Smith, T.J., Grunfeld, E., Muss, H.B., Vogel, V.G., Halberg, F., Somerfield, M.R. & Davidson, N.E. (2006). American Society of Clinical Oncology 2006 Update of the Breast Cancer Follow-Up and Management Guidelines in the Adjuvant Setting. /J Clin Oncol, /Vol. 24, No. 31, (November 2006), pp. (1-7), ISSN

Kokko, R., Holli, K. &Hakama, M. (2002). Ca 15-3 in the follow-up of localized breast cancer: a prospective study. /Eur J Cancer, /Vol. 38, No. 9, (June 2002), pp. (1189-93), ISSN

Kovner, F., Merimsky, O., Hareuveni, M., Wigler, N. & Chaitchik, S. (1994). Treatment of disease-negative but mucin-like carcinoma-associated antigen-positive breast cancer patients with tamoxifen: preliminary results of a prospective controlled randomized trial. /Cancer Chemother Pharmacol, /Vol. 35, No.1, (May 1994), pp. (80-83). ISSN

Lamy, P.J., Comte, F. & Eberlè, M.C. (2005). Combined role of tumour markers and FDG PET in follow-up of cancer patients. /Bull Canc, /Vol. 92, No. 10, (October 2005), pp. (858-864), ISSN

Liu, C.S., Shen, Y.Y., Lin, C.C., Yen, R.F. & Kao, C.H. (2002). Clinical impact of 18F-FDG in patients with suspected recurrent breast cancer based on asymptomatically elevated tumour marker serum levels: a preliminary report. /Jpn J Clin Oncol, /Vol. 32, No. 7, (July 2002), pp. (244-247), ISSN

Lonneux, M., Borbath, I.I., Berlière, M., Kirkove, C. & Pauwels, S.Liu. (2000). The Place of Whole-Body PET FDG for the Diagnosis of Distant Recurrence of Breast Cancer. /Clin Positron Imaging, /Vol. 3, No. 2, (March 2000), pp. (45-49), ISSN

Lumachi, F. & Basso, S.M. (2004). Serum tumor markers in patients with breast cancer. /Expert Rev Anticancer Ther, /Vol. 4, No. 5, (October 2004), pp. (921-931), ISSN

Mariani, L., Miceli, R., Michilin, S. & Gion, M. (2009). Serial determination of CEA and CA 15.3 in breast cancer follow-up: an assessment of their diagnostic accuracy for the detection of tumour recurrences. /Biomarkers, /Vol. 14, No. 2, (March 2009), pp. (130-136), ISSN

Molina, R., Barak, V., van Dalen, A., Duffy, M.J., Einarsson, R., Gion, M., Goike, H., Lamerz, R., Nap, M., Sölétormos, G. & Stieber, P. (2005). Tumor markers in breast cancer-European Group on Tumor Markers recommendations. /Tumour Biol, /Vol. 26, No. 6, (November-December 2005), pp. (281-293), ISSN

Montagna, E., Bagnardi, V., Rotmensz, N., Viale, G., Renne, G., Cancello, G., Balduzzi, A., Scarano, E., Veronesi, P., Luini, A., Zurrida, S., Monti, S., Mastropasqua, M.G., Bottiglieri, L., Goldhirsch, A. & Colleoni, M. (2011). Breast cancer subtypes and outcome after local and regional relapse. /Ann Oncol, /(April 2011), ISSN.

Musolino, A., Ciccolallo, L., Panebianco, M., Fontana, E., Zanoni, D., Bozzetti, C., Michiara, M., Silini, E.M. & Ardizzoni, A. (2011). Multifactorial central nervous system recurrence susceptibility in patients with HER2-positive breast cancer: epidemiological and clinical data from a population-based cancer registry study. /Cancer,/ Vol. 117, No. 9, (May 2011), pp. (1837-46), ISSN

Nakamura, T., Kimura, T., Umehara, Y., Suzuki, K., Okamoto, K., Okumura, T., Morizumi, S. & Kawabata, T. (2005). Periodic measurement of serum carcinoembryonic antigen and carbohydrate antigen 15-3 levels as postoperative surveillance after breast cancer surgery. /Surg Today, /Vol. 35, No. 1, (2005), pp. (19-21), ISSN

National comprehensive Cancer Network (NCCN) Clinical Practice Guidelines in Oncology, Breast Cancer Version 2, 2010. www.nccn.org/professionals/physician-gls/f guidelines.asp

Nicolini, A., Colombini, C., Luciani, L., Carpi, A. & Giuliani, L. (1991). Evaluation of serum CA15-3 determination with CEA and TPA in the post-operative follow-up of breast cancer patients. /Br J Cancer, /Vol. 64, No. 1, (July 1991), pp. (154-158), ISSN

Nicolini, A., Anselmi, L., Michelassi, C. & Carpi, A. (1997). Prolonged survival by 'early' salvage treatment of breast cancer patients: a retrospective 6-year study. /Br J Cancer, /Vol. 76, No. 8, (1997), pp. (1106-11), ISSN

Nicolini, A., Carpi, A., Nichelassi, C., Spinelli, C., Conte, M., Miccoli, P., Fini, M. & Giardino, R. (2003). "Tumour marker guided" salvage treatment prolongs survival of breast cancer patients: final report of a 7-year study. /Biomed Pharmacother, /Vol. 57, No. 10, (December 2003), pp. (452-9), ISSN

Nieweg, O.E., Kim, E.E., Wong, W.H., Broussard, W.F., Singletary, S.E., Hortobagyi, G.N. & Tilbury, R.S. (1993). Positron emission tomography with fluorine-18-deoxyglucose in the detection and staging of breast cancer. /Cancer, /Vol. 71, No. 12, (June 1993), pp. (3920-25), ISSN

Pecking, A.P., Mechelany-Corone, C. & Pichon, M.F. (2000). 1959-1999: from serum markers to 18F-FDG in oncology. The experience of Renè-HugueninCenter. /Pathol Biol (Paris), /Vol. 48, No. 9, (November 2000), pp. (819-24). ISSN

Pecking, A.P., Mechelany-Corone, C., Bertrand-kermorgant, F., Alberini, J.L., Floiras, J.L., Goupil, A.& Pichon, M.F. (2001). Detection of occult disease in breast cancer using Fluorodeoxyglucose Camera-Based Positron Emission Tomography. /Clinical Breast Cancer, /Vol. 2; No. 3, (October 2001), pp. (229-34), ISSN

Radan, L., Ben-Haim, S., Bar-Shalom, R., Guralnik, L. & Israel, O. (2006). The role of FDG-PET/CT in suspected recurrence of breast cancer. /Cancer, /Vol. 107, No. 11, (December 2006), pp. (2545-51), ISSN

Repetto, L., Onetto, M., Gardin, G., Costanzi, B., Giudici, S., Vitello, E., Merlini, L., Naso, C., Tannini, C., Paganizzi, M., & at. (1993) Serum CEA, CA 15-3, and MCA in breast cancer patients: a clinical evaluation. /Cancer Detect Prev, /Vol. 17, No. 3, (1993), pp. (411-5), ISSN

Robertson, J.F., Jaeger, W., Syzmendera, J.J., Selby, C., Coleman, R., Howell, A., Winstanley, J., Jonssen, P.E., Bombardieri, E., Sainsbury, J.R., Gronberg, H., Kumpulainen, E. & Blamey, R.W. (1999). The objective measurement of remission and progression in metastatic breast cancer by use of serum tumour markers. European Group for Serum Tumour Markers in Breast Cancer. /Eur J Cancer, /Vol. 35, No. 1, (January 1999), pp. (47-53), ISSN

Rosselli Del Turco, M., Palli, D., Cariddi, A., Ciatto, S., Pacini, P. & Distante, V. (1994). Intensive diagnostic follow-up after treatment of primary breast cancer. A randomized trial. National Research Council Project on Breast Cancer follow-up. /JAMA, /Vol. 271, No. 20, (May 1994), pp. (1593-97), ISSN

Saad, A., Kanate, A., Sehbai, A., Marano, G., Hobbs, G. & Abraham, J. (2008). Correlation among (18F) Fluorodeoxyglucose Positron Emission Tomography/Computed Tomography, Cancer Antigen 27.29, and Circulating Tumor Cell Testing in Metastatic Breast Cancer. /Clinical Breast Cancer, /Vol. 8, No. 4, (August 2008), pp. (357-61), ISSN

Safi, F., Kohler, I., Röttinger, E., Suhr, P.& Beger, H.G. (1989). Comparison of CA 15-3 and CEA in diagnosis and monitoring of breast cancer. /Int J Biol Markers,/ Vol. 4, No. 4, (October-December 1989), pp. (207-14), ISSN

Shen, Y.Y., Su, C.T., Chen, G.J., Chen, Y.K., Liao, A.C. & Tsai, F.S. (2003). The value of 18F fluorodeoxyglucose positron emission tomography with the additional help of tumor markers in cancer screening. /Neoplasma, /Vol. 50, No. 3, (2003), pp. (217-21), ISSN

Siggelkow, W., Zimny, M., Faridi, A., Petzold, K., Buell, U. & Rath, W. (2003). The value of positron emission tomography in the follow-up for breast cancer. /Anticancer Res, /Vol. 23, No. 2C, (March-April 2003), pp. (1859-67), ISSN

Siggelkow, W., Rath, W., Buell, U. & Zimny, M. (2004). FDG PET and tumor markers in the diagnosis of recurrent and metastatic breast cancer. /Eur J Nucl Med Mol Imaging, /Vol. 31; No. 1, (June 2004), pp. (118-24), ISSN

Sölétormos, G., Nielsen, D., Schiøler, V., Skovsgaard, T., Winkel, P., Mouridsen, H.T. & Dombernowsky, P. (1993). A novel method for monitoring high-risk breast cancer with tumor markers: CA 15.3 compared to CEA and TPA. /Ann Oncol, /Vol. 4, No. 10, (December 1993), pp. (861-9), ISSN

Sölétormos, G., Nielsen, D., Schioler, V., Mouridsen, H. & Dombernowsky, P. (2004). Monitoring different stages of breast cancer using tumour markers CA 15.3, CEA and TPA. /Eur Journal of Cancer, /Vol. 40, No. 4, (March 2004), pp. (481-6), ISSN

Strauss, L.G. & Conti, P.S. (1991). The application of PET in clinical oncology. /J Nucl Med, /Vol. 32, (1991), pp. (623-48), ISSN

Suarez, M., perez-Casteion, M.J., Jimenez, A., Domper, M., Ruiz, G., Montz, R. & Carreras, J.L. (2002). Early diagnosis of recurrent breast cancer with FDG PET in patients with progressive elevation of serum tumor markers. /Q J Nucl Med, /Vol. 46, No. 2, (June 2002), pp. (113-21), ISSN

Sutterlin, M., Bussen, S., Trott, S. & Caffler, H. (1999). Predictive value of CEA and Ca 15.3 in the follow-up of invasive breast cancer. /Anticancer Res, /Vol. 19, No. 4A, (July-August 1999), pp. (2567-70), ISSN

Tampellini, M., Berruti, A., Gerbino, A., Buniva, T., Torta, M., Gorzegno, G., Faggiuolo, R., Cannone, R., Farris, A., Destefanis, M., Moro, G., Deltetto, F. & Dogliotti, L. (1997). Relationship between CA 15-3 serum levels and disease extent in predicting overall survival of breast cancer patients with newly diagnosed metastatic disease. /Br J Cancer, /Vol. 75, No. 5, (1997), pp. (698-702), ISSN

Tampellini, M., Berruti, A., Bitossi, R., Gorzegno, G., Alabiso, I., Bottini, A., Farris, A., Donadio, M., Sarobba, M.G., Manzin, E., Durando, A., Defabiani, E., De Matteis, A., Ardine, M., Castiglione, F., Danese, S., Bertone, E., Alabiso, O., Massobrio, M. & Dogliotti, L. (2006). Prognostic significance of changes in CA 15-3 serum levels during chemotherapy in metastatic breast cancer patients. /Breast Cancer Res Treat, /Vol. 98, No. 3, (August 2006), pp. (241-8), ISSN

The GIVIO Investigators. (1994). Impact of follow-up testing on survival and health-related quality of life in breast cancer patients. A multi-centre randomized controlled trial. /JAMA, /Vol. 271, No. 20, (May 1994), pp. (1587-92), ISSN

Trampal, C., Maldonado, A., Sancho Cuesta, F., Morales, S., Senor de Uria, C., Panades, G. & Ortega, F. (2000). Role of the positron emission tomography (PET) in suspected tumor recurrence when there is increased serum tumor markers. /Rev Esp Med Nucl, /Vol. 19, No. 4, (August 2000), pp. (279-87), ISSN

Ugrinska, A., Bombardieri, E., Stokkel, M.P., Crippa, F.& Pauwels, E.K. (2002). Circulating tumour markers and nuclear medicine imaging modalities: breast, prostate and ovarian cancer. /Q J Nucl Med, /Vol. 46, No. 2, (June 2002), pp. (88-104), ISSN

Van Dalen, A., Heering, K.J., Barak, V., Peretz, T., Cremaschi, A., Geroni, P., Kurebayashi, J., Nishimura, R., Tanaka, K., Kohno, N., Kurosumi, M., Moriya, T., Ogawa, Y. & Taguchi, T. (2004). Significance of serum tumor markers in monitoring advanced breast cancer patients treated with systemic therapy: a prospective study. /Breast Cancer, /Vol. 11, No. 4, (2004), pp. (389-95), ISSN

Vranjesevic, D., Filmont, J.E., Meta, J., Silverman, D.H., Phelps, M.E., Rao, J., Valk, P.E. & Czernin, J. (2002). Whole-body 18F-FDG PET and conventional imaging for predicting outcome in previously treated breast cancer patients. /J Nucl Med, /Vol. 43, No. 3, (March 2002), pp. (325–9), ISSN

Wahl, R.L., Cody, R.L., Hutchins, G.D. & Mudgett, E.E. (1991). Primary and metastatic breast carcinoma: initial clinical evaluation with PET with the radiolabeled glucose analogue 2-[F-18]-fluoro-2-deoxy-D-glucose. /Radiology, /Vol. 179; No. 3, (June 1991), pp. (765-70), ISSN

Warburg O. (1931). The Metabolism of Tumors. New York, NY: RR Smith, Inc: 129-169. ISSN

Yasasever, V., Dinçer, M., Camlica, H., Karaloğlu, D. & Dalay, N. (1997). Utility of CA 15-3 and CEA in monitoring breast cancer patients with bone metastases: special emphasis on "spiking" phenomena. /Clin Biochem, /Vol. 30, No. 1, (February 1997), pp. (53-6), ISSN

Yu, E.Y. &Mankoff, D.A. (2007). Positron Emission Tomography imaging as a cancer biomarker. /Expert Rev Mol Diag, /Vol. 7, No. 5, (September 2007), pp. (659-67), ISSN

Zangheri, B., Messa, C., Picchio, M., Gianolli, L., Landoni, C. & Fazio, F. (2004). PET/CT and breast cancer. /Eur J Nucl Med Mol Imaging, /Vol. 31, No. 1, (June 2004), pp. (135-42), ISSN

13

Glucose Uptake During Exercise in Skeletal Muscles Evaluated by Positron Emission Tomography

Hiroyuki Shimada
Section for Health Promotion, Department of Health and Medical Care,
Center for Development of Advanced Medicine for Dementia,
National Center for Geriatrics and Gerontology
Japan

1. Introduction

Traditionally, *in vivo* skeletal muscle function has been investigated with noninvasive techniques such as magnetic resonance (MR) imaging that can characterize the motion and mechanics of contracting skeletal muscle (Axel & Dougherty, 1989; Drace & Pelc, 1994; Pipe et al., 1991). Other techniques include kinetic analyses to examine muscle activity during walking and electromyography (EMG) to evaluate muscle activity as amplitude-based algorithms. However, these techniques are limited because MR cannot be used to measure the metabolic activity of skeletal muscle, and kinetic analyses cannot measure isolated synergistic muscular activities or provide information on the etiology of the metabolic cost of exercise. Moreover, EMG quantification requires normalization of EMG amplitude to the EMG amplitude of maximal voluntary contractions, which some elderly are unable to achieve (Stevens et al., 2003). In addition, surface EMG is inappropriate for evaluating the activities of deep muscles such as the gluteus minimus.

Recently, the use of positron emission tomography (PET) and [^{18}F]fluorodeoxyglucose (FDG) has emerged as a more satisfactory method for investigating cumulative muscle activity during exercise and providing images of the spatial distribution of skeletal muscle metabolism (Fujimoto et al., 2000; Kemppainen et al., 2002; Oi et al., 2003; Shimada et al., 2007; Tashiro et al., 1999). FDG PET analysis is a metabolic imaging modality that involves the detection of intracellular FDG-6-P using gamma ray emission (Phelps et al., 1979). FDG is a glucose analog that is taken up by glucose using cells from the circulation through glucose transporters 1–4. FDG enters the glycolysis pathway and is phosphorylated into FDG-6-phosphate by hexokinase (Sokoloff et al., 1977). Intracellular FDG-6-P accumulates as it is a poor substrate for glucose-phosphate isomerase which converts glucose to fructose, and it therefore escapes dephosphorylation (Bessell & Thomas, 1973). FDG can be used to assess cumulative muscle activity over an extended period of time because the half-life of ^{18}F is relatively long (109.8 min) compared with that of other positron-emitting tracers; however, transient measurements are impossible.

FDG PET is useful for comparing task-specific muscle activity because FDG uptake is closely correlated with exercise intensity (Fujimoto et al., 2003; Kemppainen et al., 2002; Pappas et al., 2001). Results of regression analyses between normalized biceps FDG uptake and the number of repetitions of elbow flexion performed with 2 and 10 lb weights showed statistically significant positive correlations for both the 2 lb and 10 lb weights. The ratio of the slopes of the regression lines for the 10 lb and 2 lb weights was 4.94, indicating an almost fivefold difference between the external forces produced by the elbow flexors for these two loads (Pappas et al., 2001).

In this chapter, we review the findings of previous studies to demonstrate the importance of FDG PET for exercise studies and the development of rehabilitation programs for the elderly.

2. Glucose uptake in skeletal muscles during walking

2.1 Characteristics of gait function in older adults

Healthy elderly people exhibit decreased muscle mass, strength, and power production compared with healthy young people (Gallagher et al., 1997; Klitgaard et al., 1990; Larsson et al., 1979; Lynch et al., 1999; Metter et al., 1997; Porter et al., 1997; Poulin et al., 1992; Thelen et al., 1996). These decreases result in a slower gait speed, shorter step length, shorter swing phase and less range of motion at the hip, knee, and ankle joints during walking (Crowinshield et al., 1978; Elble et al., 1991; Finley et al., 1969; Hageman & Blanke, 1986; Judge et al., 1993, 1996; Kerrigan et al., 1998; Murray et al., 1969; Ostrosky et al., 1994; Winter et al., 1990). Reduced gait function in older people is associated with a decreased ability to undertake the activities of daily living (Brach & VanSwearingen, 2002; Guralnik et al., 2000).

Kinesiological studies show that older adults perform locomotor tasks nearer their maximal torque-producing capabilities than young adults. This greater effort is associated with increased neural drive to the muscles responsible for walking and enhanced coactivation of opposing muscles (Hortobagyi & DeVita, 2000; Hortobagyi et al., 2003). In addition, increased age is associated with a redistribution of joint torques and power as older adults use their hip extensors more and their knee extensors and ankle plantar flexors less when walking than the young. Data suggests that healthy older adults produce 279% more work at the hip, 39% less work at the knee, and 29% less work at the ankle compared with healthy young adults during gait (DeVita & Hortobagyi, 2000). The localized increase in muscular activation in the elderly during sustained walking may cause decreased physical activity, not because of generalized exhaustion, but due to the onset of fatigue in particular muscles. Therefore, localized muscle energy expenditure is more important than global expenditure when considering control of movement in older people (O'Dwyer & Neilson, 2000). The older adults also exposed gait instability due to enhanced coactivation of opposing muscles during walking.

2.2 Differences in glucose metabolism between young and older adults during walking

Shimada et al. (2009b) compared the differences between the glucose uptakes of skeletal muscles during walking in young and older adults using FDG PET. In this study, 10 healthy young and older men walked on a treadmill for 50 min. Walking speed was maintained at 4.0 km/hr for younger subjects and between 1.86 and 3.54 km/h as achievable limits for older subjects. FDG (360 MBq) was injected 30 min after the start of walking. PET scans of the crista iliaca-planta region were conducted in six overlapping bed positions using a 7-min emission time per position and simultaneous attenuation correction. Glucose metabolism in the regions of interest (ROIs) was evaluated from the standardized uptake value (SUV) for FDG defined as follows:

$$SUV = C/D/w \tag{1}$$

where C (Bq/ml) represents the concentration of radioactivity in the tissue, D (Bq) is the injected dose, and w is body mass (Sadato et al., 1998).

SUV was significantly increased in the semitendinosus, biceps femoris, iliacus, gluteus minimus, gluteus medius, and gluteus maximus muscles of older adults. FDG uptake ratios of older adults to young adults were 3.02 in the semitendinosus, 3.19 in the biceps femoris, 1.66 in the iliacus, 1.64 in the gluteus minimus, 3.68 in the gluteus medius, and 3.05 in the gluteus maximus muscles (Shimada et al., 2009b). The data indicate there was inefficient activity of these muscles during walking in the older adults. Figure 1 shows representative FDG PET images in a young and an older adult.

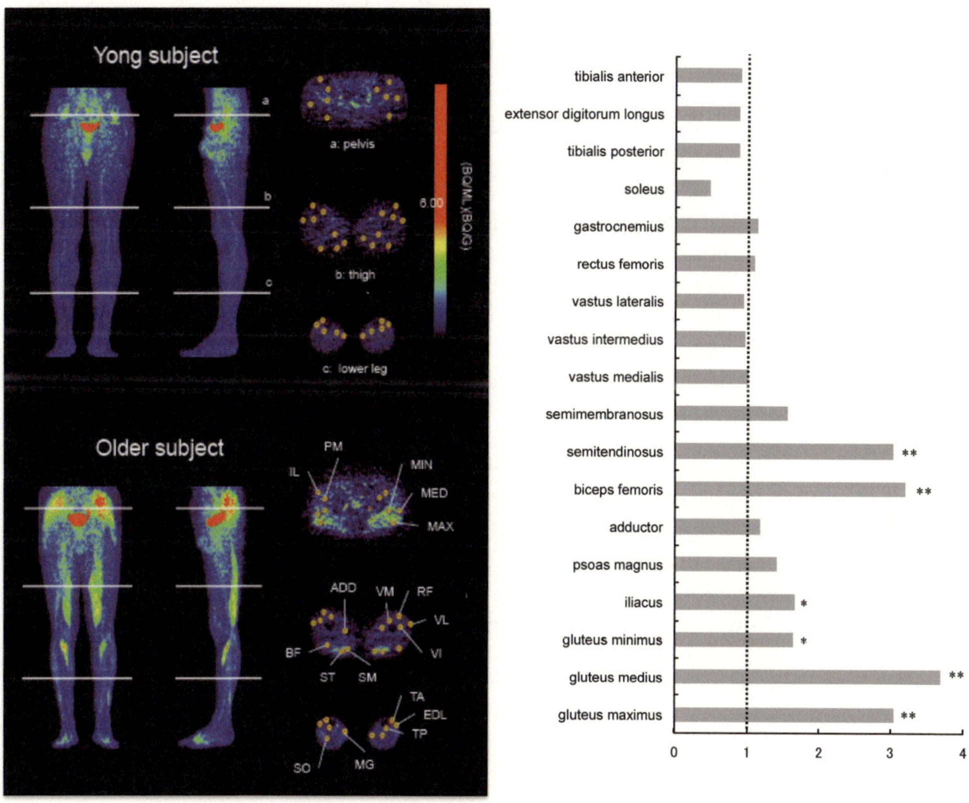

Fig. 1. FDG PET images taken after walking in a young and older subject.

Left panel: Projection and sectional images. The yellow circles indicate the following regions of interest: Section a (pelvis): 30 mm above the femoral head PM, psoas magnus; IL, iliacus; MIN, gluteus minimus; MED, gluteus medius; MAX, gluteus maximus. Section b (tight): 50% of the distance from the femoral head to the knee joint RF, rectus femoris; VL, vastus lateralis; VI, vastus intermedius; VM, vastus medialis; SM, semimembranosus; ST, semitendinosus; BF, biceps femoris; AD, hip adductor. Section c (lower leg): 30% of the distance from the knee joint to the external malleolus TA, tibialis anterior; EDL, extensor digitorum longus; TP, tibialis posterior; SO, soleus; MG, medial gastrocnemius. The red color at the center of the pelvis resulted from the accumulation of FDG in the bladder. Right panel: Graph showing FDG uptake ratios of older adults to young adults. Significant difference: $^*P < 0.05$ and $^{**}P < 0.01$.

During walking, the hamstrings are most active from the period just before to just after heel contact. Before heel contact, the hamstrings decelerate knee extension to prepare for the placement of the foot on the ground. The hamstrings are active during the initial 10% of the stance phase in walking to assist with hip extension and to provide stability to the knee through coactivation. Strong activation of the gluteus maximus allows the hip to extend and prevents forward jackknifing of the torso at heel contact. The gluteus maximus remains active from heel contact to mid stance to support the weight of the body and produce hip extension. The iliacus becomes active before toe off to decelerate hip extension. Concentric muscle activation follows eccentric muscle activation to bring the hip into flexion just before toe off and during transition into initial swing. The gluteus medius and minimus, the primary hip abductors, are most active during single-limb support to stabilize the pelvis in the frontal plane (Neumann, 2002).

A previous study showed that hip, knee, and ankle joint muscles produce 44, 5, and 51% and 16, 11, and 73% of the total extensor work during the stance phase in older and younger adults, respectively (DeVita & Hortobagyi, 2000). These data suggest that older adults perform similar amounts of work at the hip and ankle, but young adults perform the majority of work at the ankle (DeVita & Hortobagyi, 2000). In addition, coactivation time of the thigh muscles is higher in older people than in young people, and there is a linear correlation between the coactivation time and the metabolic cost during walking (Mian et al., 2006). The redistribution of joint power during walking in older adults increases glucose metabolism in the hip extensors (gluteus maximus, hamstrings) and coactivation increases glucose metabolism of the hamstrings.

The hip joint is stabilized by the gluteus medius in the initial phase of the gait cycle and by the gluteus minimus during the mid- and late-phases (Gottschalk et al., 1989). However, the degree of activation of the gluteus minimus muscle during walking is unclear because activities of deep muscles such as the iliacus and gluteus minimus cannot be evaluated by EMG. By contrast, FDG PET can measure the activity of deep muscles. FDG PET analyses showed glucose metabolism in the gluteus minimus during walking in young adults was 2.1 times higher than that at rest and higher than that of the gluteus maximus, gluteus medius, and thigh muscles (Oi et al., 2003).

3. Oxygen consumption and FDG uptake in skeletal muscles during exercise

3.1 Physical activity and oxygen consumption in older adults

Many studies have shown that there is an association between restricted outdoor activities and the deterioration of physical function in healthy and frail older people (Bruce & McNamara, 1992; Clarfield & Bergman, 1991; Fujita et al., 2006; Ganguli et al., 1996; Kono &

Kanagawa, 2001; Kono et al., 2004). A two-year prospective study in initially able-bodied older individuals showed an association between a low frequency of baseline outdoor activity and incident disability (Fujita et al., 2006). In older individuals who went outdoors once a week or less, the adjusted risks of incident mobility impairment (odds ratio = 4.02) and disability in instrumental activities of daily living (odds ratio = 2.65) were significantly higher compared with an active group who went outside once a day or more. Outdoor activity may be restricted in individuals who have difficulty walking for extended periods (Simonsick et al., 2005).

Muscle activity during exercise results in a mechanical energy cost, which is reflected by whole body metabolic cost. During physical activity, there is relatively greater muscle activity and increased levels of coactivation of opposing muscles in older people (Hortobagyi & DeVita, 2000; Hortobagyi et al., 2003). Furthermore, oxygen consumption (VO_2), which provides an index of walking efficiency, is greater in older adults even when there are no gait impairments (Malatesta et al., 2003; Martin et al., 1992; McCann & Adams, 2002; Waters et al., 1988). These data suggest that older adults may have difficulties in performing the activities of daily living as they have to work at a higher level of effort relative to their maximum capability (Hortobagyi et al., 2003).

3.2 Muscular activity and oxygen consumption

Unlike other techniques, FDG PET allows the observation of continuous activities such as extended walking and can measure cumulative muscle metabolism during unrestricted physical activities. Furthermore, FDG uptake closely correlates with exercise intensity in healthy adults and can be used to compare task-specific muscle activity (Fujimoto et al., 2003; Kemppainen et al., 2002; Pappas et al., 2001).

3.3 Relationship between FDG uptakes and VO_2

Few studies have investigated the relative contribution of different muscle groups to whole body energy consumption during walking. In one study, 10 community-dwelling older women participated in FDG PET and VO_2 analyses during exercise on separate days within one week (Shimada et al., 2010). VO_2 during walking was determined using an automated open-circuit gas analysis system (Cosmed K4b^2, Rome, Italy). The gas analyzers were calibrated immediately before each test using ambient air comprising certified standard gases at 15.94% oxygen and 4.97% carbon dioxide (Sumitomo Seika Chemicals Co., Ltd., Osaka, Japan). The subjects walked for 12 min at a comfortable speed on a circular 16 m indoor course and breath-by-breath data were obtained from the gas analyzers during walking, which was stored in the analyzer's memory. The mean VO_2 values from the 3rd to the 12th min were used to assess constant whole body energy metabolism (McArdle et al., 1997). All SUV values were adjusted for the distance walked during the 50 min FDG PET trial as:

$$\text{Adjusted SUV} = x \,/\, a \qquad (2)$$

where x represents the measured SUV, and a represents the walking distance in km.

The left and right panels show representative projection images of FDG PET uptake taken after walking. The scatterplot shows correlations between VO_2 and adjusted SUV for different muscle groups.

The VO_2 during walking was significantly and positively correlated with the adjusted SUV in the biceps femoris, gluteus minimus, gluteus medius, and the pelvis muscle group (Fig. 2; Shimada et al., 2010). This shows that these muscle groups contribute to the increase in VO_2 during walking in older adults. Evidence suggests the hamstrings, including biceps femoris, are most active from a period just before to just after heel contact during walking (Neumann, 2002). Furthermore, older adults display higher levels of antagonist coactivation during gross locomotor tasks (Hortobagyi & DeVita, 2000; Mian et al., 2006). Indeed, there is greater antagonist thigh muscle coactivation during walking in older men than young men and a linear relationship between muscle coactivation and whole body metabolic cost of walking (Mian et al., 2006).

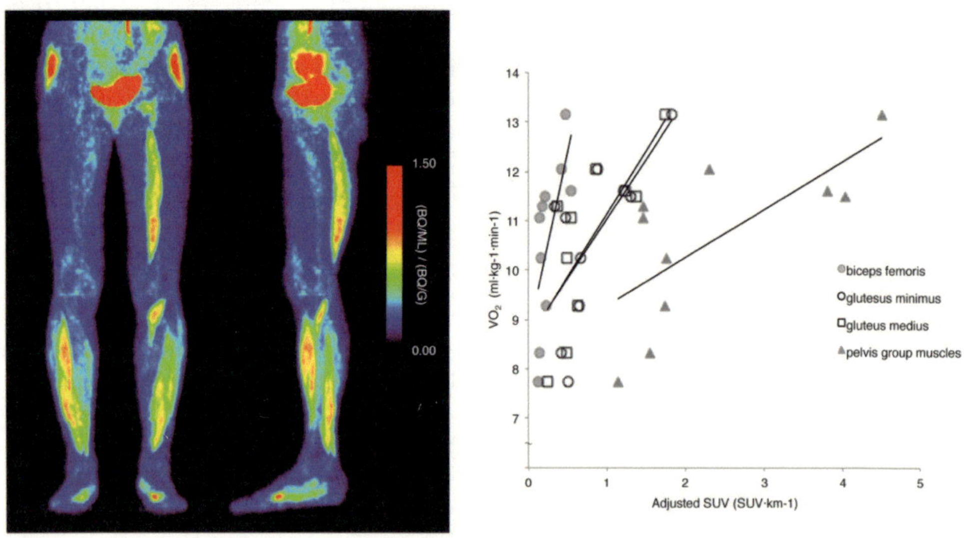

Fig. 2. Relationship between glucose uptake and VO_2 in older subjects.

Gait endurance contributes to the ability to perform the activities of daily living; however, information describing the fatiguing effect of daily activities on gait is limited. Previous studies indicate there is a relationship between muscle fatigue and physical function (Gribble & Hertel, 2004a,b; Helbostad et al.,2007; Kavanagh et al., 2006) as there are changes in gait step width, mediolateral trunk acceleration amplitude, step-length variability, and trunk acceleration variability in the vertical direction following physical fatigue induced by an atypical daily activity (i.e., sit-to-stand task), even in the absence of a change in gait speed (Helbostad et al.,2007). These gait variables are related to the incidence of falling in older people (Hausdroff et al., 2001; Maki, 1997; Mbourou et al, 2003).

The primary hip abductors, the gluteus medius and minimus, stabilize the pelvis in the frontal plane and are important for single-limb support (Neumann, 2002). During walking, the body is unstable for most of the stride cycle as its center of mass is outside the base of support 80% of the time (Winter, 1991). During walking in older people, mediolateral stability is generally reduced resulting in greater activation of the hip abductors compared with the young (Dean et al., 2007). Reduced mediolateral stability in older people can lead to an increased step width to avoid falling while walking at a preferred speed; a wider step width increases both mechanical work and metabolic energy expenditure (Donelan et al., 2001). A previous study showed older subjects selected a narrower step width when walking at a preferred speed on a treadmill with external lateral stabilization, and the energy cost with lateral stabilization was reduced in a zero step width condition i.e., tandem-like walking, compared with without stabilization (Dean et al., 2007). These findings are supported by observations of a significant relationship between the adjusted SUV in the hip abductors and VO_2.

A previous study showed that FDG uptakes by the biceps femoris, semitendinosus, iliacus, gluteus minimus, gluteus medius, and gluteus maximus muscles were significantly increased in older adults compared with young subjects (Shimada et al. 2009b). However, lower leg muscles such as tibialis anterior, tibialis posterior, and soleus had a ratio of less than one. These results suggest that the excess muscle activity of the larger thigh muscles contributes to the increase in VO_2 during walking in older adults.

Moreover, subjects with proportionally greater activity in their hip muscles had a higher VO_2 while walking compared with those with proportionally lower hip muscle activity. There may be a redistribution of muscle activity with aging; studies show increased work by the hip musculature in older adults is associated with decreased work by the musculature of the more distal joints (e.g. reduced power in plantar flexor) in both healthy older adults (DeVita & Hortobagyi, 2000; Judge et al., 1996) and older adults with a lower extremity disability (McGibbon & Krebs, 2002; McGibbon et al., 2001). FDG PET findings provide further evidence describing increased output by the hip musculature and introduce new information indicating that this increased output increases VO_2 in older adults during walking.

4. Evaluation of a walking aid using FDG PET

4.1 Importance of walking aids in older adults

Physical function is associated with the ability to perform the activities necessary for independent living without substantial risk of injury (Guralnik & Simonsick, 1993). Evidence suggests that impaired gaits in the elderly strongly affect their ability to perform daily activities (Brach & VanSwearingen, 2002; Guralnik et al., 2000); therefore, evaluation of gaits is an essential part of geriatric health and intervention programs. Kinesiological and epidemiological studies have shown that changes in gait scores such as decreased walking speed and stride length are associated with advanced age (Elble et al.,1991; Judge et al., 1996; Murray et al., 1969; Nagasaki et al., 1996; Nigg et al., 1994; Ostrosky et al., 1994; Winter et al., 1990). The age-related change in gait is characterized by a reduction in ankle power output during the terminal stance phase probably due to an age-related impairment in the power-generating capacity of the ankle which limits walking speed and stride length (McGibbon, 2003). In addition, the metabolic cost of walking is greater for the elderly than for young adults, even when there are no gait impairments (Malatesta et al., 2003; Martin et al., 1992; McCann & Adams, 2002; Waters et al., 1988). The increased metabolic cost of walking can impair the activity and quality of life of elderly people as a decrease in physical activity rapidly degrades physical and psychological functions (Backmand et al., 2006; Young et al., 1995).

There are many interventions that improve gait performance in non-disabled and disabled elderly people. Almost all these interventions include exercise programs to improve muscle strength or balance (Gillespie et al., 2003; Latham et al., 2003). Endurance in elderly people can also be improved by assisted devices such as canes or braces which affect gait speeds, stride lengths, and stability (Alexander, 1996; Joyce & Kirby, 1991; Kuan et al., 1999; Roomi et al., 1998; Van Hook et al., 2003). Shimada et al. developed an automated stride assistance system (Shimada et al., 2009a) (SAS) (Honda R & D Co. Ltd., Wako, Japan) (Figure 3), which uses robotic engineering to control walk ratios (stride length/cadence) and add supporting power to the thigh during walking. The SAS weighs 3.5 kg and it was developed to teach walking efficiency and improve gait endurance in elderly people with age-related short stride length. However, the SAS is limited because it supports movement of the hip joint during walking, which can lead to deterioration of muscle activity in the lower extremities during long-term intervention studies or practical applications.

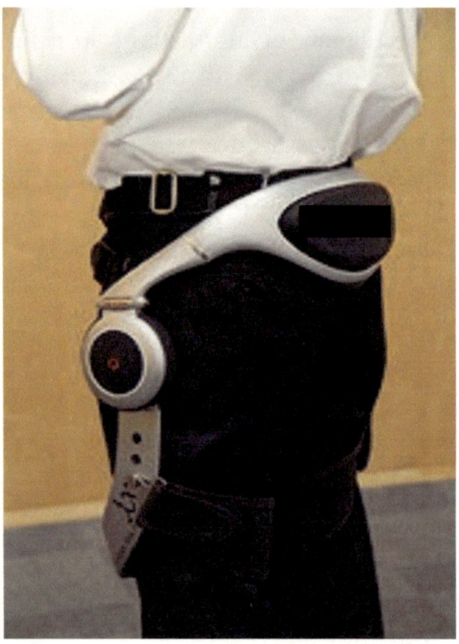

Fig. 3. Stride assistance system that can control walk ratios (stride length/cadence) and support the thigh during walking.

4.2 Muscular metabolism during walking using a robotic stride assistance system

FDG PET has been used to evaluate muscular activity during exercise with a stride assistance system (Shimada et al., 2007, 2008). In this research, 10 healthy younger men (mean age, 24.1 years) and 7 healthy older men (mean age, 76.0 years) completed FDG PET measurements twice after walking with and without the SAS. The sequence of the experiments was randomized to negate the confounding effect of prior experience of walking on a treadmill. Subjects were asked to walk for 50 min at 4.0 km/h on a treadmill (MAT-5500; Fukuda Denshi Co. Ltd., Tokyo, Japan). All young subjects walked at the target speed of 4.0 km/h. The speed of the treadmill was adjusted to 2.89–3.82 km/h without the SAS and 3.03–4.03 km/h with the SAS for the older subjects who could walk at a constant speed.

Figure 4 shows representative FDG PET images taken in young and older subjects after walking with or without the SAS. Glucose utilization in the lower-extremity muscles was evident after walking. In young subjects, walking with the SAS significantly increased FDG uptakes by the tibialis posterior and the medial gastrocnemius compared with walking without it (Shimada et al., 2007). FDG uptake ratios (SUV after walking with the SAS: SUV after walking without the SAS) of the tibialis posterior and medial gastrocnemius were 2.13 and 2.36, respectively. Walking with the SAS did not have significant effects on any other muscles. In older adults, there were no significant differences between the SUVs with and without the SAS in all lower-extremity muscles. However, walking speeds (mean walking speed without SAS, 3.46 km/h; mean walking speed with SAS, 3.56 km/h) and stride lengths (mean stride length without SAS, 54.9 cm, mean stride length with SAS, 58.2 cm) were

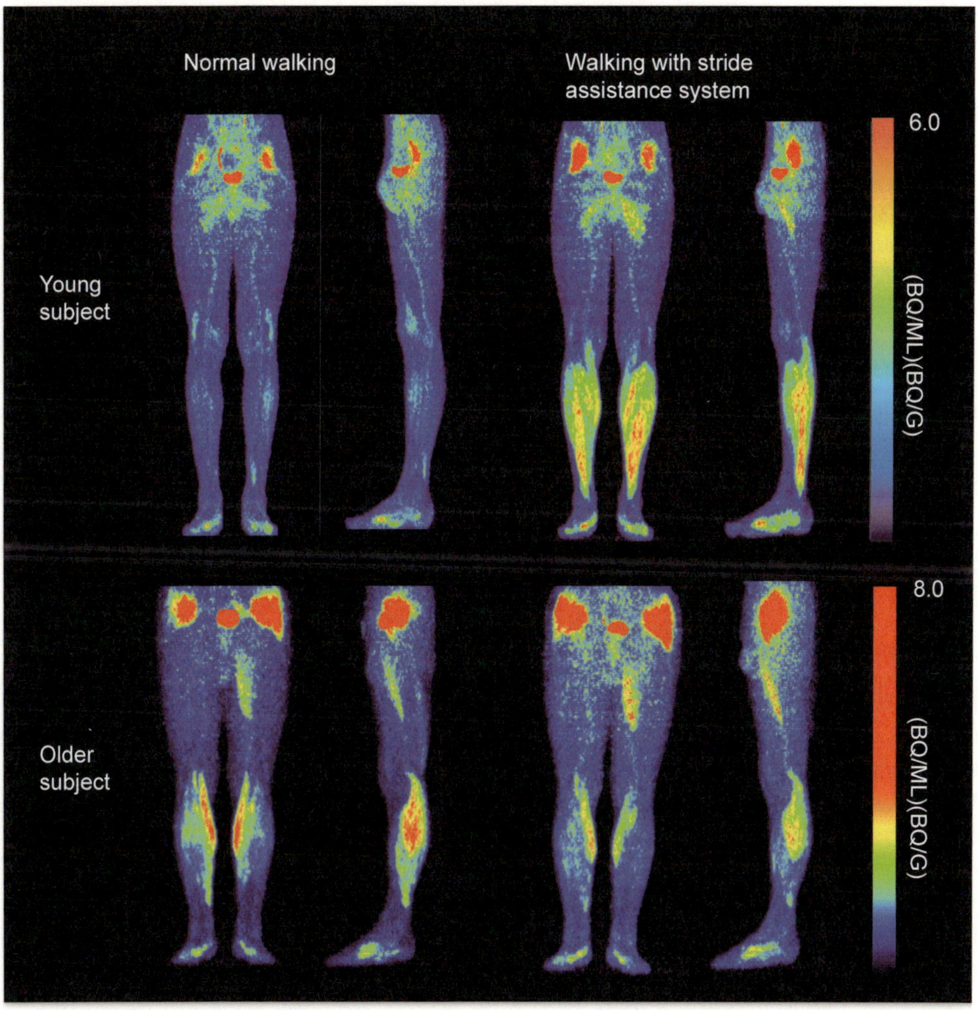

Fig. 4. FDG PET images taken after walking without or with the SAS.
The left and right panels show projection images taken after walking without or with the SAS, respectively.

significantly increased when walking on the treadmill with the SAS in the older subjects. These results suggest that the SAS can facilitate efficient walking patterns irrespective of muscle activity. The SAS may have provided assistance to the thigh and increased the torque of the hip of the older subjects resulting in improved walking scores. Therefore, stride length and walking speed increased without activating lower-extremity muscle activity.

5. Evaluation of exercise intervention using FDG PET

5.1 Effects of exercise in older adults

Older people enjoy walking exercise because it is familiar and more convenient than many other sports and recreational activities (Morris & Hardman, 1997; Mutrie & Hannah, 2004). Intervention studies show that strength or endurance training in older people can improve measures of gait such as walking speed (Binder et al., 2004; Brown & Holloszy, 1993; Buchner et al., 1997a; Ettinger et al., 1997; Judge et al., 1993). Endurance training also improves physical fitness, particularly cardiovascular fitness, as well as cognitive functions (van Uffelen et al., 2008). The development of targeted exercise programs may be facilitated by exercise intervention studies that allow a better understanding of the effects of muscle activity during walking. However, results from previous intervention studies investigating the effects of strength or endurance training on walking speed and gait are inconclusive (Buchner et al., 1997b; Ettinger et al., 1997). Walking is a near-perfect exercise for healthy and frail older people (Morris & Hardman, 1997); therefore, if walking induces walking-specific adaptations, interventions involving walking may be an efficient and appropriate means of improving walking function in older people (Shimada et al., 2003). However, knowledge of the effects of walking exercise on the physical performance of older people is limited. Most walking exercise interventions are prescribed in combination with exercises aimed at increasing muscle strength, neuromuscular coordination, and balance (Morris et al., 1999), and physical performance is not always assessed in intervention studies (Ebrahim et al., 1997).

5.2 Comparison of FDG uptakes in skeletal muscles before and after intervention

The functionality of walking may be improved by increasing the stride length of older people, which in turn may result in benefits such as improved walking efficiency. These benefits may supersede those derived from improved aerobic fitness alone. Shimada et al. (2009a) assessed the effects of a walking program for the elderly using the SAS. Fifteen subjects participated in a three-month walking program of two 90-min supervised sessions per week using the SAS. For FDG PET analysis, subjects walked for 50 min at a comfortable speed on a circular indoor walking track without the SAS. Figure 5 shows representative FDG PET images taken before and after the exercise intervention (Shimada et al., 2009a). FDG uptakes by the gluteus minimus, gluteus medius, and rectus femoris were significantly lower after the intervention than before, although walking speed during FDG PET measurements increased after the intervention. In contrast, the medial gastrocnemius and soleus (the lower distal muscles) showed higher FDG uptakes after the intervention than before, although the difference was not statistically significant.

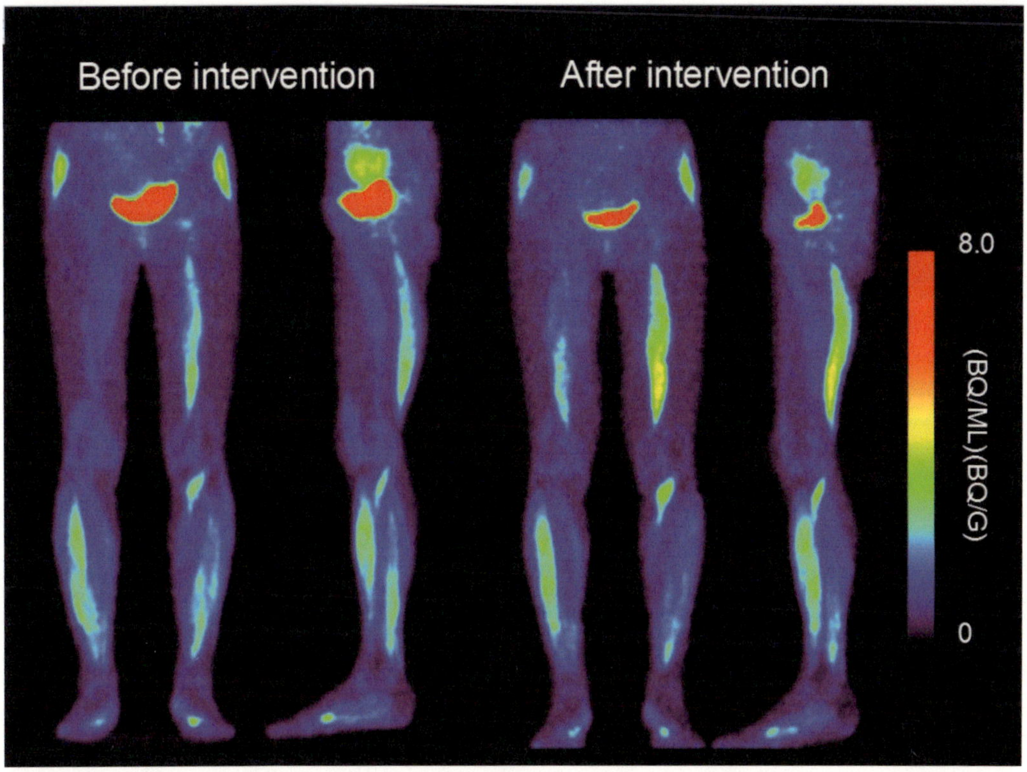

Fig. 5. FDG PET images of an older woman before and after the intervention.
The left and right panels show before and after intervention images, respectively. FDG uptakes by the gluteus minimus, gluteus medius, rectus femoris and pelvic muscles after the intervention were significantly lower than before.

The gluteus medius and gluteus minimus are the two primary hip abductors. They are most active during the first 40% of the gait cycle and they stabilize the pelvis in the frontal plane (Neumann, 2002). It is possible that the activity of the hip abductors decreases to improve mediolateral stability during long-distance walking. Further studies must be carried out using kinematic and kinetic analyses to fully understand the mechanisms involved in the change in cumulative muscle activity during prolonged walking.

Previous data indicate that the activity of hip-related muscles and hamstrings is greater than that of other lower extremity muscles in elderly people during walking. Shimada et al. 2009a found a significant decrease in the activity of the pelvic muscles (iliacus and gluteus muscles) during intervention with the SAS. However, the intervention did not increase FDG uptake of the soleus and gastrocnemius muscles, suggesting that the walking intervention improved the efficiency of muscle activity but did not redistribute muscular effort. This indicates that a walking intervention with the SAS has potential to increase walking endurance in the elderly. Indeed, the distance walked in 50 min after the intervention (median, 3579.0 m) was greater than that before the intervention (median, 3051.0 m); however, this difference was not statistically significant.

The quadriceps femoris controls knee flexion and acts as a shock absorber after heel contact; it then supports the weight of the body in mid-stance. The rectus femoris differs from that of other knee extensors as it is a hip flexor and its activity increases immediately after the toe-off phase (Neumann, 2002). A previous study showed that antagonist thigh muscle coactivation (e.g., activation of the vastus medialis, vastus lateralis, and biceps femoris) is 31% greater in older than in younger adults, and coactivation is moderately correlated with the metabolic cost of walking (Mian et al., 2006). The SAS automatically lends horizontal force to the thigh to facilitate an optimal walk ratio and may teach elderly people to use their muscles more efficiently. The consecutive stimuli provided by the SAS may help elderly people adopt an efficient walking pattern.

6. Functional FDG PET imaging as evaluating of frailty

Frail elderly people are particularly vulnerable for developing disabilities (Boyd et al., 2005; Gill et al., 2004; Hardy et al., 2005) and are at an increased risk for falls, disabilities, hospitalization, institutionalization and death, compared with their age-matched non-frail counterparts (Espinoza & Walston, 2005). Disability is closely related to medical spending; therefore, prevention of disability can lead to reduced health care costs (Cutler, 2001). Physical frailty indicators include mobility, strength, endurance, nutrition, physical inactivity, balance, and motor processing (Ferrucci et al., 2004). Gait disorder is a particularly important indicator of frailty and an independent predictor of disability. The findings of research using FDG PET has revealed a cycle of gait disorder (Figure 6).

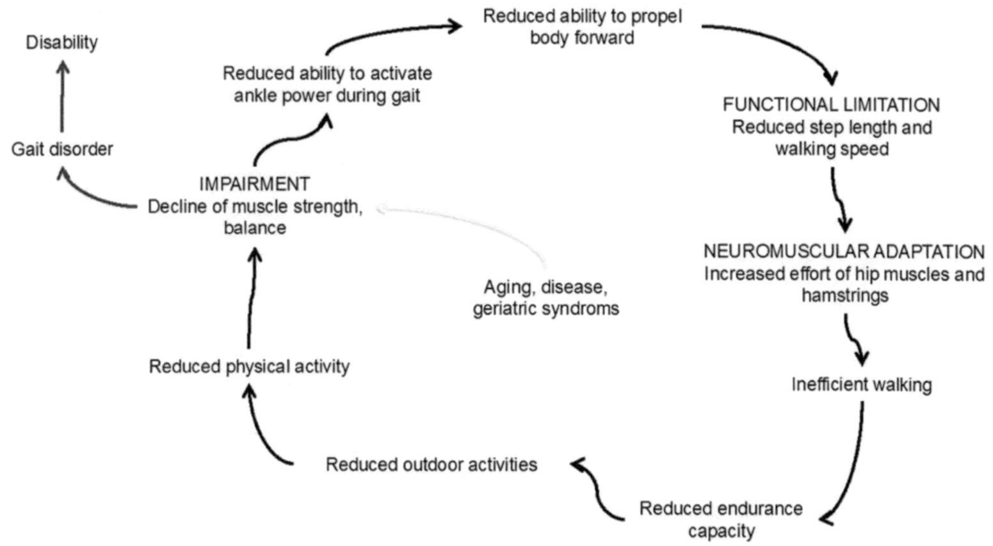

Fig. 6. Schematic diagram of the incidence of gait disorder in older adults.

Aging results in impaired muscle strength and balance, which reduces the ability to activate the ankle plantar muscles during gait and propel the body forward. These impairments manifest as functional limitations including reduced step length and walking speed, which are compensated for by neuromuscular adaptations such as increased effort of the hip muscles and hamstrings. Walking becomes inefficient and there is reduced endurance capacity. This leads to decreased involvement in outdoor activities and therefore physical activity, which worsens the impaired muscle strength and balance. Ultimately, the cycle can lead to gait disorder and disability.

7. Conclusions

FDG PET has proved useful for understanding the ability of older adults to perform physical activities. Because FDG uptake is closely correlated with exercise intensity, it can be used for comparing task-specific muscle activity. FDG PET and VO_2 analyses indicate that older adults may have difficulties in performing the activities of daily living as they have to work at a higher level of effort relative to their maximum capability due to a redistribution of muscle activity with aging. Automated exercise intervention, such as the automated stride assistance system (SAS), may help slow the cycle of events that ultimately can lead to gait disorder and disability. FDG PET evaluation of glucose metabolism in the muscles of the elderly following intervention with the automated SAS indicates that the SAS has the potential to increase walking endurance. We suggest that FDG PET is a useful method to evaluate the effects of interventions and therefore develop rehabilitation programs.

8. Acknowledgments

This work received financial support from a Grant-in-Aid for Scientific Research (B) (Tokyo, Japan). The funding source had no role in the study design, data collection, analysis, or writing of this manuscript.

9. References

Alexander, N.B. Gait disorders in older adults. *J Am Geriatr Soc*. 1996;44: 434-451.

Axel, L., & Dougherty, L. MR imaging of motion with spatial modulation of magnetization. *Radiology*. 1989;171: 841-845.

Backmand, H., Kaprio, J., Kujala, U.M., Sarna, S., & Fogelholm, M. Physical and psychological functioning of daily living in relation to physical activity. A longitudinal study among former elite male athletes and controls. *Aging Clin Exp Res*. 2006;18: 40-49.

Bessell, E.M., & Thomas P. The effect of substitution at C-2 of D-glucose 6-phosphate on the rate of dehydrogenation by glucose 6-phosphate dehydrogenase (from yeast and from rat liver). *Biochem J*. 1973;131: 83-89.

Binder, E.F., Brown, M., Sinacore, D.R., Steger-May, K., Yarasheski, K.E., & Schechtman, K.B. Effects of extended outpatient rehabilitation after hip fracture: A randomized controlled trial. *JAMA*. 2004;292: 837-846.

Boyd, C.M., Xue, Q.L., Simpson, C.F., Guralnik, J.M., & Fried, L.P. Frailty, hospitalization, and progression of disability in a cohort of disabled older women. *The American Journal of Medicine*. 2005;118: 1225-1231.

Brach, J.S., & VanSwearingen, J.M. Physical impairment and disability: relationship to performance of activities of daily living in community-dwelling older men. *Phys Ther*. 2002;82: 752-761.

Brown, M., & Holloszy, J.O. Effects of walking, jogging and cycling on strength, flexibility, speed and balance in 60- to 72-year olds. *Aging (Milano)*. 1993;5: 427-434.

Bruce, M.L., & McNamara, R. Psychiatric status among the homebound elderly: an epidemiologic perspective. *J Am Geriatr Soc*. 1992;40: 561-566.

Buchner, D.M., Cress, M.E., de Lateur, B.J., *et al.* A comparison of the effects of three types of endurance training on balance and other fall risk factors in older adults. *Aging (Milano)*. 1997a;9: 112-119.

Buchner, D.M., Cress, M.E., de Lateur, B.J., *et al.* The effect of strength and endurance training on gait, balance, fall risk, and health services use in community-living older adults. *J Gerontol A Biol Sci Med Sci*. 1997b;52: M218-224.

Clarfield, A.M., & Bergman, H. Medical home care services for the housebound elderly. *CMAJ*. 1991;144: 40-45.

Crowinshield, R.D., Brand, R.A., & Johnston, R.C. The effects of walking velocity and age on hip kinematics and kinetics. *Clin Orthop Relat Res*. 1978: 140-144.

Cutler, D.M. Declining disability among the elderly. *Health Aff (Millwood)*. 2001;20: 11-27.

Dean, J.C., Alexander, N.B., & Kuo, A.D. The effect of lateral stabilization on walking in young and old adults. *IEEE Trans Biomed Eng*. 2007;54: 1919-1926.

DeVita, P., & Hortobagyi, T. Age causes a redistribution of joint torques and powers during gait. *J Appl Physiol*. 2000;88: 1804-1811.

Donelan, J.M., Kram, R., & Kuo, A.D. Mechanical and metabolic determinants of the preferred step width in human walking. *Proc R Soc Lond B*. 2001;268: 1985-1992.

Drace, J.E., & Pelc, N.J. Measurement of skeletal muscle motion in vivo with phase-contrast MR imaging. *J Magn Reson Imaging*. 1994;4: 157-163.

Ebrahim, S., Thompson, P.W., Baskaran, V., & Evans, K. Randomized placebo-controlled trial of brisk walking in the prevention of postmenopausal osteoporosis. *Age Ageing*. 1997;26: 253-260.

Elble, R.J., Thomas, S.S., Higgins, C., & Colliver, J. Stride-dependent changes in gait of older people. *J Neurol*. 1991;238: 1-5.

Espinoza, S., & Walston, J.D. Frailty in older adults: insights and interventions. *Cleveland Clinic Journal of Medicine*. 2005;72: 1105-1112.

Ettinger, W.H., Jr., Burns, R., Messier, SP., *et al.* A randomized trial comparing aerobic exercise and resistance exercise with a health education program in older adults with knee osteoarthritis. The Fitness Arthritis and Seniors Trial (FAST). *JAMA*. 1997;277: 25-31.

Ferrucci, L., Guralnik, J.M., Studenski, S., Fried, L.P., Cutler, G.B., Jr., & Walston, J.D. Designing randomized, controlled trials aimed at preventing or delaying functional decline and disability in frail, older persons: a consensus report. *Journal of the American Geriatrics Society*. 2004;52: 625

Finley, F.R., Cody, K.A., & Finizie, R.V. Locomotion patterns in elderly women. *Arch Phys Med Rehabil*. 1969;50: 140-146.

Fujimoto, T., Itoh, M., Tashiro, M., Yamaguchi, K., Kubota, K., & Ohmori, H. Glucose uptake by individual skeletal muscles during running using whole-body positron emission tomography. *Eur J Appl Physiol*. 2000;83: 297-302.

Fujimoto, T., Kemppainen, J., Kalliokoski, K.K., Nuutila, P., Ito, M., & Knuuti, J. Skeletal muscle glucose uptake response to exercise in trained and untrained men. *Med Sci Sports Exerc*. 2003;35: 777-783.

Fujita, K., Fujiwara, Y., Chaves, P.H., Motohashi, Y., & Shinkai, S. Frequency of going outdoors as a good predictor for incident disability of physical function as well as disability recovery in community-dwelling older adults in rural Japan. *J Epidemiol.* 2006;16: 261-270.

Gallagher, D., Visser, M., De Meersman, R.E., *et al.* Appendicular skeletal muscle mass: effects of age, gender, and ethnicity. *J Appl Physiol.* 1997;83: 229-239.

Ganguli, M., Fox, A., Gilby, J., & Belle, S. Characteristics of rural homebound older adults: A community-based study. *J Am Geriatr Soc.* 1996;44: 363-370.

Gill, T.M., Allore, H., Holford, T.R., & Guo, Z. The development of insidious disability in activities of daily living among community-living older persons. *The American Journal of Medicine.* 2004;117: 484-491.

Gillespie, L.D., Gillespie, W.J., Robertson, M.C., Lamb, S.E., Cumming, R.G., & Rowe, B.H. Interventions for preventing falls in elderly people. *Cochrane Database Syst Rev.* 2003: CD000340.

Gottschalk, F., Kourosh, S., & Leveau, B. The functional anatomy of tensor fasciae latae and gluteus medius and minimus. *J Anat.* 1989;166: 179-189.

Gribble, P.A., & Hertel, J. Effect of lower-extremity muscle fatigue on postural control. *Arch Phys Med Rehabil.* 2004a;85: 589-592.

Gribble, P.A., & Hertel, J. Effect of hip and ankle muscle fatigue on unipedal postural control. *J Electromyogr Kinesiol.* 2004b;14: 641-646.

Guralnik, J.M., Ferrucci, L., Pieper, C.F., *et al.* Lower extremity function and subsequent disability: consistency across studies, predictive models, and value of gait speed alone compared with the short physical performance battery. *J Gerontol A Biol Sci Med Sci.* 2000;55: M221-231.

Guralnik, J.M., & Simonsick, E.M. Physical disability in older Americans. *J Gerontol.* 1993;48 Spec No: 3-10.

Hageman, P.A., & Blanke, D.J. Comparison of gait of young women and elderly women. *Phys Ther.* 1986;66: 1382-1387.

Hardy, S.E., Dubin, J.A., Holford, T.R., & Gill, T.M. Transitions between states of disability and independence among older persons. *American Journal of Epidemiology.* 2005;161: 575-584.

Hausdorff, J.M., Rios, D.A., & Edelberg, H.K. Gait variability and fall risk in community-living older adults: A 1-year prospective study. *Arch Phys Med Rehabil.* 2001;82: 1050-1056.

Helbostad, J.L., Leirfall, S., Moe-Nilssen, R., & Sletvold, O. Physical fatigue affects gait characteristics in older persons. *J Gerontol A Biol Sci Med Sci.* 2007;62: 1010-1015.

Hortobagyi, T., & DeVita, P. Muscle pre- and coactivity during downward stepping are associated with leg stiffness in aging. *J Electromyogr Kinesiol.* 2000;10: 117-126.

Hortobagyi, T., Mizelle, C., Beam, S., & DeVita, P. Old adults perform activities of daily living near their maximal capabilities. *J Gerontol A Biol Sci Med Sci.* 2003;58: M453-460.

Joyce, B.M., & Kirby, R.L. Canes, crutches and walkers. *Am Fam Physician.* 1991;43: 535-542.

Judge, J.O., Davis, R.B., 3rd, & Ounpuu, S. Step length reductions in advanced age: the role of ankle and hip kinetics. *J Gerontol A Biol Sci Med Sci.* 1996;51: M303-312.

Judge, J.O., Underwood, M., & Gennosa, T. Exercise to improve gait velocity in older persons. *Arch Phys Med Rehabil.* 1993;74: 400-406.

Kavanagh, J.J., Morrison, S., & Barrett, R.S. Lumbar and cervical erector spinae fatigue elicit compensatory postural responses to assist in maintaining head stability during walking. *J Appl Physiol.* 2006;101: 1118-1126.

Kemppainen, J., Fujimoto, T., Kalliokoski, K.K., Viljanen, T., Nuutila, P., & Knuuti, J. Myocardial and skeletal muscle glucose uptake during exercise in humans. *J Physiol.* 2002;542: 403-412.

Kerrigan, D.C., Todd, M.K., Della Croce, U., Lipsitz, L.A., & Collins, J.J. Biomechanical gait alterations independent of speed in the healthy elderly: Evidence for specific limiting impairments. *Arch Phys Med Rehabil.* 1998;79: 317-322.

Klitgaard, H., Mantoni, M., Schiaffino, S., *et al.* Function, morphology and protein expression of ageing skeletal muscle: A cross-sectional study of elderly men with different training backgrounds. *Acta Physiol Scand.* 1990;140: 41-54.

Kono, A., Kai, I., Sakato, C., & Rubenstein, L.Z. Frequency of going outdoors: a predictor of functional and psychosocial change among ambulatory frail elders living at home. *J Gerontol A Biol Sci Med Sci.* 2004;59: 275-280.

Kono, A., & Kanagawa, K. Characteristics of housebound elderly by mobility level in Japan. *Nurs Health Sci.* 2001;3: 105-111.

Kuan, T.S., Tsou, J.Y., & Su, F.C. Hemiplegic gait of stroke patients: the effect of using a cane. *Arch Phys Med Rehabil.* 1999;80: 777-784.

Larsson, L., Grimby, G., & Karlsson, J. Muscle strength and speed of movement in relation to age and muscle morphology. *J Appl Physiol.* 1979;46: 451-456.

Latham, N., Anderson, C., Bennett, D., & Stretton, C. Progressive resistance strength training for physical disability in older people. *Cochrane Database Syst Rev.* 2003: CD002759

Lynch, N.A., Metter, E.J., Lindle, R.S., *et al.* Muscle quality. I. Age-associated differences between arm and leg muscle groups. *J Appl Physiol.* 1999;86: 188-194.

Malatesta, D., Simar, D., Dauvilliers, Y., *et al.* Energy cost of walking and gait instability in healthy 65- and 80-yr-olds. *J Appl Physiol.* 2003;95: 2248-2256.

Maki, B.E. Gait changes in older adults: Predictors of falls or indicators of fear. *J Am Geriatr Soc.* 1997;45: 313-320.

Martin, P.E., Rothstein, D.E., & Larish, D.D. Effects of age and physical activity status on the speed-aerobic demand relationship of walking. *J Appl Physiol.* 1992;73: 200-206.

Mbourou, G.A., Lajoie, Y., & Teasdale, N. Step length variability at gait initiation in elderly fallers and non-fallers, and young adults. *Gerontology.* 2003;49: 21-26.

McArdle, D.W., Katch, I.F., & Katch, L.V. (1997). *Exercise Physiology: Energy, Nutrition, and Human Performance.* 4th ed. Williams & Wilkins, Baltimore, Maryland.

McCann, D.J., & Adams, W.C. A dimensional paradigm for identifying the size-independent cost of walking. *Med Sci Sports Exerc.* 2002;34: 1009-1017.

McGibbon, C.A. Toward a better understanding of gait changes with age and disablement: Neuromuscular adaptation. *Exerc Sport Sci Rev.* 2003;31: 102-108.

McGibbon, C.A., & Krebs, D.E. Compensatory gait mechanics in patients with unilateral knee arthritis. *J Rheumatol.* 2002;29: 2410-2419.

McGibbon, C.A., Krebs, D.E., & Puniello, M.S. Mechanical energy analysis identifies compensatory strategies in disabled elders' gait. *J Biomech.* 2001;34: 481-490.

Metter, E.J., Conwit, R., Tobin, J., & Fozard, J.L. Age-associated loss of power and strength in the upper extremities in women and men. *J Gerontol A Biol Sci Med Sci.* 1997;52: B267-276.

Mian, O.S., Thom, J.M., Ardigo, L.P., Narici, M.V., & Minetti, A.E. Metabolic cost, mechanical work, and efficiency during walking in young and older men. *Acta Physiol (Oxf)*. 2006;186: 127-139.

Morris, J.N., Fiatarone, M., Kiely, D.K., *et al.* Nursing rehabilitation and exercise strategies in the nursing home. *J Gerontol A Biol Sci Med Sci*. 1999;54: M494-500.

Morris, J.N., & Hardman, A.E. Walking to health. *Sports Med*. 1997;23: 306-332.

Murray, M.P., Kory, R.C., & Clarkson, B.H. Walking patterns in healthy old men. *J Gerontol*. 1969;24: 169-178.

Mutrie, N., & Hannah, M-K. Some work hard while others play hard. The achievement of current recommendations for physical activity levels at work, at home, and in leisure time in the west of Scotland. *Int J Health Promot Educ*. 2004;42: 109-107.

Nagasaki, H., Itoh, H., Hashizume, K., Furuna, T., Maruyama, H., & Kinugasa, T. Walking patterns and finger rhythm of older adults. *Percept Mot Skills*. 1996;82: 435-447.

Neumann, D.A. (2002). *Kinesiology of the musculoskeletal system: foundations for physical rehabilitation*. St. Louis, Missouri, Mosby.

Nigg, B.M., Fisher, V., & Ronskey, J.L. Gait characteristics as a function of age and gender. *Gait Post* 1994;2: 213-220.

O'Dwyer, N.J., & Neilson, P.D. (2000). Metabolic energy expenditure and accuracy in movement: Relation to levels of muscle and cardiorespiratory activation and the sense of effort. In: *Energetics of human activity. Human Kinetics*. W.A. Sparrow, (Ed.), 1-42, Champaign, IL.

Oi, N., Iwaya, T., Itoh, M., Yamaguchi, K., Tobimatsu, Y., & Fujimoto, T. FDG-PET imaging of lower extremity muscular activity during level walking. *J Orthop Sci*. 2003;8: 55-61.

Ostrosky, K.M., VanSwearingen, J.M., Burdett, R.G., & Gee, Z. A comparison of gait characteristics in young and old subjects. *Phys Ther*. 1994;74: 637-644; discussion 644-636.

Pappas, G.P., Olcott, E.W., & Drace, J.E. Imaging of skeletal muscle function using 18FDG PET: Force production, activation, and metabolism. *J Appl Physiol*. 2001;90: 329-337.

Phelps, M.E., Huang, S.C., Hoffman, E.J., Selin, C., Sokoloff, L., & Kuhl, D.E. Tomographic measurement of local cerebral glucose metabolic rate in humans with (F-18)2-fluoro-2-deoxy-D-glucose: Validation of method. *Ann Neurol*. 1979;6: 371-388.

Pipe, J.G., Boes, J.L., & Chenevert, T.L. Method for measuring three-dimensional motion with tagged MR imaging. *Radiology*. 1991;181: 591-595.

Porter, M.M., Vandervoort, A.A., & Kramer, J.F. Eccentric peak torque of the plantar and dorsiflexors is maintained in older women. *J Gerontol A Biol Sci Med Sci*. 1997;52: B125-131.

Poulin, M.J., Vandervoort, A.A., Paterson, D.H., Kramer, J.F., & Cunningham, D.A. Eccentric and concentric torques of knee and elbow extension in young and older men. *Can J Sport Sci*. 1992;17: 3-7.

Roomi, J., Yohannes, A.M., & Connolly, M.J. The effect of walking aids on exercise capacity and oxygenation in elderly patients with chronic obstructive pulmonary disease. *Age Ageing*. 1998;27: 703-706.

Sadato, N., Tsuchida, T., Nakaumra, S., *et al.* Non-invasive estimation of the net influx constant using the standardized uptake value for quantification of FDG uptake of tumours. *Eur J Nucl Med*. 1998;25: 559-564.

Shimada, H., Uchiyama, Y., & Kakurai, S. Specific effects of balance and gait exercises on physical function among the frail elderly. *Clin Rehabil.* 2003;17: 472-479.

Shimada, H., Kimura, Y., Suzuki, T., *et al.* The use of positron emission tomography and [18F]fluorodeoxyglucose for functional imaging of muscular activity during exercise with a stride assistance system. *IEEE Trans Neural Syst Rehabil Eng.* 2007;15: 442-448.

Shimada, H., Suzuki, T., Kimura, Y., *et al.* Effects of an automated stride assistance system on walking parameters and muscular glucose metabolism in elderly adults. *Br J Sports Med.* 2008;42: 922-9.

Shimada, H., Hirata, T., Kimura, Y., *et al.* Effects of a robotic walking exercise on walking performance in community-dwelling elderly adults. *Geriatr Gerontol Int.* 2009a;9: 372-381.

Shimada, H., Kimura, Y., Lord, S.R., *et al.* Comparison of regional lower limb glucose metabolism in older adults during walking. *Scand J Med Sci Sports.* 2009b, 19: 389-397.

Shimada H, Sturnieks D, Endo Y, *et al.* Relationship between whole body oxygen consumption and skeletal muscle glucose metabolism during walking in older adults: FDG PET study. *Aging Clin Exp Res.* 2010.

Simonsick, E.M., Guralnik, J.M., Volpato, S., Balfour, J., & Fried, L.P. Just get out the door! Importance of walking outside the home for maintaining mobility: findings from the women's health and aging study. *J Am Geriatr Soc.* 2005;53: 198-203.

Sokoloff, L., Reivich, M., Kennedy, C., *et al.* The [14C]deoxyglucose method for the measurement of local cerebral glucose utilization: theory, procedure, and normal values in the conscious and anesthetized albino rat. *J Neurochem.* 1977;28: 897-916.

Stevens, J.E., Stackhouse, S.K., Binder-Macleod, S.A., & Snyder-Mackler, L. Are voluntary muscle activation deficits in older adults meaningful? *Muscle Nerve.* 2003;27: 99-101.

Tashiro, M., Fujimoto, T., Itoh, M., *et al.* 18F-FDG PET imaging of muscle activity in runners. *J Nucl Med.* 1999;40: 70-76.

Thelen, D.G., Schultz, A.B., Alexander, N.B., & Ashton-Miller, J.A. Effects of age on rapid ankle torque development. *J Gerontol A Biol Sci Med Sci.* 1996;51: M226-232.

Van Hook, F.W., Demonbreun, D., & Weiss, B.D. Ambulatory devices for chronic gait disorders in the elderly. *Am Fam Physician.* 2003;67: 1717-1724.

van Uffelen, J.G., Chinapaw, M.J., van Mechelen, W., & Hopman-Rock, M. Walking or vitamin B for cognition in older adults with mild cognitive impairment? A randomised controlled trial. *Br J Sports Med.* 2008;42: 344-351.

Waters, R.L., Lunsford, B.R., Perry, J., & Byrd, R. Energy-speed relationship of walking: Standard tables. *J Orthop Res.* 1988;6: 215-222.

Winter, D.A. (1991). *The biomechanics and motor control of human gait: normal, elderly and pathological.* University of Waterloo Press, Waterloo.

Winter, D.A., Patla, A.E., Frank, J.S., & Walt, S.E. Biomechanical walking pattern changes in the fit and healthy elderly. *Phys Ther.* 1990;70: 340-347.

Young, D.R., Masaki, K.H., & Curb, J.D. Associations of physical activity with performance-based and self-reported physical functioning in older men: The Honolulu Heart Program. *J Am Geriatr Soc.* 1995;43: 845-854.